OCCUPATIONAL HEALTH NURSING

CONCEPTS AND PRACTICE

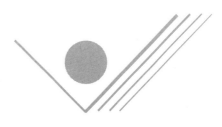

OCCUPATIONAL
HEALTH NURSING
CONCEPTS AND
PRACTICE

BONNIE ROGERS, RN, DrPH, COHN, FAAN
Associate Professor of Nursing and Public Health
Director, Occupational Health Nursing Program
School of Public Health
University of North Carolina
Chapel Hill, North Carolina

W.B. SAUNDERS COMPANY
A Division of Harcourt Brace & Company
Philadelphia   London   Toronto   Montreal   Sydney   Tokyo

W.B. Saunders Company
A Division of
Harcourt Brace & Company
The Curtis Center
Independence Square West
Philadelphia, PA 19106

Library of Congress Cataloging-in-Publication Data

Rogers, Bonnie.
    Occupational health nursing : concepts and practice / Bonnie
Rogers.—1st ed.
      p.   cm.
    ISBN 0-7216-7588-3
    1. Industrial nursing.   I. Title.
RC966.R64   1994
610.73'46—dc20   93-48841

OCCUPATIONAL HEALTH NURSING: ISBN 0-7216-7588-3
Concepts and Practice

Printed in United States of America.

Last digit is the print number: 9 8 7 6 5 4 3 2 1

About the Author

Bonnie Rogers is an Associate Professor of Nursing and Public Health and Director of the Occupational Health Nursing Program at the University of North Carolina, School of Public Health, Chapel Hill, North Carolina. Dr. Rogers received her diploma in nursing from the Washington Hospital Center School of Nursing in Washington, D.C.; her baccalaureate in nursing from George Mason University, Fairfax, Virginia; and her master of public health degree and doctorate in public health with a major in occupational health nursing from Johns Hopkins University, Baltimore, Maryland. She holds a postgraduate certificate as an adult health clinical specialist and is certified in occupational health nursing and community health nursing. She was invited to study ethics as a visiting scholar at the Hastings Center in New York and was granted a NIOSH career award to study ethical issues in occupational health. In addition to the managerial, consultant, and educator/researcher positions Dr. Rogers has held, she also practiced for many years as a public health nurse, occupational health nurse, and occupational health nurse practitioner. She has published numerous articles and book chapters and is the senior author of the book *Occupational Health Nursing Guidelines for Primary Clinical Conditions*. She is a strong advocate of occupational health nursing research, and her research interests focus primarily on hazards to health care workers, particularly nurses, and ethical issues in occupational health nursing. She serves on numerous editorial panels and as an ethics consultant.

To my husband, Jonathan Edan Klein,
who encouraged me to get the book started
and supported me through the process.

To our beautiful daughter, Lara,
who helped me get the text finished in the year of her birth, 1993.

To the memory of my dad,
who taught me to always do my best.

Preface

From its early beginnings, occupational health nursing practice has been grounded in the concepts and principles of public health practice, focusing on prevention, health teaching, health maintenance, and the control and elimination of workplace health hazards. Early occupational health nurses provided health care to workers and their families not only at the worksite but also in their homes and at hospitals.

Occupational health nursing practice has expanded considerably in the last few decades and has evolved into a highly specialized field with major emphasis on health promotion and prevention of illness and injuries in worker populations and on role expansion in clinical education, entrepreneurial management, and research areas.

Occupational Health Nursing: Concepts and Practice provides a framework for occupational health nursing practice and relevant discussion of the practical application of the concepts. The reader is exposed to the complexity and rich diversity of occupational health nursing and is stimulated to think critically about the challenges and opportunities that exist for practice expansion. The text

- Discusses factors affecting occupational health nursing practice related to individual and collective workforce health and problems and the promotion of health and quality living;
- Provides a conceptual framework for assessing, planning, implementing, and evaluating occupational health services and programs to improve the health of the workforce; and
- Addresses skills and capabilities needed in managing occupational health programs within the context of legal-ethical parameters and external influences.

Chapter 1 presents an overview of the meaning and relevance of work and health status indicators of the general and working population. The historical evolution of occupational health nursing is presented in Chapter 2 along with key milestones. The nature and scope of occupational health nursing practice is thoroughly discussed in Chapter 3 within the context of philosophical and public health underpinnings and the application of prevention principles. A conceptual model for practice is presented that emphasizes the relationship of internal and external influences on worker health and the nurse's interaction with these influences. Various occupational health nursing roles including clinician, manager, educator, researcher, and consultant are fully described in Chapter 4.

The work setting is the usual practice setting for the occupational health nurse. Because exposure to toxins in the workplace can produce significant stress in the worker and for the family, the occupational health nurse must possess relevant epidemiologic knowledge and skills to assess and monitor work-related health hazards, evaluate health status indicators, and analyze and interpret data regarding illness and injury trends. This is dealt with in Chapter 5. The team approach to problem identification and resolution cannot be overemphasized. Knowledge concepts, industrial hygiene, toxicology, safety, and ergonomics are discussed in Chapter 6 to provide a context for the interdisciplinary approaches to occupational health and safety programming.

Using a conceptual approach to initiate and expand occupational health services can serve as a systematic guide for program development. A model is presented in Chapter 7 that will challenge the occupational health nurse to consider a variety of parameters in establishing a comprehensive approach to service delivery. In Chapter 8 the occupational health nurse will find useful practical guides to help assess both the organization and the work setting in a discussion of organizational culture and comprehensive worksite assessment.

Health assessment, monitoring, surveillance, and clinical management are important components of the occupational health nurse's practice. Chapters 9 to 11 provide a thorough discussion of these activities and also discuss the importance of independent nursing actions as well as clinical guidelines for practice, with several examples provided.

An in-depth discussion of health promotion, health protection, levels of prevention, and health promotion models is presented in Chapter 12. A model for designing a health promotion program is described, and examples of health promotion programs are given along with several tools to assess work health needs.

Occupational health nurses are assuming a much greater role in management, and this topic is addressed from both a leadership and an administrative perspective in Chapter 13. Managerial functions, quality, and change are discussed. In addition, occupational health nurses will need to become more skilled and involved in research, which provides the foundation for practice. Chapter 14 provides a general overview of the research process and also addresses critical areas needing occupational health nursing research.

Besides knowing the legal parameters for practice encompassed in nurse practice acts, the occupational health nurse must be fully cognizant of occupational health and safety laws impacting worker health and nursing practice. Several examples of recent occupational health and safety legislation are discussed in Chapter 15, along with general content related to workers' compensation. The ethical practice of occupational health nursing is addressed in Chapter 16 within the framework of ethical theories, principles, and a model for ethical decision making.

Chapter 17 addresses future issues important to occupational health nursing practice including expansion in primary care, case management, research, and environmental health and various models for health care delivery at the worksite. Developing and maintaining a concept of health at the worksite is emphasized. Throughout the text, occupational health nurses "making a difference" is shown through creative ventures to promote health and prevent illness and injury and through the demonstration of care for those we serve.

Bonnie Rogers

Acknowledgments

Many occupational health nurses contributed their spirit and supplied me with the enthusiasm to write this book. I thank them for that. Special appreciation is given to the many occupational health nurses I have had the privilege to work with as students whose vitality, curiosity, and perseverance gave me the encouragement to get the text finished. I also want to recognize members of my own local North Carolina Tarheel Association of Occupational Health Nurses whose professionalism repeatedly inspired me.

A sincere thank you is given to Agape Blackley for her secretarial assistance through all the revisions of the manuscript. Finally, I am indebted to my family and friends who gave me continuous support and prodded me with fond impatience saying "when will the book be done?"

The author and publisher would like to thank the following reviewers, whose supportive comments and criticism helped to make this a better book: **Kathleen C. Brown, RN, PhD,** University of Alabama, Birmingham, Alabama; **Jane Lipscomb, RN, PhD,** University of California, San Francisco, California; **Darlene Meservy, RN, Dr PH,** University of Utah, Salt Lake City, Utah; **Jane Parker-Conrad, RN, PhD,** Knoxville, Tennessee; and **Linda A. Shortridge, RN, PhD,** University of Cincinnati, Cincinnati, Ohio.

Contents

1

WORK AND HEALTH: TRENDS AND CHALLENGES

■ **THE MEANING OF WORK**

In America, work is considered a basic part of life's experience. Most adults spend approximately one fourth to one third of their time at work and often perceive work as part of their self-identity. In addition, almost three quarters of employed men and the majority of employed women indicate they would prefer to work even if they had no financial need to do so (Kahn, 1981). Therefore, work is considered by most an integral component of life in a productive society.

Kahn (1981) points out that work involves an exchange between the worker and employer wherein a contractual relationship exists (written or unwritten) in which the worker agrees to perform certain tasks in exchange for a monetary commitment. However, for many, the value of work is characterized not solely by extrinsic rewards such as compensation, benefits, and status, but often, and more importantly, by intrinsic rewards such as self-satisfaction, achievement, pride, joy, self-enhancement, self-direction, and improved self-esteem (Bezold et al., 1986; PBS, 1992). The increased focus on intrinsic variables emphasizes the importance of a trust and supportive relationship between management and workers resulting in enhanced productivity, which is often viewed by the employer as an indicator of quality.

In addition to productivity, the quality of the work environment can be viewed in terms of the organization's relationship to meeting the needs and abilities of the workers (Graham, 1991). Significant changes in the characteristics of the population and workforce have caused the employer to reexamine the goodness of fit between the worker and the job in developing worker potential, enhancing health and safety at the worksite, increasing organizational flexibility in terms of job design, and addressing issues of critical importance such as child care, elder care, family stressors, and disability. To this end, work impacts all aspects of the worker's well-being (i.e., physical, psychological, emotional, social), and extends beyond the working walls to affect one's overall quality of life. The occupational health nurse needs to be fully cognizant of changing demographic trends and employer and employee perceptions of work, health, and other influences (e.g., family) in order to be an effective team member in the design of programs to promote and protect the health of all workers.

1

This chapter will describe the changing face of America's workforce, factors impacting worker health, and issues related to health care costs. The *Healthy People 2000: Occupational Safety and Health Objectives* are presented.

■ CHANGING POPULATION AND WORKFORCE CHARACTERISTICS

aging population

The population of the United States is expected to increase from approximately 250 million people in 1990 to an estimated 270 million people by the year 2000 (NCHS, 1990; Spencer, 1989; U.S. Bureau of Census, 1984). The U.S. population will be older with a median age of more than 36 years, compared to 29 years in 1975. The greatest growth will be among people over age 65 (representing 13% of the population) with a diminishment of the under 25-year-olds (Spencer, 1989). This will be reflected in the workforce with a decrease in the number of young job seekers. It is estimated that by the year 2000, 49% of the workforce will be between the ages of 35 and 54 and 8 million persons will be older than 80 (Johnson, 1988).

↑ minority

The racial and ethnic population in the United States is changing. Spencer (1986, 1989) estimates that the white population, not including Hispanic Americans, will decline from 76% to 72%. The fastest growing population group will be Hispanic Americans with an increase from 8% to 11.3%; the black or African-American population will increase its proportion from 12.4% to 13.1%; and native and Asian-Americans will increase their population proportion from 3.5% to 4.3%. Economic expansion will create approximately 18 million new jobs and racial/ethnic populations will enter the workforce at higher rates than whites, reflective of the population changes (USDHHS, 1990).

more women

Workforce changes also include a shift in the proportion of men and women in the workplace and the types of jobs available to and occupied by each group. According to data collected by the Bureau of Labor Statistics (1985) and the National Center for Health Statistics (1989), in 1985 approximately 110 million people comprised the American workforce, of which 56% were men and 44% were women. These statistics compare to 74% men and 29% women workers in 1948.

Of the civilian female adult population, 53% were in the labor force, which represented a 20% increase since 1948. More than half the female labor force was concentrated in three areas: administrative support/clerical (26%), service (14%), and professional specialty (14%); 12% were employed in fields such as labor, transportation and moving, machine operation, precision products, crafts, and farming, forestry, or fishing. In the male labor force nearly 20% worked in precision production, crafts, or repair occupations, 13% in executive positions, 11% in professional specialty occupations, and 10% in sales. There has been a shift from employment in the manufacturing to the service sector (including government), with approximately 75% of workers employed in the latter (NCHS, 1989).

Women will be the major source of new entrants into the job market, comprising 47% of the total workforce by 2000, compared to 45% in 1988. Half the women in the workforce will be between the ages of 35 and 54, a change from 1986 when the majority was between the ages of 25 and 44. White men will account for only 25% of the labor force growth (Kutscher, 1987).

■ HEALTH STATUS OF THE NATION AND WORKFORCE

The health of the American workforce can best be improved through health promotion and risk reduction strategies. However, in order to do this, the occupational health nurse must be familiar with current literature describing relevant health status indicators of the nation, in addition to occupational health and safety problems. One important document, *Healthy People 2000: National Health Promotion and Disease Prevention Objectives,* provides a thorough discussion of the nation's health, including occupational health and safety issues, and sets forth national health objectives to enhance health and reduce disease. Health professionals are encouraged to obtain this document as an important reference and resource.

The Nation's Health

Although not always recognized, many problems apparent in the nation's health, such as hypertension, diabetes, depression, substance abuse and other chronic and debilitating diseases, are mirrored in the workforce and impact on productivity. In order to enlarge one's perspective about the health of the nation and its interrelatedness to the health of the workforce, it is important to examine some of these factors.

Healthy People 2000 (USDHHS, 1991, p. 3) reports that much progress was made in the 1980s in the decline of mortality rates for three of the leading causes of American deaths: heart disease, stroke, and unintentional injuries (Fig. 1–1). Much of this progress mirrors reductions in risk factors, such as control of high blood pressure, decrease in cigarette smoking and intake of cholesterol and dietary fats, the effective use of seat belts, and the decline in alcohol abuse.

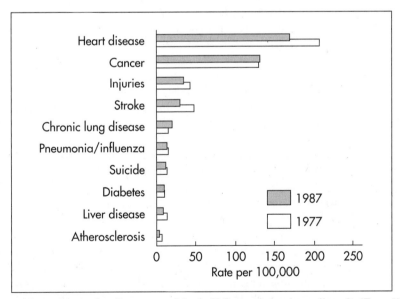

■ **Figure 1–1**   Leading causes of death, U.S. population (age-adjusted). (From *Health, United States, 1989, and Prevention Profile and National Center for Health Statistics, Centers for Disease Control.*)

Despite these health improvements, lung cancer and breast cancer rates remain consistently high, and the nation continues to be burdened by preventable illness, injury, and disability with a high health care cost bill for society.

Many of the leading causes of death between the ages of 25 and 65 are preventable through lifestyle changes. It is estimated that 30% of cancer deaths, 21% of all coronary heart disease deaths, and 87% of lung cancer deaths are linked to smoking (Office on Smoking and Health, 1989). If tobacco use stopped entirely today, an estimated 390,000 Americans would survive each year (Office on Smoking and Health, 1989).

It is estimated that 35% of cancer deaths may be related to dietary habits (Eddy, 1986). Certain eating patterns such as high fat consumption are associated with the risk of heart disease, breast cancer, and colon cancer. Being overweight is a problem for one quarter of American adults, and this is associated with high blood pressure, high cholesterol, diabetes, heart disease, stroke, some cancers, and gall bladder disease. It is apparent that more emphasis needs to be placed on developing and enhancing effective nutrition programs at the worksite, not only for workers but their families.

Substance abuse, of course, contributes not only to the social ills of society and the workforce but also affects the economy of the company. News stories about drug-related crime, crack-addicted babies, drunk-driving tragedies, and the family legacy of alcoholism—as well as mounting evidence on the health effects of passive smoking—make it painfully clear that substance abuse has a negative impact on all of society, not just on users. The per capita consumption of alcohol dropped in 1987, which may in part be attributed to the aging of the population, the public's preoccupation with fitness and health, and a greater preference for beverages with lower alcohol content. However, the number of alcoholic persons is expected to increase from 10.5 million in 1985 to 11.2 million in 1995 (RWJF, 1991). Alcohol is a major risk factor for motor vehicle fatalities, homicides and suicides, liver cirrhosis and some cancers, and birth defects (NIDA, 1989). Deaths related to alcohol use are shown in Figure 1–2.

The use of illicit drugs is of major concern and the high rate of use is expected to continue for some years. In 1989, cocaine-related emergency room visits constituted 39% of all visits related to drugs (NIDA, 1987). Alcohol, cigarettes, and marijuana are usually the first substances teenagers try, with the year of entering high school a peak period for experimentation. In a 1989 survey of high school seniors, most who had ever used drugs or alcohol reported doing so by the ninth grade: alcohol (65%), marijuana (55%), cocaine (23%) and cigarettes (79%) (RWJF, 1991). Deaths related to drug use, highest between the ages of 25 and 44, and mortality from alcohol abuse each year could be reduced by 100,000 unnecessary deaths (USDHHS, 1991).

In fiscal year 1989, private insurance, mostly supplied through U.S. businesses, provided 31% of the reimbursement for alcohol and drug treatment. In addition, claims for substance abuse and mental health are accelerating faster than routine health benefit payments (NIDA, 1989). Employee assistance and rehabilitation programs, as well as family counseling and prevention programs for substance abuse, are sorely needed at the worksite, from both a clinical management and cost-containment perspective.

Chronic problems such as arthritis, osteoporosis, visual and hearing impair-

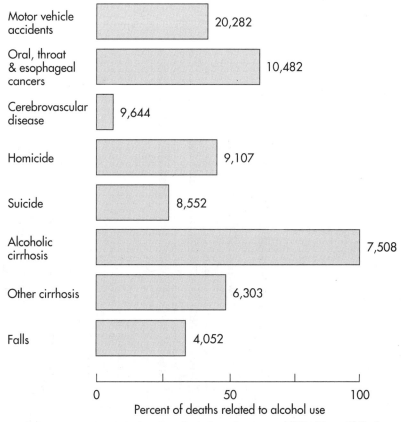

■ **Figure 1–2**   Deaths related to alcohol use by cause, 1987. (From *U.S. Centers for Disease Control. Morbidity and Mortality Weekly Report. 39*(11), 1990. Table 1, p. 174.)

ment, and hypertension are responsible for a significant portion of people's health care needs, and impact everyday living for individuals and family members on and off the job. Figure 1–3 shows the prevalence of the four most common chronic conditions—arthritis, hypertension, diabetes, and respiratory diseases such as asthma, emphysema, and bronchitis—which varies among population groups (RWJF, 1991). For example, diabetes is more common among blacks, and arthritis is much more common among women. All four chronic conditions shown in the figure are more common in older people. A key ingredient to healthy aging and reduction in chronic problems is physical activity, yet more than 40% of people over 65 report no physical activity related to leisure time (CDC, 1989).

In addition, the chance of having an activity limitation or disability rises with increasing age, and are reported more frequently among low-income persons. About 20% of people under 65 who earn less than $10,000 annually have disabilities, compared to only 7% to 8% of people earning at least $30,000 (NCHS, 1991). Some reasons postulated for this contrast are that low-income people may be at higher disability risk because of hazardous occupations or

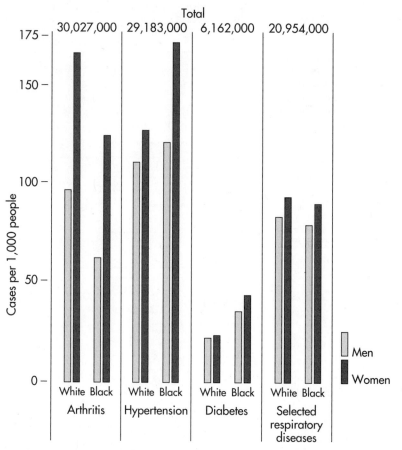

■ **Figure 1–3** Prevalence of selected chronic conditions by race and gender, 1988. *Note:* Data are not age adjusted. (From *unpublished data from the U.S. National Center for Health Statistics, Division of Health Interview Statistics, with analysis by the Environmental Studies Branch.*)

unsafe living conditions, inability to obtain appropriate medical care, or lack of higher earning power due to their disability (RWJF, 1991).

The control and prevention of infectious diseases remains a priority. There is no question that HIV/AIDS is the principal viral problem today with new cases of infection and disease rising rapidly over the past few years. In addition, infectious diseases such as hepatitis, tuberculosis, and Lyme disease, to name a few, need careful attention (Wenzel, 1992), and improved methods for surveillance, control, and prevention need emphasis.

Worker Health

Premature deaths, diseases, disabilities, injuries, and other unhealthful conditions resulting from occupational exposures pose important problems to the nation as a whole. Over the years, several pieces of legislation have been enacted to provide protection for the worker and the environment. However, in terms of occupational health, by far the strongest legislation enacted was the William-

■ **TABLE 1–1**   The 10 Leading Work-Related Diseases and Injuries, United States, 1982*

1. Occupational lung diseases: asbestosis, byssinosis, silicosis, coal workers' pneumoconiosis, lung cancer, occupational asthma
2. Musculoskeletal injuries: disorders of the back, trunk, upper extremity, neck, lower extremity; traumatically induced Raynaud's phenomenon
3. Occupational cancers (other than lung): leukemia; mesothelioma; cancers of the bladder, nose, and liver
4. Amputations, fractures, eye loss, lacerations, and traumatic deaths
5. Cardiovascular diseases: hypertension, coronary artery disease, acute myocardial infarction
6. Disorders of reproduction: infertility, spontaneous abortion, teratogenesis
7. Neurotoxic disorders: peripheral neuropathy, toxic encephalitis, psychoses, extreme personality changes (exposure-related)
8. Noise-induced loss of hearing
9. Dermatologic conditions: dermatoses, burns, contusions (abrasions)
10. Psychologic disorders: neuroses, personality disorders, alcoholism, drug dependency

*The conditions listed under each category are to be viewed as selected examples, not comprehensive definitions of the category.

From NIOSH, "Leading Work-Related Disease and Injuries–United States," *Morbidity and Mortality Weekly Report,* January 21, 1983.

Steiger Act, better known as the Occupational Safety and Health Act of 1970. The purpose of the Act is "to assure so far as possible every working man and woman in the nation safe and healthful working conditions." This is accomplished through establishment and enforcement of health and safety standards. Within the Act, the National Institute for Occupational Safety and Health (NIOSH) was established to focus primarily on education and research. NIOSH has identified the leading work-related illnesses and injuries (Table 1–1) and related prevention strategies to help eliminate or minimize workplace hazards (Millar, 1988; NIOSH, 1984; NIOSH, 1987).

As reported in *Healthy People 2000* (USDHHS, 1991), the state of worker health and safety bears improvement in several areas. The prevention of accidents and injuries at the worksite must remain a priority. While some surveys indicate a decline in work-related deaths, fatal injuries remained consistently high in mining (30.3 deaths per 100,000) and construction (25 per 100,000), based on a 1983–87 average (NSC, 1988). In addition, the National Safety Council has estimated a rate as high as 52.1 deaths per 100,000 among agricultural workers, and nonfatal injuries often result in extensive rehabilitation and permanent disability (NCASH, 1989).

Although the number of fatal occupational injuries has decreased in recent years, work-related illnesses and injuries appear to be rising. NIOSH estimates that at least 10 million injuries occur on the job each year, of which 3 million are severe. Nearly 50% of reported injuries require off-work time or restricted duty (BLS, 1988a), particularly in construction, nursing, farm work, transportation, and mining (Fig. 1–4). During 1987 alone, permanent job-related impairments grew from 60,000 to 70,000, total disabling injuries numbered 1.8 million, and there was an increase by 12.5% in the number of illness/injuries in the manufacturing sector (BLS, 1988b).

Persons with disabilities face many of the same health risks as other people, such as inadequate nutrition, physical inactivity, alcohol and drug abuse, and

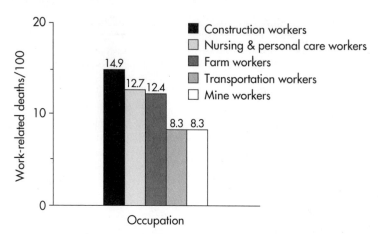

■ **Figure 1–4**   Work-related injuries 1983–87 average. (From *Bureau of Labor Statistics: Handbook of labor statistics, Bulletin 2217.* Washington, DC: U. S. Department of Labor, 1985.)

stress. However, reducing risks may be a particular challenge, such as fitness programs where people must develop new skills, gain access to special equipment, and be part of a special network to enable participation.

Other important problems occurring at the worksite include cumulative trauma disorders from repetitive motion or repeated noise exposure; occupational skin diseases and disorders from exposure to chemical toxins, abrasive materials, and sun, which constituted 28% of all reported occupational illnesses in 1987; infection of health care workers with hepatitis B virus, estimated to be as high as 12,000 cases annually; occupationally induced hearing loss with an estimated 3 million workers exposed daily to levels exceeding 85 dBA; and exposure of men and women to lead resulting in neurologic deficits, hypertension, and reproductive toxicity (CDC, 1988). In addition, shiftworkers, who constitute more than 10 million American workers, may have significant health problems related to disturbed sleep and increased fatigue, which may result in increased injuries and illness such as stress or gastrointestinal disorders (Phillips and Brown, 1992).

Exposure to environmental or occupational toxins is of paramount importance. An estimated one tenth of congenital anomalies are caused by environmentally related factors, such as viruses, chemicals, and radiation (USDHHS, 1991). Industrial toxins appear to lead to reproductive toxicity, yet their relationships and interactions are still unclear and controversial. As new chemicals continue to proliferate and saturate the market and workplace, priority efforts will need to focus on vigilant monitoring and the development of new methods to create nonhazardous substances, and to educate workers about existing substances that remain potentially toxic.

One of the most important challenges facing American industry today is keeping the worker on the job and maximizing cost containment. To meet this challenge requires not only devising safe and healthful approaches to returning the injured worker to work but also meeting the needs of pregnant women and parents at work. Currently, 33% of workers are between the ages of 16 and 44, and nearly half of them are women. With more women in the workforce, pregnancy and newborn care are becoming serious issues. More than 250,000 low-birth-weight infants are born each year with an associated increased mortality risk and a wide range of disorders, including neurodevelopmental conditions, learning disorders, behavior problems, and lower respiratory tract infections (National Commission to Prevent Infant Mortality, 1988). In addition, providing health care coverage for two to three premature infants in a short time could deplete medical coverage funds in a self-insured company. The average cost of a premature infant at birth is $55,000 with $10,000 for each hospital readmission (Chenoweth, 1988).

The motivation for providing women's health programs at work, such as prenatal care, is not only to provide health promotion and support but to control costs. Factors related to high risk pregnancies can often be eliminated or modified through education and screening. In addition, illness during pregnancy can increase absenteeism, and concerns or guilt regarding breastfeeding or day care could prompt mothers to quit. Childhood illness coupled with a large percentage of single parent households may also increase absenteeism and decrease productivity. The occupational health nurse has an important role in the establishment of preconception counseling, prenatal, postnatal, child health, and day care programs, and counseling regarding workplace hazards that may affect pregnancy outcomes.

■ HEALTH CARE COSTS

The health share of the Gross National Product (GNP) in 1960 was 5%, in 1990 it reached 12.4% (HCFA, 1990), and estimates for 1992 indicate the United States will spend $817 billion, or 14% of the GNP, on health care (APHA, 1992). Lost economic productivity for morbidity and premature mortality equalled nearly 18% of the GNP in 1980, and injuries alone accounted for well over $100 billion annually, cancer more than $70 billion, and cardiovascular disease $35 billion (Rice et al., 1989). Sophisticated technology for the diagnosis and treatment of disease conditions has outstripped society's ability to pay for it. However, while some of these expenditures are related to conditions of aging (Hart & Moore, 1992), many of these expenses may be avoidable. For example, 7 million Americans are affected by coronary artery disease, with 1.5 million heart attacks and 500,000 deaths annually. Nearly 300,000 bypass surgeries, each costing an average of $30,000, are performed yearly, and treatment for a single case of lung cancer is about $29,000. Hospital expenditures accounted for 44% of personal health care costs in 1988 reaching $212 billion, followed by physician services at 22% (HCFA, 1990).

Health insurance costs for employers have skyrocketed. During the 1980s, spending for employer-based health insurance premiums increased 164%, rising from $66 billion to $174 billion per year (APHA, 1992). One way to show the significance of this expense is to compare it to another important measure— corporate profits. In 1965, U.S. businesses paid $14 for health services and supplies for every $100 of their after-tax corporate profits. By 1988, health expenses were almost $86 for every $100 of after-tax profits and peaked at $110/ $100 in 1986 (Fig. 1–5).

Companies not only pay health insurance premiums for their employees but also the employer share of public payroll taxes for Medicare, the medical portion of workers' compensation, temporary disability insurance premiums and, in some

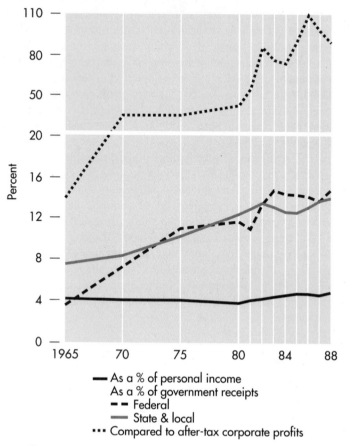

■ **Figure 1–5** Expenditures for health services and supplies in relation to personal income, government receipts and after-tax corporate profits, selected years, 1965-1988. (From *unpublished data from the U.S. Health Care Financing Administration, Office of the Actuary, Office of National Cost Estimates.*)

cases, the costs of on-site health services, as well. These costs to companies are passed along in higher prices for goods and services and in lower wages.

Even while most Americans (212 million) have some form of public or private health insurance, approximately 36 million remain uninsured (NCHS, 1989; AHCPR, 1990). The continued increase in health care costs will place an even greater economic burden on society. Ultimately, consumers pay for rising health care costs through higher taxes, higher prices for goods and services, and reductions in wages and salaries (RWJF, 1991).

■ **NATION'S HEALTH OBJECTIVES: OCCUPATIONAL SAFETY AND HEALTH**

Within the framework of the nation's health objectives, *Healthy People 2000,* prevention of occupational health hazards through changes in work practices, engineering controls, use of protective devices, monitoring the workforce and workplace surveillance for health risks, and increased education of the working population, guide the framework of the occupational health and safety goals for the nation's workforce. Improvement in monitoring and surveillance activities to identify high risk groups, and implementation of prevention focused initiatives are critically needed within a quality driven and cost-effective framework. Fifteen objectives as well as priorities for increasing training and education opportunities for occupational health and safety personnel, improving surveillance activities, and increasing research in the field of occupational health and safety are delineated and follow:

Health Status Objectives

1. Reduce deaths from work-related injuries to no more than 4 per 100,000 full-time workers (baseline: 6 during 1983–87).
2. Reduce work-related injuries resulting in medical treatment, lost time from work, or restricted work activity to no more than 6 per 100 workers (baseline: 7.7 for 1987).
3. Reduce cumulative trauma disorders to no more than 60 per 100,000 workers (baseline: 100 in 1987).
4. Reduce occupational skin diseases and disorders to an incidence of no more than 55 per 100,000 workers (baseline: 64 during 1983–87).
5. Reduce hepatitis B infection among any occupationally exposed workers to an incidence of 1,200 cases (baseline: estimated 6,200 cases in 1987).

Risk Reduction Objectives

6. Increase to at least 75% the proportion of worksites with 50 or more employees that mandate employee use of occupant protection systems, such as seat belts, during all work-related motor vehicle travel (baseline: 82.4% in 1992). NOTE: Target of 75% was established before baseline data were available; hence target has been exceeded.
7. Reduce to no more than 15% the proportion of workers exposed to average daily noise levels exceeding 85 dBA (baseline data not available).
8. Eliminate exposure that results in workers having blood lead concentrations greater than 25 μg/dl of whole blood (baseline: 4,505 workers with blood level levels greater than 25 μg/dl in six states in 1988).
9. Increase hepatitis B immunization levels to 90% among any occupationally exposed workers (baseline: 37% in 1989).

Service and Protection Objectives

10. Implement occupational safety and health plans in 50 states for the identification, management, and prevention of leading work-related diseases and injuries within the state (baseline: 10 states in 1989).
11. Establish in 50 states exposure standards adequate to prevent the major occupational lung diseases to which their worker populations are exposed (byssinosis, asbestosis, coal workers' pneumoconiosis, and silicosis) (baseline data not available).
12. Increase to at least 70% the proportion of worksites with 50 or more employees that have implemented programs on worker health and safety (baseline: 63.8% in 1992).
13. Increase to at least 50% the proportion of worksites with 50 or more employees that offer back injury prevention and rehabilitation programs (baseline: 28.6% in 1985).
14. Establish in 50 states either public health or labor department programs

that provide consultation and assistance to small businesses to implement safety and health programs for their employees (baseline: 26 states in 1991).

15. Increase to 75% the proportion of primary care providers who routinely elicit occupational health and safety exposures as a part of patient history and provide relevant counseling (baseline: <15% in 1992—various types of providers).

Priorities are recommended for the following:

• **Personnel:** ensure an adequate supply of personnel to accomplish the practice, education, and research objectives; provide relevant curricular and continuing education content on occupational health and safety across disciplines; and increase the number of faculty development programs and fellowships in occupational health and safety.

• **Surveillance:** allow accurate assessment data related to incidence, prevalence, severity, and so forth of occupational injuries and illnesses; provide data on the nation's 10 leading work-related illnesses and injuries; identify groups at specific risk (e.g. women, minorities).

• **Research:** continue to work toward the education of work-related illnesses/injuries through identifying workplace stressors, developing new measurement tools and biomarkers of exposure; and identifying at-risk populations for work-related disease or injury and mechanisms that result in insult.

■ SUMMARY

Much has been accomplished in the control of work-related injuries and illnesses, particularly during the past two decades; however, much more needs to be done. Implementation of what is already known about promoting health and preventing disease is the challenge health care professionals face, not only in terms of saving lives and dollars but reducing unnecessary suffering, illness and disability, and improving working and environmental conditions. Efforts need to focus not only on health enhancement and protection in the workplace, but on improving the health and quality of life in general with a cost-containment conscience. Health promotion and protection are perhaps our best weapons.

References

Agency for Health Care Policy and Research. Estimates of the uninsured population, calendar year 1987; National Medical Expenditure Survey; Data Summary 2. Rockville, MD: DHHS. Pub. No. (PHS90/3469), p. 7, 1990.

American Public Health Association. A national health program for all of us. American Public Health Association Guide to Health Care Reform Debate, 1992, pp. 1–16.

Bezold, C, Carlson, RJ, & Peck, JC. The future of work and health. Institute for Alternative Futures. Dover, MA: Auburn House, 1986.

Bureau of Labor Statistics. Handbook of labor statistics, Bulletin 2217. Washington, DC: U.S. Department of Labor, 1985.

Bureau of Labor Statistics. Annual survey of occupational injuries and illnesses. Washington, DC: Department of Labor, 1988(a).

Bureau of Labor Statistics. Occupational injuries and illnesses in the U.S. by industry, 1986 Bulletin 2308. Washington, DC: Department of Labor, 1988(b), pp. 3,7.

Centers for Disease Control. The nature and extent of lead poisoning in children in the United States: A Report to Congress. Atlanta: Department of Health and Human Services, 1988.

Centers for Disease Control. Behavioral risk factor surveillance system. Atlanta: Author, 1989.

Centers for Disease Control. Update: Surveillance of outbreaks. Morbidity and Mortality Weekly Report 40(16): 173–176, 1991.

Chenoweth, DH. Health care cost management. Indianapolis: Benchmark Press, 1988.

Eddy, DM. Setting priorities for cancer control programs. Journal of the National Cancer Institute, 76: 187–189, 1986.

Graham, KJ. Quality of life in the working environment. Public Health Nursing, 8(2): 67, 1991.

Hart, B & Moore, P. The aging workforce. AAOHN Journal, 40(1): 36–40, 1992.

Health Care Financing Administration, Office of the Actuary. National health care expenditures, 1988. Health Care Financing Review 11(4): 1–41, 1990.

Johnson, E. Older workers help meet employment needs. Personnel Journal, 5: 100–105, 1988.

Kahn, RL. Work and health. New York: John Wiley & Sons, 1981.

Kutscher, RE. Projections 2000: Overview and implications of the projections to 2000. Monthly Labor Review, September, 1987.

Millar, JD. Summary of proposed national strategies for the prevention of leading work-related diseases and injuries, Part I. American Journal of Industrial Medicine 13: 223–240, 1988.

National Coalition for Agricultural Safety and Health. A Report in the nation: Agriculture at risk. Iowa City: The University of Iowa, 1989.

National Center for Health Statistics, J.G. Collins & O.T. Thomberry. Health Characteristics of workers by occupation and sex: United States, 1983–85. Advance Data From Vital and Health Statistics, No. 168, DHHS Pub. No. (PHS) 89-1250. Public Health Service, Hyattsville, MD, 1989.

National Center for Health Statistics. Prevention profile. Health, United States, 1989. DHHS Pub. No. (PHS)90-1232. Hyattsville, MD: U.S. Department of Health and Human Services, 1990.

National Center for Health Statistics. People with disabilities. Unpublished data, 1991.

National Commission to Prevent Infant Mortality. Indirect costs of infant mortality and low birth weight. Washington, DC: Author, May, 1988.

National Institute on Drug Abuse. Data from the Drug Abuse Warning Network (DAWN): Annual Data 1986. DHHS Pub. No. (ADM)87-1530. Washington, DC: U.S. Department of Health and Human Services, 1987.

National Institute on Drug Abuse. Highlights from the 1989 national drug and alcoholism treatment unit survey. Rockville, MD: Author, 1989.

National Institute for Occupational Safety and Health. Prevention of the leading work-related diseases and injuries. Morbidity and Mortality Weekly Report 33(16), 1984.

National Institute on Occupational Safety and Health. National occupational hazard survey, Vol. III. Atlanta: Department of Health and Human Services. NIOSH Pub. No. 78-114, 1987.

National Safety Council. Accident facts, 1988. Chicago: Author, 1988.

Office of Smoking & Health. Reducing the health consequences of smoking: 25 years of progress. A Report of the Surgeon General. DHHS Pub. No. (CDC) 89-8411. Washington, DC: U.S. Department of Health & Human Services, 1989.

Phillips, JA & Brown, KC. Industrial workers on a rotating shift pattern. AAOHN Journal, 40(10): 468–475, 1992.

Public Broadcasting System. The Deming of America, 1992.

Rice, DP, MacKenzie, EJ, Jones, AS, Kaufman, SR, deLissovoy, GV, Max, W, McLoughlin, E, Miller, TR, Robertson, LS, Salkever, DS, & Smith, GS. Cost of injury in the United States: A report to Congress, 1989. San Francisco: Institute for Health and Aging, University of California, and Injury Prevention Center, Johns Hopkins University, 1989.

Robert Wood Johnson Foundation. Challenges in health care. Princeton, NJ: Author, 1991.

Spencer, G. Projections of the Hispanic population: 1983–2080. Current Population Reports, Population Estimates and Projections. Series P-25, No. 995. Washington, DC: U.S. Department of Commerce, Bureau of the Census, 1986.

Spencer, G. Projections of the population of the United States by age, sex, and race: 1988–2080. Current Population Reports, Population Estimates and Projections. Series P-25, No. 1018. Washington, DC: U.S. Government Printing Office, 1989.

U.S. Bureau of the Census. Projections of the population of the United States by age, sex, and race: 1983–2080. Current Population Reports, Population Estimates and Projections. Series P-25, No. 952. Washington, DC: U.S. Government Printing Office, 1984.

USDHHS. Healthy People 2000: National Health Promotion & Disease Prevention Objectives (DHHS Pub No 91-50212, 94–110). Washington, DC: U.S. Government Printing Office, 1991.

Wenzel, P. Control of communicable disease. In J. Last & R. Wallace, Eds. Public Health and Preventive Medicine (ed. 13). Norwalk, CT: Appleton & Lange, pp 57–60, 1992.

2

HISTORICAL PERSPECTIVES IN OCCUPATIONAL HEALTH NURSING

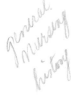

Nursing is older than civilization. Whenever and wherever persons first began to care for the injured, the sick, and the wounded, then nursing began. Medicine and nursing have often been represented in language by the same person; however, in more recent years a distinction has been made between the two. The emergence of modern nursing has brought with it a thirst and quest for knowledge in a practice-based discipline with strong emphasis on research as the foundation for practice. However, the importance of historical events cannot be understated as they provide evidence of advancement, change, and stability. This chapter will provide an overview of key historical events that have influenced occupational health and occupational health nursing practice (Table 2–1).

Nursing in the Middle Ages was primarily conducted by religious orders. From the 16th to the 18th centuries, nursing had largely deteriorated to a job of housework, laundry, and scrubbing (Dock, 1938). Women were subjugated during these centuries and the deprivation of education was a deliberate attempt to keep them in an inferior status. However, during this time the work of St. Vincent de Paul and the Sisters of Charity brought enthusiasm and a fresh zeal into nursing. They performed both hospital and visiting nursing, were considered earnest and dedicated by the society they served, treated the sick with respect and humility, and gave medicines according to the prescriptions of the physician (Bullough & Bullough, 1964). Modern nursing began with reforms initiated at the end of the 18th century, and developed in parallel to the industrial revolution. Centered in England in the 18th century and to a lesser degree in France, the Industrial Revolution gradually spread to Germany, the United States, and the rest of the world in 19th and 20th centuries. This parallel development of nursing and industry provided a natural link to offer nursing services to workers and their families at the worksite.

In England, the Industrial Revolution, by substituting mechanically powered and paced machinery for manual labor, gave rise to many problems that affected workers' health. The factory system developed to house new and expensive machines, which had to be located near sources of power, primarily water power. Families were disrupted by having to move to where factories were located, and away from their farms, which had always been a source of income and pride.

■ **TABLE 2–1** Historical Milestones in Occupational Health and Occupational Health Nursing in the United States

1633-1714	Bernardino Ramazzini generally accepted as Father of Industrial Medicine
1884	Bureau of Labor established, which later became the Department of Commerce and Labor (1903), then the U.S. Department of Labor (1913)
1888	Betty Moulder of Pennsylvania worked with coal miners
1895	Vermont Marble Company initiated Industrial Nursing Service with Ada Mayo Stewart as the industrial nurse
1897	John Wanamaker Company hired Anna B. Duncan as industrial nurse
1899-1906	Several U.S. businesses hired industrial nurses:
	Frederick Loeser Department Store (NYC)
	The Emporium (San Francisco)
	Plymouth Cordage Company (Massachusetts)
	Anaconda Mining (Montana)
	Broadway Store (Los Angeles)
	Macy's Department Store (NYC)
	Filene's (Boston)
	Carson, Pirie, Scott (Chicago)
	Fulton Cotton Mills (Georgia)
	Bullock's (Los Angeles)
1903	First nurse practice acts enacted
1909	Metropolitan Life Insurance provided nursing services for workers through efforts of Lillian Wald
1911	Workers' Compensation laws enacted
	National Organization for Public Health Nursing was formed
	Fire at the Triangle Shirt Waist Factory in New York City resulted in 146 worker deaths
1912	38 nurses employed by business firms
	National Council for Industrial Safety established, which became the National Safety Council in 1913
1913	Industrial nurses registry established in Boston
1914	World War I begins
1915	Boston Industrial Nurses Club founded, which grew into the New England Association of Industrial Nurses
1916	Factory Nurses Conference established (later called itself AAIN, then merged with the NEAIN in 1933)
	American Association of Industrial Physicians and Surgeons formed, later called the American Occupational Medicine Association, then the American College of Occupational Medicine, and the American College of Occupational and Environmental Medicine in 1991
1917	First industrial nursing course offered at Boston University, College of Business Administration
1918	1,213 nurses employed in 871 business firms
1919	First book on industrial nursing written by Florence Wright
1929	Stock market crash and beginning of Depression
1930	3,189 nurses employed by industry
1935	Wagner Act—National Labor Relations Act—enacted
	Social Security Act enacted
1936	Walsh-Healey Act for worker health and safety standards enacted
1937	2,200 nurses employed by industry
1938	Regional annual industrial nurses conferences began
	Fair Labor Standards Act (Wage and Hour Act) enacted
1939	American Industrial Hygiene Association formed

Table continued on following page.

■ **TABLE 2–1** Historical Milestones in Occupational Health and Occupational Health Nursing in the United States *Continued*

1941	Beginning of World War II with an estimated 6,000 nurses working in industry
	First industrial nurse employed by the federal government, Olive Whitlock
1942	American Association of Industrial Nurses founded—Catherine Dempsey, first president
	Estimated 11,000 nurses working in industry
1947	Taft-Hartley Act enacted
1953	*Industrial Nursing Journal* began which later became the *Occupational Health Nursing Journal* and then *AAOHN Journal*
1956	Textbook in occupational health nursing published by Mary Louise Brown
1964	Civil Rights Act enacted
1966	Federal Metal and Non-Metalic Safety Act enacted
1969	Federal Coal Mine and Safety Act enacted
1970	Occupational Safety and Health Act enacted
	Occupational Safety and Health Administration
	National Institute for Occupational Safety and Health
	Occupational Safety and Health Review Commission
	Environmental Protection Agency established
1970s	Graduate programs in occupational health nursing offered with the University of North Carolina at Chapel Hill, Yale, and New York University being the forerunners
1972	Equal Employment Opportunity Act enacted
	Noise Control Act enacted
	Black Lung Benefits Act enacted
	Clean Water Act enacted
	American Board for Occupational Health Nurses established
1973	Health Maintenance Organization Act enacted
	Rehabilitation Act enacted
1976	Toxic Substances Control Act enacted
1977	AAIN renamed as the American Association of Occupational Health Nurses
1983	AAOHN established research awards
	Hazard Communication Standard enacted
1986	National Center for Nursing Research established at the National Institutes for Health
1988	OSHA hires first occupational health nurse
1990	Americans with Disabilities Act enacted
1991	Bloodborne Pathogens Standard enacted
1993	National Center for Nursing Research became the 17th institute at NIH: the National Institute of Nursing Research
	Office of Occupational Health Nursing established at OSHA

The primary motive for the factory owners was profit, and employees were not only required to work 14-hour days, but were often laid off when product demand declined. In addition, employers began to replace male employees with women and children, who would work cheaper. With the lack of farm revenue previously enjoyed, the result was not only a decrease in overall income but an increase in family tension and difficult living conditions. Reforms were demanded and laws were enacted that regulated working conditions in factories including the length of the working day for women and children. Eventually laws prohibited child labor under a certain age (Bullough & Bullough, 1964; Hunter, 1978).

Nursing reform began in England under the direction of Florence Nightingale, whose determination and visionary outlook laid the foundation for the profession and discipline of nursing as we view and practice it today (Bullough & Bullough, 1964; Dock, 1938). Many events influenced her thinking and modern approach to nursing science. Born in 1820, Nightingale came from a well-to-do English family and had all the benefits and comforts of genteel privilege. Though intense in her desire to enter nursing and help the helpless, she encountered stern opposition from her family. Much of her nursing knowledge was self-taught, gained from care of her relatives.

Through friends, she learned of the work of the Fliedners who had established a deaconess house at Kaiserwerth, Germany in 1836. The intention of the Fliedners was to organize an order of deaconesses to care for the sick. Nurse deaconesses were given instruction in both medicine and pharmacy by qualified physicians and pharmacists. They bathed patients, gave them medications, fed the weaker ones, and did the necessary mending, darning, and ward work (Bullough & Bullough, 1964). Deaconesses were trained in four areas, including hospital and private nursing, relief of the poor, care of children, and work with unfortunate women; their primary thrust, however, was religious (Dock, 1938). Hearing of the work of the Fliedners, Nightingale visited Kaiserwerth against her family's wishes, and stayed for three months in 1851. In later writings she described the nursing there as poor and crude.

After her return to England she was even more determined to become a nurse. In 1853 she spent one month of study with the Sisters of Charity in Paris, having to return home to care for a dying grandmother. Nightingale subsequently became the superintendent of a hospital system in London where she was widely known for her quality of patient care, executive abilities, and visionary ideas in the practice of nursing.

Nightingale is probably best known, however, for her reform methods in the provision of nursing care to a workforce of soldiers in the British Army during the Crimean War (Woodham-Smith, 1950). In 1854 she was asked by Sidney Herbert, the Secretary of War, to command a party of nurses to provide care to the ill and injured soldiers. It was reported that hospital conditions were horrid. There were no supplies to care for the ill and injured, the men were devoured by vermin, and the mortality rate was approximately 50% (Cohen, 1984). Nightingale and her nurses systematized a nursing service for the first time for the British Army, brought about extensive sanitary and engineering controls, and provided humanistic and rigorous care that resulted in a decrease in the death rate at the hospital in Scutari from 42.7% of the cases treated to 2.2% (Cohen, 1984). It was reported, however, that she was dictatorial in her methods with both nurses and physicians, causing moderate dissension; despite these difficulties, the mission was successful. Her sanitary reform methods improved the environmental/occupational work conditions for the soldiers, which drastically reduced the mortality that occurred primarily from disease rather than battle wounds.

After the Crimean War the popular image of the nurse had been transformed. In gratitude to Miss Nightingale, the British nation established the Nightingale Fund, which the now-acclaimed nursing leader used to start a nursing training school at St. Thomas' Hospital in 1860. As a result of this revolutionary process in nursing education, Nightingale nurses were educated nurses. This model was soon emulated by many other countries including the United States (Nightingale, 1946).

As had been the case in Europe, nursing in the United States during colonial times was provided mostly by religious orders. However, ties with England had always been close and the English example was very influential. By 1731,

Bellevue Hospital in New York and Philadelphia General Hospital (formerly called Blockley) were established. Almshouses were prevalent in many cities, but the nursing care, which required no special training, was poor. Both religious and secular groups were interested in reforms, and in 1861 the Women's Hospital in Philadelphia opened a school for nurses under the direction of the medical staff, who were all women. However, the teaching was considered too elementary, and the educational standards had to be revised. In the United States, another "first school" at the New England Hospital for Women and Children was organized by a physician, Marie Zabrzewska, who reportedly began teaching nurses as early as 1860. However, when the Civil War broke out in 1861 there were practically no trained nurses in the country and most war nurses were self-taught volunteers. After the war, these experiences helped focus attention on the weaknesses of the nursing system and the need for reform. Three nursing schools in America to be organized on the lines of the Nightingale system, each with a nurse superintendent, opened in 1873. The first school was at Bellevue Hospital in New York City, followed by the Connecticut Training School in New Haven and Massachusetts General Hospital in Boston. Soon thereafter, nursing schools in the United States proliferated rapidly. The women who brought nursing reform to the forefront in this country were dedicated, strong, and determined not only in the training and education of nurses, but in the development of sound nursing practice and a strong nursing profession (Bullough & Bullough, 1964).

■ OCCUPATIONAL HEALTH AND DISEASE

The occurrence of diseases as they relate to occupations has been studied for more than 2000 years (Hunter, 1978). As early as 400 B.C., Hippocrates wrote of various occupational diseases involving tradesmen and craftsmen, and the earliest record of the use of protective masks for miners exposed to inhalation dusts is found in the writings of Pliny the Elder (ca, A.D. 23–79). This apparatus consisted of a bladder tied over the mouth to prevent inhalation of poisonous dusts and vapors. Until the 16th century, little was known about occupational disease and less about occupational health. Georgius Agricola (1494–1555), a physician and mineralogist, and Aureolus von Hohenheim, M.D., known as Paracelsus (1493–1541), were leaders in the field of occupational medicine and spent many years studying the effects of mining, smelting, and the toxicology of certain metals. Agricola reported on the hazards of dust exposure, poor ventilation, and resultant harmful effects including asthma, silicosis, and tuberculosis. He also stated that:

If the dust has corrosive qualities, it eats away the lungs and implants consumption in the body. In the mines of the Carpathian Mountains women are found who have married seven husbands, all of whom this terrible consumption has carried off to a premature death.

Bernardino Ramazzini (1633–1714) published the first complete, systematic, and classic book on occupational diseases, *De Morbis Artificum Diatriba (The Diseases of Workmen)* in 1700, which earned him the title of the Father of Occupational Medicine. The scope of the text covers more than 100 different occupations and associated hazards and the significance of faulty posture, want of ventilation, unsuitable temperatures, personal cleanliness, and protective clothing. Regarding exposure of miners to metals he wrote:

The first and most potent is the harmful character of the materials that they handle, for these emit noxious vapors and very fine particles inimical to human beings and induce particular diseases; the second cause I ascribe to certain violent and irregular motions and unnatural postures of the body, by reason of which the natural structure of the vital machine is so impaired that serious diseases gradually develop therefrom.

The latter reflects his awareness of the discipline now called ergonomics. In addition to his classical work on occupational diseases, Ramazzini counseled that when obtaining information concerning illness from a patient, particularly one from the working class, it was of utmost importance to ask "What occupation does he follow?" and to consider this a potential cause for the illness or condition at hand (Goldwater, 1985).

The introduction of machinery into the textile industries of England began not with cotton but silk, with the first factory being built in 1718 (Hunter, 1978). The machinery was complicated, yet the operational processes were relatively simple. Again, the industrial revolution (1760–1830) transformed the situation, changing the face of England with many new inventions and developments including the spinning wheel, the power loom, the advent of steam power into mill factories, the upgrading of the steam engine, and the development of a railway system. The rapidity of these developments found Great Britain unprepared and disorganized. With the sudden and rapid population growth in urban areas, epidemics of cholera broke out in the town; however, social reform and regulation of public hygiene later in the early 19th century succeeded in making town life healthy and tolerable. With the advent of a new power source it became possible to build many factories in convenient spots, preferably near population centers.

Social consequences of the industrial revolution fell with particular severity on women and children. Orphaned or unwanted children were often virtually sold into slavery to the mill owners for cheap labor. Children were often abused and made to work up to 18 hours per day, and there was no legal provision for their welfare. Gradually, public opinion began to regard the excessive toil of children in the factory system as a monstrous exploitation. In 1819, The Factory Act was passed, which stipulated 9 years as a minimum age for child employment and also limited the number of working hours. Social reform was a continuous movement and The Factory Act of 1833 forbade night work for those under 18 and restricted their hours to 12 per day not to exceed 69 per week; factory schools were established, and children under 13 were required to attend at least two hours a day. This Act applied to all textile factories, whereas the previous Act (1819) did not (Hunter, 1978).

Mining was not affected by this Factory Act. The employment of women and girls was confined to certain mining districts where they were paid lower wages than men. Women were often harnessed, like horses, to coal trucks for hauling coal, or they carried coal in baskets on their backs up steep ladders and work passages. In some cases, girls of age 6 were found carrying 50 pounds of coal on their backs up ladders. In 1842 the Mines Act was passed, which forbade employment of girls and women for underground mining and of boys under 10. Reforms were also being advanced in the United States with the passage of the first child labor law in Massachusetts in 1836, stipulating that children under 15 were to receive at least three months of school during the work year. Six years later, an amendment to the law mandated that children under 12 could not work more than 10 hours daily in manufacturing establishments.

Related to society's concerns about child labor and occupational safety, the first paper on occupational medicine was produced by Benjamin McCready in 1837 titled "On the Influence of Trades, Professions, and Occupations in the United States, in the Production of Disease." It warned about the dangers of child labor, long working hours, and improper ventilation (McCready, 1837). However, it was more than 30 years before the first federal legislation was passed in 1968 regarding the eight-hour work day for certain groups of workers.

In the late 19th century, several companies and associations, including the Northern Pacific Railway Beneficial Association, the Macy Mutual Aid Association, the Domestake Mining Company of Lead, South Dakota, and the Pennsylvania Steel Company, began to establish programs for industrial medical services through hiring or contracting with physicians and surgeons (Felton, 1990). In 1916, with nearly 200 members, the American Association of Industrial Physicians and Surgeons was formed. It was later renamed the American Occupational Medicine Association, still later the American College of Occupational Medicine, and in 1991 the American College of Occupational and Environmental Medicine.

As industry continued to flourish in the United States, the concern for the health and safety of the workforce also increased. Massachusetts was the first state to study occupational safety, later requiring the reporting of industrial accidents in 1886. Several states soon followed and several State Bureaus of Labor Statistics were formed between 1872 and 1884. At the federal level the Bureau of Labor was established in 1884, which later became the Department of Commerce and Labor (1903), and then the United States Department of Labor (1913) (Grossman, 1973). One of the major industrial catastrophes of this time was a fire causing the deaths of 146 workers at the Triangle Shirt Waist Factory in New York City in 1911 (Stein, 1962). Working conditions in many factories were deplorable and deteriorated even further in the face of an industrial ethic that placed property rights above human rights. The proponents of this ethic maintained that industrial accidents were inevitable and were simply the cost of progress (LaDou, 1981). The United States lagged far behind Europe in protecting its workers. By 1897, Great Britain and several other countries had instituted safeguards for workers and workers' compensation systems to compensate workers injured as a result of their employment. It was not until 1911 that workers' compensation was instituted in the United States. By 1920, 40 states had workers' compensation laws, which for the most part were inadequate and rarely enforced. The Depression of the 1930s contributed to worker injuries; however, workers often overlooked the hazards of the workplace in order to keep their jobs (LaDou, 1981). In 1912 the National Council for Industrial Safety, which became the National Safety Council in 1913, was organized to collect data and promote accident prevention programs.

In the early 1900s, Dr. Alice Hamilton, a pioneer in the field of occupational health, began studying toxic industrial exposures, particularly lead. Her work on lead received notoriety and resulted in her appointment, as the first woman, to the faculty of the Harvard School of Medicine.

Little activity in occupational health was seen during World War I. However, delayed effects of cancer among radium watch dial painters (who in the course of their work dipped their brushes in radium, then to their lips with subsequent absorption) were brought to the public eye (Levy & Wegman, 1988). In addition, silicosis was becoming a more visible problem as a result of work in the "dusty trades," which brought to the forefront job-related lung disease.

In 1936 the Walsh-Healey Act, which set worker safety and health standards for employers receiving federal contracts over $10,000, was passed just before the advent of World War II. The Second World War witnessed an increased need for workers in defense plants and other manufacturing operations. In addition, increasing numbers of physicians, nurses, and other types of health professionals became engaged in the field of occupational health. After World War II and into the 1950s and early 1960s, little attention was directed toward occupational health, excepting the establishment of radiation safety standards under the Atomic Energy Act of 1954 (Levy & Wegman, 1988).

In the late 1960s and early 1970s several laws were enacted to protect worker health and safety. The Federal Metal and Non-Metalic Safety Act of 1966 was passed, followed by the Federal Coal Mine Safety and Health Act of 1969 as a result of fatal accidents in those industries, such as the deaths of 78 miners in a 1968 coal mine explosion in West Virginia. Shortly thereafter the Black Lung Benefits Act was passed in 1972.

The Environmental Protection Agency was formed in 1970 to protect air and water, while the first comprehensive occupational safety and health law, the Occupational Safety and Health Act (OSH Act) of 1970 was enacted to mandate a safe and healthful work environment for all employees. The OSH Act created three bodies including the Occupational Safety and Health Administration (OSHA) within the Department of Labor to set and enforce standards; the National Institute for Occupational Safety and Health (NIOSH) in the Department of Health and Human Service for research and education; and the Occupational Safety and Health Review Commission (OSHRC) to dispute arbitration (OSH Act 1970; Goldstein, 1971). OSHA's responsibilities include the promulgation and enforcement of occupational health and safety standards and require most employers to maintain records of work-related illnesses and injuries to be reported.

The chemical industry proliferated rapidly with the development of such compounds as dyes, synthetic dyestuffs, explosives, perfumes, plastics, and soaps, which brought with it new work processes and hazards that society was unprepared to handle. In 1976, the Toxic Substances Control Act was enacted to require testing of certain chemicals, thereby providing individual and environmental protection from the harmful effects of these substances.

In the 1980s, federal budget cuts and deregulation weakened OSHA. However, community and activists' concern for the workplace and environment resulted in the passage of the Hazard Communication Standard in 1983. The Standard was promulgated to require manufacturers and importers to determine if hazards are associated with products they produce or import, to evaluate those hazards, and to develop a written hazard communication program including hazardous substance labeling and employee training. This standard was later expanded to include all industries (Babbitz, 1986).

With the entrance of HIV / AIDS into society, more awareness has been created about the health and safety of at-risk individuals such as health care workers who may be potentially exposed to blood and other body fluids. This resulted in the establishment of the Bloodborne Pathogens Standard in 1991, designed to protect workers from potential and actual exposures to contaminated body fluids.

In 1990, the Americans With Disabilities Act (ADA) was passed to become effective in 1992. The ADA is designed to protect disabled individuals from discrimination, and Title I of the Act specifically addresses employment discrimination. The Act requires that employers treat disabled individuals fairly and equally with respect to employment practices. Health care professionals play a major role within these provisions with respect to such areas as understanding job functions, recommending reasonable accommodations, and job placement activities.

■ OCCUPATIONAL HEALTH NURSING

The emergence of occupational health nursing, formerly called industrial nursing, was gradual. The current practice of occupational health nursing is the result of an evolutionary process that began late in the 19th century. Health hazards related to workplace exposures and working conditions resulted in illnesses and injuries that in large measure could have been prevented. This gave rise to a new field of nursing practice. The first nurses in industry stemmed their practice from a prevention/public health nursing model and provided family and community health services as well as industrial health services focused on prevention and treatment of work-related illness and injury. Today the occupational health nurse's role has expanded considerably in scope to include such practice areas as health promotion, management, research, and policy development and has been influenced by and is a reflection of the growth and type of industry in contemporary society. However, the historical underpinnings of the practice remain grounded in preventive health care efforts and public health principles.

The earliest recorded evidence of industrial nursing was the employment of Phillipa Flowerday by the firm of J. & J. Colman of Norwich, England, in 1878 (Slaney, 1984). Miss Flowerday, who had trained for more than a year at the Norfolk and Norwich Hospital, was engaged at the mustard company by Mrs. Colman to assist the doctor in the dispensary and to visit sick employees and their families in their homes (Godfrey, 1978). Miss Flowerday made work-related home visits until her marriage in 1888. The Colman Company continued to employ nurses to provide health service to employees, established three shelters for those suffering from tuberculosis, and provided an ambulance service for ill or injured employees to be transported to the hospital. The company espoused prevention as being better than cure and provided employees with a recreational club house and the availability of rental houses, which were to ensure good, clean living conditions. Soon other companies began to appoint nurses to care for the ill and injured at work. World War I gave a great impetus toward the prevention of illness as it was thought that workers in ammunition factories were dying as a result of exposure to and absorption of toxic materials used in the work processes (Slaney, 1984). In addition, tuberculosis was rampant, and industrial nurses provided a large measure of health education with respect to sanitation and hygiene.

In the United States, the beginning of industrial or occupational health nursing dates back to the late 19th century. It has been reported that in 1888 a group of coal mining companies in Pennsylvania hired a nurse named Betty Moulder, a graduate of Philadelphia's Blockley Hospital, to care for ailing miners and their families (AAIN, 1976; Markolf, 1945; McGrath, 1945; Wright, 1919). The Vermont Marble Company is often credited with the first employment of an industrial health nurse, Ada Mayo Stewart in 1895 (Felton, 1985; Markolf, 1945). Felton (1985) gives an interesting description of the industrial operations in Vermont, from the 18th to the 20th century.

During the 18th century, Vermont, a state with promising economic potential in agriculture and lumber, became the site of a major marble industry when important deposits were discovered. The first commercial quarry opened in Dorset, Vermont around 1784, and the quarry at Sutherland Falls opened in 1836. The Sutherland Falls Marble Company did not prosper and subsequently dissolved; however, Colonel Redfield Proctor, who saw great promise in quarrying, acquired the company in 1869 and reorganized it into a viable business enterprise in 1870. In the early 1880s the rival Rutland Marble Company merged with the Sutherland Falls Company to become the Vermont Marble Company with Colonel Proctor as its president.

In 1889, Redfield Proctor, then governor of Vermont, became the Secretary of War and followed that with a tenure as United States Senator in 1891. He was succeeded at the Vermont Marble Company by his son Fletcher Proctor in 1889 until his death in 1911. The company continued to acquire other quarry properties and focused on the sale of sawed marble for monument use; finishing processes were added later. The Proctors were concerned about the welfare of their employees and their families, and Fletcher Proctor, who later also became governor of Vermont, had become familiar with the work of district nurses in several cities. He persuaded the board of directors of the Vermont Marble Company to employ a district nurse, Ada Mayo Stewart in 1895, a graduate of the Waltham School of Nursing in Massachusetts, who was skilled in surgical and dispensary nursing. Waltham School was also unique in its provision of training in visiting nursing.

Safety devices were nearly nonexistent in the quarrying process, resulting in what would now be considered preventable injuries, such as lacerations, contusions, and fractures. The worker population was ethnically varied, which made communication all the more challenging. Miss Stewart, whose primary mode of transportation was a bicycle, visited sick employees in their homes, provided emergency care, taught habits for healthy living, and taught mothers about child care. She learned much about the customs and methods of the sick used in the native countries of the workers and their families. Miss Stewart also gave talks on health and hygiene to school children, initially at the request of the school teacher, a personal friend.

A second nurse, Harriet Stewart, sister of Ada M. Stewart, was hired by the Vermont Marble Company in late 1895 to provide nursing services primarily to employees in the West and Center Rutland areas. With the success of the nursing service, the Vermont Marble Company opened a company hospital in August 1896 for the benefit of the employees and their families. Community residents could also be admitted as pay patients. Ada M. Stewart, who served as the first matron for two years, and Katherine Feld constituted the entire nursing staff and provided both hospital and home care services. Miss Stewart left Rutland and worked in several states doing private duty nursing, office nursing, massage therapy, and teaching of student nurses. She married in 1918 after returning to Rutland; however, little more is known of her activities. She died in Eastern Star nursing home in Randolph, Vermont, in 1945.

In the 19th century in America only two other accounts of nurses known to be employed by industries were recorded. In 1897, Anna B. Duncan was hired by the Benefit Association of the John Wanamaker Company, New York City, to visit sick employees, distribute funds fairly, provide emergency care, make referrals for ill and injured employees, conduct follow-up visits and carry out a communicable disease program aimed at prevention and rehabilitation (AAIN, 1976; Cahall, 1981). In 1899, Frederick Loeser established a nursing service for employees of his department store in Brooklyn, New York (AAIN, 1976; McGrath, 1945).

In the early 1900s employee health services proliferated rapidly throughout the country from Maine to California. Industrial products were reflective of the geographical areas; for example, in 1905 a Georgia nurse was employed by the Fulton Cotton Mills, and in Maine, nursing services were offered to employees of Great Northern Paper Company in 1913 (Obuchowski, 1963). By this time several employers in the New England states had hired industrial nurses, recognizing that the provision of organized, comprehensive, and well-managed health services to employees resulted in a more productive workforce as well as decreased absenteeism. In 1909, Metropolitan Life Insurance Company of New York City began offering a home visiting service to industrial workers insured through company policies. This type of service was extremely successful and spread to other regions of the country and Canada (AAIN, 1976; McGrath, 1946).

The rise of industrial nursing from 1910–1920 was accelerated by the advent of workers' compensation laws, World War I, and the emphasis on prevention of communicable diseases, especially tuberculosis (McGrath, 1945). The first organized movement in American industrial health nursing began in New England with the establishment of the first industrial nurse registry in 1913. In 1915, the Boston Industrial Nurses' Club was organized under the leadership of Anna Stabler, and gave nurses working in industry an opportunity to study and discuss common problems. This group soon evolved into the Massachusetts Industrial Nurses' Association and adjoining state associations soon developed and merged to form the New England Industrial Nurses' Association in 1918 (McGrath, 1946).

Another organization, the Factory Nurses Conference, composed only of graduate, state-registered nurses affiliated with the American Nurses' Association, originated in Boston in 1916. Meetings of this group resulted in an identified need for specialty education in industrial nursing, in addition to that of customary hospital training. As a result, arrangements were made with the Boston University College of Business Administration to offer a course titled Industrial Service for Nurses, which began in 1917 and continued annually for five years (McGrath, 1945). The course consisted of four hours of lecture per week for 16 weeks plus a two-week practice experience. Course content seemed to focus on industrial health issues and economics. In 1919 the first industrial nursing book was published (Wright, 1919).

During this period several prominent organizations that affected industrial nursing came into existence, including the American Nurses' Association (ANA) in 1911 (formerly organized as the Association Alumni, 1908), the National Organization for Public Health Nursing (NOPHN) in 1912, and the National League of Nursing Education (NLNE) in 1913 (formerly the Society of Superintendents, 1890) (Best, 1940). Both the NOPHN and ANA subsequently established Industrial Nursing Sections in 1920 and 1944, respectively. By 1922, branches of the Factory Nurses Conference had formed in several locations in the United States and Canada and the organization changed its name to the American Association of Industrial Nurses (AAIN), although its activities were never national in scope (McGrath, 1946).

During the 1920s several colleges and universities offered short courses in principles of industrial hygiene in which industrial nurses participated (Heimann, 1964; Klem, 1950). The NOPHN was quite interested and instrumental in the development of quality education in nursing and undertook, through a survey, an examination of the state of the art. The study resulted in the Winslow-Goldmark Report (1923), which in part emphasized the need for reform in industrial nursing education and recommended that all nursing education be in colleges or universities. The NLNE disagreed with the recommendation to close diploma schools and instead developed revised curricula for these schools; however, industrial nursing was not given much emphasis (Rood, 1941).

During the Great Depression, industrial growth ceased, unemployment increased, and worker health and safety programs became less important. As a result, the need for industrial nurses decreased. This reduction in force also had its impact on association memberships and AAIN merged with the more viable New England Association of Industrial Nurses in 1933 (McGrath, 1946).

In the late 1930s, the American Public Health Association and the National Organization of Public Health Nursing conducted a study of the duties and functions of 85 nurses working in 42 companies. The results of the study indicated a lack of uniformity in industrial nursing practices; unawareness of the importance of community resources on the part of the industrial nurses; lack of public health standards in this area; and finally, lack of training courses in the profession of industrial nursing (NOPHN, 1940).

The report emphasized that the responsibility for the status, image, education, professionalism, and setting of standards for practice rested with nursing and encouraged nursing to meet the challenge and accept the responsibility. However, nursing leaders both in service and education were slow to respond.

By 1928, there was a sufficient number of nurses employed by industry to support an independent specialty nursing association, and the First Joint Conference of the New England, New Jersey, New York, and Philadelphia Industrial Nurses Associations was held in New York City (AAIN, 1976). With the advent of World War II in 1940, industries grew and the demand for nurses increased dramatically. State nurse consultants were used to help meet the needs of new nurses in industry, with the first industrial health nurse consultant, Ruth Scott, employed in Indiana in 1939 (McGrath, 1945). The Industrial Hygiene Division of the United State Public Health Service added nurse consultants to their staff to expand their advisory services (Roberts, 1964). Annual conferences continued with more regional and local constituent associations joining as conference members, and it was soon recognized that a broader-based organizational structure was needed. In 1942, at the Fourth Joint Conference, members voted to create a national association, the American Association of Industrial Nurses, with Catherine Dempsey as its first president; annual dues were set at 50 cents (AAIN, 1976). The purposes of AAIN were to improve industrial nursing practice and education, increase interdisciplinary collaborative efforts, and act as the professional voice for industrial health nurses. Bylaws were adopted in 1943. (Note that the national organization, AAIN, was not the same organization previously identified as AAIN as an outgrowth of the Factory Nurses' Conference.)

Well into the 1940s, industrial nurses continued to work in isolation with no standardized practice approaches and limited course and field work available in industrial nursing in university settings. The NOPHN sought to correct the situation through development of a staff training course in industrial nursing (NOPHN, 1942). In 1944, AAIN published an Outline of Basic College Courses for Industrial Nurses, which was circulated for use among interested colleges and universities. In addition, five universities—Columbia, Harvard, Johns Hopkins, University of Michigan, and Yale—offered graduate programs in industrial hygiene to nurses.

In 1945 at least 15 colleges and universities offered industrial nursing courses at the baccalaureate level (Roberts, 1964). The NOPHN Industrial Nursing Section, the AAIN and the NLNE established an advisory committee to study the issue of preparing nurses at the baccalaureate level for industrial nursing positions (ANA, 1945). The committee believed this was a specialty area that should be taught at the graduate level. The report of the Advisory Committee on Industrial Nursing resulted in the discontinuance of the industrial nursing courses in baccalaureate schools of nursing excepting the University of Pittsburgh (Roberts, 1964). Schools that offered additional specialties at the baccalaureate level were not accredited by NLNE. During this same year AAIN opened its first headquarters in New York City and published the Qualifications of Nurses in Industry, which it distributed to corporate managers (AAIN, 1976).

AAIN began participation in a structure study of the six existing national nursing organizations. (In addition to AAIN were the American Nurses' Association, National League for Nursing Education, Association of Collegiate Schools of Nursing, National Association of Colored Graduate Nurses, and the National Organization of Public Health Nursing.) The purpose of the study was to explore the possibility of incorporating all six groups into one national nursing organization, and during the next six years the directors of each of these groups met and considered the proposal.

In 1952, at the annual AAIN conference in Cincinnati, members voted to remain an independent and autonomous voice for the nation's industrial nurses. This historic decision came in response to the study undertaken in 1946 by AAIN and the other national nursing organizations to explore merging into one national group. (As a result of that study, three of the associations—the National League for Nursing Education, the Association of Collegiate Schools of Nursing, and the National Organization of Public Health Nursing—merged to form the National League of Nurses, and the National Association of Colored Graduate Nurses merged with the American Nurses' Association.)

The decision by AAIN to remain independent was perhaps the most carefully considered decision in the Association's entire history. It was based on the belief that the interest of the nation's industrial nurses would best be served if they focused their power, thought, and effort in one single group organized by and for industrial nurses. At the same time, however, AAIN reaffirmed its intention of working closely with other nursing organizations, which continues today.

AAIN was incorporated in 1953, and the first issue of the *Industrial Nurses Journal,* AAIN's new official publication, was published. During the 1950s, the

AAIN, NLN, ANA and PHS formed a committee that established the functions of industrial health nurses and also identified the educational needs of nurses in the specialty. During this period several separate studies on the role, function, and educational preparation of the industrial health nurse were conducted. Recommendations included increasing industrial health nursing content into nursing curricula and encouraging industrial managers to employ qualified industrial health nurses. In 1958 the ANA Industrial Nursing Section voted to change their section name to occupational health nursing, the rationale being that the term was broader, more inclusive, and better described the role of the nurse in the specialty (AJN, 1958).

In the 1960s, occupational health and safety became a public issue via the media and environmental and civil rights movements. Of particular concern were mining accidents, cave-ins, and black lung disease. The importance of adequate education and training for professional disciplines was gaining increasing congressional support. In 1962, AAIN appointed a committee to study the possibility of establishing the American Board for Certification of Industrial Nurses, which was later established in 1972 (AAOHN, 1976). However, education for occupational health nurses in the 1960s continued to wax and wane and additional studies were conducted to examine occupational health nursing content in baccalaureate programs and recommendations for additional content to be included. In 1965, the ANA recommended that all nursing education be taught in colleges and universities and that diploma schools be closed. The NLN again opposed this position and reversed its position for approval of public health nursing in both baccalaureate and master's programs (ANA, 1965).

By the beginning of the 1970s, nursing education and practice were in a transitional state and more emphasis was placed on the clinical expanded role for the nurse. The landmark Occupational Health and Safety Act of 1970 provided a new stimulus and interest among both the practice and academic communities to prepare occupational health nurses and nurse practitioners at the graduate level to work in occupational health settings. Under the auspices of NIOSH, Occupational Safety and Health Educational Resource Centers were established to provide education and research opportunities in occupational health and safety for nurses, physicians, engineers, and industrial hygienists. Undergraduate, graduate (master's and doctoral level), and continuing education are provided for within the mission of the Act; however, much more emphasis is placed on graduate level training and providing continuing education courses. A listing of NIOSH-funded Educational Resource Centers can be found in Appendix 2–1.

In 1977, the AAIN changed its name to the American Association of Occupational Health Nurses. The term occupational health nurse has replaced industrial nurse to reflect the broad scope of practice of the occupational health nurse. In 1994, organizational membership exceeded 12,000, representing more than 50% of the estimated number of practicing occupational health nurses.

The 1980s witnessed an expansion of the role of the occupational health nurse with more involvement in health promotion, management and policy development, cost containment, research and regulatory issues affecting practice (Babbitz, 1983; Rogers, 1988). As mentioned previously, the Hazard Communication Standard was promulgated in 1983. In order to protect the "trade secret" of a chemical, the original standard stated that the identity of a chemical would only be disclosed to a physician or nurse in emergency situations or in nonemergency situations, to a health care professional upon written need to know. The definition of health professional was limited to physician, epidemiologist, toxicologist, or industrial hygienist. Occupational health nurses were blatantly excluded. Through intense negotiations with OSHA and lobbying activities by AAOHN and occupational health nurses nationwide, access to trade secret chemical identity was extended to occupational health nurses in order to treat them the same as other health professionals. In addition, employees and their designated representatives who could demonstrate a "need to know" were granted access with the provision that confidentiality be maintained. The importance of this standard is not only reflected by its notification to workers and others as to the hazards related to chemical exposure, but the rightful recognition of registered nurses as health care professionals.

Efforts by AAOHN contributed to the hiring of the first occupational health nurse consultant by OSHA in 1988 to provide technical assistance in occupational health standards development, and field consultation regarding OSHA regulatory statutes. This provided further recognition of the importance of the nurse's contribution to the health of the American workforce and ultimately resulted in the establishment of the Office of Occupational Health Nursing at OSHA in 1993.

As with other fields of nursing practice, research in occupational health nursing has become more important. In 1983, the AAOHN established the first research award, named for Mary Louise Brown, an occupational health nurse consultant, educator, and author of the textbook *Occupational Health Nursing* (1956), given to recognize research that advances occupational health nursing practice. In 1986, Congress recognized the important role nurses play in health care, and that nursing research contributes to the delivery of more effective, efficient, and humane health care. Hence, the National Center for Nursing Research (NCNR), which was designated the National Institute for Nursing Research (NINR) in 1993, was established to promote the growth and quality of research related to nursing and patient care, and to help focus the nation's nursing research activities (Rogers, 1986). In 1989, the first AAOHN research priorities in occupational health nursing (see Chapter 14) were established and published in order to identify the most pertinent areas needing investigation, and to encourage private and public sources such as NINR and NIOSH to recognize the need for funding occupational health nursing research (Rogers, 1989).

■ CONCLUSION

For approximately a century, occupational health nurses have been providing health care at the worksite in order to promote, protect, and preserve the health of America's workforce. During this time occupational health nursing practice has expanded considerably and nurses have embraced newer areas of health promotion, research, and policy making. The history of occupational health nursing is rich and provides the underpinnings for our practice, which is sound and will continue to evolve.

References

American Association of Industrial Nurses. The nurse in industry. New York: The American Association of Industrial Nurses, 1976.

American Nurses' Association. A position paper. New York: Author, 1965.

American Nurses' Association. Industrial nursing in the basic curriculum. American Journal of Nursing, *45:* 478, 1945.

Babbitz, M. The practice of occupational health nursing in the U.S. Occupational Health Nursing, *31:* 23–25, 1983.

Babbitz, M. Hazard communication: Workers' right to know, nurses' need to know. AAOHN Journal, *34*(6): 260–263, 1986.

Best, E. Brief historical review and information about current activities of the American Nurses' Association including certain facts relative to the National League for Nursing Education. New York: American Nurses' Association, 1940.

Bullough, B & Bullough, VL. The emergence of modern nursing. New York: Macmillan, 1964.

Cahall, JB. The history of occupational health nursing. Occupational Health Nursing, *29:* 11–13, 1981.

Cohen, B. Florence Nightingale. Scientific American, *250:* 128–137, 1984.

Dock, LL & Stewart, IM. A short history of nursing. New York: G.P. Putnam's Sons, 1938.

Felton, J. The genesis of American occupational health nursing: Part I. Occupational Health Nursing, *33:* 615–621, 1985.

Felton, JS. Occupational medical management. Boston: Little, Brown, & Company, 1990.

Godfrey, H. One hundred years of industrial nursing. Nursing Times, Nov. 30, 1978, pp. 1966–1969.

Goldstein, DH. The occupational safety and health act of 1970. American Journal of Nursing, *71:* 1535–1538, 1971.

Goldwater, L. Historical highlights in occupational medicine. Readings and Perspectives in Medicine, *9:* 1–42, 1985.

Grossman, J. The Department of Labor, New York: Praeger, 1973.

Heimann, H. Occupational health 1914–1964. Public Health Reports, *79:* 941–947, 1964.

Hunter, D. The diseases of occupations (6th ed.). London: Hodder & Stroughton, 1978.

Klem, M. Industrial health and medical programs. Washington, DC: Government Printing Office, 1950.

LaDou, J. Occupational health law. New York: Marcel Dekker, 1981.

Levy, B & Wegman, D. Occupational health: Recognizing and preventing work-related disease. Boston: Little, Brown & Company, 1988.

Markolf, AS. Industrial nursing begins in Vermont. Public Health Nursing, *37:* 125–129, 1945.

McCready, B. On the influence of trades, professions and occupations in the United States in the production of disease, 1837. Johns Hopkins Press, Baltimore: 1943.

McGrath, BJ. Fifty years of industrial nursing. Public Health Nurse, *37:* 119–124, 1945.

McGrath, BJ. Nursing in commerce and industry. New York: The Commonwealth Fund, 1946.

National Organization for Public Health Nursing. A study of industrial nursing services. Public Health Nursing, *32:* 631–636, 1940.

National Organization for Public Health Nursing. A program for staff education. Public Health Nursing, *34:* 39–47, 1942.

Nightingale, F. Notes on nursing: What it is and what it is not. New York: Appleton-Century-Crofts, 1946.

Obuchowski, M. The industrial nurse in New England. New England Association of Industrial Nursing, 13–14, 1963.

Occupational Safety and Health Act of 1970. Public Law 91-596. Washington, DC: U.S. Government Printing Office, 1987.

Roberts, MM. American nursing: History and interpretation. New York: Macmillan, 1964.

Rogers, B. National Center for Nursing Research. AAOHN Journal, *34:* 196–197, 1986.

Rogers, B. Establishing research priorities in occupational health nursing. AAOHN Journal, *37:* 493–500, 1989.

Rogers, B. Perspectives in occupational health nursing. AAOHN Journal, *36:* 151–155, 1988.

Rood, D. The university and the industrial nurse. American Journal of Nursing, *41:* 201–205, 1941.

Slaney, B. The development of occupational health nursing. Nursing (Lond.), *2:* 1–3, 1984.

Stein, L. The Triangle Fire. Philadelphia: Lippincott, 1962.

The 1958 Convention, American Journal of Nursing, *58:* 980, 1958.

Woodham-Smith, C. Florence Nightingale. London: Constable, 1950.

Wright, FS. Industrial nursing. New York: Macmillan, 1919.

2–1

National Institute for Occupational Safety and Health Educational Resource Centers

ALABAMA EDUCATIONAL RESOURCE CEN-
TER
University of Alabama at Birmingham
School of Public Health
Birmingham, AL 35294-0008
(205) 934-7032

CALIFORNIA EDUCATIONAL RESOURCE
CENTER NORTHERN
University of California, Berkeley
School of Public Health
322 Warren
Berkeley, CA 94720
(510) 642-0761

CALIFORNIA EDUCATIONAL RESOURCE
CENTER SOUTHERN
University of Southern California
Inst. of Safety & Systems Management
University Park
Los Angeles, CA 90089-0021
(213) 740-4038

CINCINNATI EDUCATIONAL RESOURCE
CENTER
University of Cincinnati
Department of Environmental Health
3223 Eden Avenue
Cincinnati, OH 45267-0056
(513) 558-5701

HARVARD EDUCATIONAL RESOURCE
CENTER
Harvard School of Public Health
Department of Environmental Health
665 Huntington Avenue
Boston, MA 02115
(617) 432-3325

ILLINOIS EDUCATIONAL RESOURCE CENTER
University of Illinois at Chicago
School of Public Health
P.O. Box 6998, M/C 922
Chicago, IL 60680
(312) 996-7887

JOHNS HOPKINS EDUCATIONAL RESOURCE
CENTER
Johns Hopkins University
School of Hygiene and Public Health
615 North Wolfe Street
Baltimore, MD 21205
(301) 955-3602

MICHIGAN EDUCATIONAL RESOURCE
CENTER
University of Michigan
School of Public Health
Dept. of Environmental and Industrial Health
Ann Arbor, MI 48109
(313) 936-0753

MINNESOTA EDUCATIONAL RESOURCE
CENTER
University of Minnesota
School of Public Health
1158 Mayo Memorial Bldg.
420 Delaware Street, S.E.
Minneapolis, MN 55455
(612) 626-0900

NEW YORK/NEW JERSEY EDUCATIONAL
RESOURCE CENTER
Department of Community Medicine
Mt. Sinai School of Medicine
P.O. Box 1057
10 E. 102nd St.
New York, NY 10029
(212) 241-4804

NORTH CAROLINA EDUCATIONAL RE-
SOURCE CENTER
University of North Carolina
School of Public Health
Rosenau Hall, CB 7400
Chapel Hill, NC 27599-7410
(919) 966-5001

TEXAS EDUCATIONAL RESOURCE CENTER
The University of Texas Health Science Center at
Houston
School of Public Health
P.O. Box 20186
Houston, TX 77225
(713) 792-4638

UTAH EDUCATIONAL RESOURCE CENTER
University of Utah
Rocky Mountain Center for Occupational and En-
vironmental Health
Bldg. 512
Salt Lake City, UT 84112
(801) 581-8719

WASHINGTON EDUCATIONAL RESOURCE
CENTER
University of Washington
Department of Environmental Health, SC-34
Seattle, WA 98195
(206) 543-6991

3

THE NATURE AND PRACTICE OF OCCUPATIONAL HEALTH NURSING

The field of occupational health nursing has changed substantially in recent decades. Although the basic philosophy of occupational health nursing has not changed, that is, to maintain a health orientation, protect worker health, keep workers healthy, and provide a safe and healthful work environment, contemporary occupational health nursing philosophy incorporates increased emphasis on health promotion, research-based practice, interdisciplinary collaboration, improved quality of life in general and work life in specific, and program and policy development. The occupational health nurse functions in many roles including clinician, manager, educator, researcher, and consultant as described later in Chapter 4. Within the scope of these roles, the nurse functions as an employee advocate and as a liaison with management to influence the concept of health at the worksite.

▪ PRACTICE UNDERPINNINGS

From its early beginnings in the 19th century, occupational health nursing practice has been grounded in the concepts and principles of public health practice, focusing on prevention, health teaching, and the control and elimination of health hazards in the workplace and community. For example, early occupational health nurses provided health-oriented nursing services not only to employees at the worksite, but also to workers and families in the community. Community surveillance observations and school-based health talks to children were also part of the occupational health nurse's activities in the late 19th century (Felton, 1985; McGrath, 1946; Wright, 1919). Occupational health nurses worked to provide public health agency-sponsored nursing services to industries, particularly aimed at controlling communicable diseases. In addition, in 1909 the first home nursing service program, established by Lillian Wald, was offered through the Metropolitan Life Insurance Company to provide public health nursing services to holders of industrial policies (Christy, 1970). Parker-Conrad (1988) states that "out of the home nursing services provided by early occupational health nurses, employers recognized that nurses could save them money by teaching good health habits, monitoring and following up on medical care, and assuring that employees were following medical advice and that they returned for necessary care."

The specialty of occupational health nursing has always been closely linked to community health and public health nursing, which provides the underpinnings for the practice base. Community and public health nurses utilize knowledge synthesized from public health and nursing fields to improve the health of the population, through prevention and health promotion strategies. Consistent with historical and contemporary public health philosophy, Williams (1988) describes public health nursing as aggregate or population-focused, which provides the distinguishing characteristic from other nursing specialties (e.g., medical-surgical, oncology). Occupational health nurses also utilize public health and nursing knowledge as cornerstones for practice in addition to more specific knowledge fields such as occupational health, toxicology, and safety. Although definitions will be presented later, it is important to appreciate these underpinnings of practice, as they provide the foundations upon which occupational health nursing practice builds.

This chapter focuses on a discussion of the philosophy, nature, and scope of practice in occupational health nursing and describes a conceptual model for nursing practice. Foundational underpinnings and prevention concepts will be explored as major contributions to the practice base.

■ PHILOSOPHY

The purpose of a philosophy is that it helps to clarify and establish beliefs and values about one's orientation to and direction in life including relationships with other people, society, and the environment in which one lives and works. It assists in understanding why certain decisions and choices are made. One's personal philosophical beliefs extend to and are integrated in a philosophy of professional nursing practice.

The heritage of occupational health nursing is reflected in a degree of independence in practice often not shared by other nursing colleagues in acute care settings. This is complemented by an interdependent role with other professionals and groups, which not only is integral to occupational health nursing practice but also enhances the health care provided at the worksite. In the delivery of occupational health nursing services it is important to provide comprehensive professional health care to individuals, groups, and workforces with respect to human dignity and self-worth while promoting accountability. The occupational health nurse has the primary responsibility for the management of worker health and safety with consideration to ethical, cultural, spiritual, and corporate beliefs.

The worksite is a community with health needs requiring attention to health promotion and protection, prevention of disease and disability, and treatment of illness and injury. However, for many industries, health services may be considered of secondary importance, inasmuch as they do not generate income, but rather cost the company money. The nurse helps management to recognize the economic and human benefits of occupational health programs and helps maximize productivity by promoting employee mental and physical well-being while ensuring cost-effectiveness.

Within a values framework, the occupational health nurse functions autonomously, maintains self-integrity, and demonstrates leadership in decision-making. Uustal (1978) defines values as general guides to behavior and standards of conduct that one endorses and tries to live up to or maintain. Values provide a basic frame of reference to guide individuals as they deal with issues involving decision-making, and in professional lives, how decisions regarding the delivery of health care to worker clients are made. The occupational health nurse will be involved in many issues in the workplace that will have a direct effect on the health and well-being of the individual worker and workforce. For example, issues related to access of health records may present problems or conflicts if the premise of confidentiality is not shared by others. When conflicts arise, the occupational health nurse will need to make decisions that involve some risk-taking (Rogers, 1988). Management, occupational health nurses, and other health care professionals must strive to understand and respect each others' roles, and must confront issues which threaten worker health and safety.

Brown (1981) states that the smooth administration of the occupational health unit is in part contingent upon the occupational health nurse's commitment to a philosophy of providing quality services to workers, and that this philosophy should be in writing. A philosophy of occupational health nursing service should be a clear, concise statement that reflects one's fundamental beliefs and forms the basis for practice and professional activities. A philosophy of occupational health nursing practice and service should emphasize the conviction that the health and safety of the worker and workforce is the concern of the occupational health nurse. It should reflect statements of beliefs and values about:

1. the promotion and protection of health throughout the work community;
2. a commitment to a concept of quality health as reflected in the goals and objectives of the occupational health service, including resource appropriation and utilization;
3. respect for worker rights and treatment related to principles of self-determination and non-discrimination, and the receipt of quality health care while protecting employee confidentiality;
4. dynamics of the work environment and diversity of the worker population;
5. employer and employee responsibility for health and safety;
6. the benefits of the occupational health service to the worker population and company;
7. the competence and continuing professional development of the staff including recognition of legal and ethical considerations and accountability for practice; and
8. collaborative multidisciplinary relationships that support and enhance worker health and safety, and the relationship of the occupational health service to the community.

Knowledge of the company and workers, including the history, company culture, policies, programs, workplace hazards, and workforce trends will be helpful, as this may provide information regarding congruence between the occupational health nurse's philosophy and the organization's philosophy of health and safety. If there are conflicting differences, they will need to be discussed and resolved with management. The Code of Ethics of the American Association of Occupational Health Nurses (AAOHN), which was revised and adopted in 1991, can serve as a guide for developing a philosophy statement for the occupational health nursing service (AAOHN, 1991). An example of a philosophy statement is shown in Table 3–1.

■ **TABLE 3–1**   Philosophy of Occupational Health Nursing Service

The occupational health service contributes to a safe and healthful work environment through programs aimed at reducing and eliminating work-related hazards and enhancing health promotion. Occupational health services are provided to individual workers and the collective workforce within an environment that considers and meets the needs of a diverse workforce.

The occupational health nursing service is central and integral to an effective occupational health program. The occupational health nurse professional is an advocate for the worker and often manages the occupational health service. As such the occupational health nurse is concerned not only with how the worker's health is affected or influenced by the worksite and organization but also by how the worker, her or his family, the community, and the environment interact to affect worker health and productivity.

To protect worker rights, workers are given information regarding work-related hazards so that informed decisions can be made. In addition, confidentiality of health records and information is safeguarded.

The occupational health nurse professional is part of a collaborative team that has the responsibility to inform the employer of unsafe and unhealthful working conditions and practices and of the need for workplace controls. The employer has the responsibility to provide a safe and healthful work environment and to recognize and support the occupational health nurse as a professional with specialized knowledge and skills.

The occupational health nurse professional has an obligation to maintain and improve knowledge and skills relative to her or his position and to keep current with research and legislation affecting occupational health and nursing practice; the occupational health nurse professional is accountable for interventions, judgments, and decisions made according to practice standards.

The occupational health nursing service encourages a mutually supportive relationship with the community through referrals and utilization of resources and by being a productive part of the larger ecosystem that enhances the environment.

High-quality occupational health care is provided in a cost-effective manner that promotes productivity through good health.

In the work environment a philosophy statement can aid in the orientation of employees to the corporate and health mission, and provide a foundation for the delivery of quality services (Brown, 1984). The formulation of a written philosophy will help to establish the beliefs about the health care of the workforce, provide the foundation for putting those beliefs into practice, and guide the activities of the occupational health nurse. Over time, an individual's philosophy will evolve through new experiences, and those considered meaningful will be integrated into one's own belief system.

■ **SCOPE OF OCCUPATIONAL HEALTH NURSING PRACTICE**
Definitions

The definition of occupational health nursing has evolved over time and reflects the changing role of the occupational health nurse with more emphasis on autonomous decision making, independent functioning, health promotion, prevention, analytical and investigative skills, and management of health care services. Many factors have influenced the evolution of occupational health nursing practice, such as the changing population and workforce; the introduction of new chemicals and work processes into the work environment; a concomitant increase in hazards in the workplace; technological advances and regulatory mandates; an increased interest in health promotion and illness/injury prevention; and an increase in health care costs and workers' compensation claims. Because of the nature of occupational health nursing, it is important that the nurse utilize a multidisciplinary approach to address the health problems of the workforce.

Adapted from the scope of practice document of the American Association of Occupational Health Nurses (1993) and embodied within the standards for practice, occupational health nursing practice is defined as:

The specialty practice that provides for and delivers health care services to workers and worker populations. The practice focuses on promotion, protection and restoration of workers' health within the context of a safe and healthy work environment. Occupational health nursing practice is autonomous, and occupational health nurses make independent nursing judgements in providing occupational health services. The foundation for occupational health nursing practice is research-based with an emphasis on optimizing health, preventing illness and injury, and reducing health hazards.

Occupational health nursing practice is derived from a synthesis of knowledge gained primarily from the nursing, medicine, public health, occupational health, social/behavioral sciences, as well as from management/administration theories and concepts and legal/regulatory principles.

As previously discussed, occupational health nursing is closely linked to community health and public health nursing philosophically and through theoretical and practice applications; thus, the occupational health nurse will also want to be familiar with these definitions. Using the terms community health nursing and public health nursing synonomously, the American Nurses Association (ANA) (1986) defines community health nursing as follows:

Community health nursing practice promotes and preserves the health of populations by integrating skills and knowledge relevant to both nursing and public health. The practice is comprehensive and general, and is not limited to a particular age or diagnostic group; it is continual, and is not limited to episodic care. Community health nursing practice promotes the public's health. The programs, services, and institutions involved in public health emphasize promotion and maintenance of the population's health, and the prevention and limitation of disease. Public health activities change with changing technology and social values, but the goals remain the same; to reduce the amount of disease, premature death, discomfort, and disability.

The American Public Health Association (APHA) (1981), Public Health Nursing Section, has defined public health nursing as follows:

Public health nursing synthesizes the body of knowledge from the public health sciences and professional nursing theories for the purpose of improving the health of the entire community. This goal lies at the heart of primary prevention and health promotion and is the foundation for public health nursing practice. To accomplish this goal, public health nurses work with groups, families, and individuals as well as in multidisciplinary teams and progams. Identifying the subgroups (aggregates) within the population which are at high risk of illness, disability, or premature death, and directing resources toward these groups is the most effective approach for accomplishing the goal of public health nursing. Success in reducing the risks and in improving the health of the community depends on the involvement of consumers, especially groups experiencing health risks, and others in the community, in health planning, and in self-help activities.

Both the ANA and APHA definitions emphasize prevention and health promotion efforts as strategic for health improvement and reducing the risk of illness, which is consistent with the guiding precepts for occupational health nursing practice.

The Prevention Foundation

Consistent with public health philosophy, prevention marks the cornerstone for occupational health nursing practice. Within this health-orientation framework of prevention, the primary goals of occupational health nursing practice are to:

- promote, maintain, and restore the physical and psychosocial well-being of the workers in order to enhance optimal functioning;
- protect the worker from hazards that may occur as a result of the work experience;
- encourage and participate in a company culture supportive of health; and
- collaborate with workers, management and other disciplines, and health care professionals to ensure a safe work environment.

While health promotion, protection, and prevention are discussed in much greater detail in Chapter 12, conceptual definitions as they apply to the occupational health nurse's scope of practice will be discussed here.

As shown in Figure 3–1, Leavell and Clark (1965) first classified levels of prevention in three phases—primary, secondary, and tertiary, as follows:

Prevention may be accomplished in the prepathogenesis period by measures designed to promote general optimum health or by the specific protection of human beings against disease agents or the establishment of barriers against agents in the environment. These procedures have been termed primary prevention.

As soon as the disease is detectable, early in pathogenesis, secondary prevention may be accomplished by early diagnosis and prompt and adequate treatment. When the process of pathogenesis has progressed and the disease has advanced beyond its early stages, secondary prevention may also be accomplished by means of adequate treatment to prevent sequelae and limit disability. Later, when defect and disability have been fixed, tertiary prevention may be accomplished by rehabilitation (1965, p. 20).

Within this framework, primary prevention incorporates both health promotion and protection, secondary prevention is aimed at early diagnosis/treatment and disability limitation, and rehabilitation is the main strategy for tertiary prevention. This model has provided a useful guide for public health professionals in recognizing health intervention strategies prior to developing or at different stages of a disease.

The occupational health nurse practices at all levels of prevention. Using the Leavell and Clark framework, Wachs and Parker-Conrad (1990) identify programmatic activities that relate to prevention strategies in the occupational health setting (Table 3–2). Delivery of primary prevention services to employees is directed toward promoting health and averting a problem. In the occupational health setting, the purpose of health promotion is to maintain or enhance the well-being of individuals or groups of employees, and the company in general. Activities are designed to bring about changes in knowledge, attitudes, and behaviors of workers and management as they relate to health and safety practices at work, and in the larger sense, lifestyle patterns. This may include programs

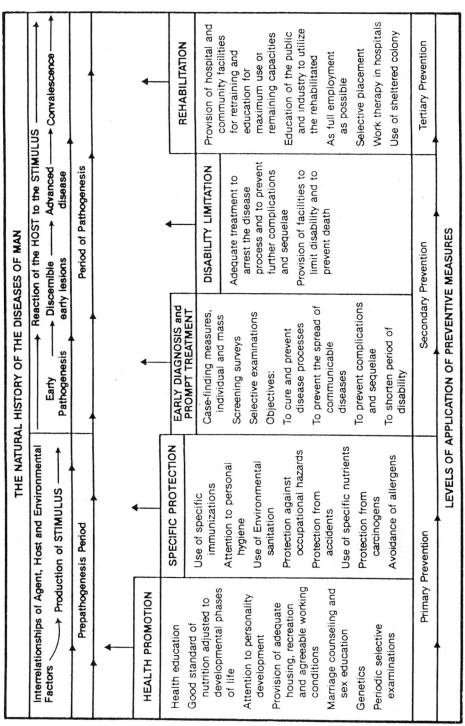

■ **Figure 3–1** Three levels of disease prevention (From Leavall, HR & Clark, EG. Preventive medicine for the doctor and his community (3rd ed.). New York: McGraw-Hill, 1965.)

■ **TABLE 3-2**   Examples of Comprehensive Occupational Health Program Elements

Primary Prevention		Secondary Prevention	Tertiary Prevention
Health Promotion	*Disease Prevention*	Preplacement; yearly and termination exams	Early back to work
Nutrition	Injury prevention	Health surveillance	Modified duty
Fitness/exercise	Accident investigation	Triage system	Work hardening
Coping enhancement	Disease prevention	Employee record system	Onsite therapy
ment	Health risk appraisal	Accident reporting	Chronic illness
Recreation	Health education	Injury diagnosis and treatment	Monitoring
Parenting skills	Smoking cessation		
	Weight control		
	Stress management		

From Wachs, J & Parker-Conrad, J. Applied Occupational and Environmental Hygiene, 5: 200–203, 1990.

designed to enhance coping skills or good nutrition and knowledge about potential health hazards both in and outside the workplace.

Health protection measures are designed to eliminate or reduce the risk of disease in order to prevent the development of an illness or injury. Walk-throughs by the occupational health nurse and/or other team members to identify workplace hazards are aimed at health protection. Environmental monitoring strategies to contain and control toxic substances in the workplace, so workers are not harmed, are health protection strategies.

Specific protection programs or interventions often require active participation on the part of the employee. Participation in an immunization program, utilization of personal protective equipment, such as respirators or gloves, or actual smoking cessation are examples of specific health protection measures.

Secondary prevention occurs after a disease process has already begun and is aimed at early detection, prompt treatment, and prevention of further limitations. For employees, early detection involves health surveillance and periodic screening to identify an illness at the earliest possible moment in its course, and elimination or modification of the hazard-producing situation. The provision of screening services such as high blood pressure monitoring or periodic breast screening/examinations, and reporting and analysis of injury trend data are further examples of early detection measures. Interventions aimed at disability limitation are intended to prevent further harm or deterioration. For example, referral for counseling and treatment of an employee with an emotional/mental health problem whose work performance has deteriorated, or removal of workers from heavy metal exposure who manifest neurologic symptoms, would provide an avenue for prevention of a potentially harmful or serious disorder.

Tertiary prevention is intended to restore health as fully as possible and assist individuals to achieve their maximum level of functioning. Rehabilitation strategies such as return-to-work programs after a heart attack or limited duty programs after a cumulative trauma injury are examples of tertiary prevention. Continued rehabilitation of employees with substance abuse problems through hospitalization or outpatient referral, counseling an employee with chronic obstructive lung disease regarding smoking cessation, or chronic illness monitoring would constitute tertiary preventive measures.

Pender (1987) distinguishes health promotion from prevention with the former directed toward increasing one's level of well-being and moving toward a state of optimal health including activities such as regular exercise and good nutrition. Prevention and health protection activities are directed toward risk avoidance (e.g., smoking cessation), disease detection and disability limitation (e.g., screening and periodic examinations), and health rehabilitation or restoration (e.g., chronic disease monitoring). Pender's model and the occupational health nurse's role in health promotion, protection, and prevention will be described more in-depth in Chapter 12.

■ CONCEPTUAL MODEL FOR PRACTICE

Various components of the scope of occupational health nursing practice have been described by several authors (AAOHN, 1987; Babbitz, 1983; Brown, 1981; Hannigan, 1984; Lee, 1978; McKechnie, 1983; Wachs & Parker-Conrad, 1990; Rogers, 1990). Figure 3–2 depicts a conceptual model for occupational health nursing practice. The occupational health nurse is considered a key figure in the management and delivery of occupational health services and practices within a legal/ethical framework. The ultimate goal of occupational health nursing is to improve, protect, maintain, and restore the health of the worker and workforce. This is accomplished through a scope of practice that is expansive and is impacted by both external and internal or work setting influences. Thus, areas representative of the scope of occupational health nursing practice (Fig. 3–2) are dis-

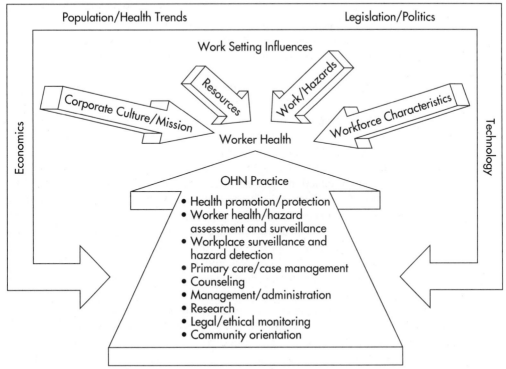

■ **Figure 3–2**   Conceptual model for occupational health nursing practice. (Adapted from Rogers, B. AAOHN Journal, *38*(11): 536–543, 1990. By permission of the American Association of Occupational Health Nurses.)

cussed within the context of this conceptual model for occupational health nursing practice.

External Influences

The work setting and ultimately worker health are impacted by external factors including population and health trends, legislation and politics, technology, and the economy.

- Population and health trends to be considered include such areas as an increase in socio-cultural diversity, an aging society with concomitant chronic diseases, health and social consequences of societal substance abuse and violence, and infectious/communicable diseases (e.g., TB, HIV). Furthermore, in years to come, bipolar population trends with respect to age (i.e., the very old and the very young group) will be apparent, which will bring with it a need for varying types of health programs specific to population needs. As the workplace is a microcosm of the larger society, trends such as these will be reflected in the workplace. In addition, more single family households resulting in more women in the workforce will require workplace changes such as the availability of or accommodation for child care and consideration for alternative work scheduling.
- Legislation and resulting regulations regarding worker health and safety will specifically impact the workplace in terms of required health and safety program initiatives and expansion, implementation of administrative and control mechanisms, available resources, and associated costs. Recent examples include initiatives associated with the Americans With Disabilities Act, the Bloodborne Pathogens Standard, the Hazard Communication Standard, and potential implications related to the OSHA Reform Act. In addition, any proposed health care reform legislation will have a significant impact on the business community with respect to related health care costs and service delivery.

   Political influence affects the passage of legislative acts; thus, efforts of professional societies and special interest groups currently play a major role in health legislation and worker health and safety regulations. Concern regarding fairness, equality and undue influence with respect to political decision-making has been repeatedly expressed by society.
- Technological advances in work processes may provide avenues for increased productivity and efficiency, but also may create situations where workers are displaced with new machines, computers, or robotics. As a result, workers may need to be retrained to assume different or expanded job responsibilities or may be terminated. This, in turn, may create increased stress and anxiety not only for workers but for families. Computer technology in terms of information processing and management will also present a challenge in recordkeeping, data management, and issues pertaining to confidentiality.

   In addition, new work processes may involve various exposures and hazards not previously encountered. Methods and techniques to identify, monitor, and control potential exposures will need to be implemented and evaluated.
- Economic factors will impact the health of the company in terms of product/services growth and expansion, and will ultimately affect the growth and expansion of the workforce. What this means is that if the company is

profitable, the workforce will probably be at least stable if not increase in size. However, with decreases in profits, companies often turn to "downsizing" or "resizing" to fit or balance the bottom line, resulting in higher levels of unemployment and more individuals uninsured with regard to health benefits. In addition, increased health care costs related to medical technological advances and debilitating illnesses will be paid for by the employer through higher health care insurance premiums as well as escalating costs related to workers' compensation. While measures directed toward cost containment remain a priority, concern for quality health care services should not be compromised.

Internal Influences

Internal or work setting influences include such areas as corporate culture, mission and goals, the workforce, work and related hazards, and resources both human and operational.

- Corporate culture, mission, and goals influence the framework for the health and safety program. Management's attitude toward worker health and productivity, health and safety programming including worker participation in decision making, wellness and health promotion, and a corporate commitment to a concept of health are factors that will significantly influence worker health through role modeling, resource allocation for occupational health and safety, and regulatory compliance. Occupational health and safety goals and objectives will provide the blueprint for program success and will need to be congruent with the corporate or company mission and goals.
- Workforce characteristics including size, health status and behaviors, worker health needs and perceptions about health and health risk, and demographic/composition (e.g., age, gender, ethnicity, education) will influence the types of programs and services developed. Family, co-worker, and other peer influences should also be considered.
- The type of work, work processes, and related hazards require thorough consideration, as these may result in actual or potential health problems. The interaction of the worker with the work may require preventive programs necessary to maintain and effect healthy outcomes. Availability and utilization of appropriate control strategies are important for hazard elimination and/or hazard relief.
- Adequate resources are essential to establish an effective occupational health and safety program. This includes human resources such as occupational health nurses, physicians, industrial hygienists, and safety specialists, and operational resources such as facilities, equipment, supplies, travel, and so forth. Collaboration with management and between and among disciplines is essential in order to assure effective and efficient resource management.

It is important for the occupational health nurse to be fully cognizant of external and internal workplace factors as these factors will impact the nurse's scope of practice. The occupational health nurse will need to utilize negotiation skills to acquire appropriate and adequate resources to engage an effective and comprehensive occupational health and safety program.

■ SCOPE OF PRACTICE

The scope of practice in occupational health nursing, as shown in the conceptual model (Fig. 3-2), is broad and comprehensive and is directed toward improving and promoting worker health. The practice encompasses several areas.

Health Promotion and Protection

A major component of occupational health nursing practice includes activities related to health promotion and protection for both individuals and groups of workers incorporating primary, secondary, and tertiary prevention strategies previously discussed. This might include developing strategies or programs to increase employees' awareness and knowledge related to toxic and hazardous exposures and their mitigation; discussing the meaning and application of results from personal and group health risk appraisals; promoting positive lifestyle interventions such as smoking cessation and improved exercise and nutrition; designing strategies to help alter attitudes and behaviors to improve health; and encouraging self-responsibility for utilization of health resources (personal and organizational). In addition, information obtained from workers' needs assessments may help to target health promotion programs or activities such as diabetes or cardiovascular risk factor screening, aimed at early detection of employee health problems. The occupational health nurse may also initiate special health activities or programs based on regulatory mandates and/or hazards related to the work environment, such as hearing conservation, respiratory surveillance, or ergonomic enhancement.

Rehabilitation is part of the prevention program for the worker aimed at health restoration and maintenance. This includes returning the impaired or injured worker to a productive worklife. Rehabilitation of the ill or injured worker begins at the time the injury occurs or when the health problem (e.g., chronic disease) becomes known to the health care provider. The rehabilitation plan should include attention to the physical and/or psychosocial needs of the affected worker, including a work adaptation plan, handling co-workers' concerns, and encouraging active participation of management in the process.

In collaboration with the physician or other health care professionals, the occupational health nurse will seek to prevent further disability, to identify barriers to health restoration early, and, as part of the treatment plan, to recommend job restructuring, modified work schedules, and worker retraining. Helping workers to understand the concept of health in order to reduce morbidity and mortality and improve one's quality of life, and encouraging workers to utilize health protection strategies designed to reduce risks in the work environment, such as recognizing toxic substances and appropriately using protective equipment, is integral to enhancing the health state of the worker.

Worker Health/Hazard Assessment and Surveillance

To identify health problems and determine the state of health of the worker, the occupational health nurse may perform several types of assessments, examinations, monitoring, and surveillance activities including occupational health histories, preplacement, and periodic examinations. For example, the preplacement assessment helps to match prospective employees with their jobs and to identify health problems or conditions that may be aggravated by job duties for which appropriate accommodations may be recommended. In addition, preplacement assessments help establish base-line data indexes for future health monitoring. Knowledge of the job demands is necessary in order to match the capabilities of the worker with the job.

Periodic health assessments are performed to determine if adverse health effects have occurred as a result of work conditions and hazards in order to recommend appropriate corrective measures and for early identification of chronic health conditions. The periodic evaluation may be part of the medical/health surveillance program to monitor employees who may be at risk of exposure to toxic substances. Other types of assessments may include return to work, pre-retirement, or termination from employment.

Workplace Surveillance and Hazard Detection

The occupational health nurse must be involved with the workplace monitoring and surveillance program in order to identify potential hazards harmful to workers' health. Through conducting walk-throughs, the nurse becomes familiar with the work environment, all production processes and methods, and equipment handling practices.

If a hazard is identified, services of the industrial hygienist or safety specialist will probably be needed to measure levels of exposure of specific substances, or help with job task analyses. In collaboration with the physician and other health care professionals, the occupational health nurse reviews data obtained in order to recommend health surveillance activities and participate in control recommendations and implementation strategies. Multidisciplinary collaboration is key to development and implementation of a successful workplace surveillance and hazard control program.

The walk-through assessment of the workplace provides an opportunity for the occupational health nurse to observe workers at work, their work practices and habits, use of personal protective equipment, health characteristics of the workforce such as smoking and social interaction, employee morale and productivity, and to identify actual and potential workplace health and safety hazards. The joint conduct of walk-throughs and participation on health and safety committees will enhance the overall health mission.

Primary Care/Case Management

Health care given at the worksite is primarily for work-related illnesses and injuries including treatment, follow-up, referral for medical care, and emergency care.

Many occupational health nurses also provide nonoccupational health care, generally limited to minor health care problems, or monitoring and follow-up of employees with stable chronic health problems. In addition, in some work settings, nurse practitioner-managed primary care services, including diagnosis and treatment of minor health problems, referral, and counseling, are offered to family members (Touger & Butts, 1989). The emphasis is on comprehensive care, early investigation, and wellness strategies to improve health and lower costs. Written medical and nursing protocols or guidelines collaboratively developed as appropriate should be in place in accordance with state legal requirements. In addition, case management may be offered to provide coordinated health care for early intervention and to help workers return to work sooner. Case management is a complex set of activities designed to coordinate and manage services and resources pertinent to the outcome of the individual's health problem (Leigh, 1993). Services depend on worker needs; however, intensive case management is indicated for a severe illness or injury, a chronic physical or mental health condition likely to result in loss time or permanent change in employee status, or when an employee has extended work absence.

Counseling

Counseling is designed to help employees clarify problems and make informed decisions and choices and to give positive reinforcement. It provides strategic interventions and appropriate referrals to deal with a crisis situation and time to reflect on impending decisions and to evaluate actions taken. The occupational health nurse may be involved in counseling workers with respect to prevention and management of work-related and nonoccupational illnesses and injuries, as well as counseling managers regarding special problems of the workforce such as substance abuse.

Employees may be initially referred to the occupational health nurse by the supervisor for performance-related problems. These problems can be caused by many factors such as behavioral, marital, social, and work-related events and may result in increased absenteeism, accidents, or stress-related illnesses. Employees may be referred to employee assistance programs provided in-house or offered through community agencies. The occupational health nurse may be directly involved in managing the employee assistance program or may be the referral liaison. Employee assistance programs are designed to identify troubled employees early, to help them seek appropriate assistance to manage the problem and remain productive, and to help management recognize and appropriately deal with workers' problems.

Management and Administration

The occupational health nurse assumes a major role in the management and administration of the occupational health unit. In order to effectively manage the occupational health unit and contribute to the overall health goals of the company, the nurse must be fully aware of the corporate mission, culture, and business goals, as well as the characteristics of the workforce and related health and safety priorities and needs. The scope of management responsibilities includes program planning and goal development; budget planning and management; organizing, staffing, and coordinating activities, including the development of policy, procedure, and protocol manuals; and evaluation of unit performance, based on achievement of goals and objectives.

The occupational health nurse should be involved in quality improvement and assurance, which requires specific activities such as satisfaction determinations, audits, and record reviews. Quality performance should take into consideration the match between effectiveness and efficiency. Cost-effectiveness and cost containment of health care services must be a health management imperative.

Increasingly, the nurse is becoming a key figure in the development of policies that affect the health and safety of the workforce. Policy development should be a collaborative effort between company management, the occupational health nurse manager, the physician, if one is employed, and other appropriate health care professionals. At the very least, the occupational health nurse should have input into strategic and operational policy decisions affecting the occupational health program and should have management responsibility for operation of the occupational health nursing service. Employee input regarding occupational health and safety policies should be elicited.

Research

The importance of the role the occupational health nurse plays in research related to worker health conditions cannot be overstated. The provision of a safe and healthful work environment is contingent upon knowledge of the relationship between the worker and elements in the work field and related environments. For example, understanding the effects of toxic exposures, designing strategies to prevent work-related accidents/injuries or illnesses, evaluating the cost-effectiveness of health interventions, or understanding human behavior and motivation related to health promotion activities are important occupational health nursing investigations.

The occupational health nurse is always in a position to collect data through accurate and detailed recordkeeping, which can be an invaluable source to identify trends in illness and injury patterns and other events in the workforce. As part of the research team, the occupational health nurse can participate in the design of research studies and data collection about occupational health and related problems. Data can be used to determine which types of programs or interventions are most effective in promoting health and minimizing risk.

Legal-Ethical Management

Company management has the responsibility to ensure a safe and healthful work environment for all employees through implementation of programs to support this effort. The occupational health nurse must be aware and knowledgeable of laws and regulations that govern the occupational health and safety of workers (e.g., OSH Act, Hazard Communication Standard) and recommend and implement programs responsive to mandated health and safety requirements. The importance of good recordkeeping cannot be overemphasized with respect to legal documentation.

Occupational health nursing practice is regulated by state nurse practice acts and guided by standards of occupational health nursing practice. The occupational health nurse should have copies of and be familiar with these documents in order to ensure adequate and appropriate nursing care.

There are many issues in the work environment that may create ethical conflicts, such as confidentiality of employee health records, hazardous exposures to vulnerable populations, and threats to worker health. The occupational health nurse's framework for practice is guided by ethical treatment of workers as expressed in the Code of Ethics. Ethical decision making is integral to the nurse's practice and is discussed in Chapter 16.

Community Orientation

Collaboration with community groups and organizations enables the occupational health nurse to develop a network of resources to more efficiently and effectively provide services to employees and the company. The nurse can also help the industry to focus a health relationship with the community through modeling environmental health awareness and providing or sponsoring health-related activities to workers' families and the community at large. The community/industry relationship should be mutually beneficial. In addition, the nurse will be involved in disaster preparedness of the workforce, which may entail articulation with environmental, emergency, and other public agencies.

■ PRACTICE SETTINGS

As reported by AAOHN membership surveys, approximately 70% of occupational health nurses work in single-nurse units in workplaces that employ more than 1,000 employees. More than one third of these nurses work in settings with at least 2,000 workers and nearly 20% are employed where there are 5,000 or more workers (Cox, 1989). However, there is an increasing trend for companies to contract for part-time or full-time occupational health nursing services in an effort to conserve dollars (Brown, 1988).

Occupational health nursing services are provided in a variety of workplace settings such as textile mills, pharmaceutical companies, furniture factories, banks, department stores, food processing, cosmetic and meat packing companies, construction sites, government and insurance agencies, automotive and telephone industries, hospitals, airline industries, and wherever there is a workforce in need of occupational health services. Often the workforce and work processes at a singular worksite are quite diverse, thereby requiring the nurse to have broad and substantive knowledge related to various hazards, populations, health care, and service management and delivery.

The types of services and programs provided will be dependent on the characteristics and size of the workforce, actual and potential hazards, available resources, company culture, and worker and management attitudes about health and safety and regulatory mandates. For example, hazard reduction programs in a textile mill will in part focus on cotton dust exposure and hearing conservation, whereas programs for office environment hazards will focus primarily on ergonomics and stress. Occupational health services at a construction site or area will vary depending on factors such as location of a jobsite, availability of equipment and health facilities, which by necessity may be a mobile unit, and the make-up of the workforce population and its needs. Construction work is one of the most dangerous types of employment with hazards such as noise from blasting and heavy machinery; exposure to whole body vibration, solar radiation, and cold; dermatitis from irritants such as rubber, epoxy fixatives, and degreasing agents; lacerations, contusions, amputations; and exposure to potential carcinogens such as paints, plastics, resins, and a variety of chemicals (Felton, 1990). Even with all these hazards, health services for construction workers, including surveillance, job placement, and care for traumatic injuries, have not been provided consistently, to say nothing of health promotion, education, and restoration activities. However, more recently, contractual services with occupational medicine clinics and outreach hospital services have been of some aid.

Hospitals and related health care facilities sometimes employ occupational health nurses to provide and manage health care services to employees, and the number is growing. The hospital environment is filled with hazards of all types, including infectious diseases, chemical and physical agents, and ergonomic and psychosocial stressors. The risks are numerous, ubiquitous, and affect all occupational groups. Employee health services are provided to only a small segment of the hospital/health care facility community and the types of services provided vary greatly (Rogers & Haynes, 1991). Hospital settings may employ thousands of workers who are at risk every day from serious health threats, and many of these workers have minimal or no occupational health services, monitoring, or surveillance activities. Occupational or employee health nurses are the health care professionals most frequently employed to deliver these services and many more are needed.

■ SUMMARY

The bulk of health care services provided at the worksite are delivered by occupational health nurses. The occupational health nurse is the primary health care manager at the worksite and works with management to provide cost-effective health services. In recent decades the scope of practice has expanded with more emphasis on health promotion. The nurse utilizes a prevention framework with a philosophy of practice aimed at promoting and protecting the health of the workforce and maintaining a healthy work environment with interdisciplinary collaboration.

REFERENCES

American Association of Occupational Health Nurses. A guide to establishing a comprehensive occupational health service. Atlanta: Author, 1987.

American Association of Occupational Health Nurses. Code of Ethics. Atlanta: Author, 1991.

American Association of Occupational Health Nurses. Standards of occupational health nursing practice. Atlanta: Author, 1994.

American Nurses Association. Standards of community health nursing. Washington, DC: Author, 1986.

American Public Health Association. The definition and role of public health nursing in the delivery of health care. Washington, DC: Author, 1981.

Babbitz, M. The practice of occupational health nursing in the U.S. Occupational Health Nursing, 31: 23–25, 1983.

Brown, C. AAOHN membership survey final report. Rochester, NY: Associated Research Group, 1988.

Brown, K. Development of philosophy, policies, and procedures for an occupational health nursing service. AAOHN Update Series, 1(1), 1984.

Brown, ML. Occupational health nursing. New York: MacMillan Company, 1981.

Christy, T. Portrait of a leader: Lillian Wald. Nursing Outlook, 18: 50–54, 1970.

Cox, A. Planning for the future of occupational health nursing. AAOHN Journal, 37: 356–360, 1989.

Felton, JS. Occupational medical management. Boston: Little, Brown & Company, 1990.

Felton, JS. The genesis of American occupational health nursing. Occupational Health Nursing, 33: 615–621, 1985.

Hannigan, L. Occupational health nursing practice: A state of the art. Occupational Health Nursing, 32: 17–20, 1984.

Leavell, HR & Clark, EG. Preventive medicine for the doctor and his community (3rd ed.). New York: McGraw-Hill, 1965.

Lee, J. The new nurse in industry. Cincinnati: U.S. Department of Health, Education & Welfare, NIOSH, 1978.

Leigh, B. Case management in a health maintenance organization. AAOHN Journal, 41 (4): 170–173, 1993.

McGrath, BJ. Nursing in commerce and industry. New York: The Commonwealth Fund, 1946.

McKechnie, M. A descriptive study of the scope of practice of occupational health nurses in one-nurse units. Occupational Health Nursing, 31: 18–22, 1983.

Parker-Conrad, J. A century of practice in occupational health nursing. AAOHN Journal, 36(4): 156–161, 1988.

Pender, N. Health promotion in nursing practice. Appleton-Century-Crofts, 1987.

Rogers, B. Ethical dilemmas in occupational health nursing. AAOHN Journal, 37: 100–105, 1988.

Rogers, B. Occupational health nursing practice, education and research: Challenges for the future. AAOHN Journal, 38: 536–543, 1990.

Rogers, B & Haynes, C. A study of hospital employee health programs. AAOHN Journal, 39(4): 157–166, 1991.

Touger, GN & Butts, J. The workplace: An innovative and cost-effective practice site. The Nurse Practitioner, 14(1): 35–42, 1989.

Uustal, DB. Values clarification in nursing: Application to practice. American Journal of Nursing, 78: 2058–2063, 1978.

Wachs, J & Parker-Conrad, J. Occupational health nursing in 1990 and the coming decade. Applied Occupational and Environmental Hygiene, 5: 200–203, 1990.

Williams, CA. Population focused practice. In Community Health Nursing, J. Lancaster & M. Stanhope, eds. Washington, DC: Mosby, pp. 292–303, 1988.

Wright, FS. Industrial nursing. New York: MacMillan, 1919.

4

ROLES OF THE OCCUPATIONAL HEALTH NURSE

Susan A. Randolph, RN, MSN, COHN

Over the years the scope of occupational health nursing practice has been constantly evolving and expanding. Occupational health nurses, besides providing direct care for work-related injuries and illnesses, are committed to the client's wellness and incorporate health promotion, disease prevention, injury prevention, health education, case management, and safety into their practice. This increasing focus on prevention has been partially responsible for the advancement of occupational health nursing roles. More important, the growth of graduate programs in occupational health nursing has contributed to the development of advanced practice roles.

Occupational health nurses function in a variety of roles and work in diverse settings such as industry, hospital employee health units, occupational health clinics, and government facilities. Increasingly, theory and research are integrated with occupational health nursing practice. A sound theoretical base for practice contributes to clear role definition and scope of practice. This chapter will examine and define the five major roles of the occupational health nurse. The purpose and function of each role will be described in detail utilizing a theoretical base for practice.

■ ROLE DEVELOPMENT

A role is defined as a part or character to be played or as the proper or customary function of a person. Role can also refer to both the expected and the actual behaviors associated with a job either by the person or by someone else (Hardy & Conway, 1978). Whenever a person changes an existing role or takes on a new role, she or he goes through several phases of role development. In the role development process, common themes are evident: the nurse must clearly identify the role purpose and function, implement the role through goal-directed interactions, and achieve positive recognition and support of the role (Oda, 1977). Role definition can assist the occupational health nurse in examining and clarifying the role(s); and then communicating that role to peers, workers, management, and society.

Several factors influence the role or roles the occupational health nurse will

Susan Randolph is the Occupational Health Nursing Consultant with the North Carolina Department of Environment, Health, and Natural Resources, Occupational Health Section, Raleigh, North Carolina.

develop in the workplace. These factors include the commitment of the company's management, skill level of the occupational health nurse, role perception, and industry size and type. Commitment of management to the occupational health service is of major importance. To ascertain the degree of commitment, the philosophy of management toward health must be examined. The philosophy will determine the scope of the occupational health service, and to some extent, the role of the occupational health nurse. Is the company's emphasis episodic in that only emergency care and first aid services are provided, or is the philosophy of health more comprehensive, encompassing all three levels of prevention? Will only occupationally related injuries and illnesses be treated, or will nonoccupational health problems be managed as well? In the former, the occupational health nurse will have a difficult time implementing worker health education and disease prevention programs, thus limiting the nurse's role. In addition to the philosophy, the goals and objectives of the occupational health service will help to further clarify the scope of services to be provided.

A second factor that influences the occupational health nurse's role is the position for which the nurse is hired. Ideally, the right occupational health nurse will be selected for the position. The occupational health nurse should meet the requirements of the position based on the philosophy of health as well as on the goals and objectives of the occupational health service. There should be congruence between the goals and objectives of the company, the needs of the employees, and the abilities and knowledge base of the occupational health nurse. Some occupational health nursing positions require specific educational preparation and skills, such as an occupational health nurse practitioner or an occupational health nurse educator. If a nurse administrator is needed to manage the occupational health service, then a person with those skills and educational background should be hired. The nurse is generally hired for one main role, with the position title designating certain functions and responsibilities. However, in actual practice, the nurse functions in a more comprehensive, multifaceted manner encompassing other roles. For instance, an occupational health nursing consultant provides consultation to other occupational health nurses and management in industry. The same consultant also functions as an educator when lecturing to nursing students and as a researcher when conducting research.

The third factor is the perception of the role by the nurse and by the company. The occupational health nurse has certain expectations about the role and management may have some differing opinions about that same role. This discrepancy may lead to role conflict. For example, a nurse hired by a company to develop a health promotion program for employees discovered, once on the job, that management really wanted the nurse to develop an occupational health program to meet selected health needs of the employees, namely first aid and safety. Consequently, the health promotion program was delayed until these employees' needs could be met.

Another source of potential conflict in role expectations is management's prior experience with an occupational health nurse. Has the experience been positive or negative? How might that affect management's perception of the nurse? For example, one occupational health nurse was having difficulty in maintaining the confidentiality of employee health records because management was demanding access to these records. The nurse later determined that the previous nurses at the industry allowed management access to employee health records. Since she refused management this option, the occupational health nurse was reprimanded by management as insubordinate. The nurse is now trying to educate management about her profession, the Code of Ethics (AAOHN, 1991), and her responsibility to maintain employees' trust. Both examples illustrate the need for clarity of occupational health nurse functions and accurate communication between the nurse and management.

A well-written position description will help delineate clear position functions and responsibilities as well as clarify role expectations. Basic elements of a position description include title, purpose and scope, job summary, organizational placement, personal requirements, and salary range. The title should accurately reflect the skills required and importance of the position in the organization. The job summary describes the functions or duties and the responsibilities of the job, including the breadth and depth of the work involved. Organizational placement is essential to determine the lines of communication and authority. It also describes to whom the nurse is accountable and for whom the nurse is responsible. Personal requirements delineate the knowledge and skill, as well as physical and mental energy required to perform the work. The challenge is matching the human capacities and resources available to the needs of the position.

The size of the industry or agency is the fourth factor. As the size of the industry increases, so does the need for nursing staff. The number of nursing staff needed also depends on the type of industry and the nature of the hazards. A steel mill or chemical industry with 300 employees is more likely to employ at least one or more nurses than an insurance company with 1,200 employees. In addition, the roles and functions of the occupational health nurse will vary based on the size of the nursing staff. The occupational health nurse who works in a one-nurse unit (solo practice) has different roles, functions, and responsibilities than an occupational health nurse who works in a multi-nurse unit. The occupational health nurse who works alone typically takes on many roles: manager of the occupational health service; clinician in providing direct care for workers' injuries; educator in planning, implementing, and evaluating health promotion/education programs; and consultant in sharing pertinent information with managers, supervisors, and other members of the occupational health team. The nurse must possess skills in decision making, problem solving, communication, and independent nursing judgment. In essence, the nurse is responsible for the operation of the occupational health service. On the other hand, an occupational health nurse who works in a multi-nurse unit may have more distinct role responsibilities. She or he may be hired as a clinician to treat workers' injuries, as a health educator to plan, implement, and evaluate disease prevention programs, or as an administrator of the health service.

■ ROLE DEFINITION

Regardless of position or work setting, the occupational health nurse must be knowledgeable about nursing practice from several perspectives: legally as dictated in the Nursing Practice Act and other related laws; professionally through standards of practice, Code of Ethics, and certification (COHN); and academically through educational preparation and continuing education. All of these enable the occupational health nurse to function in the variety of roles encountered in occupational health nursing practice.

Theory and research influence role definition, scope of practice, and the knowledge base of nursing. Nursing theory as well as other theories assist the nurse in using relevant knowledge to guide actions. They also provide direction for day-to-day practice. Several nursing theories apply to the occupational health setting and have been utilized in nursing research. Roy's Adaptation Model, (Thompson, 1986), Orem's Theory of Self-Care, (Javid & Lester, 1983), and Newman's Health Care Systems Model (Heasley & Hughes, 1985), are some examples. Non-nursing theories such as Antonovsky's Theory of Salutogenesis, Systems Theory, and the Health Belief Model have also been tested successfully in the work setting (Fiorentino, 1986; Javid & Lester, 1983; Dickson et al., 1986).

■ ROLES

Five major practice roles exist in occupational health nursing: clinician/practitioner, administrator, educator, researcher, and consultant (Randolph, 1988). Each of the five roles will be discussed separately.

Clinician/Practitioner

The occupational health nurse clinician/practitioner is an essential role encompassing the application of the nursing process to direct care for occupational and often nonoccupational injuries and illnesses. In addition, the clinician/practitioner collaborates with other members of the occupational health team to maintain a safe and healthful work environment.

In closer examination of the role, a distinction can be made between the clinician and the practitioner, although commonalities exist. As the commonalities between the clinician and practitioner roles increase due to changes in the health care delivery system, a future merger of the two roles exists (Kitzman, 1989). For the purposes of this chapter, a clinician is defined as a registered professional nurse who provides care to employees. The practitioner is also a registered professional nurse who has specialized training in physical assessment and management of health conditions. She or he is educationally prepared in a nurse practitioner certificate program or, more recently, in an advanced degree nursing program with an emphasis on occupational health. Both the clinician and the practitioner use expert clinical knowledge in assessing and evaluating the worker. They maintain a high degree of professionalism through continuing education, certification, and adherence to a Code of Ethics in providing occupational health nursing services.

The theoretical base for the clinician/practitioner is the nursing process. This systematic approach to nursing care provides the framework for decision making. The main steps of the nursing process are assessment, nursing diagnosis, planning, implementation, and evaluation.

The clinician/practitioner assesses the health problem by gathering data about the worker and the work environment. What does the worker state about his chief complaint? What signs and symptoms does the worker exhibit? Could the health problem be related to his job? What actual or potential health hazards are present in the work environment? In answering these questions, appropriate interdisciplinary collaboration is essential. Other members of the occupational health team can contribute additional information about the worker and the work environment. The occupational physician offers medical information about the worker; the industrial hygienist provides area and/or personal sampling data about actual or potential health hazards in the work environment; and the safety professional investigates the work environment for safety hazards or potentially unsafe conditions and provides information about job tasks.

Once all the relevant data are collected and analyzed, nursing diagnoses are formed. The nursing diagnoses are the basis for planning and managing employee health care through the development of a nursing care plan. Goals and objectives are mutually identified by the occupational health nurse and the worker, and actions/methods to achieve them are then determined.

The care plan is implemented through direct nursing care, worker and perhaps family education, and communication. Appropriate referral and follow-up are initiated to insure continuity of care. To accomplish this effectively, the clinician/practitioner communicates with a variety of community resources, health services, health care providers, as well as with members of the occupational health team.

Finally, the goals and objectives are evaluated. Were they met? Why or why not? What could be improved? Were the desired behaviors, actions, or outcomes achieved? Reassessment occurs and the nursing process continues, illustrating its cyclic and dynamic nature.

Specific functions of the occupational health nurse clinician/practitioner include, but are not limited to, the following activities:

1. Assesses the work environment for actual or potential health and safety hazards.
2. Assesses the health status of workers.
   a. health history
   b. occupational health history
   c. lifestyle–health risk appraisal
3. Performs physical examinations.
   a. job placement
   b. periodic
   c. return to work
   d. health surveillance
   e. termination/retirement
4. Conducts appropriate laboratory tests.
5. Provides direct nursing care for occupational and nonoccupational injuries and illnesses.
6. Conducts health education and counseling.
7. Establishes mutual goals and objectives with the worker for her or his care plan.
8. Collaborates, communicates, and consults with other members of the occupational health team.
9. Maintains accurate and complete health records of the workers.
10. Develops and implements programs designed to correct or minimize the identified health and safety hazards.
11. Institutes appropriate personal protection programs.
    a. safety glasses
    b. safety shoes
    c. hearing protection
    d. respiratory protection
    e. personal protective clothing

12. Initiates referrals to community specialists.
13. Conducts screening programs.
14. Develops and implements health promotion and/or disease prevention programs.
15. Evaluates the various programs.
16. Develops and maintains rapport with workers and management.
17. Collaborates and communicates with other health care providers in the community.
18. Manages workers' compensation claims.
19. Conducts training for cardiopulmonary resuscitation (CPR) and first aid.
20. Serves as a preceptor for nursing students.
21. Maintains professionalism and ethical conduct (AAOHN, 1987).

Administrator

The occupational health nurse administrator serves an important function in the total operation of the occupational health service by providing the structure and direction for the development, implementation, and evaluation of an effective, high-quality nursing program. Furthermore, the occupational health nurse administrator communicates and interprets the occupational health program to management and other members of the occupational health team.

While functioning in a comprehensive executive role, the administrator sets goals, formulates policy, and manages the health service. The ability to reach a decision and then translate that thought into action is essential. All of these activities refer to the basic functions of the management framework: planning, organizing, directing, coordinating, and controlling (Gillies, 1989).

Planning can be defined as assessing the future and making provisions for it, which is the most important but most difficult function to accomplish. It also involves considering problems or unmet needs and figuring out solutions or ways to meet those needs. An example is the development of a limited duty/return-to-work program for injured workers (Randolph & Dalton, 1989). The occupational health nurse administrator plans for both long range and short term goals. Long range goals are necessary to anticipate and meet the needs of the organization or industry as well as the employees. For instance, based on plans for remodernization and expansion of the company, the administrator anticipates that additional or different health services may be needed as the number of employees changes, environmental exposures alter, and stress levels increase. Short term goals reflect more ongoing or current needs, and result in such decisions as plans for additional staffing in the occupational health service or plans for a specific program, such as a pre-retirement seminar for workers and their spouses.

Organizing involves developing a framework so that people and things relate to each other in such a manner as to reach an objective. It can also be necessary in defining the tasks and time frames necessary to achieve the solution. The occupational health nurse administrator organizes the occupational health service using all available resources to meet the defined program objectives. This involves appropriate utilization of the occupational health staff, training of staff to maintain or acquire new skills or abilities, as well as delegation of tasks to personnel along with the needed responsibility and authority. Besides people, the administrator organizes the budget, equipment, supplies, facilities, and anything else related to the efficient operation of the program. In the example of the pre-retirement seminar, goals and objectives are defined by the staff along with a tentative timetable such as one session per week for six weeks. Resources for successful implementation of the program must also be identified.

Another management function is directing. Directing is defined as the face-to-face interaction between managers and subordinates in accomplishing the goals of the organization. It includes supervising and instructing staff as well as making assignments and structuring their responsibilities. To be able to direct effectively, the administrator must have excellent communication skills, both oral and written. For instance, it is at this point that the nurse administrator delegates the responsibility for the pre-retirement seminar implementation to one of the staff.

Coordinating refers to any harmonizing activities aimed at achieving the desired outcome. Key questions the administrator may ask are, Do I have the information and data to accomplish the services, outcomes, and measurements? To reach this goal, what is needed to be successful? What barriers, if any, exist that might prevent goal attainment and how do I overcome them? For any program, the occupational health nurse administrator must coordinate these resources and activities including management approval and support. In the seminar example, the occupational health nurse must determine and coordinate the number of workers close to retirement age and their spouses, the budget allocated for the seminar, a staff member to implement the seminar, and community resource people and company representatives such as personnel needed to participate, as well as handout materials and equipment. The preretirement seminar represents the goal.

Controlling is the last management function. It is defined as verifying whether everything occurred in conformity with the plan adopted, instructions issued, and principles established. Controlling implies providing the necessary motivation throughout the process and evaluating results. The occupational health nurse administrator has the ability to monitor and adjust the occupational health work according to standards, such as standards of occupational health nursing practice. This is necessary in order to advance nursing practice and the profession. Evaluation is another mechanism to determine if the plan, program, or occupational health service was successful. Were the objectives of the pre-retirement seminar met? How did the workers like it? Did it meet their needs or answer their questions? What could be done to improve the seminar when it is offered again? Quality assurance using peer review, audit criteria, and performance appraisal are all tools that the occupational health nurse administrator may use to evaluate the program as well as the staff.

The occupational health nurse administrator improves interpersonal relations with staff and workers, along with work conditions using planning, organizing, directing, coordinating, and controlling. With everyone working toward a common goal, anything is possible. To function efficiently and effectively, the administrator is a registered professional nurse who has education in occupational health nursing, safety, management and/or nursing administration, communications, and group dynamics. Ideally, the person has had administrative experience.

Specific functions of the occupational health nurse administrator follow the management functions or the nursing process. They include, but are not limited to, the following activities:

1. Defines goals (long and short term) and objectives of the occupational health service.
2. Develops, implements, and evaluates the occupational health service.
3. Formulates policies.
4. Manages the budget to provide for efficient occupational health nursing services and effective employee health services.
5. Plans, develops, and promotes the necessary facilities, equipment, supplies, and record system needed to operate the employee health service.
6. Determines the nursing staff required, participates in staff selection, and determines minimum qualifications and functions for various positions.
7. Coordinates in-service education and professional growth opportunities for staff.
8. Assesses program needs in consultation with other members of the occupational health team.
9. Implements new programs and program changes, and manages ongoing programs consistent with goals and objectives.
10. Evaluates quantitative outcomes of employee health and safety programs.
11. Assumes responsibility for adequate data collection for quantitative evaluation of program outcomes of worker health and safety while maintaining confidentiality.
12. Initiates quality assurance, audits, and peer review of the occupational health staff.
13. Participates as an active member of the central management team.
14. Uses community resources appropriately.
15. Maintains awareness of technological, legal, and professional changes associated with occupational health and safety.
16. Serves as a preceptor for nursing students.
17. Maintains professionalism and ethical conduct.

Educator

With the development of undergraduate, graduate, and doctoral programs in occupational health nursing, the occupational health nurse educator has emerged as a role of growing importance. The occupational health nurse educator teaches and prepares nursing students to function as occupational health specialists, nurse practitioners, administrators, educators, researchers, or consultants at the worksite. The responsibility parallels the educator's goal, which is to prepare occupational health nurses to assume leadership positions to improve, maintain, and account for quality nursing care provided to workers.

In order to serve as faculty in a school of nursing and/or school of public health, the educator must be a registered professional nurse who is academically and professionally prepared to teach occupational health nursing. In addition, the occupational health nurse educator must be familiar with concepts in industrial hygiene, safety, loss prevention, toxicology, epidemiology, management, occupational/environmental health, health promotion, human behavior and motivation, research, and statistics. At least two years' experience in occupational health and safety is helpful. Experience in occupational health nursing is important so that the educator can integrate theory with practice. Most baccalaureate and master's level nursing programs require that nursing faculty have a doctoral degree, or be in the process of obtaining such a degree (Bernhardt, 1986). The educator must also be knowledgeable of various worksites in the geographic area for appropriate clinical placement of students with nursing preceptors who will serve as expert role models. Furthermore, the occupational health nurse educator designs curriculum content and learning strategies to ensure that graduates can develop and implement new roles (Snyder, 1989) in occupational health nursing.

Changes in nursing education generally reflect changes in nursing practice. The educator must keep current on issues affecting both nursing practice in general and occupational health nursing practice in particular. Areas such as government, legal and ethical concerns, the health care delivery system, malpractice and liability issues, and company mergers, takeovers, or bankruptcies should be considered topics of interest as they relate to worker health care. Information about these topics can be obtained from newspapers, journal articles, key informants, and other sources. In addition, the occupational health nurse educator is encouraged to continue occupational health nurse practice, thus blending education and service. The educator can then illustrate how theory-based practice is applied in real world situations.

In some schools of nursing, limited content on the role of the occupational health nurse and general concepts of occupational health nursing practice are integrated within a community health nursing course. However, since occupational health nursing is considered a specialty area and should therefore be taught at the graduate level, most occupational health nurses learn about the field through on-the-job training and continuing education programs.

Continuing education is another fundamental area in which occupational health nurse educators play an invaluable role. By conducting continuing education programs, the educator has the opportunity to expand and/or update occupational health nurses' knowledge and skills in delivering quality nursing care to workers. In addition, continuing education courses taught by qualified educators are needed to help occupational health nurses qualify for or maintain certification in occupational health nursing or in another area of nursing practice. The educator should have adult education/adult learning courses in order to teach occupational health nurses who have varied educational levels, different career goals, and different attitudes toward education.

Specific functions of the occupational health nurse educator include, but are not limited to, the following activities:

1. Develops, implements, and evaluates curricula appropriate to various levels of educational preparation.
2. Promotes integration of occupational health nursing content into undergraduate nursing education.
3. Uses research findings and conducts research relevant to occupational health nursing and occupational health and safety.
4. Disseminates research findings to other nurses, health care professionals, and occupational health specialists by publication and/or presentation.
5. Promotes occupational health nursing as a challenging area of nursing practice.
6. Uses experts in occupational health and safety in planning and coordinating relevant education programs.
7. Plans and conducts continuing education programs relevant to occupational health nursing and occupational safety and health.

8. Maintains occupational health nursing practice expertise.
9. Collaborates with other occupational health nurses regarding practice issues and student practicum sites.
10. Serves as a role model for students.
11. Maintains professionalism and ethical conduct.

Researcher

The role of the occupational health nurse researcher is growing rapidly. This area of practice has evolved in recent years due to the commitment to research by the American Association of Occupational Health Nurses and the development of graduate programs in occupational health nursing (Rogers & Spencer, 1984). In 1985 a "Research Corner" was implemented in the *AAOHN Journal* and research awards in occupational health nursing were supported by AAOHN. Occupational health nursing research may help to bridge the gap between the development and implementation of nursing theory and the application of theory in the occupational health practice setting (Silberstein, 1983; Rogers, 1990).

A researcher develops researchable questions, conducts research, and communicates the research findings to occupational health nurses, other researchers, and to the public. The importance of identifying answerable research questions to which appropriate statistical techniques are applied cannot be overemphasized as this will make the conduct of the research easier and more meaningful (Rogers, 1991). As occupational health nurses become aware of research findings and the implications of these findings, they will start to apply them in their own practice at the worksite. The intent, then, of research-based practice is to promote, maintain, protect, and restore the health of the workers as well as improve the work environment.

Two examples of research studies that have made a significant contribution to occupational health nursing follow. Wild et al. (1987) conducted a retrospective epidemiological study to analyze the problem of wrist injuries among the total population of female employees in the finishing department of a paper products company. A self-administered questionnaire was used to collect data on age, sex, height, weight, length of time on the job, smoking habits, employment history, feelings toward the job, medications, medical and surgical history, and symptoms/conditions experienced. The workplace design of the finishing department was also assessed. It was found that the younger, shorter, less experienced worker was most susceptible to wrist injuries or problems associated with repetitive motion tasks. Implications for the occupational health nurse are clear. Health personnel must be alert and responsive to the occurrence of signs and symptoms of forearm, wrist, and hand injuries during early periods of employment. Workers need to be aware of those signs and symptoms and what to do if they occur. An ergonomic workplace assessment may be warranted. By modifying or redesigning the worksite, wrist injuries may be prevented and safe work practices can be implemented.

Reith (1987) conducted a descriptive survey of healthy adult workers to determine their perceptions concerning personal control over their own health status. The Multidimensional Health Locus of Control Scale (MHLC) was applied to Pender's Modified Health Belief Model. It is thought that people who perceive more personal control over their own health are more likely to practice preventive health behaviors. The results indicated that the sample of adult workers surveyed perceived themselves to have a high degree of internal control over their health status. This information is important for nurses as they plan health promotion programs, establish care plans for workers, and initiate worker education.

Characteristics of the occupational health nurse researcher include curiosity, open-mindedness, and tenacity (McKechnie & Rogers, 1985). Instead of just accepting things the way they are, the researcher wonders "Why . . . ? What if . . . ? Is there a better way? How can this program or my practice be improved?" With this quest for knowledge or improvement in practice, the researcher initiates a study. Open-mindedness means being receptive to new ideas or freedom from bias. Once the study is completed, the researcher must be able to interpret the data and draw accurate conclusions from the findings. In addition, the researcher demonstrates tenacity in that she or he continues the research until an acceptable answer/solution is found.

The occupational health nurse researcher, from an academic perspective, is a registered professional nurse with an advanced degree. Graduates from a master's program in occupational health nursing generally complete a research study or thesis in partial fulfillment of the requirements for their degree. They have had courses in research, statistics, and epidemiology as a foundation for research. Doctoral programs have a strong research emphasis that is essential in the development of the researcher/investigator role.

However, many occupational health nurses utilize research findings and can identify possible research questions. Basic research techniques are often used to solve occupational health problems, techniques that the occupational health nurse can implement (McKechnie & Rogers, 1985). Examples of researchable topics that could be examined by occupational health nurses include the effects of wearing contact lenses in industry, assessment of safety hazards and correlations with injury data, factors influencing return to work, effectiveness of ergonomic strategies to reduce worker injury and illness, and identification of nursing interventions that have the most favorable impact on worker health promotion (Randolph, 1987; AAOHN, 1990; Rogers & Spencer, 1984). For more complex problems or answers to research design questions, the beginning researcher is encouraged to contact an experienced researcher for assistance.

Specific functions of the occupational health nurse researcher include, but are not limited to, the following activities:

1. Participates in the development and implementation of research in occupational health nursing.
2. Disseminates research findings to others through presentation, publication, and practice.
3. Incorporates research results into own practice.
4. Promotes, assists, and collaborates with occupational health nurses in developing and conducting research.
5. Collaborates with other members of the occupational health team in developing and conducting research.
6. Protects the participants' (employees' and employers') rights while the research is conducted.
7. Maintains professionalism and ethical conduct.

Consultant

The last major role of the occupational health nurse is that of the occupational health nurse consultant. In this role, the consultant serves as a resource person to other occupational health nurses, management, members of the occupational health team, as well as to related organizations and agencies. The consultant assists in evaluating and developing occupational health services by recommending specific actions and alternatives. Services are often provided in the areas of administration, education, research, and community resources. However, the consultant generally does not have direct responsibility for implementing or enforcing the recommendations.

"For the nurse, a 'position of consultant' is likely to involve not only specific consultative duties, but also some functioning as a teacher, supervisor, administrator, coordinator, etc." (Lange, 1979). To obtain the skills necessary for this multifaceted and complex role, the consultant is a registered professional nurse who has knowledge and experience in occupational health nursing. The consultant should be able to communicate effectively, both orally and in writing, as well as possess good administrative, consultative, and listening skills.

Nurse consultants in occupational health are either internal or external to the company. The internal consultant is someone within the company who is given the responsibility to plan and implement constructive change, whereas the external consultant is brought into the company from the outside (Lange, 1987). An example of an internal consultant could be a Corporate and/or Regional Director of Nursing who provides consultation to occupational health nurses within the company. External occupational health nurse consultants may be self-employed, employed by an insurance company, hired by a private consulting firm, or located in the occupational health section of a governmental agency, such as a state health department or department of labor (AAOHN, 1987). The place of employment determines the focus of the consultant's services (advisory versus enforcement), the fee schedule if applicable, and the types of services available. An occupational health nurse consultant in a state health department offers free consultative services to occupational health nurses and management but does not have the authority to implement the recommendations. On the other hand, a consultant hired from a consulting firm charges a fee for specified services but is not responsible for carrying out the suggestions. However, a consultant hired by the department of labor may have enforcement as well as consultative responsibilities that can be a potential source of conflict for the consultant and the client.

The consultation process is the theoretical base for practice. Although different phases or steps of the process have been identified (Stevens, 1978; Oda, 1982), commonalities exist that parallel the nursing process (Table 4–1). This is illustrated below as three key questions are addressed: What is the problem? What can be done about it? Was the problem resolved? (Forti, 1981).

In an example cited previously, a state occupational health consultant was contacted by an occupational health nurse (entry and initial contact) for assistance regarding confidentiality of employee health records. The consultant gathered the following information (data gathering): the occupational health nurse's management was demanding access to employee health records without appropriate justification, and the occupational health nurse refused management's request. The occupational health nurse was reprimanded as being insubordinate. Previous

■ **TABLE 4–1** Common Phases in the Consultative Process Paralleled with the Nursing Process

Nursing Process	Consultation Process
Assessment	**ENTRY AND INITIAL CONTACT; DATA GATHERING** Recognize own needs and motives Establish relationship Define roles/expectations Determine client motivation and agenda Define the client's relationship to the problem Define areas for data gathering Build support Gather data
Nursing Diagnosis	**DIAGNOSIS; FEEDBACK AND DECISION TO RISK** Define areas of stress Define the problem Define the objectives Acknowledge the problem to be explained Agree on next step Determine client responsibility Initiate a contract
Planning/ Implementation	**PLANNING AND IMPLEMENTATION** Determine timing and readiness Identify resources Identify areas of power and legitimacy Determine priorities and goals Determine types of intervention Identify consequences and impacts of the interventions Build understanding and proceed
Evaluation	**EVALUATION AND RECYCLE; CLOSURE AND TERMINATION** Use client criteria for success Evaluate outcome Complete contract Determine if follow-up is needed Write report/summary

occupational health nurses at the company allowed management access to employee health records, and there was no policy, written or otherwise, addressing confidentiality. After listening to the occupational health nurse, the consultant determined the occupational health nurse's areas of stress, which included how to maintain confidentiality of the records and still keep her job; how to maintain her credibility among employees and keep the employees' trust; and how to maintain an effective occupational health service.

The defined problems (diagnosis) were two-fold: 1) management's lack of understanding regarding confidentiality of employee health records, and 2) lack of a written policy on that issue. Obviously, the occupational health nurse has a responsibility as a registered professional nurse to practice nursing according to the standards of occupational health nursing and the profession's Code of

Ethics. Both the consultant and the occupational health nurse agreed that the problems were valid and of concern, and that prompt action was needed (feedback and decision to risk). The consultant discussed with the occupational health nurse strategies (planning) to deal with the problems (education, policy development, continued refusal of access by management to records) as well as resources, such as professional associations (AAOHN, ANA), pertinent articles, references (Code of Ethics, Standards of Practice), and so on. One identified consequence of the interventions may be that the occupational health nurse could lose her job. The implementation of the recommendations is up to the occupational health nurse, not the consultant, although the consultant will support the occupational health nurse's decision. The occupational health nurse is currently still working with and educating management about the role of the nurse and her responsibility in maintaining the confidentiality of employee health records. A policy on confidentiality has yet to be written. The consultant continues to monitor the occupational health nurse's progress and will visit the nurse on site as needed.

Consultation may be requested by the client, such as the occupational health nurse, management, hospital, university, or local health department. Sometimes the consultant may initiate contact with the client to learn about the health services offered to employees. Depending on the expertise of the consultant, assistance may be provided in the following areas:

- planning and development of a new occupational health service
- facility design, equipment, and supplies
- policy and procedure manual
- job descriptions
- orientation of new occupational health nurses
- record and reporting systems
- environmental and/or health surveillance programs
- safety
- immunization
- confidentiality
- program development
- certification
- specific problems that concern the occupational health nurse and/or management
- health promotion and health education programs
- staffing ratios
- protocols
- budgeting
- legislation
- disaster planning
- job opportunities
- continuing education
- community resources
- references and resources
- publications
- research and development

Specific functions of the occupational health nurse consultant include, but are not limited to, the following activities:

1. Advises clients on the recommended scope and content of employee health services based on needs assessment and analysis.
2. Consults with management to stimulate the development of new occupational health programs.
3. Assists with orienting nurses new to occupational health and safety.
4. Encourages and supports opportunities for continuing education to help update the occupational health nurse.
5. Serves as a resource on acceptable occupational health nursing practice issues.
6. Promotes interdisciplinary health management of toxic or hazardous situations in the work environment.
7. Serves as a preceptor for nursing students.
8. Stimulates the introduction of some occupational health content into the basic curricula within a school of nursing/public health.
9. Participates in research activities and disseminates the research findings.
10. Serves as a resource person for matching occupational health nurses looking for employment with employers having available positions.
11. Maintains professionalism and ethical conduct.

■ SUMMARY AND FUTURE DIRECTIONS

Each of the five major roles in occupational health nursing practice (clinician/practitioner, administrator, educator, researcher, and consultant) is essential to the further development, refinement, and advancement of occupational health nursing. Although a nurse is hired for one of these advanced practice roles, certain aspects of the other four roles are often intertwined in her or his practice. For this reason, occupational health nurses must clarify and communicate their individual roles to themselves, their peers, the workers they care for, the management they report to, and the public.

Graduate programs in occupational health nursing prepare students to function in these roles. In fact, many of the graduates from the programs have been successfully recruited by industry, agencies, municipalities, or universities for advanced clinical, administrative, educational, research, and/or consultative positions.

Other roles are inherent in occupational health nursing. The occupational health nurse is also a change agent, a role model, an innovator, a risk taker, and a policy maker. In these capacities, the ability and the foresight to lead, motivate, and influence others regarding occupational health nursing, health, wellness, disease prevention, quality health care, and professionalism are important characteristics. Furthermore, the occupational health nurse strives to promote fellow occupational health nurses as well. This is enhanced by networking and mentoring. Success of an occupational health nurse in an advanced role is a positive reflection upon all others (Nail & Singleton, 1986). Opportunities for networking and mentoring occur at professional meetings, such as the annual American Occupational Health Conference, state and regional meetings, and special interest groups. There is a commitment to the profession and to professionalism.

Nurses are "responsible and accountable for professional behavior that involves application of the nursing process and cooperation with appropriate others, within current legislation affecting the practice of nursing, according to the profession's code of ethics and of practice, within the context of the policies and practices of the employing agency, and within the customs and values of the society in which the nursing care is being provided" (Curtin & Flaherty, 1982). This has direct application to occupational health nursing practice. Regardless of role, each occupational health nurse is committed to wellness of workers, research and education, standards of practice, personal and professional accountability, quality care, and advancement of occupational health nursing practice (Randolph, 1988).

REFERENCES

American Association of Occupational Health Nurses. A comprehensive guide for establishing an occupational health service. Atlanta: Author, 1987.

American Association of Occupational Health Nurses. Code of ethics. Atlanta: Author, 1991.

American Association of Occupational Health Nurses. Research priorities in occupational health nursing. Atlanta: Author, 1990.

Babbitz, MA. Enhancing the roles of the occupational health nurse. Occupational Health and Safety, 49(2): 39–40, 1980.

Bernhardt, JH. Education: Current factors affecting nursing practice and occupational health nursing. AAOHN Journal, 34(5): 210–215, 1986.

Curtin, L & Flaherty, MJ. Nursing ethics: Theories and pragmatics. Bowie, MD: Robert J. Brady Co., p. 74, 1982.

Dickson, G, Parsons, MA, Greaves, P, Jackson, KL, Kronenfeld, JJ, Ward, WB, & Ureda, JR. Breast self-examination: Knowledge, attitudes and practice behaviors of working women. AAOHN Journal, 34(5): 228–232, 1986.

Fiorentino, LM. Stress: The high cost to industry. AAOHN Journal, 34(5): 216–220, 1986.

Forti, TJ. Advice: A well-intentioned ineffectual notion. Nurse Practitioner, 6(1): 25–27, 1981.

Gillies, DA. Nursing management: A systems approach (2nd ed.). Philadelphia: WB Saunders, 1989.

Hardy, ME & Conway, ME. Role theory: Perspectives for health professionals. New York: Appleton-Century-Crofts, 1978.

Heasley, PM & Hughes, ST. A comparison study of coronary artery disease in employed women and housewives. Occupational Health Nursing, 33(10): 487–490, 1985.

Javid, LB & Lester, MM. Occupational health nursing: A model for practice. Occupational Health Nursing, 31(3): 38–40, 1983.

Kitzman, HJ. The CNS and the nurse practitioner. In AB Hamric & JA Spross (Eds.), The

clinical nurse specialist in theory and practice (2nd ed.) (pp. 379–394). Philadelphia: WB Saunders, 1989.

Lange, FC. The nurse as an individual, group, or community consultant. Norwalk, CT: Appleton-Century-Crofts, 1987.

Lange, FM. The multifaceted role of the nurse consultant. Journal of Nursing Education, 18(9): 30–34, 1979.

McKechnie, M & Rogers, B. Developing research skills in occupational health nursing: Where to begin? Occupational Health Nursing, 33(10): 515–516, 1985.

Nail, FC & Singleton, EK. The corporate nurse consultant. Journal of Nursing Administration, 16(7,8): 13–20, 1986.

Oda, D. Specialized role development: A three-phase process. Nursing Outlook, 25(6): 374–377, 1977.

Oda, DS. Consultation: An expectation of leadership. Nursing Leadership, 5(1): 7–9, 1982.

Randolph, SA. Contact lens survey: Implications for the occupational health nurse, 35(1): 6–12, 1987.

Randolph, SA. Occupational health nursing: A commitment to excellence. AAOHN Journal, 36(4): 166–169, 1988.

Randolph, SA & Dalton, PC. Limited duty work: An innovative approach to early return to work. AAOHN Journal, 37(11): 446–453, 1989.

Reith, L. The multidimensional health locus of control applied to four classifications of working adults. AAOHN Journal, 35(1): 41–48, 1987.

Rogers, B. Occupational health nursing practice, education, and research: Challenges for the future. AAOHN Journal, 38(11): 536–543, 1990.

Rogers, B. The question and the answer, Part II: Planning for data analysis. AAOHN Journal, 39(1): 42–44, 1991.

Rogers, B & Spencer, GA. Nursing research in occupational health. Occupational Health Nursing, 32(10): 552–553, 1984.

Silberstein, C. Nursing research in occupational

health. Occupational Health Nursing, *31*(3): 9, 1983.

Snyder, M. Educational preparation of the CNS. In AB Hamric & JA Spross (Eds.), The clinical nurse specialist in theory and practice (2nd ed.) (pp. 325–342). Philadelphia: WB Saunders, 1989.

Stevens, BJ. The use of consultants in nursing service. Journal of Nursing Administration, *8*(8): 7–15, 1978.

Thompson, M. Role enactment: A model for pre-retirement planning. AAOHN Journal, *34*(5): 221–227, 1986.

Wild, E, Gerberich, SG, Hunt, K, & Coe, K. Analyses of wrist injuries in workers engaged in repetitive tasks. AAOHN Journal, *35*(8): 356–366, 1987.

5

EPIDEMIOLOGY

As a health care professional in an occupational environment, the occupational health nurse needs to be familiar with epidemiologic concepts and principles in order to determine the nature, relevance, and impact of workplace exposures. Employees may present themselves to the occupational health unit with headaches, skin rashes, or any number of complaints and the occupational health nurse will need to know how to investigate potential exposures. The nurse may want to examine health and illness trends in the worker population and knowledge and application of epidemiologic methods to analyze and interpret data will be required. This chapter will provide a review of epidemiologic concepts and principles that are used in assessing and evaluating health-related events so that measures can be instituted to control and prevent health problems, and promote health in worker populations. However, the reader is referred to an epidemiologic text such as Mausner and Kramer (1985) or Hennekens and Buring (1987) for a more in-depth discussion.

The term epidemiology is derived from the Greek language (epi, upon; demos, people; and logos, science), with early epidemiologic investigations concerned primarily with the study of diseases and disease states that were observed to be "upon the people." Epidemiology, as defined by Mausner and Kramer (1985), is the study of the distribution and determinants of diseases and injuries in human populations. Tyler and Last (1992) provide a recent definition of epidemiology as agreed upon by an international panel: epidemiology is the study of the distribution and determinants of health-related states and events in specified populations and the application of this study to the control of health problems. This definition provides a conceptual expansion to recognize health determinants and prevention.

Until the early 1900s infectious diseases such as smallpox, tuberculosis, typhoid, and diphtheria constituted the primary causes of mortality in populations. For example, the average life expectancy for newborns in 1900 in the United States was about 50 years (Gwatkin & Brandel, 1982) compared to an average of nearly 75 years in 1987 (USDHHS, 1990a). Much of the increase in life extension is attributable to significant improvements in living and working conditions, nutrition, sanitation and hygiene, and the introduction of antibiotics and vaccines that have helped curb the spread of infectious diseases in at-risk groups.

■ **TABLE 5–1**   Age-Adjusted Leading Causes of Death in the United States, 1900 and 1990

1900		1990	
Pneumonia/influenza	11.8%	Heart disease	33.5%
Tuberculosis	11.2%	Cancer	23.5%
Heart disease	9.4%	Stroke	6.7%
Stroke	7.6%	Accidents	4.3%
Diarrhea/enteritis	6.3%	Chronic lung disease	4.0%
Nephritis	5.9%	Pneumonia/influenza	3.7%
Cancer	4.5%	Diabetes mellitus	2.2%
Accidents	4.2%	Suicide	1.4%
Diphtheria	1.9%	Chronic liver disease	1.2%
Other	37.2%	HIV	1.2%
		Other	18.3%

From National Center for Health Statistics, 1991.

With the increased control of infectious diseases in the 20th century, a shift to chronic diseases as the major causes of death in the United States has emerged (Table 5–1). Of the nation's 10 leading causes of death in 1990, the top two causes, coronary heart disease and cancer, accounted for nearly 60% of all deaths. By comparison, pneumonia and influenza, which constituted the chief mortality causes in 1900 (12%), contributed only 3.7% of all U.S. deaths (NCHS, 1991).

Workplace exposures are also recognized as contributing to the development of acute and chronic health problems. The concern about the adverse health effects of occupational exposures dates back to Hippocrates, who urged physicians to explore patients' vocational, environmental, and lifestyle influences as potential determinants for disease etiology (Lilienfeld & Lilienfeld, 1980). Occupational epidemiology is concerned with the study of the effects of these workplace exposures on the frequency distribution of diseases and injuries in worker populations (Checkoway, 1989).

The recognition of occupational hazards has often begun with anecdotal reports of debilitating conditions or acute traumatic events related to the job, which has then led to epidemiologic investigations. For example, Agricola reported premature mortality among miners in the 16th century, while later mortality surveys described excessive rates of respiratory disease and cancer among underground metal miners (Hunter, 1978; Lorenz, 1944; Peller, 1939; Pirchan & Sikl, 1932).

Percival Pott (1775) described the exposure of chimney sweeps to soot as the cause for scrotal cancer, and is credited with providing the first substantiated evidence of chemical carcinogenesis from an occupational exposure (Waldron, 1983). Other studies have demonstrated morbidity and mortality patterns of asbestos insulation workers (Selikoff et al., 1964; 1979), and bladder cancer among dyestuff factory workers (Case et al., 1954; Goldwater et al., 1965; Wendell et al., 1974).

Studies in occupational health and disease have expanded to examine work practices and behaviors of workers in order to determine associated risks of exposure, and to identify factors that may contribute to or minimize the risk. Behavioral risk factors are important determinants of some diseases that also have occupational etiologies and therefore require investigation within the framework of occupational epidemiologic research.

The natural history of disease is an evolving, interactive process that occurs over time, and in the case of chronic and many occupational diseases occurs in stages that may take years to become apparent. Thus, determining the causes of chronic and many occupational diseases, and thereby the development of preventive strategies to reduce exposure or disease risk, can be difficult. In addition, depending on the particular condition, several factors may collectively be involved, including lifestyle and environmental influences, which may result in conflicting or confounding evidence as to the etiology of the problem. However, the development of new and refinement of existing methodologies, including data collection techniques and analyses, provide for improved quantification of the magnitude of the exposure-disease relationship in humans; alteration of the risk through interventions; and information to serve as the foundation for public health policy decisions (Hennekens & Buring, 1987).

In the work setting, observations of conditions and exposures associated with symptom or disease occurrence, and the analysis of recorded data about illness or injury, the environment, work practices, occupational health unit visits and such, provide the basis for designing health protection, promotion, and surveillance programs. It is important for the occupational health nurse to be involved not only in the accurate collection of data but in evaluating outcomes and determining effective control procedures to minimize risk exposure. Through increased understanding of epidemiologic concepts and principles such as the dynamics of health/disease processes and determinates, environmental relationships and interactions, and approaches to measurement and study design, the occupational health nurse will be in a position to collaborate more effectively in decisions affecting the health and safety of workers.

■ EPIDEMIOLOGIC CONCEPTS

The unit of concern in the field of epidemiology is the population and its subgroups. Illness and injury conditions are unevenly dispersed throughout the population; therefore, studying the frequency characteristics of illnesses and injuries in groups, and trying to tie together related associations between health and illness patterns provide the basis to determine if causal relationships exist or can be inferred.

The basic concept underlying epidemiologic approaches is related to the theory of multiple causation, wherein the development of disease is dependent on the interaction of several factors and cannot be attributed to any single factor alone. Several models have been used to illustrate this interaction, all of which specify a relationship between the host (living species/individual human) and the environment and related elements (external factors that influence the host health state). One model, referred to as the epidemiologic triangle, depicts a relationship between three variables, the host, the environment, and the agent (a factor such as a virus or chemical necessary to produce the condition or disease). This model (Fig. 5–1) implies a dynamic equilibrium among each of the three variables or factors, with any change in this equilibrium resulting in either positive or negative infuences toward health or illness (Lilienfeld & Lilienfeld, 1980). This model continues to be widely used.

MacMahon (1970) offers a classic and conceptually similar model, referred

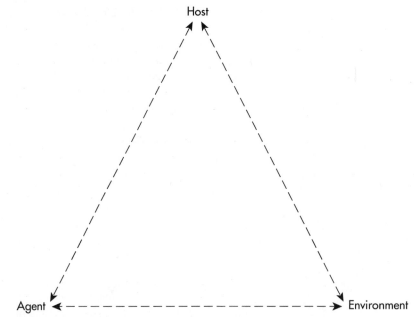

■ **Figure 5–1**   Epidemiologic triangle depicting dynamic agent-host-environment relationship.

to as the "web of causation," which relates a multiplicity of factors and linkages involved in a particular health condition or problem (in this example hepatitis) in which the agent is an integral part of the environment (Fig. 5–2). Another example is the development of coronary heart disease, which is influenced by both intrinsic host factors, such as age, genetics, and previous medical history, and extrinsic factors, such as occupation, diet, medication, smoking, and exercise. Mausner and Kramer (1985) deemphasize the agent as separate from the environment and stress the multiplicity of interactions between host and environment. However, considering these two models, examples of selected agent, host, and environmental factors adapted in part from Lilienfeld & Lilienfeld (1980) are shown in Table 5–2 and are briefly discussed.

Agent Factors

An agent may be thought of as a substance that must be present for a disease or condition to occur. Examples are shown in Table 5–2,I. Transmission of an agent to a host may be accomplished in a variety of ways: toxic vapors may be inhaled, poisons ingested, chemicals absorbed through the skin, and infectious agents spread by direct contact such as through sneezing or sexual intercourse. Exposure to biological agents, such as the human immunodeficiency virus, hepatitis B virus, and cytomegalovirus poses threats for disease development in health care and laboratory workers; transmission of the hepatitis B virus serves as an example. The agent of hepatitis B is a virus, and the reservoir that perpetuates the agent is an individual infected with the virus. The mode of conveyance of the organism is through contact with infected body fluids, and the route or portal of entry is through intimate sexual contact, perinatally, permucosally, or percutaneously via injection with a contaminated needle (such as with

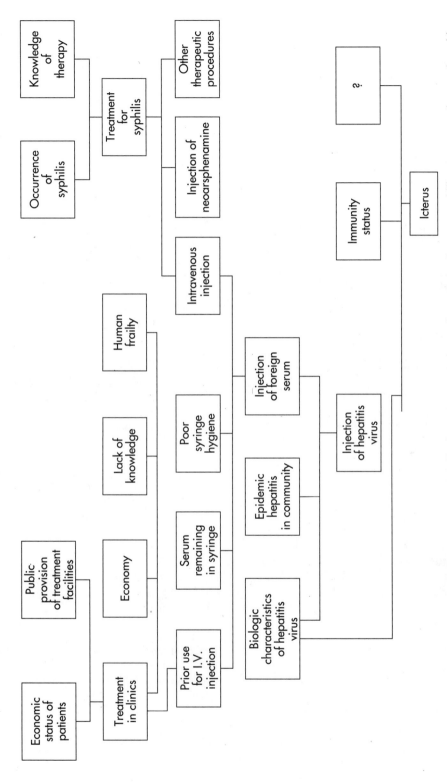

■ **Figure 5–2** Classic example of "web of causation" indicating some components of association between syphilis treatment and serum hepatitis. (Reprinted with permission from MacMahon, B & Pugh, TF. Epidemiologic principles and methods. Boston: Little, Brown & Company, copyright 1970.)

■ **TABLE 5–2** Classification by Selected Agents, Host Factors, and Environmental Factors that Influence the Health and Distribution of Diseases in Human Populations

I. AGENTS OF DISEASE (NECESSARY ETIO-LOGIC FACTORS)

EXAMPLES

A. Biological agents

Bacteria — Gonorrhea, Lyme disease, pneumonia, staphylococcal/streptococcal infections, syphilis, tuberculosis

Fungi — Candidiasis, dermatophyte infections, histoplasmosis

Rickettsia — Rocky Mountain spotted fever

Viruses — AIDS, hepatitis, herpes, influenza, rabies, rubella, upper respiratory tract infections

B. Chemical agents

Poisons — Asbestos, arsenic, carbon monoxide, hydrogen sulfide, drugs

Allergens — Medications, poison ivy, ragweed

C. Physical agents — Cold, heat, ionizing radiation, noise

D. Psychosocial — Family stress, personal or work conflicts, work overload

II. HOST FACTORS (INTRINSIC FACTORS)—INFLUENCE EXPOSURE, SUSCEPTIBILITY, OR RESPONSE TO AGENTS

EXAMPLES

A. Genetic — Sickle cell disease

B. Age — —

C. Sex — —

D. Ethnic group — —

E. Physiologic state — Fatigue, nutritional state, pregnancy, puberty, resistance, stress

F. Prior immunologic experience

Active — Hypersensitivity, immunization, prior infection

Passive — Gamma globulin prophylaxis, maternal antibodies

G. Intercurrent or preexisting disease — —

H. Human behavior — Diet, exercise, food handling, health resources, occupation, personal hygiene, recreation, interpersonal relations, substance abuse, utilization of health resources

III. ENVIRONMENTAL FACTORS (EXTRINSIC FACTORS)—INFLUENCE EXISTENCE OF AGENT, EXPOSURE, OR SUSCEPTIBILITY TO AGENT.

EXAMPLES

A. Physical environment — Climate, geology wastes

B. Biologic environment

Human populations — Density

Flora — Sources of food; influence on vertebrates and arthropods as a source of agents

Fauna — Food sources, vertebrate hosts, arthropod vectors

C. Socioeconomic Environment

Occupation

Urbanization and economic development — Exposure to hazardous agents, urban crowding, literacy, health care access

Disruption — Disasters, wars

Adapted from Lilienfeld, A & Lilienfeld, D. Foundations of epidemiology. New York: Oxford University Press, 1980.

a needlestick injury) or contact with a contaminated sharp (CDC, 1990a). Routes of entry, including direct contact, inhalation, ingestion, injection, and skin absorption, and modes of transmission, such as airborne droplet spray or via a contaminated needle, are important factors related to both the virulence and resultant pathogenicity of the agent.

Chemical agents are well-recognized hazardous substances and take the form of dusts, fumes, gases, liquids or vapors. Thousands of chemicals are prevalent in the workplace, many of which cause acute, chronic, and local effects in the human system. Examples include asbestos and asbestosis and lung cancer; benzene and aplastic anemia and leukemia; cotton dust and byssinosis; vinyl chloride and liver cancer; and various contact agents causing dermatoses. As a chemical agent example, lead is commercially produced by mining, smelting, refining, and secondary recovery. Lead is primarily used in the manufacture of storage batteries, and in numerous other applications, such as paints, plastics, ceramics, electrical cables, and shielding. Workers in these fields are at greatest risk of exposure (Lewis, 1990; WHO, 1986).

Lead and its components enter the body through inhalation and ingestion from exposure to lead dust and fumes in operating processes such as grinding, welding, and spray painting and in the manufacture of such products as paints, pigments, and lead batteries. Absorption through the skin is limited to certain organic compounds. Once absorbed, lead is transported through the bloodstream to several organ systems (e.g., brain, kidney, liver, skin, and skeletal muscle); however, the bone constitutes the major site of deposition. Acute and chronic clinical effects may be manifested in disturbances in related body systems, such as the gastrointestinal, hematopoietic, nervous, renal, musculoskeletal, and reproductive systems.

Physical agents may interact with the susceptible host to cause some form of tissue trauma. For example, high levels of noise or exposure to radiation may produce noise-induced hearing loss or leukemia, respectively (Levy & Wegman, 1988).

Psychosocial agents or stressors such as interpersonal conflicts, excessive workloads, depersonalization and shiftwork may create highly stressful conditions leading to both physiological and psychological problems (Cronin-Stubbs & Rooks, 1985). For example, shiftwork is associated with the disruption of circadian rhythms and decrement in human performance, which may increase errors and injuries (Monk, 1990).

Host Factors

Host factors such as age, sex, ethnicity, and health status are intrinsic to the individual and are listed in Table 5–2,II. An agent-host interaction occurs once an agent is transmitted to a susceptible host. Susceptibility is dependent on host defenses and inherent resistance, virulence of the agent, and environmental conditions. Immunity is the host's resistance to a specific infectious agent and it can be active or passive. Active immunity occurs as an antigen-antibody induced response, is long lasting, and may protect an individual for life. It can be attained naturally by actual infection (e.g., measles, rubella) or artifically by inoculation of vaccine designed to stimulate an antibody response (e.g., hepatitis B vaccine). Active immunity forms the basis for mass vaccination programs such as for influenza virus. Passive immunity is temporary and is provided by an antibody produced in another host. It may be acquired naturally through maternal-fetal antibody transfer or artifically by administration of an antibody-containing preparation, such as gamma globulin (Benenson, 1990).

Inherent resistance refers to the host's ability to resist disease unassociated with antibody production and response, and thereby reflects the host's ability to respond not only to infectious but other types of agents such as chemical exposures and stress. Resistance is related to the physiological and health state of the individual. Factors such as good nutrition, regular exercise, proper rest, and activities aimed at general health promotion will probably affect one's resistance to infection or a disease process even though immunity may be lacking or not a factor. For example, the relationship between coronary heart disease and the influences of preexisting high blood pressure, smoking, exercise, diet, and occupational stress are well documented (Blackburn, 1989; Dorian & Taylor, 1984; Doll & Hill, 1964; Feinleib, 1983; Leon et al., 1987; NRC, 1989; Pooling Project, 1978; Slattery et al., 1989; Wilhelmsen, 1988). Evidence regarding the interplay of personality factors have yet to be proven (Shekelle et al., 1983; Leon et al., 1988).

In relationship to the spread of infectious diseases between people or in populations, two concepts—generation time and herd immunity—are particularly important. Generation time refers to the period between the receipt of infection by and maximal communicability of the host (Mausner & Kramer, 1985; Sartwell, 1973). Maximum communicability may precede or occur concurrently with the incubation period (time between receipt of infection and illness onset). A classic example is the mumps virus, whose maximum communicability occurs approximately 48 hours before its clinical manifestation. Hepatitis B virus blood infectivity has been shown to occur many weeks before the onset of first symptoms, through the acute clinical course of the disease, and during the carrier state (Benenson, 1990).

The concept of what is called herd immunity is particularly important and has been defined in an older but relevant reference by Fox and Hall (1970) as the "resistance of a group to invasion and spread of an infectious agent, based on the immunity of a high proportion of individual members of the group." This concept is based on the principle that the halt or spread of infection in a particular community or group will be related to the proportion of susceptible (or resistant) hosts at risk of infection. In other words, there must be a relatively large pool of persons susceptible, or at risk of acquiring infection, in order for a disease to continue to spread. If a sufficient number of individuals in the population are immune, the spread of disease will be interrupted because of lack of infectious reservoirs or hosts. It is generally believed that for most infectious agents, it is not necessary to achieve 100% population immunity in order to prevent an epidemic or control disease spread; however, it is unclear as to how much below the 100% level is sufficient to disrupt the spread of disease (Mausner & Kramer, 1985).

In recent years, significant outbreaks of measles have occurred in the United States, with approximately 40% of the cases occurring in individuals with a history of previous vaccination. As measles is one of the most highly communicable infectious diseases, a herd immunity of at least 94% may be needed to prevent additional disease spread. In addition to routine revaccination at school entry, revaccination should also be required of those entering educational institutions beyond high school, or workers entering hospital employment, unless measles history or two-dose measles vaccination is documented (Benenson, 1990).

Genetic influences are now thought to play a more prominent role in either increased or decreased host susceptibility to certain diseases. For example, persons with sickle cell trait seem to have a decreased risk of malaria, and individuals with xeroderma pigmentosum have a genetically determined inability to repair ultraviolet light–induced damage, thereby placing them at greater risk of skin cancer related to sun exposure. The latter would pose a potential hazard to workers with this condition who are occupationally exposed to the sun, such as construction workers, gardeners, and aircraft workers (Zenz, 1993). In addition, human behavior, in terms of lifestyle practices, is important to consider, as this will contribute to the impact of risk factors on one's health status.

Environmental Factors

The environment, which may be classified as physical, biological, or social, represents external conditions that interact with the host and the agent (Table 5–2,III). The physical environment involves the geological and atmospheric structure of an area and the source of such elements as water, temperature, and radiation, which may serve as positive or negative stressors. Humans generally have a great deal of control over the physical environment through the provision of adequate shelter against extremes of weather, purification of drinking water, treatment of sewage, and control of ventilation. However, new environmental problems continue to arise such as an increase in industrial wastes and toxins and indoor and outdoor environmental pollution, which present opportunities for significant health threats to the working and general population.

The biological environment includes animals, living plants, and humans that serve as vectors or reservoirs for transmission of the infectious agents. For example, food may serve as the vehicle source for bacteria from infected food handlers and human body fluids serve as a reservoir for the transmission of various types of organisms.

The social aspects of the environment encompass the economic and political forces affecting society and its health. This includes factors such as sanitation/hygiene practices, housing conditions, level and delivery of health care services, development and enforcement of health-related codes (e.g., occupational health and safety, pollution), employment conditions, population crowding, literacy, ethnic customs, extent of support for health-related research, and equitable access to health care. Addictive behaviors such as alcohol and substance abuse and various forms of psychosocial stress may be an outgrowth of negative social environments.

The occupational environment, within the context of the social environment, is represented by the workplace and work setting, and the interactive effects of this environment on the worker. One must consider the hazards and threats posed by this enviornment, and the commitment of the employer to providing a safe and healthful workplace through use of preventive strategies and controls (i.e., engineering, substitution).

■ DESCRIPTIVE EPIDEMIOLOGY

Within an epidemiologic framework, investigations generally begin with observations and recording of information related to the condition or event of interest, such as disease or injury. Data are then derived relative to patterns of health and illness and expressed quantitatively as frequencies, percentages, rates, and so forth. To describe the occurrence of illness or injury in a population, such as a group of workers, certain questions must be answered, such as who is affected and where and when do cases occur. These types of questions specify the interelationship between person, place, and time, which provides descriptive information from which hypotheses can be generated for future analytical epidemiologic investigations.

Person

Although there are numerous variables that characterize individuals, the personal variables—age, gender, and ethnic group or race—are generally the most important to consider in epidemiologic study. Examination of personal characteristics will help to determine risk factors associated with individuals who get a particular disease. Increasingly, occupation is recognized as a variable which has significant impact on the health outcome of exposed populations and provides important data regarding the determinants of health/illness relationships.

Age is probably the most important personal variable and is strongly tied to morbidity (illness/injury) and mortality (death) rates of most conditions. With respect to morbidity, acute infectious processes occur most commonly in children, while accidents occur more frequently in older children, teenagers, and young adults. Adults may be plagued with conditions related to occupational exposure (e.g., musculoskeletal injuries, respiratory disorders, dermatoses, cancer, and stress), and chronic disease conditions such as arthritis and hypertension increase in frequency as one gets older. Death rates are fairly high in infancy, decrease during childhood, begin to rise gradually until middle age, and then increase sharply.

Gender plays a significant role in morbidity and mortality patterns where morbidity rates are generally higher for females but mortality rates are higher for males than females at every age. Coronary heart disease, lung cancer, homicide, cirrhosis of the liver, and chronic obstructive lung disease are more common among men, whereas arthritis and depression are more common in women (Harper, 1986). Life expectancy has consistently been highest for white females and lowest for nonwhite males. For 1988, these rates were 78.9 and 64.9 years, respectively (NCHS, 1991).

Racial and ethnic differences exist with respect to both morbidity and mortality and may be related to differences in socioeconomic status, education, and access to health care. Blacks have higher rates of hypertension, cerebrovascular accidents, homicide, and accidental deaths. Whites have higher rates of death from atherosclerotic heart disease, suicide, and leukemia (Harper, 1986). Inherited diseases such as sickle cell anemia are primarily restricted to blacks while cystic fibrosis occurs mostly in whites. The nonwhite population in the United States has an average life expectancy of six years less than that of whites (NCHS, 1990).

Since people spend a substantial portion of their lives in the workplace, occupationally related experiences and the work environment itself can contribute significantly to both morbidity and mortality. These influences may occur through a variety of exposures (e.g., chemicals, noise, stress, infectious agents). Personal work practices and habits play an important role in health maintenance and protection particularly as they relate to workplace exposures. Observations of these behaviors will contribute to the assessment of workplace exposures further discussed in the next section.

In addition to the aforementioned factors, other influences such as lifestyle behaviors, personality traits, and the degree, quality and utilization of health care will affect, at least in part, morbidity and mortality rates.

Place

The occurrence and frequency of disease in individuals often vary by place. For example, natural boundaries may play a role in the frequency distribution of certain diseases such that certain epidemics may be contained in populations due in part to geographic contours such as mountain ranges. Some cancers show distinct geographic patterns such as higher rates of melanoma in the South, which suggest that sun rays contribute to the pathogenesis of malignant melanoma. Lead poisoning also displays a geographic pattern where airborne lead particulates occur in communities surrounding lead smelters. Multiple sclerosis is much more prevalent in northern latitudes than in southern regions; however, the etiologic association for this has yet to be identified (Hennekens & Buring, 1987). Examining disease rates in groups within specific geographic areas is helpful in etiologic reasoning, such as within defined population areas, specific industries, and areas surrounding industrial sites.

Health differences are noted between urban and rural populations. Persons living in urban areas are faced with overcrowding, social problems including homicide, and increasing problems of substance abuse and related crimes of violence. The concentration of industrial worksites has led to increased problems with air pollution and toxic waste dumping.

In the past 50 years there has been a significant shift in the population distribution from farms to urban areas (approximately 70% in 1980). However, for many persons remaining in rural areas, illiteracy, lack of job opportunities, malnutrition, and limited access to health care continue. Health problems of the farm community remain largely unrecognized and understudied. For example, the Bureau of Labor Statistics (1988) reported the average death rate (1983-87) of farmers as 14 per 100,000; however, the National Safety Council has estimated a death rate as high as 52 per 100,000 (NCASH, 1989). Farm accidents remain a serious cause of death and disability from exposure to dangerous equipment, pesticides and other chemicals, and microorganisms.

Migrant workers face difficult living and working conditions, and their health problems remain serious. Cultural and language differences have been shown to be barriers to health care for these workers, particularly related to primary care access. The stresses of the job may vary with the type of crop involved in the work; however, the range of agent exposures is broad, including pesticide exposure, snake bites, mechanical trauma, sun exposure, and difficult environmental conditions.

Epidemiologic studies have related many diseases to occupational hazards or exposures such as heavy lifting and back injury (Bigos et al., 1986; Cato et al., 1989); reproductive toxicity (Hemminki et al., 1985; Whorton & Foliart, 1983); noise-induced hearing loss (OSHA, 1983); neurologic and behavioral disorders related to metal and solvent exposure (Elofsson, 1980; Feldman et al., 1980); kidney impairment due to cadmium exposure (Roels, 1989; Thum, 1993); cor-

■ **TABLE 5–3** Agents Related to Occupationally Induced Cancer

Agent	Site or Type of Cancer	Occupation
Aromatic amines 4-Aminobiphenyl Benzidine 2-Naphthylamine	Bladder	Dye manufacturers, rubber workers, coal gas manufacturers
Arsenic	Skin, lung	Copper and cobalt smelters, arsenical pesticide manufacturers, some gold miners
Asbestos	Lung, pleura, peritoneum	Asbestos miners, asbestos textile manufacturers, asbestos insulation workers, certain shipyard workers
Benzene	Marrow, leukemia	Workers with glues and varnishes
Bischloromethyl ether	Lung	Makers of ion-exchange resins
Cadmium	Prostate	Cadmium workers
Chromium	Lung	Manufacturers of chromates from chrome ore, pigment manufacturers
Ionizing radiations	Lung	Uranium and some other miners
	Bone	Luminizers
	Marrow, all sites	Radiologists, radiographers
Isopropyl oil	Nasal sinuses	Isopropyl alcohol manufacturers
Mineral oils, untreated and mildly treated	Skin	Metal working, printing
Mustard gas	Larynx, lung	Poison gas manufacturers
Nickel	Nasal sinuses, lung	Nickel refiners
Polycyclic hydrocarbons in soot, coal tar, oil	Skin, scrotum, lung, bladder	Coal gas manufacturers, roofers, asphalters, aluminum refiners, many groups selectively exposed to certain tars and oils
Talc containing asbestiform fibers	Lung	Miners
UV light	Skin	Farmers, seamen
Vinyl chloride	Liver	PVC manufacturers

Data from Harper, 1986; and Thomas, 1992.

onary artery disease and carbon monoxide exposure (Stern & Steenland, 1993); and lung and cancer disorders previously described. Occupational substances that have been shown to be carcinogenic are listed in Table 5–3. Workers in mining, construction, transportation, and agriculture are among the occupations with the highest rates of injury-related deaths from trauma (USDHHS, 1990) (Fig. 5–3).

As a health care professional in an occupational environment, the occupational health nurse needs to be familiar with epidemiologic concepts in order to evaluate workplace exposures. For example, an employee may be concerned about reproductive effects related to chemical exposure on the job. Assessing the nature and scope of workplace exposures, including information recorded about types of jobs, length of employment, potential and specific exposures, including intensity and duration, and actual agent sampling measurements, are important in helping to quantify exposure. Variation in exposure due to differences in work performed, work habits and practices, use of personal protective equipment, and

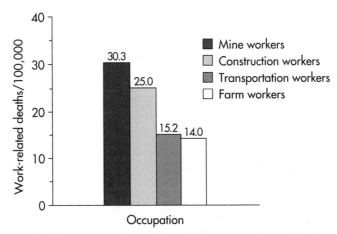

■ **Figure 5–3**   Work-related deaths 1983–1987 average. (From U.S. Department of Health and Human Services. Healthy People 2000, 1990.)

general workplace environmental hygiene are important determinants in making risk estimates about disease occurrence.

Time

The study of disease related to time of occurrence is basic to epidemiologic investigation; morbidity and mortality events should be examined not only as a precedent to disease occurrence but as trends occurring over time. For example, although there has been little change in the death rate from breast cancer over time, lung cancer deaths in women have steadily increased from 6 per 100,000 in the 1960s to 28 per 100,000 in 1987 and are attributed to an increase in cigarette smoking in this group (Kelsey & Gammon, 1991; Garfinkel & Silverberg, 1991). Time trends of disease patterns may also occur in cycles such as seasonal epidemics of variant types of influenza virus and other types of infectious diseases such as pneumonia, the common cold, and respiratory infections. However, some of this may be explained by crowding of groups of people into confined spaces in winter months (including the workplace) and other lifestyle habits such as lack of exercise and poor nutrition.

Considerable interest lies in exploring factors related to clustering of events or diseases. For example, the occurrence of dermatitis in a group of workers or increased reproductive insults should be investigated with respect to the relationship of an exposure to time and place, taking into consideration the personal variables of those exposed such as exposures in the home.

■ MEASURES OF DISEASE FREQUENCY

In order to describe the distribution and patterns of occurrence of illness, injury, or health outcome in a population it is necessary to quantify the occurrence of the event outcome of interest. (For ease of discussion the term "disease" will be used primarily.) The most basic measure of disease occurrence is the frequency, number, or simple count of affected individuals or events. However, the number of health/illness events itself has limited utility in making statements about the determinants and distribution of disease without a reference point. Yet when the frequency is expressed in relation to the size of the affected or at-risk population and the time frame of occurrence, it is called a rate and is of great value in comparing groups with the disease or the outcome under consideration. A rate is defined as:

$$\frac{\text{Number of events (cases or deaths) in a specific period}}{\text{Population at risk of these events in a specified period}} \times k$$

The numerator of the rate includes all those with the disease or event being counted, and the denominator is the population at risk for the disease or event. Rates of disease are called morbidity rates and rates of death are called mortality rates. For ease of comparing two rates, a population constant (k) is used and expressed in terms of multiples of 10, such as 100, 1,000, 10,000, or 100,000. Most vital statistics are reported per 100,000 population. For example, the population death rate (NCHS, 1993) for all persons in the United States in 1990 was 863.8 per 100,000 population, which is expressed as follows:

$$\frac{\text{Deaths in U.S. residents in 1990 (2,148,463)}}{\text{U.S. population in 1990 (248,722,273)}} \times 100,000$$

Examples of common rate measures are shown in Table 5–4.

Incidence and Prevalence Rates

Two basic types of rates are used in epidemiology: incidence and prevalence rates.

Incidence Rates.   The incidence rate measures the number of new cases of disease or event outcome occurring during a specified period of time (Table 5–4). It is a measure of the probability of risk for which new disease develops in previously disease-free individuals. To determine the incidence it is necessary to know the actual number of persons or cases with disease (numerator data), the time period of disease occurrence, and the population at risk of exposure or disease development. The at-risk population needs to be accurately enumerated and theoretically should not include those who already have disease (or those who are not susceptible because of immunity in the case of infectious diseases).

For example, to determine the incidence of hypertension in a population of workers at a telecommunications company, it is necessary to know the number of workers actually diagnosed with hypertension during a definite time period, usually one year (although it may be any length of time), and the total number of workers employed, but excluding those previously diagnosed with hypertension. If the disease frequency is low and the population is large, this correction to the population denominator would make little statistical difference. However, if the condition is common or if precise information is desired, the denominator should only include those at risk (those without disease) (Mausner & Kramer, 1985). The number of persons at risk is likely to change over time; therefore the population at midpoint of the period would be used to represent the average population at risk.

In this example, suppose the total population of workers in 1992 was 2,050. From a health record review, 214 individuals were identified with a preexisting diagnosis of hypertension. During 1992, all employees were screened for high blood pressure and ultimately 21 employees were newly diagnosed with hyper-

■ **TABLE 5–4**   Rates Most Frequently Used as Indices of Population Health

Rates	Usual Population Factor
GENERAL MORTALITY	
Crude death rate $= \dfrac{\text{Number of deaths in a year}}{\text{Average (midyear) population}}$	per 100,000 population
Cause-specific death rate $= \dfrac{\text{Number of deaths from a stated cause in a year}}{\text{Average (midyear) population}}$	per 100,000 population
Age-specific death rate $= \dfrac{\text{Number of deaths among persons in given age group in a year}}{\text{Average (midyear) population in specified age group}}$	per 100,000 population
Proportional mortality rate $= \dfrac{\text{Number of deaths from specific cause in specified time period}}{\text{Total deaths in a same time period}}$	percent of deaths
Case-fatality rate $= \dfrac{\text{Number of deaths due to specified disease}}{\text{Number cases of specified disease}}$	per 100 cases
MORBIDITY	
Incidence $= \dfrac{\text{Number of new cases of disease/condition during a specified time period}}{\text{Population at risk for same time period}}$	per 100,000 population
Point prevalence $= \dfrac{\text{Number of existing cases/conditions at a point in time}}{\text{Total population at same time point}}$	per 100,000 population

tension. The incidence rate is calculated to be 11.4 per 1,000 employees ([21 × 1000]/[2050 − 214]).

As another example, the reporting of three cases of infectious hepatitis in Industry A, nine cases in Industry B, and ten cases in Industry C might lead one to believe that hepatitis is a more common and serious problem in both Industries B and C. However, as shown in Table 5–5 the annual rate of occurrence in Industry A is higher than either B or C. The populations in both Industries B and C are larger, and to compare the actual incidence in all populations, it is necessary to account for both the difference in population sizes and lengths of reporting periods. In this example, the annual rate of occurrence of hepatitis is 3 per 10,000 for one year in Industry A and 9 per 30,000 for three years or 3 per 30,000 for one year in Industry B, and the comparable rate for Industry C is 10 per 25,000 for two years or 5 per 25,000 for one year.

To compare the rates more directly, the same denominator population unit is used, such as a common unit of 100,000. Hence, in this example in Table 5–5, the annual rates of 3 per 10,000, 3 per 30,000, and 5 per 25,000 can be

■ **TABLE 5–5** Comparison of Incidence Rates

Location	New Cases Hepatitis	Reporting Period	Industry Population
Industry A	3	1990	10,000
Industry B	9	1989-1991	30,000
Industry C	10	1989-1990	25,000

ANNUAL RATE OF OCCURRENCE

Industry A:	3/10,000/1 year =	3:10,000/year =	30/100,000/year
Industry B:	9/30,000/3 years =	3:30,000/year =	10/100,000/year
Industry C:	10/25,000/2 years =	5:25,000/year =	20/100,000/year

expressed as 30, 10, and 20 per 100,000 in Industries A, B, and C, respectively.

Incidence rates are useful in monitoring the occurrence of disease or health-related events in defined populations for a period of time. For example, a sudden increase in spontaneous abortions may reflect the introduction of a new chemical substance or exposure into the work environment. Comparisons over time or with another population can be done to determine any rate increase.

Prevalence Rates.   The prevalence rate measures the number of people in a population (cases) who have the disease or event outcome at a given time. Unspecified prevalence rates usually refer to point prevalence (i.e., a specific point in time) (Table 5–4). For example, one might conduct a one-time survey of all workers in the company to determine the prevalence of smoking in the population. Another type of prevalence, period prevalence, includes all cases existing at a point in time, plus any new or recurring cases during a specified time period. Prevalence measures are most useful for planning health care programs and tracking changes in disease patterns over time through a series of cross-sectional surveys. In this way, period prevalence is a helpful predictor of workload and program costs.

Crude and Specific Rates

Rates may be expressed as crude or specific. Crude rates represent actual numbers of events during a time period, such as births or deaths in a total population; whereas, specific rates are detailed for selected, usually demographic, characteristics such as age, sex, or subgroups of the population. Crude rates require only the number of events in a year being measured and the total population (which was previously demonstrated by showing the crude death rate in the United States in 1990 as 863.8/100,000).

Crude rates are limited because they may not show an accurate picture of the risks in population subgroups; that is, they reflect both the probability of dying and the age of the population. Age is an important consideration, as the very young and very old are much more likely to die in a given year than those in other age groups. For example, a geographic region of the country or state, such as Florida, which houses many retirees, is likely to present a biased mortality picture reflected in the crude death rate. Because of the significant effect of age on mortality, age-specific rates are recommended rather than crude rates when comparing mortality experiences (Hennekens & Buring, 1987). Examples are given in Tables 5–6 and 5–7.

■ **TABLE 5–6**   Crude and Age-specific Mortality Rates from Cancer in the United States, 1980

Age (Years)	Number of Cancer Deaths	Population as of July 1, 1980	Mortality Rate per 100,000
Under 5	686	16,348,000	4.2
5-9	777	16,700,000	4.7
10-14	720	18,242,000	3.9
15-19	1,145	21,168,000	5.4
20-24	1,538	21,319,000	7.2
25-29	2,041	19,521,000	10.5
30-34	3,040	17,561,000	17.3
35-39	4,684	13,965,000	33.5
40-44	7,786	11,669,000	66.7
45-49	14,230	11,090,000	128.3
50-54	26,800	11,710,000	228.9
55-59	41,600	11,615,000	358.2
60-64	53,045	10,088,000	525.8
65-74	127,430	15,581,000	817.9
75+	130,959	9,969,000	1,313.7
TOTAL	416,481	226,546,000	183.8·

Data from U.S. Bureau of the Census, 1984; and NCHS, 1985.

The data in Table 5–6 represent the number of cancer deaths in the United States in 1980 along with estimates of the midyear population. The crude death rate from cancer equals the total number of cancer deaths divided by the total number of individuals in the population: 416,481/226,546,000 = 183.8/ 100,000. Age-specific cancer death rates are measured by the number of cancer deaths occurring among individuals in each age stratum divided by the total number of individuals in that stratum. Thus, the cancer death rate for ages 5 to 9 years is calculated as 777/16,700,000 = 4.7 per 100,000.

■ **TABLE 5–7**   Comparison of Death Rates in Two Industry Populations by Age

Population	Age (Years)	Population Number	Population Proportion	Annual Number of Deaths	Annual Age-specific Death Rate (per 1,000)	Crude Death Rate (per 1,000)
		(1)	(2)	(3)	(4)	(5)	(6)
Industry A	<15	1,500	0.30	3	2	
	15-44	2,000	0.40	12	6	
	≥45	1,500	0.30	30	20	
	All ages	5,000	1.00	45		$\frac{45}{5,000} = 9.0$
Industry B	<15	2,000	0.40	4	2	
	15-44	2,500	0.50	15	6	
	≥45	500	0.10	10	20	
	All ages	5,000	1.00	29		$\frac{29}{5,000} = 5.8$

Adapted from Mausner, J & Kramer, S. Epidemiology: An introductory text. Philadelphia: W. B. Saunders, 1985.

Table 5–7 presents data that compares death rates for two industries (Mausner & Kramer, 1985). While the crude death rates differ because of the difference in age distribution in the industry populations (column 6), the age-specific death rates are the same for both industries (column 5), indicating no true difference in the risk of death. Industry A has relatively more older people (i.e., 30% over 45 years in Industry A compared to only 10% in Industry B), and as death rates are higher for older people, the crude death rate for Industry A is higher. However, the true risk of dying in each age group is the same for both populations (column 5). Although of limited utility, crude rates provide at least summary information and are relatively easy to compute.

Specific rates provide valuable and more accurate information about the health of the population, as groups may differ with respect to characteristics such as age, race, and sex, which affect the overall rates of disease and death. Notably, males and blacks have higher mortality rates than females and whites do; therefore, calculating rates specific to these variables of interest is important. For example, if one wants to determine the breast cancer death rate for women for a specified time period, it would be calculated as follows:

$$\frac{\text{Number of women dying from breast cancer (1992)}}{\text{Number of women in the population midyear 1992}} \times k \text{ (e.g., 1,000)}$$

■ SOURCES OF DATA

Accurate measures of mortality and morbidity in occupational groups are essential for occupational health nurses to help plan prevention and health promotion and protection programs for workers; however, data are not always readily available. Even notifiable diseases may not always be reported, and for most chronic diseases such as hypertension, cancer, and coronary heart disease, no nationwide notification system exists. Yet there are many sources of data that the occupational health nurse may use, which provide prevalence estimates of health and illness indices in occupational settings. Examples are given in Table 5–8.

Census data are necessary for an accurate picture of the health status of the population as these data serve as denominator data for births and deaths. Vital statistics, for a variety of events, are collected by governmental entities and processed by the National Center for Health Statistics. Of major interest to health care providers are births and deaths in the United States, of which more than 99% are reported. Deaths are classified and recorded according to the International Classification of Diseases, thereby allowing for international comparisons. Epidemiologic studies are often based on mortality data.

The Centers for Disease Control and Prevention maintains a system for collecting various kinds of data. Examples include demographic, clinical, and laboratory data from state agencies on notifiable diseases such as AIDS, diphtheria, malaria, sexually transmitted diseases, tetanus, tuberculosis, many childhood infectious diseases, and other conditions that may have a preventable component.

Other sources for morbidity data that may be of interest to the occupational health nurse include hospital records, health records from private physicians, insurance records, disease registries, and health survey data such as the National Health and Nutrition Examination Survey (NHANES). The latter is a continuing

■ **TABLE 5–8**   Data Sources Useful in Occupational Health

Agency	Database	Purpose
CENSUS DATA		
Bureau of the Census/ CDC	Decennial Census	Total enumeration of the U.S. population by demographic characteristics, such as age, race, sex, marital status, education, and employment characteristics.
Bureau of the Census/ CDC	Current Population Survey	Annual household sample survey of the population for basic demographic variables.
CDC/Bureau of Labor Statistics (DOL)	Occupational Employment Statistics (1970, 1984, 1986)	Sample survey of all occupations and industries except active duty military to examine current and projected occupational demands to the year 2000.
VITAL RECORDS		
NCHS	Vital Statistics: Mortality	Underlying cause of death and demographic data for all deaths in the United States: state-specific data from death certificates such as age, sex, race, residence, place of death.
NCHS	National Death Index	Computerized index of death records from state vital statistics offices for research purposes.
NCHS/CDC	Vital Statistics: Fetal Mortality	Sample of registered U.S. fetal death certificates and information associated with the deaths obtained from mothers, physicians, and hospitals.
NCHS/CDC	Vital Statistics: Natality	Number of registered U.S. live births from birth certificates; includes age, race, education, marital status, and geographic area.
FOOD CONSUMPTION/CONTAMINATION		
FDA	Diet and Health Survey	National probability sample of households; measures public attitudes, knowledge, and practices about food and nutrition relative to chronic disease.
FDA	Pesticides, Industrial Chemicals, Toxic Elements	Pesticides, industrial chemicals, and toxic elements in samples of food.
FDA	Industrial Chemical Contaminants	Sample analyses of fish to determine the level of industrial chemical contaminants.
EPIDEMIOLOGY		
NCHS/CDC	National Health Interview Survey	Household interviews of a representative sample of the U.S. population; includes data on illnesses, injuries, chronic conditions, utilization of health resources, and demographic characteristics; occupational health supplement (1988).
NCHS/CDC	National Health Interview Supplement	Investigations on topics of concern such as child health, elderly disease prevention, health promotion, nutrition, dental health, epidemiology (cancer).

Table continued on following page

■ **TABLE 5–8** Data Sources Useful in Occupational Health *Continued*

Agency	Database	Purpose
EPIDEMIOLOGY *Continued*		
NCHS	National Health and Nutrition Examination Survey	National probability sample of the U.S. civilian population to determine prevalence of specific diseases and nutritional deficiencies based on physical exams, medical history, biochemical tests and dietary intake.
CDC	Behavioral Risk Factor Surveillance System	Prevalence of behavioral risk factors such as cigarettes, alcohol, and obesity, contributing to 10 leading causes of premature death and disability.
INFANT/MATERNAL		
CDC	Birth Defects Monitoring Program	Hospital discharge on birth defects by county among participating hospitals.
CDC	National Infant Mortality Surveillance (NIMS)	U.S. infant deaths from extracts of birth death records; includes birth weight, maternal age, race, and maternal risk factor.
NCHS	National Maternal and Infant Health Survey	National representative data on fetal loss, low birth weight, and infant death.
NCHS	National Hospital Discharge Survey	Sample of discharged U.S. hospital inpatients that contains diagnoses, surgical procedures, and characteristics of inpatients.
OCCUPATIONAL MORBIDITY/FATALITIES		
CDC	Industry-wide Studies Program	Results of industry-wide studies conducted to identify the occupational causes of disease in working populations from work-related exposure to toxic substances.
NIOSH/CDC	Surveillance Program	Data from OSHA, EPA, the National Occupational Survey (1974), and the Survey on National Occupational Exposure (1982) on occupational hazards; used to identify potential hazards in the workplace and related diseases, disability, and mortality.
Bureau of Labor Statistics	Annual Survey of Illness and Injury	National estimates of the number and incidence rates of occupational fatalities, nonfatal illness, and injuries.
NIOSH/CDC	National Occupational Health Survey of Mining	Assessment of the potential exposure of mine workers to chemical and physical agents.
NIOSH/CDC	Workers' Compensation Supplementary Data System	Occupational injury and illness data from state workers' compensation claims in 30 states compiled by the Bureau of Labor Statistics.
NIOSH/CDC	National Electronic Injury Surveillance System (NEISS)	Sample of U.S. hospitals with emergency rooms, which provides national estimates of the number and severity of injuries associated with occupations.
NIOSH	National Traumatic Occupational Fatality Database	Ongoing census through 1990 of any traumatic occupational injury fatality based on vital records.

■ **TABLE 5–8**   Data Sources Useful in Occupational Health *Continued*

Agency	Database	Purpose
NIOSH/CDC	Fatal Accident Circumstances and Epidemiology (FACE)	Data from fatal accidents to identify risk factors that influence fatal injuries for employees.
NIOSH	Sentinel Event Notification System for Occupational Risks (SENSOR)	Surveillance of selected occupational conditions.
USDOL	Dictionary of Occupational Titles	Description of job categories, work process by industrial codes.

Data from Baker, Supplement, 1989; and Gable, 1990.

National Center for Health Statistics survey, based on a sample of the population, that provides information about the health needs of the entire country. Components of the survey include physical examinations and laboratory tests and household interviews on health and nutrition status.

Occupational disease surveillance is an important measure in efforts to control and prevent work-related illness and injury; however, surveillance efforts in occupationally related diseases and injuries lag far behind those of infectious diseases. The Bureau of Labor Statistics reported an incidence of occupational illness and injury for 1984 of 8.0 cases and 63.4 lost workdays per 100 full-time workers (CDC, 1990b), which is most likely an underestimate. Reportable occupational illness and injury-related events vary by state; however, only seven states mandatorily require the reporting of "any occupational disease" (CDC, 1990b). Efforts to improve both the recognition of occupational illness and injury events and surveillance activities have been heightened through the establishment of the Sentinel Health Events-Occupational and the NIOSH-sponsored Sentinel Event Notification System for Occupational Risks (SENSOR), which is in place in several states and is designed to establish reporting mechanisms for certain occupational conditions selected by NIOSH, including carpal tunnel syndrome, lead poisoning, noise-induced hearing loss, occupational asthma, pesticide poisoning, and silicosis.

There are many commercially prepared directories for public health data sources as well as federal directories such as the Health and Human Services Data Inventory (Gable, 1990). Gable has prepared an excellent compendium on public health data sources and accessing information. In addition, the "Surveillance in Occupational Health and Safety" supplement (Baker, 1989) also provides a detailed description of these databases relevant to occupational health. The reader is referred to these sources for further information.

■ **EPIDEMIOLOGIC METHODS AND ANALYSIS**

Case reports often provide the first clues in the identification of new diseases or adverse effects of exposures which ultimately lead to analytical epidemiologic investigations. Case reports are commonly reported in the medical science journals and describe the experience of a single patient or group with a similar problem or diagnosis. For example, early case reports of *Pneumocystis carinii* pneumonia and Kaposi's sarcoma led the Centers for Disease Control & Prevention to initiate an epidemiologic surveillance program and design analytic studies to identify specific risk factors associated with the development of AIDS (CDC, 1987). The limitation of case reports is that they are based on the experience of one person; however, they do lead the way for further investigative studies.

Occupational epidemiology involves investigating the frequency of occurrence and causal factors for health effects that have nonoccupational as well as potential occupational etiologies. Lung cancer, for example, can be induced by occupational and nonoccupational exposures; in fact, in all industrialized countries the predominant risk factor for lung cancer is cigarette smoking, not occupational exposures. The practice of occupational epidemiology becomes increasingly complex when the diseases of interest are delayed effects of exposure that become manifest many years after first exposure (latency period), or when the health outcomes are subtle physiologic responses rather than overt diseases.

Once groups have been identified with a specific disease or problem through descriptive studies, analytic studies can be designed to determine associated risk factors and potential reasons for disease occurrence. For example, if a survey was conducted to elucidate respiratory complaints among workers in a certain department, further studies could be conducted to determine potential exposures that might contribute to the problem. Once such identification has been made, the next step is to determine why the rate is high (or low) in a particular group. Observations of differences in occurrence of disease between populations lead to the formulation of hypotheses (i.e., testable propositions that can be accepted or rejected through investigations). The results of these analytic (i.e., hypothesis-testing) studies generate ideas for additional descriptive studies as well as new hypotheses. This sequence of events may be schematized as a feedback system in an epidemiologic study cycle (Fig. 5–4).

Types of Designs

Four types of epidemiologic designs are commonly used to determine relationships between exposure and disease or health outcome events: cross-sectional

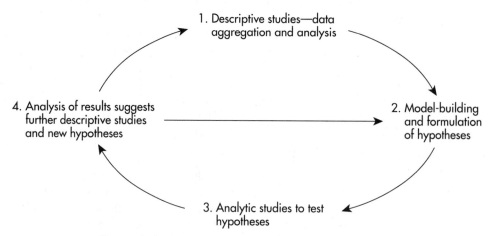

■ **Figure 5–4** Schema for an epidemiologic study cycle. (From Mausner, J & Kramer, S. Epidemiology: An introductory text. Philadelphia: W.B. Saunders, 1985.)

■ **TABLE 5–9**   Types of Epidemiologic Study Designs

Type of Design	Equivalent Name	Description
Cross-sectional	Prevalence study Correlational	A group of individuals is studied at a point in time for both the risk factor and the disease or event outcome.
Case-control	Retrospective	A group of individuals with the study disease and a group without the disease are compared for prior exposure to the study factor under investigation.
Prospective	Cohort Longitudinal	A group of individuals with a known exposure and a similar group without exposure are followed into the future and compared with respect to the development of disease or event outcome.
Historical cohort	Retrospective cohort Nonconcurrent cohort	A cohort of workers is enumerated from previous records and the cohort is traced to the present and sometimes future with analysis of disease rates.

studies, case-control studies, prospective studies, and historical prospective/cohort studies (Meininger, 1989). These designs are contrasted in Table 5–9.

Cross-sectional surveys, also called prevalence surveys, provide information about the frequency and characteristics of a disease, or the health attributes or events in certain groups or occupations at a point in time. For example, the National Health and Nutritional Examination Survey (as previously mentioned) is a cross-sectional survey, conducted by the National Center for Health Statistics, in which data in such areas as health conditions, physiologic measurements, and health utilization patterns are collected from a random sample of the population. Comparisons can then be made among groups (e.g., men and women) about certain attributes such as blood pressure, diet, lifestyle habits, and various diseases.

Another example is a cross-sectional study, conducted by Ciesielski et al. (1991), of occupational injuries among a random sample of 287 migrant farm workers in 22 migrant camps in eastern North Carolina through use of verbally administered questionnaires. Nearly 10% of respondents reported at least one occupational injury. Frequent obstacles to receiving adequate health care were reported by the farm workers, including lack of provision of transportation (legally required) by the employer, earlier return to work than advised by the health care provider, and fear of retribution. In addition, employers covered medical expenses for only 38% of the injured workers and compensated only 20% of the workers for lost time.

A study to investigate the relationship of smoking to work absenteeism may be measured in worker groups through use of a survey to determine employee smoking habits and through examination of work employment records of attendance. While a causal relationship cannot be drawn, this data obtained may provide information about the relative impact of smoking on absenteeism. Other examples could include employee attitudinal surveys about occupational health risks or other specific issues, or determining the most prevalent reasons for visits to the occupational health unit.

Three major analytical methods available are case-control, prospective, and historical-prospective studies. These are contrasted in Figure 5–5 (Rogers & Moreland, 1986). The purpose of these kinds of studies (case-control and prospective) is to employ specific statistical comparisons to determine potential

Retrospective Approach

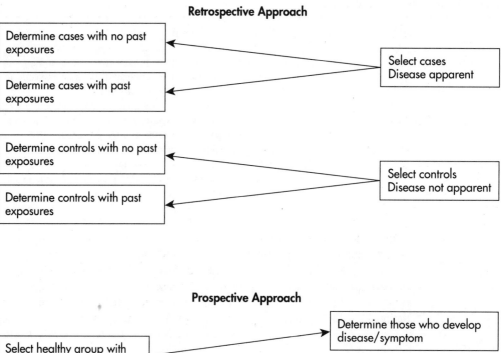

Prospective Approach

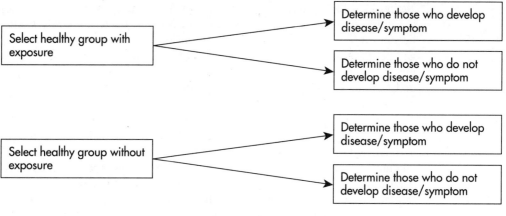

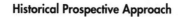

Historical Prospective Approach

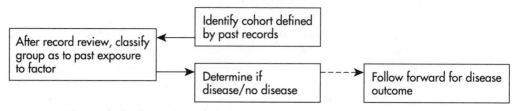

■ **Figure 5–5** Comparison of retrospective and prospective epidemiological studies.

causal relationships. Careful evaluation for the strength of the association of the health outcome with a particular risk factor, the consistency of the association, the time, sequence, any dose/response considerations, and concurrence with existing knowledge is necessary.

In a case-control study, sometimes called a retrospective study, individuals already diagnosed as having a disease (cases) are compared with individuals without the disease (controls) for the presence or absence of an antecedent risk factor, such as an exposure, which may have contributed to disease development. For example, to study the relationship between benzene exposure and aplastic anemia, a case-control study would compare a group of individuals with aplastic anemia compared to a control group of subjects without the diagnosis, and determine in each group if benzene exposure had occurred. Statistical determinations are then made by comparing cases and controls with respect to exposure versus nonexposure to the element or factor in their past experience, in this case, benzene. Selection of a representative sample of cases and controls is very important in order to avoid bias, which could lead to false conclusions; that is, cases should be representative of the cases and controls should be representative of the general population.

Another example is a case-control study by Selevan and colleagues (1985), who examined the relationship between fetal loss and occupational exposure to antineoplastic agents of nurses in Finland. Each nurse with a fetal loss was matched with three nurses who gave birth. Data on health and exposure were obtained from study participants through mailed questionnaires. The study found that women who experienced fetal loss were more than twice as likely to have had occupational exposures to antineoplastic drugs during the first trimester as were women who gave birth (odds ratio = 2.30).

In contrast, a prospective or cohort study starts with a group of people (cohort) considered to be free of disease or health problems but who vary in exposure to a suspected element or factor (i.e., those with differing degrees of exposure and those with no exposure). The cohort is monitored forward in time to determine differences in the rate at which disease develops in relation to the exposure or nonexposure to the suspected agent (Mausner & Kramer, 1985). Evidence for causal relationships can be obtained because there is a temporal relationship between presumed cause and outcome. For example, data from the classic study by Doll and Hill (1956) on the mortality experience of British physicians are shown in Table 5–10. Annual death rates from lung cancer and coronary heart

■ **TABLE 5–10**   Relative Risk of Mortality from Lung Cancer and Coronary Heart Disease for Heavy Smokers and Nonsmokers among British Physicians

	Annual Death Rates per 100,000 Persons	
EXPOSURE CATEGORY	Lung Cancer	Coronary Heart Disease
Heavy smokers	166	599
Nonsmokers	7	422
MEASURE OF EXCESS RISK		
Relative risk	$\dfrac{166}{7} = 23.7$	$\dfrac{599}{422} = 1.4$

From Doll, R & Hill, AB. British Medical Journal, 2:1071-1072, 1956.

disease for heavy smokers and nonsmokers along with relative risk measures are presented. A very high relative risk (23.7) for heavy smokers compared to nonsmokers indicates a strong association between heavy smoking and lung cancer. The relative risk (1.4) for coronary heart disease is much smaller, which suggests that other attributes such as diet or stress may be operating and require alteration.

A *historical cohort* identifies both exposed and unexposed cohorts through previously existing records that permit correct classification of the exposure status of individuals. Study subjects then are traced forward to the present and followed into the future to determine if they have or have not developed the disease or outcome of interest (Mausner & Kramer, 1985). Statistical calculations are made to determine an association between the risk of disease among those with or without exposure.

Confounding Variables

In the conduct of any causally associated study, it is important to ascertain and consider how to control for "confounding variables," that is, factors known to be associated with the exposure and disease or outcome of interest. For example, if one wants to investigate the relationship between a chemical agent exposure and birth outcomes, factors such as age, parity, cigarette smoking, and drug use would need to be determined and controlled. This can be accomplished in the design stage through restricting participation of study subjects with certain characteristics (e.g., eliminating smokers) or matching cases and controls so they are similar with respect to specific attributes (e.g., matching a case with a control subject on age, parity, and/or smoking status). Another approach to handling confounding bias is in the analysis stage through statistical techniques such as stratification on variables or other techniques such as regression analysis that can adjust for the confounding factors simultaneously (Breslow & Day, 1982). Stratification involves the analysis of data by strata, such as gender, so as to eliminate the potential bias associated with one's sex status. If, for example, gender were a potential confounder, data would be evaluated for men and women separately. Similar strata-specific evaluations can be calculated for other potential confounding variables such as race, age, education, smoking status, and parity.

Epidemiologic Analysis

Once data are derived, they must be expressed as a risk estimate in order to evaluate the effects of the exposure. Data are usually presented in a two-by-two table with columns and rows indicating the presence or absence of the disease or exposure (Fig. 5–6). Four cells are created (a,b,c,d) which represent the following:

a = the number of individuals exposed who have disease
b = the number of individuals exposed who do not have disease
c = the number of individuals unexposed who have disease
d = the number of individuals unexposed who do not have disease

The margins of the table represent the totals in each column and row:

a + b = the total number of individuals exposed
c + d = the total number of individuals unexposed

Disease

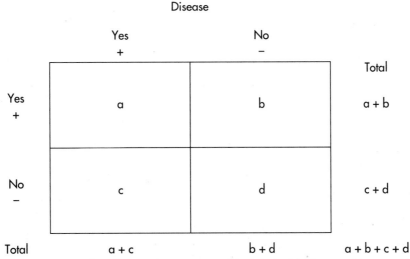

■ **Figure 5–6**   Presentation format for epidemiologic data for use with prospective or case-control designs.

a + c = the total number of individuals with disease
b + d = the total number of individuals without disease

The total sample size is represented by the sum of all four cells (a + b + c + d).

Two major types of risk estimates are the relative risk for cohort studies and the odds ratio (OR) for case-control studies, which is an estimate of the relative risk. The relative risk, also called the rate ratio, provides an estimate of the likelihood of developing the disease in the exposed group relative to the unexposed group (i.e., the ratio of the rate in the exposed to the unexposed group) and is a measure of the strength of the association between exposure and disease (Hennekens & Buring, 1977). Relative risk is calculated as:

$$\frac{\text{Disease rate in the exposed}}{\text{Disease rate in the unexposed}}$$

or

$$(a/[a + b])/(c/[c + d])$$

The data presented in Table 5–10 demonstrate the relative risk for cigarette smokers in developing lung cancer and coronary heart disease.

A relative risk of 1.0 indicates that the disease incidence among the exposed and nonexposed is the same; that is, no association exists between the exposure and disease. A value greater than 1.0 equals an increased risk, whereas a value less than 1.0 indicates a decreased risk among those exposed.

In case-control studies, incidence rates cannot be derived directly because participants are selected on the basis of disease status and the total population of those exposed/unexposed and diseased/nondiseased are unknown. Therefore, a relative risk of disease associated with exposure cannot be calculated. However, an estimate of the relative risk, known as the OR (i.e., the odds of having the disease with and without exposure) is a useful measure. From Figure 5–6 it can

■ **TABLE 5–11**   Odds Ratio (OR) from a Case-control Study of Cigarette Smoking and Lung Cancer

	Lung Cancer Cases	**Controls**	**Total**
Smokers	75(a)	425(b)	500
Nonsmokers	25(c)	900(d)	925
	100	1,325	1,425

$$OR = \frac{ad}{bc} \quad = \quad \frac{(75)(900)}{(425)(25)} = 6.4$$

be seen that $a/(a + b)$ is representative of the disease rate in the exposed group, whereas $c/(c + d)$ represents disease in the unexposed group. Since we assume that "a" is a small portion of "a + b" and "c" a small portion of "c + d," then the odds ratio becomes ($[a/b]/[c/d]$) or $(ad)/(bc)$, which yields an approximation or estimate of the relative risk. Table 5–11 presents hypothetical data from a case-control study relating cigarette smoking to lung cancer showing the OR. Since the OR is an estimate of the relative risk, one can conclude that the data show an increased risk of lung cancer in smokers versus nonsmokers.

■ SUMMARY

This chapter has provided a discussion of selected concepts, principles, and methodologies in epidemiology including agent-host-environmental relationship, descriptive and analytical methods, and approaches to measurement, design, and causal inferences. However, more in-depth information is provided through other sources (see references). The occupational health nurse will find this information useful in understanding the dynamic processes and interrelationships between health, illness, and injury events in worker populations.

Using epidemiologic tools the occupational health nurse will be able to more effectively identify workers at risk of exposure and risk factors that contribute to disease development. Collaborative efforts can then be developed to design preventive and control strategies to minimize risk conditions.

References

Baker, E (Ed.). Surveillance in occupational health and safety. American Journal of Public Health, *79:* Supplement, 1989.

Benenson, AS (Ed.). Control of communicable diseases in man, 15th Ed. American Public Health Association, 1990.

Bigos, SJ, Spangler, DM, Martin, NA, Zeh, J, Fisher, I, & Nachemson, A. Back injuries in industry: A retrospective study/employee related factors. *Spine, 11:* 252–256, 1986.

Blackburn, H. Trends and determinants of CHD mortality: Changes in risk factors and their effects. International Journal of Epidemiology *18*(suppl 1): S210–S215, 1989.

Breslow, NE. The variance of the Mantel-Haenszel estimator. Biometrics, *38*: 943–952, 1982.

Bureau of Labor Statistics. Annual survey of occupational injuries and illnesses. Washington, DC: Department of Labor, 1988.

Case, RAM, Hosker, ME, McDonald, DB, & Pearson, JT. Tumors of the urinary bladder in workmen engaged in the manufacture and use of certain dyestuff intermediates in the British chemical industry. British Journal of Industrial Medicine, *11:* 75–104, 1954.

Cato, C, Olson, D, & Studer, M. Incidence, prevalence, and variables associated with low back pain in staff nurses. AAOHN Journal, *37:* 321–328, 1989.

Centers for Disease Control. Human immunodeficiency virus infection in the United States: A review of current knowledge. Morbidity and Mortality Weekly Report, *36* (suppl): 1–48, 1987.

Centers for Disease Control. Mandatory reporting of infectious diseases by clinicians and mandatory reporting of occupational diseases by clinicians. Morbidity and Mortality Weekly Report, *39:* 19–28, June 22, 1990a.

Centers for Disease Control. Protection against viral hepatitis. Morbidity and Mortality Weekly Report, *39:* 1–26, February 9, 1990b.

Checkoway, H, Pearce, N, & Crawford-Brown, D. Research methods in occupational epidemiology. New York: Oxford University Press, 1989.

Ciesielski, S, Hall, SP, & Sweeney, M. Occupational injuries among North Carolina migrant farmworkers. American Journal of Public Health, *81:* 926–928, 1991.

Cronin-Stubbs, D & Rooks, C. Stress, social support and burnout of critical care nurses: Results of research. Heart and Lung, *14:* 31–39, 1985.

Doll, R & Hill, AB. Mortality in relation to smoking: Ten years' observations of British doctors. British Medical Journal, *1*(5395): 1399–1410, 1964.

Doll, R & Hill, AB. Lung cancer and other causes of death in relation to smoking. British Medical Journal, *2:* 1071–1072, 1956.

Dorian, B & Taylor, CB. Stress factors in the development of coronary artery disease. Journal of Occupational Medicine, *26:* 747–756, 1984.

Elofsson, S-A. Exposure to organic solvents. Scandinavian Journal of Work and Environmental Health, *6:* 239–273, 1980.

Feinleib, M. Risk assessment, environmental factors and coronary heart disease. Journal of the American College of Toxicology, *2:* 91–104, 1983.

Feldman, R, Ricks, N, & Baker, E. Neuropsychological effects of industrial toxins: A review. American Journal of Industrial Medicine, *1:* 211, 1980.

Fox, JP & Hall, CE. Epidemiology: Man and disease. New York: Macmillan, 1970.

Gable, C. A compendium of public health data sources. American Journal of Epidemiology, *131:* 381–394, 1990.

Garfinkel, L & Silverberg, E. Lung cancer and smoking trends in the United States over the past 25 years. CA-A Cancer Journal for Clinicians, *41:* 137–145, 1991.

Goldwater, LJ, Rosso, AJ, & Kleinfeld, M. Bladder tumors in a cool tar dye plant. Archives of Environmental Health, *11:* 814–817, 1965.

Gwatkin, DR & Brandel, SK. Life expectancy and population growth in the Third World. Scientific American, *246:* 62, 1982.

Harper, A. The health of populations. New York: Springer Publishing, 1986.

Hemminki, K, Kyronen, P, & Lindbohm, M. Spontaneous abortions and malformations in the offspring of nurses exposed to anaesthetic gases, cytostatic drugs, and other potential hazards in hospitals, based on registered information of outcome. Journal of Epidemiology and Community Health, *39:* 141–147, 1985.

Hennekens, CH & Buring, JE. Epidemiology in medicine. Boston: Little, Brown & Company, 1987.

Hunter, D. Diseases of occupations. London: Hodder & Stoughton, 1978.

Kelsey, J & Gammon, M. The epidemiology of breast cancer. CA-A Cancer Journal for Clinicians, *41:* 146–165, 1991.

Leon, AS, Connett, J, Jacobs, DR Jr, Rauramaa, R. Leisure time physical activity levels and risk of coronary heart disease and death: The Multiple Risk Factor Intervention Trial. Journal of the American Medical Association, *258:* 2388–2395, 1987.

Leon, GR, Finn, SE, Murray, D, & Bailey, JM. Inability to predict cardiovascular disease from hostility scores of MMPI items related to type A behavior. Journal of Consulting Clinical Psychologists, *56:* 597–600, 1988.

Lewis, R. Metals. In Occupational Medicine, J. LaDou, Ed. Norwalk, CT: Appleton & Lange, pp. 297–326, 1990.

Levy, B & Wegman, D. Occupational health: Recognizing and preventing work-related disease. Boston: Little, Brown & Company, 1988.

Lilienfeld, A & Lilienfeld, D. Foundations of epidemiology. New York: Oxford University Press, 1980.

Lorenz, E. Radioactivity and lung cancer: A critical review of lung cancer in miners of Schneeberg and Joachimisthal. Journal of the National Cancer Institute, *5:* 1–5, 1944.

MacMahon, B & Pugh, TF. Epidemiologic principles and methods. Boston: Little, Brown & Company, 1970.

Mausner, J & Kramer, S. Epidemiology: An introductory text. Philadelphia: W.B. Saunders, 1985.

Meininger, J. Epidemiologic designs. In Brink & Woods, Advanced design in nursing research. Newbury Park: Sage, 1989.

Monk, TH. Shiftworkers performance. Occupational Medicine: State of the Art Reviews, *5*(2): 183–198, 1990.

National Center for Health Statistics. Annual Report of Final Mortality Statistics, 1990. Monthly Vital Statistics Report, *41*(7): 1–52, 1993.

National Center for Health Statistics. Annual summary of births, marriages, divorces, and deaths: United States, 1990. Monthly Vital deaths: United States, 1990. Monthly Vital Statistics Report, *39*(13): 1–28, August 28, 1991.

National Center for Health Statistics. Vital statistics of the U.S., Pub. No. 85–1102, Washington, DC, 1985.

National Coalition for Agricultural Safety and Health. A report to the Nation: Agriculture at risk. Iowa City: The University of Iowa, 1989.

National Research Council. Diet and health: Implications for reducing chronic disease risk. Report of the Committee on Diet and Health, Food and Nutrition Board. Washington, DC: National Academy Press, 1989.

Occupational Safety and Health Administration. Occupational noise exposure: Hearing conservation final amendment. Federal Register, *48:* March 8, 9738–9785, 1983.

Peller, S. Lung cancer among miners in Joachmisthal. Human Biology, *11:* 130–143, 1939.

Pirchan, A & Sikl, H. Cancer of the lung of miners. American Journal of Cancer, *15:* 681–722, 1932.

The Pooling Project Research Group: Relationship of blood pressure, serum cholesterol, smoking habits, relative weight and ECG abnormalities to incidence of major coronary events: Final report of the Pooling Project. Journal of Chronic Diseases, *31:* 201–306, 1978.

Pott, P. Chirurgical observations. London: Hawes, Clark & Collins, 1775.

Roels, H, Lauwerys, R, Buchet, J. Health significance of cadmium-induced renal dysfunction: A five-year follow-up. British Journal of Industrial Medicine, *46:* 755–764, 1989.

Rogers, B & Moreland, R. Principles of epidemiology in occupational health nursing. Princeton, NJ: Continuing Professional Education Center, 2(22): 1–7, 1986.

Selevan, S, Lindbohm, M, Hornung, R, & Hemminki, K. A study of occupational exposure to antineoplastic drugs and fetal loss in nurses. New England Journal of Medicine, *313:* 1173–1178, 1985.

Selikoff, IJ, Churg, J, & Hammond, EC. Asbestos exposure and neoplasia. Journal of the American Medical Association, *188:* 22–26, 1964.

Selikoff, IJ, Hammond, EC, & Seidman, H. Mortality experience of insulation workers in the U.S. and Canada. Annals of the New York Academy of Sciences, *330:* 91–116, 1979.

Shekelle, RB, Gale, M, Ostfeld, AM, & Paul, O. Hostility, risk of coronary heart disease,

and mortality. Psychosomatic Medicine *45:* 109–114, 1983.

Slattery, ML, Jacobs, DR Jr, & Nichaman, MZ. Leisure time physical activity and coronary heart disease death: The U.S. Railroad Study. Circulation, *79:* 304–311, 1989.

Stern, F & Steenland, K. Heart disease mortality among workers exposed to carbon monoxide in New York City. In Case Studies in Occupational Epidemiology, K. Steenland, Ed., New York: Oxford University Press, 21–34, 1993.

Thomas, DB. Cancer. In Public Health and Preventive Medicine, J. Last & R. Wallace, Eds. Norwalk, CT: Appleton & Lange, pp. 811–826, 1992.

Thun, M. Kidney dysfunction in cadmium workers. In Case Studies in Occupational Epidemiology, K. Steenland, Ed. New York: Oxford University Press, 21–34, 1993.

Tyler, CW, & Last, JM. Epidemiology. In Public Health and Preventive Medicine, J. Last & R. Wallace, Eds. Norwalk, CT: Appleton & Lange, 11–40, 1992.

U.S. Bureau of the Census, Statistical Abstracts of the United States: 1983, Washington, DC, 1984.

U.S. Department of Health and Human Services. Prevention 89/90: Federal programs and progress. Washington, DC: U.S. Government Printing Office, 1990a.

U.S. Department of Health and Human Services. Healthy People 2000. Washington, DC: Government Printing Office, 1990b.

Waldron, HA. A brief history of scrotal cancer. British Journal of Industrial Medicine, *40:* 390–401, 1983.

Wendell, RG, Hoegg, UR, & Zavon, MR. Benzidine: A bladder carcinogen. Journal of Urology, *111:* 607–610, 1974.

Wenzel, P. Control of communicable disease. In J. Last & R. Wallace, Eds. Public Health and Preventive Medicine (ed. 13). Norwalk, CT: Appleton & Lange, pp. 57–60, 1992.

Whorton, M & Foliart, D. Mutagenicity, carcinogenicity and reproductive effects of DBCP. Mutation Research, *123:* 13–30, 1983.

Wilhelmsen, L. Coronary heart disease: epidemiology of smoking and intervention studies of smoking. American Heart Journal, *115:* 242–249, 1988.

World Health Organization. Early detection of occupational diseases. Geneva: Author, pp. 85–90, 1986.

Zenz, C. Occupational medicine. Chicago: Yearbook Medical Publishers, pp. 463–464, 1993.

6

INTERDISCIPLINARY KNOWLEDGE IN OCCUPATIONAL HEALTH NURSING PRACTICE

Monitoring workplace hazards is a complex process that requires the knowledge and skills of multidisciplines. Thus, the occupational health nurse will find it essential to collaborate with other health and science professionals to better understand the effects of work and workplace exposures on human health. An understanding of the principles underlying the fields of industrial hygiene, toxicology, safety, and ergonomics and nursing's collaborative and interdependent relationship with medicine adds to the knowledge base in occupational health nursing and will serve to foster increased collaboration among professional disciplines. This chapter will focus on interdisciplinary fields of knowledge fundamental to occupational health nursing practice, which will enhance the nurse's knowledge of workplace hazards, mechanisms of exposures, and methods to control or minimize associated risks.

■ INDUSTRIAL HYGIENE

Because of the nature and complexity of hazards in the work environment, the occupational health nurse must work closely with many other health care professionals such as physicians, industrial hygienists, safety specialists, and ergonomists who are familiar with workplace exposures and health effects, in order to develop an effective risk management program. By definition, specific skills directed toward the recognition, evaluation, and control of workplace hazards fall within the discipline of industrial hygiene (Kayafas, 1989; Smith, 1988; Verma & Verrall, 1985). However, occupational health nurses and other members of the occupational health and safety team play an integral role in identifying and managing workplace exposures and hazards. Further, depending on the company size and scope and nature of the workplace hazards, an industrial hygienist may or may not be employed by the company. Thus, the occupational health nurse may play a larger role in the identification and management of workplace hazards and be able to secure external industrial hygiene consultation. Therefore, the nurse needs to be familiar with all aspects of the work and work environment in order to accurately assess workplace hazards and/or provide data needed for effective consultation.

As a result of exposure to specific agents, workplace hazards can be potentiated and categorized as biological/infectious, chemical, environmental/mechanical, physical, or psychosocial and are described below.

1. **Biological/infectious hazards:** infectious/biological agents, such as bacteria, viruses, fungi, or parasites, which may be transmitted via contact with infected patients or contaminated body secretions/fluids to other individuals.
2. **Chemical hazards:** various forms of chemicals, including medications, solutions, gases, vapors, aerosols, and particulate matter that are potentially toxic or irritating to the body system.
3. **Environmental/mechanical hazards:** factors encountered in the work environment that cause or potentiate accidents, injuries, strain, or discomfort (e.g., unsafe/inadequate equipment or lifting devices, slippery floors, work station deficiencies).
4. **Physical hazards:** agents within the work environment, such as radiation, electricity, extreme temperatures, and noise that can cause tissue trauma.
5. **Psychosocial hazards:** factors and situations encountered or associated with one's job or work environment that create or potentiate stress, emotional strain, and/or interpersonal problems.

Industrial hygiene is the science of protecting human health through control of the work environment. Industrial hygienists are primarily concerned with biological, chemical, and physical agent hazards (Verma & Verrall, 1985). The American Industrial Hygiene Association (AIHA) formed in 1939 has defined industrial hygiene as that science and art devoted to the recognition, evaluation, and control of those environmental factors or stresses, arising in or from the workplace, which may cause sickness, impaired health and well-being, or significant discomfort and inefficiency among workers or among the citizens of the community (AIHA, 1959; Horstman, 1992). Within the context of this definition, the AIHA further specifies that the industrial hygienist works (1) to recognize the environmental factors and stresses associated with work and work operations and to understand their effect on man and his well-being; (2) to evaluate, on the basis of experience and with the aid of quantitative measurement techniques, the magnitude of these stresses in terms of the ability to impair man's health and well-being; and (3) to prescribe methods to eliminate, control, or reduce such stresses when necessary to alleviate their effects. Increasingly, the focus of hazard recognition is placed on the anticipation of occurrence of hazards early in the development of an industrial process in order to redesign or alter a process prior to implementation (Horstman, 1992). The importance of collaboration among professionals, including the occupational health nurse, safety specialist, physician, and management, in this process is essential to securing a safe and healthful work environment.

Hazard Recognition

The process of hazard recognition and identification involves reviewing job classifications and determining potential hazards, reviewing background and toxicologic information on processes and associated hazards, visiting the relevant work unit to observe work processes, practices, and control measures, formulating plans to determine the exposure levels through ambient/environment sampling, and evaluating worker complaints related to workplace exposures (Smith, 1988). Use of an industrial hygiene survey checklist as shown in Table 6–1 may aid in the recognition process.

Specific exposures can be identified and evaluated related to various steps involved in the work processes. The goal is to discover potential illness-producing processes and operations, record their nature, and determine approaches necessary to deal with them effectively and efficiently (Kayafas, 1989). Examples of some common work processes and related hazards are shown in Table 6–2. In addition, a full-scale worksite assessment and walk-through survey, as described in detail in Chapter 9, may be in order.

It is important to determine if all hazardous chemicals are identified, list catalogued, and if the inventory is periodically updated. One of the major tools that can be utilized to aid in the initial identification of chemical hazardous materials is the Material Safety Data Sheet (MSDS). The MSDS is a document prepared by the manufacturer that describes the physical and chemical properties of products, their physical and health-related hazards, and precautions for safe handling and use. All facilities are required by law to have an MSDS for each hazardous chemical that is used in the facility (U.S. Dept. Agriculture, 1987). While the MSDS may provide valuable information about the toxicities and health effects of material substances, it is important to note that they may be out of date or incomplete (Levy & Wegman, 1988). Thus, other sources of information should also be utilized. MSDSs may appear in different formats; however, the OSHA Hazard Communication Standard (29CFR 1910-1200 [g]) requires that certain information be supplied (Table 6–3). Appendixes 6–1 and 6–2 are examples of MSDS.

Hazard Evaluation

Evaluation of health hazards at the worksite follows recognition. Exposure measurements are intended to evaluate the dose delivered to the worker. In the evaluation process, several important questions should be considered:

1. **What are the potential or actual agents/exposures?** Determine what categories of agents or factors are present at the worksite with the potential to cause illness/injury (i.e., biological, chemical, ergonomic/environmental/mechanical, physical, psychosocial) that require evaluation.
2. **Where and when does the exposure occur?** Determine the location of the exposure and the degree or magnitude of exposure associated with a particular work process, work area or department, shiftwork, or seasonal variation.
3. **Which workers are exposed and how does exposure occur?** Identify not only those workers involved with the work processes under investigation but also determine if other workers in close proximity may also be exposed. Determine all routes of exposure (e.g., ingestion, inhalation, skin contact) and compliance with work practice and safety standards.
4. **What is the evidence of exposure?** Determine if there are obvious signs of hazards or exposures such as dusts, smoke, broken machinery, and slippery floors or if previous air sampling or other industrial hygiene

■ **TABLE 6–1**   Worksite Walk-Through Survey Checklist

1. Determine purpose of the survey:
- Comprehensive survey?
- Evaluation of exposures of limited group of workers to specific agents?
- Determination of compliance with specific recognized standards?
- Evaluation of effectiveness of engineering controls?
- Response to specific complaint?

2. Become familiar with worksite operations:
- Obtain and study process flow sheets and site layout.
- Obtain a list of job classifications and the agents/environmental stresses to which workers are potentially exposed.
- Compile an inventory of raw materials, intermediates, by-products, and products.
- Review relevant toxicologic information.
- Observe the activities associated with each job classification.
- Review the status of workers' health.
- Observe and review administrative and engineering control measures used.
- Review reports of previous studies.
- Determine the potential health hazards (e.g., chemical, physical) associated with worksite operations.
- Review adequacy of labeling and warning.

3. Prepare for the walk-through:
Although each worksite has different operations, equipment, and physical layouts, certain items are quite common to many and deserve special mention. The following types of items should generally be considered in making an inspection:
- Atmospheric conditions: dusts, gases, fumes, vapors, illumination.
- Pressurized equipment: boilers, pots, tanks, piping, hosing.
- Containers: all objects for storage of materials, such as scrap bins, disposal receptacles, barrels, carboys, gas cylinders, solvent cans.
- Hazardous supplies and materials: flammables, explosives, gases, acids, caustics, toxic chemicals.
- Buildings and structures: windows, doors, aisles, floors, stairs, roofs, walls.
- Electrical conductors and apparatus: wires, cables, switches, controls, transformers, lamps, batteries, fuses.
- Fire fighting equipment: extinguishers, hoses, hydrants, sprinkler systems, alarms.
- Machinery and parts thereof: power equipment that processes, machines, or modifies materials (e.g., grinders, forging machines, power presses, drilling machines, shapers, cutters, lathes).
- Material-handling equipment: conveyors, cranes, hoists, lifts.
- Hand tools: items such as bars, sledges, wrenches, hammers, as well as power tools.
- Structural openings: shafts, sumps, pits, floor openings, trenches.
- Transportation equipment: automobiles, trucks, railroad equipment, lift trucks.
- Personal protective clothing and equipment: items such as goggles, gloves, aprons, leggings.

4. Inspection
- Determine which agents (e.g., chemical, physical) are to be evaluated, if any.
- Arrange for appropriate personnel/professional to conduct measurements.
- Obtain personal protective equipment as required (hard hat, safety glasses, goggles, hearing protection, respiratory protection, safety shoes, coveralls, gloves).
- Sample each element referred.
- Observe fire exits: clear marking, access, obstruction.
- Inspect storage areas: clearance, obstruction, clutter, working signs, lifting.
- Observe all machinery for guarding, tagging, lockout.
- Observe all electrical equipment for proper grounding, loose wires, insulation.
- Observe housekeeping procedures and outcomes: cleanliness, safety, clutter, labeling.

■ **TABLE 6–2**   Some Common Work Processes and Related Hazards

Work Processes	Common Hazard
Abrasive blasting	Silica and metal dust
Cosmetology	Chemical exposures
	Repetitive bending, standing
Farming	Pesticide exposure
	Heat exposure
	Heavy lifting
	Hazardous equipment
Grinding, polishing, and buffing	Inhalation of toxic dusts from metals and abrasives
Painting	Inhalation of solvents as mists, vapors, toxic substances
Meat wrapping	Lifting, standing, repetitive motion, fume exposure from wrap
Welding	Inhalation of metal fumes, toxic gases, materials

surveys have been conducted and their findings. Evaluate if worker health-related complaints such as skin rash, cough, dyspnea, headaches, dizziness, anorexia, fatigue, eye irritation, or numbness/tingling of extremities are exposure related and if the complaints resolve in the absence of exposure. Conduct biological and environmental sampling and analyze and interpret results in terms of existing health standards or known effects.

5. **What control measures are present, available, and effective?** Assess if engineering controls (e.g., ventilation systems) are appropriate, operable, and effective; if appropriate personal protective equipment is available and utilized; and if hygiene and appropriate work practice measures are observed.

■ **TABLE 6–3**   OSHA Required Information for Material Safety Data Sheets

- Identity of the material as listed on the label.
- Chemical and common names of all ingredients which have been determined to be health hazards.
- Physical and chemical characteristics of the hazardous chemical.
- Physical hazards of the hazardous chemical (i.e., fire, explosion, reactivity).
- Health hazards of the hazardous chemical including signs/symptoms of exposure, and health conditions generally recognized as being aggravated by the exposure.
- Primary routes of entry.
- OSHA permissible exposure limit, ACGIH threshold limit value and any other applicable exposure limits.
- Carcinogenic status (confirmed or potential) of the hazardous chemical.
- Precautions for safe handling including measures taken during equipment repair and procedures for clean-up of spills/leaks.
- Applicable control measures (i.e., engineering, work practice, protective equipment).
- Emergency and first-aid procedures.
- Date of preparation (or last change) of the MSDS.
- Name, address, and telephone number of the chemical manufacturer, importer, employer, or other parties responsible for MSDS preparation and distribution.

Hazard evaluation must take into account the changing nature of the work environment, such as operations, processes, materials, production schedules, routes of exposure, and control measures (Travers, 1986). Decisions as to whether a hazard exists are based on three sources of information (Smith, 1988): (1) scientific literature and various exposure limit guides such as the threshold limit values (TLVs), a set of consensus standards about exposures established, revised and published yearly by the American Conference of Governmental Industrial Hygienists (ACGIH); (2) legal requirements of federal, state, and local statutes and regulations; and (3) evaluative results of the exposed worker based on examinations by qualified health care professionals.

Threshold Limit

The concept of threshold limit is important to understand in an exposure-effect relationship. The concept implies that there is a threshold limit of "effect" (and conversely "no effect") wherein a certain level or dose of exposure will produce a measurable effect in a target organ system. While it is important to emphasize that worker exposures should be held to the lowest minimum possible, in some cases workers may be exposed to ambient levels greater than zero. Thus, in the workplace threshold limit values (TLVs) are used by industrial hygienists and others trained in the science as a guide to the maximum tolerable exposure limit (Fowler, 1990). This assumes an eight-hour work day, five days per week. Exposing employees to amounts above the TLVs is believed to be potentially harmful (Kayafas, 1989; Verma & Verrall, 1985).

It is important to note that the TLVs are based on animal toxicity data and limited epidemiologic studies. Animal experiments have shortcomings in extrapolating data to the human workforce (Danse, 1991), as the dose, routes of exposure, and toxicokinetics may differ considerably in humans. In addition, they do not necessarily address the sensitive populations in the workforce, those with prior exposure or preexisting disease, or exposures from other sources such as second jobs, hobbies, or home exposures. The American Conference of Governmental Industrial Hygienists (ACGIH) expresses TLVs in three ways:

1. **Threshold limit value–time weighted average (TLV–TWA):** the time-weighted average concentrations for a normal eight-hour workday and a 40-hour workweek, to which nearly all workers may be repeatedly exposed, day after day, without adverse effects.

2. **Threshold limit value–short term exposure limit (TLV–STEL):** the concentration to which workers can be exposed continuously for a short period of time without suffering from (a) irritation, (b) chronic or irreversible tissue change, or (c) narcosis of sufficient degree to increase the likelihood of accidental injury, impair self-rescue, or materially reduce work efficiency, and provided that the daily TLV-TWA also is not exceeded.

A STEL (short term exposure limit) is defined as a 15-minute time-weighted average (TWA) exposure that should not be exceeded at any time during a workday even if the TWA is within the TLV. Exposures at the STEL should not be longer than 15 minutes and should not be repeated more than four times per day. There should be at least 60 minutes between successive exposures at the STEL. An averaging period other than 15 minutes may be recommended when this is warranted by observed biological effects.

3. **Threshold limit value–ceiling (TLV–C):** the concentration that should not be exceeded even instantaneously.

The Occupational Safety and Health Administration has adopted permissible exposure limits (PELs) for chemical exposure, most of which are based directly on the TLV list of the ACGIH in effect in 1968 (USDHHS-NIOSH, 1990). Since that time, the TLVs have been updated yearly but most PELs have not changed (Silverstein, 1988). Thus, TLVs may be more restrictive than PELs. The National Institute for Occupational Safety and Health (NIOSH) has published recommended exposure limits (RELs) that are TWA concentrations for up to a 10-hour workday during a 40-hour workweek (USDHHS-NIOSH, 1990). The occupational health nurse should be familiar with these terms and their meaning; however, evaluation of results should be done by one trained in industrial hygiene. A listing of the ACGIH-TLVs may be found in the *Threshold Limit Values and Biological Exposure Indices* (ACGIH, 1990). OSHA-PELs and NIOSH-RELs are found in the *NIOSH Pocket Guide to Chemical Hazards* (USDHHS, NIOSH, 1990).

Sampling Methods and Techniques

Quantifying exposures is usually done by the industrial hygienist through sampling methods and devices. There are two major approaches to air sampling: personal breathing zone sampling and area sampling. Personal breathing zone sampling is usually preferred and considered more accurate as exposures are measured at the worker entry point and measurement devices move with the worker. Area sampling, however, may be needed to measure source emissions, background concentrations, or to measure several worksite areas simultaneously to determine the effectiveness of engineering controls (Plog, 1989). Fowler (1990) describes several types of sampling procedures. Gas and vapor sampling may be accomplished by any of five methods:

1. Active collection, by drawing a measured volume of air through a collection system that is then analyzed
2. Passive collection, with a dosimeter that attracts gas or vapor molecules by diffusion from the atmosphere
3. Collection in a color-sensitive medium in a device in which color change is proportionate to concentration of the contaminant and which can be read directly
4. Collection in an evacuated container used to carry a sample of air to a convenient site for analysis
5. Collection in direct-reading instruments sensitive to one or several atmospheric gases or vapors

Airborne particulate matter is usually measured with filters, the choice of which is dependent on the material of interest.

When skin contact is the route of exposure, as is the case with pesticide exposure, cloth patches or wipe sampling of the exposed skin area can be used to determine the amount of contamination. Wipe sampling is also used to evaluate surface contamination and for identifying contaminated areas when a toxic spill has occurred.

Evaluation of physical agents, such as noise, may be measured with sound level meters that give a source level decibel readout, or noise dosimeters that involve placing a small microphone close to the worker's ear to record noise exposure. The latter approach is preferred as it gives a more accurate and specific measure of individual exposure.

Once sampling techniques have been selected, a sampling strategy will need to be developed in order to determine exposure routes and variations and time-weighted exposures. Exposure measurements are then compared with existing standards and guides to determine if exposures meet acceptable levels. Interpretation of results is critical to the evaluation process and should be a collaborative effort between the industrial hygienist, the occupational health nurse, and physician in order to relate the exposure to the health effect.

Control Measures

Once the hazard has been identified and evaluated, control measures, which usually require the expertise of the industrial hygienist, will need to be instituted to correct the problem. Hazard reduction can be achieved by a variety of individual methods or a combination of methods. Jones et al. (1990) recommend the following practices:

- When selecting control methods, consider the specific hazardous work, processes, and number of employees involved, the work environment, available control alternatives, and all exposure and sampling data.
- Consider all possible routes of exposure when developing and implementing prevention programs.
- Eliminate hazards where possible. In some cases, substitution of a less hazardous process or material will considerably reduce the potential for harm. Ensure that any substituted environment, method, or chemical is safer than that originally used and as safe as science/technology is able to provide.
- When possible, reduce hazards by process redesign, preventive maintenance, or equipment modification.
- When a hazard cannot be eliminated, control at the source of generation is usually the most effective means of exposure reduction. Evaluate appropriate engineering controls, such as local exhaust ventilation, to reduce airborne hazard potentials at or near the source of generation.
- Initiate special control procedures for energy sources, especially noise, radiation, lighting, heat, and vibration.
- Examine and modify employee work practices as necessary to decrease exposure and hazard potentials.
- Use personal protective devices as a last resort or as an additional control measure if the foregoing methods prove to be unsuccessful, inappropriate, infeasible, or inadequate.
- Train employees to understand hazard potentials and the importance of appropriate control methods.

Basic risk reduction approaches to controlling occupational health hazards follow in hierarchical order of effectiveness:

1. **Elimination/substitution.** Eliminating, changing, or substituting the process or materials used in the process so that toxic substances are not used. Substitution can be done only if a useful substitute is available. An example includes substituting safe manmade insulation fibers for asbestos.
2. **Isolation and containment.** Removing the hazard to a location away from the worker and enclosing the hazard by placing a barrier between the exposure source and the worker. For example, an enclosure to reduce or alter a noise source; a puncture-resistant container for needles/sharps.

3. **Engineering controls.** Designing and installing systems to limit or prevent the release of toxic materials in the worker's environment. For example, a local exhaust ventilation is designed to capture contaminants and remove them from the workplace.

4. **Work practice controls.** Educating and training workers with respect to proper use of control strategies and effective work practice procedures, which may help to minimize exposure risk. Good hygiene, safe handling of potentially contaminated devices, and good housekeeping are examples.

5. **Administrative controls.** Limiting potential or actual hazard exposure so that the amount of exposure is reduced to or below permissible levels. For example, job rotation is used so as to avoid excessive exposure of any one individual. Obviously, this approach has limited utility and should not be considered a substitute for adequate exposure control. Placing warning signs about hazardous materials, prohibiting access to restricted areas, and maintenance of equipment are other examples.

6. **Personal protection.** Providing adequate and appropriate protective devices and utilizing these devices to minimize exposure to hazardous materials. Examples include the use of protective clothing, gloves, head protection, ear plugs, goggles/glasses, safety shoes, and barrier creams appropriate to the situation. The effectiveness of personal protective equipment is dependent on many factors, such as worker understanding and compliance, proper fitting devices, and state-of-the-art equipment.

The process of identifying and controlling hazards in the workplace is essential in providing a safe and healthful work environment. This is fostered by a multidisciplinary effort among workers and key health professionals including occupational health nurses, industrial hygienists, physicians, safety professionals, and others. The occupational health nurse must be familiar with basic concepts and principles related to industrial hygiene including hazard recognition, evaluation, and control, and ensure active participation in managing workplace hazards.

■ TOXICOLOGY

Everything in our physical world—the food we eat, the water we drink, the clothes we wear, the medicines we use, all the materials of daily living (furniture, automobiles, home)—are composed of chemicals. To date, more than 6 million synthetic chemicals have been registered by the American Chemical Association, and the number of naturally occurring chemicals in the environment is unknown (Ottoboni, 1991). Workers are exposed to a variety of chemicals in the production of materials in the work environment, and the occupational health nurse may be the first person to assess the exposure. Thus, it is essential that occupational health nurses have an understanding of general principles related to toxicological concepts. However, for a more in-depth discussion, the reader should consult a toxicology reference.

Toxicology is the study of harmful effects of chemicals on biological systems, and a toxic agent is one capable of producing a harmful response in a biological system. Chemicals achieve their effect on biological systems through a series of events and reactions as depicted in Figure 6–1. This includes concentration of the agent in the environment, exposure of the host and entry into the body, and internal distribution to and effect on the target organ (Gibaldi & Perrier, 1982).

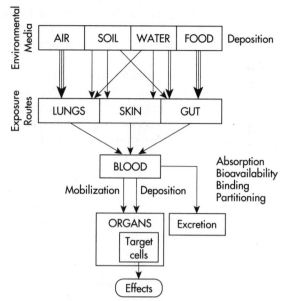

■ **Figure 6–1**   Chemical distribution: multiplicative effect. (From Gochfeld, M. Toxicology. In J. Last & R. Wallace [Eds.], Public Health and preventive medicine [13th ed.] [p. 316]. Norwalk, CT: Appleton & Lange, 1992.)

Industrial toxicology is the subdiscipline of toxicology primarily concerned with evaluating human health effects posed by chemical exposure in the workplace (Williams & Burson, 1985). The wisdom of Paracelsus (1493-1541) is important in noting that "All substances are poisons; there is none which is not a poison. It is the dose only that distinguishes a poison and a remedy." Thus, most all chemicals have the potential to create a toxic situation, wherein a toxic effect potentiates damage to an organism measured in terms of a loss, reduction, or change in function. However, it should be noted that effects that are considered adverse in one person may be desirable or therapeutic in another (Gochfeld, 1992a).

Chemical Classifications and Effects

Chemicals may be classified in several different ways. By nature of their substance, the American National Standards Institute has adopted the following definitions:

Dusts solid particles generated by handling, crushing, grinding, rapid impact, and detonation of organic or inorganic materials such as rocks, ore, metal, coal, wood, and grain. Dusts do not tend to flocculate except under electrostatic forces; they do not diffuse in air but settle under the influence of gravity.

Fumes solid particles generated by condensation from the gaseous state, generally after volatilization from molten metals, and often accompanied by a chemical reaction such as oxidation. Fumes flocculate and sometimes coalesce.

Mists suspended liquid droplets generated by condensation from the gaseous to the liquid state or by breaking up a liquid into a dispersed state, such as by splashing, foaming, or atomizing.

Vapors the gaseous form of substances that are normally in the solid or liquid state and

■ **TABLE 6–4** Classification of Toxic Agents by Exposure and Effect

Classification	Example: Welding on Zinc	Example: Carbon Tetrachloride
Acute toxicity: Adverse toxic effects occurring from a short-term, usually single high-dose exposure to a toxic chemical, resulting in often severe symptoms developing rapidly. Effect is often reversible.	Symptoms of metal-fume fever	Depression of mental capacity
Chronic toxicity: Adverse toxic effects occurring from repeated or continuous exposure, usually low level, over a relatively long period of time. Effect is often irreversible.	Latent pneumoconiosis, pulmonary fibrosis	Liver or kidney damage
Local toxicity: Effect occurring at the site of application or exposure between the toxicant and biological system.	Burn	Irritation of eyes and throat
Systemic toxicity: Effect occurring within the body as a result of absorption and distribution of the toxicant via the bloodstream to susceptible organs that are the sites of action.	Gastrointestinal symptoms, musculoskeletal aches.	Central nervous system depressant

can be changed to these states by either increasing the pressure or decreasing the temperature. Vapors diffuse.

Gases normally formless fluids that occupy the space of enclosure and can be changed to the liquid or solid state only by the combined effect of increased pressure and decreased temperature. Gases diffuse.

In addition, classification may be according to the duration of exposure, that is, acute or chronic toxicity, or by target site of action, either local or systemic as displayed in Table 6–4. Exposure to a high dose over a short time is an acute exposure, whereas chronic exposure usually involves continuous or periodic small doses over an extended period. With respect to end-point health effect, the liver is of particular concern as many substances are directly transported to the liver for intermediary metabolism. Here, harmful chemicals that are of themselves toxic may be detoxified, or benign substances may be converted into a biologically harmful metabolite (Gochfeld, 1992). The toxicity of a substance is its ability to damage an organ system, disrupt a biochemical process such as hematopoietic mechanisms, or to disturb an enzyme system. Toxic exposure may range from minor, such as an irritation, to serious, such as liver or kidney damage or cancer, or to death from organ failure (Table 6–5).

Health effects from chemical exposure may be manifested as mutagenic, carcinogenic, or teratogenic and should be differentiated. A mutagen is a substance that interacts with genetic material and causes point mutations, chromosomal damage, or interference with cell development and division (Williams & Burson, 1985). Alterations in the DNA affect the somatic, reproductive, or germ cells. Adverse effects on germ cells may be transmitted to offspring (Fig. 6–2).

A carcinogen is a substance that, through the processes of *initiation and promotion,* is capable of causing cancer. Initiation is the process by which the genetic material of the cell is altered, predisposing it to cancer, and the process to which humans are exposed all their lives. The changes that constitute initiation

■ TABLE 6–5 Selected Metals Related to Specific Target Organ Systems

Metal	Renal System	Nervous System	Liver	GI Tract	Respiratory System	Hematopoietic System	Bone	Endocrine System	Skin	Cardiovascular System
Aluminum		+			+					
Arsenic		+	+	+	+	+		+		
Beryllium					+				+	
Bromide		+							+	
Cadmium	+	+		+	+		+			+
Chromium	+	+	+		+				+	
Cobalt		+		+	+			+	+	+
Copper				+		+				
Fluoride		+			+		+		+	
Iron		+	+	+	+	+		+		
Lead	+	+		+		+			+	
Manganese		+			+					
Mercury	+	+		+	+					
Nickel		+			+				+	
Selenium	+			+	+				+	
Silver									+	
Thallium	+	+	+	+	+	+	+			
Zinc				+			+			

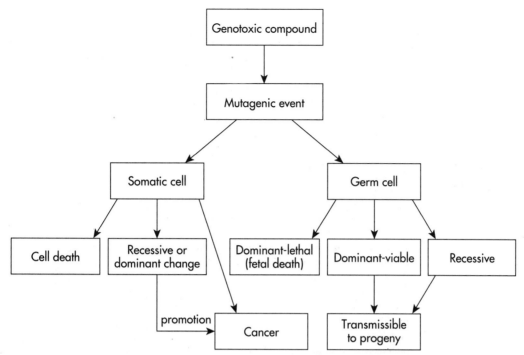

■ **Figure 6–2** Potential consequences of a mutagenic event in somatic and germinal cells. (From Williams, P & Burson, J. Industrial toxicology. New York: Van Nostrand Reinhold, 1985.)

may be reversed by repair mechanisms or may lie dormant, perhaps controlled by the immune system. This is followed by the stage of *promotion,* whereby initiated cells are stimulated or allowed to become cancerous (Armitage, 1985). Examples of substances known or suspected of being carcinogenic are shown in Table 6–6.

A teratogen is a substance that interferes with embryonic or fetal development and may cause major structural birth defects, slowed maturation, embryonic death or even behavioral or learning dysfunction postnatally (Needleman et al., 1979). Teratogenesis will be discussed in more detail later.

The scheme of classification relative to how we use substances is essential for government regulation of such items as foods, drugs, cosmetics, pesticides, industrial chemicals, and medical devices. If a substance is claimed to be a food, it is governed by the food laws. If the exact same substance is packaged and labeled a drug, it is governed by the drug laws, not by the food laws; the laws that pertain to a substance depend on what use the manufacturer specifies for the product. For example, hydrochloric acid is regulated as a household product when it is present in cleaning compounds, as a drug when it is used to treat people with low gastric acidity, as a hazardous industrial chemical when it is used in electroplating, and as a pesticide adjuvant when it is used to enhance the germicidal activity of chlorine in swimming pools. Hydrochloric acid is natural when produced by the stomach and synthetic when made in the laboratory (Ottoboni, 1991). Ottoboni lists the following properties by which chemicals can be harmful:

■ **TABLE 6–6**   Known or Reasonably Anticipated Carcinogens Listed in the Sixth Annual Report of the National Toxicology Program, 1991

---

1. Substances or groups of substances and medical treatments that are known to be carcinogenic

Aflatoxins
4-Aminobiphenyl
Analgesic mixtures containing phenacetin
Arsenic and certain arsenic compounds
Asbestos
Azathioprine
Benzene
Benzidine
Bis (chloromethyl) ether and technical-grade chloromethyl methyl ether
1, 4-Butanediol dimethylsulfonate (Myleran)
Chlorambucil
1-(2-Chloroethyl)-3-(4-methylcyclohexyl)-1-nitrosourea (MeCCNU)
Chromium and certain chromium compounds
Conjugated estrogens
Cyclophosphamide
Diethylstilbestrol
Erionite
Melphalan
Methoxsalen with ultraviolet A therapy (PUVA)
Mustard gas
2-Naphthylamine
Thorium dioxide
Vinyl chloride

2. Substances or groups of substances and medical treatments that may reasonably be anticipated to be carcinogens

Acetaldehyde
2-Acetylaminofluorene
Acrylamide
Acrylonitrile
Adriamycin
2-Aminoanthraquinone
o-Aminoazotoluene
1-Amino-2-methylanthraquinone
Amitrole
o-Anisidine hydrochloride
Benzotrichloride
Beryllium and certain beryllium compounds
Bischloroethyl nitrosourea
Bromodichloromethane
1, 3-Butadiene
Butylated hydroxyanisole
Cadmium and certain cadmium compounds
Carbon tetrachloride
Chlorendic acid
Chlorinated paraffins (C_{12}, 60% chlorine)
1-(2-Chloroethyl)-3-cyclohexyl-1-nitrosourea (CCNU)
Chloroform

■ **TABLE 6–6** Known or Reasonably Anticipated Carcinogens Listed in the Sixth Annual Report of the National Toxicology Program, 1991 *Continued*

3-Chloro-2-methylpropene
4-Chloro-o-phenylenediamine
C.1. basic red 9 monohydrochloride
Cisplatin
p-Cresidine
Cupferron
Dacarbazine
DDT
2,4-Diaminoanisole sulfate
2,4-Diaminotoluene
1,2-Dibromo-3-chloropropane
1,2-Dibromoethane (EDB)
1,4-Dichlorobenzene
3,3'-Dichlorobenzidine and 3,3'-dichlorobenzidine dihydrochloride
1,2-Dichloroethane
Dichloromethane (methylene chloride)
1,3-Dichloropropene (technical grade)
Diepoxybutane
Di(2-ethylhexyl)phthalate
Diethyl sulfate
Diglycidyl resorcinol ether
3,3'-Dimethoxybenzidine
4-Dimethylaminoazobenzene
3,3'-Dimethylbenzidine
Dimethylcarbamoyl chloride
1,1-Dimethylhydrazine
Dimethyl sulfate
Dimethylvinyl chloride
1,4-Dioxane
Direct black 38
Direct blue 6
Epichlorohydrin
Estrogens (not conjugated): estradiol-17
Estrogens (not conjugated): estrone
Estrogens (not conjugated): ethinylestradiol
Estrogens (not conjugated): mestranol
Ethyl acrylate
Ethylene oxide
Ethylene thiourea
Ethyl methanesulfonate
Formaldehyde (gas)
Hexachlorobenzene
Hexamethylphosphoramide
Hydrazine and hydrazine sulfate
Hydrazobenzene
Iron dextran complex
Kepone (chlordecone)
Lead acetate and lead phosphate
Lindane and other hexachlorocyclohexane isomers
2-Methylaziridine (propyleneimine)

Table continued on following page

■ **TABLE 6–6** Known or Reasonably Anticipated Carcinogens Listed in the Sixth Annual Report of the National Toxicology Program, 1991 *Continued*

4,4'-Methylenebis (2-chloroaniline) (MBOCA)
4-4'-Methylenebis (N,N-dimethyl) benzenamine
4,4-Methylenedianiline and its dihydrochloride
Methyl methanesulfonate
N-Methyl-N'-nitro-N-nitrosoguanidine
Metronidazole
Michler's ketone
Mirex
Nickel and certain nickel compounds
Nitrilotriacetic acid
Nitrofen
Nitrogen mustard hydrochloride
2-Nitropropane
N-Nitrosodi-n-butylamine
N-Nitrosodiethanolamine
N-Nitrosodiethylamine
N-Nitrosodimethylamine
N-Nitrosodi-*n*-propylamine
N-Nitroso-N-ethylurea
4-(Nitroso methylamino)-1-(3-pryidyl)-1-butanone
N-Nitroso-N-methylurea
N-Nitrosomethylvinylamine
N-Nitrosomorpholine
N-Nitrosonornicotine
N-Nitrosopiperidine
N-Nitrosopyrrolidine
N-Nitrososarcosine
Norethisterone
Ochratoxin A
4,4'-Oxydianiline
Oxymetholone
Phenacetin
Phenazopyridine hydrochloride
Phenoxybenzamine hydrochloride
Phenytoin
Polybrominated biphenyls
Polychlorinated piphenyls
Polycyclic aromatic hydrocarbons, 15 listings
   Benz[a]anthracene
   Benzo[b]fluoranthene
   Benzo[j]fluoranthene
   Benzo[k]fluoranthene
   Benzo[a]pyrene
   Dibenz[a,h]acridine
   Dibenz[a,j]acridine
   Dibenz[a,h]anthracene
   7H-Dibenzo[c,g]carbazole
   Dibenzo[a,e]pyrene
   Dibenzo[e,h]pyrene
   Dibenzo[a,i]pyrene

■ **TABLE 6–6** Known or Reasonably Anticipated Carcinogens Listed in the Sixth Annual Report of the National Toxicology Program, 1991 *Continued*

Dibenzo[a,l]pyrene
Indeno[1,2,3-cd]pyrene
5-Methylchrysene
Procarbazine hydrochloride
Progesterone
1,3-Propane sultone
B-Propiolactone
Propylene oxide
Propylthiouracil
Reserpine
Saccharin
Safrole
Selenium sulfide
Silica, crystalline (respirable)
　Quartz
　Cristobalite
　Tridymite
Streptozotocin
Sulfallate
2,3,7,8-Tetrachlorodibenzo-*p*-dioxin (TCDD)
Tetrachloroethylene (perchloroethylene)
Thioacetamide
Thiourea
Toluene diisocyanate
o-Toluidine and *o*-toluidine hydrochloride
Toxaphene
2,4,6-Trichlorophenol
Tris(1-aziridinyl)phosphine sulfide
Tris(2,3-dibromopropyl)phosphate
Urethane

From U.S. Department of Health and Human Services, National Toxicology Program. Sixth Annual Report on Carcinogens, 1991.

- Explosiveness and reactivity
- Flammability and combustibility
- Radioactivity
- Corrosiveness
- Irritation
- Sensitization and photosensitization
- Toxicity

A poison is differentiated from a toxin wherein a poison is a chemical that produces illness or death when taken in very small quantities (Ottoboni, 1991). Legally a poison is defined as a chemical that has an LD_{50} of 50 milligrams (mg) or less of chemical per kilogram (kg) of body weight. An LD_{50} is the quantity of a chemical administered in one dose that is lethal for 50% of test animals within a 14-day period (Ottoboni, 1991). LD refers to the lethal dose and subscript 50 to the percentage of the animals for which the dose was lethal. LD_{50} is also

■ **TABLE 6–7** Ranking System for Acute Chemical Toxicity

Toxicity Rating or Class	Probable Oral Lethal Dose for Average Adult	Example of Substance
1. Practically nontoxic	>15 g/kg (more than 1 quart)	Sugar
2. Slightly toxic	5-15 g/kg (between 1 pint and 1 quart)	Salt
3. Moderately toxic	0.5-5 g/kg (between 1 ounce and 1 pint)	2, 4-D (herbicide)
4. Very toxic	50-500 mg/kg (between 1 teaspoonful and 1 ounce)	Arsenic acid
5. Extremely toxic	5-50 mg/kg (between 7 drops and 1 teaspoonful)	Nicotine
6. Supertoxic	<5 mg/kg (a taste [<7 drops])	Botulism toxin

From Hansen, D. The work environment: Occupational health fundamentals. Chelsea, MI: Lewis Publishers, 1991. Lewis Publishers is a subsidiary of CRC Press, Boca Raton, FL.

used to express acute inhalation toxicity, which refers to the lethal concentration of an airborne contaminant. The smaller the LD_{50}, the greater the toxicity, and conversely, the larger the LD_{50}, the lesser the toxicity. LD_{50s} and LC_{50s} are obviously unknown for humans for any chemical, as humans cannot be placed in these types of experimental conditions to test lethal doses. However, it is important to understand this concept as data from animal experiments are extrapolated to humans to estimate toxicity. For toxic effects one assumes that man is at least as sensitive to the toxicity as the test species is and may be more susceptible. A relative ranking system of acute chemical toxicity is shown in Table 6–7.

Dose-Response

Lioy (1990) describes an exposure-effect relationship on a continuum from point source emission → to human contact exposure → to potential dose to the body → biologically effective/response dose to the target system → early expression of disease → health effect on endpoint. The degree of harmfulness of a substance or chemical is the dose of that chemical and the relationship of that dose to producing an adverse biologic or health effect. This is in contrast to an effective dose (ED) in which the response is a desirable one. This concept of dose-response is the hallmark of toxicology and is critically important as it is used as the basis for determining the relative safety of a chemical compound in the living organism (Hansen, 1991). Most often the response is measured as the percentage of exposed animals that show a particular effect.

Generally, higher levels of toxic exposure will invoke greater responses such as when higher concentrations of inhaled carbon monoxide produce higher carboxyhemoglobin levels (Becker, 1990). A dose-response graph as shown in Figure 6–3 quantifies the relationship of the biological or health effect as a result of dose levels. The typical dose-response curve is demonstrated by the sigmoidal shape shown.

Important to the dose-response concept is the threshold dose or level at which there is no observed effect. In the figure the lower end reflects the existence of a threshold dose (no effect noted) followed by a sharp rise in the curve, often displayed as a linear phase, where the increase in response is proportional to the dose increase. The upper end displays a flattening of the curve or ceiling level of maximal response that cannot be increased by greater doses. This level might

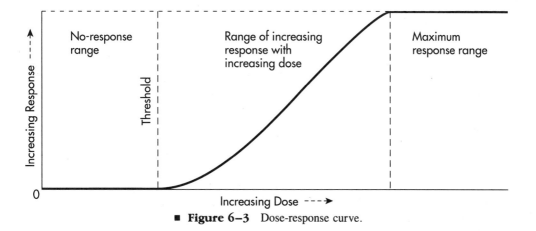

■ **Figure 6–3**   Dose-response curve.

correspond to the death of an individual. In the dose-response relationship, it is necessary to know the end-point of measurement, which may be, for example, the presence of a lesion (e.g., tumor), a biological, physiological, or behavioral alteration (response dose or effective dose), or death (lethal dose). Figure 6–4 shows a dose-response relationship between exposure to antineoplastic agents and urine mutagenicity in a population of exposed nurses (Rogers, 1987).

In addition to dose-response relationships, the concept of latency, the time between exposure and effect, is an important variable in interpreting presumed cause-effect relationships. If the latency period is very short (e.g., acute exposure to hydrogen sulfide), the effect is immediately measurable. In other situations, such as asbestos-induced mesothelioma, the latency period may be 40 years (Selikoff & Lee, 1978). For situations where the latency period may be long, the exposure may not necessarily be associated with the outcome. Thus, it is important that the occupational health nurse be familiar with and document exposures in order to investigate cause-effect relationships through epidemiologic studies.

Routes of Exposure

In the workplace, chemicals enter the body primarily through dermal absorption, inhalation, and oral ingestion. While chemicals can enter the body through other routes (e.g., injection), this is uncommon as a workplace exposure, except in the health care setting where needlestick injuries present a route of exposure (Neuberger et al., 1984).

Chemicals may be absorbed through the skin into the circulatory system. However, the skin provides a significant barrier to absorption primarily because of the layers of epidermal and dermal cells that in general are not very permeable to toxicants, although this will vary considerably depending on the chemical type and duration of exposure, and skin condition. Percutaneous absorption can be increased by damage or abrasion to the skin, increased skin wetness, or vascularization. Certain organic solvents, such as dimethylsulfoxide (DMSO), also appear to act as delipidizing agents that reduce the barrier function of the stratum corneum, the outermost layer (Framkin, 1988). Once a chemical penetrates the skin, it enters the bloodstream and is carried throughout the body.

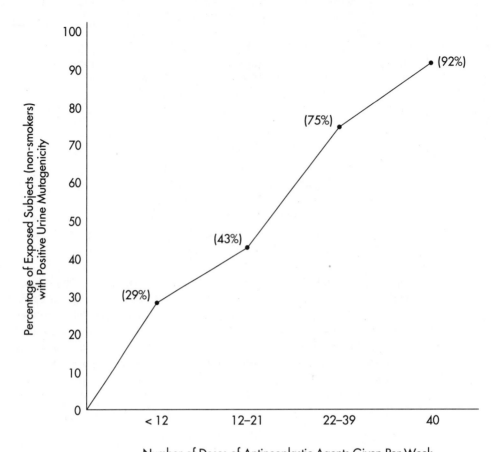

■ **Figure 6–4**   Percentage of positive urine mutagenicity results for exposed subjects (nonsmokers) by total number of doses of antineoplastic agents given.

Inhalation is the major route of entry of the gases, vapors, mists and airborne particulate matter encountered in the workplace. Gases, vapors, and mists can cause both damage to the respiratory tract, and pass through the lung to the bloodstream for distribution to other parts of the body, causing systemic poisoning. Highly soluble irritant gases, such as hydrogen fluoride, ammonia, and sulfuric acid, often produce an immediate irritation, while less soluble gases such as nitrogen dioxide and phosgene reach the alveoli and dissolve slowly, causing acute pneumonitis and pulmonary edema several hours later (Framkin, 1988).

Asphyxiants exert toxicity through interruption of oxygen to the tissues. Simple asphyxiants, such as carbon dioxide and nitrogen, cause hypoxia by displacing oxygen in the ambient air, which may be a problem in confined spaces. Chemical asphyxiants block the delivery of oxygen at the cell site. Carbon monoxide, which is a product of incomplete combustion found in coke ovens and foundries, acts to interfere with oxygen transport by binding to the hemoglobin forming carboxyhemoglobin. Cyanide and hydrogen sulfide are other examples of chemical asphyxiants (Becker, 1990).

The delivery of gases, vapors, and mists to body tissues may be enhanced by rapid deep breathing as occurs with strenuous exercise, or by a poorly designed or poorly fit respirator. In addition, those substances that are lipid-soluble cross the alveolar membrane to the bloodstream and deposit themselves in fatty depots, thus allowing the blood to clear or free itself for another pick-up as it passes again through the lung. Examples of lipid-soluble substances include chloroform, carbon disulfide, and halogenated hydrocarbons (Williams & Burson, 1985).

Inhaled particles exert their adverse effects primarily through deposition in the lung tissue. The three basic regions of the lung are the nasopharyngeal region, tracheobronchial region, and alveolar region. The location and extent of deposition are influenced by the anatomy of the respiratory tract, particle size, and ventilation (Framkin, 1988). For example, because the nasopharynx has sharp bends and nasal hairs, deposition may be enhanced, which may account, in part, for the increased incidence of nasal cancer in some groups occupationally exposed to dust-containing carcinogens, such as workers exposed to wood dusts, cork dusts, and fiberboard (Wills, 1982).

The effective anatomy of the respiratory tract changes significantly with a simple shift from nose-breathing to mouth-breathing, as occurs normally during physical exertion. This bypasses the more efficient filtration of larger particles by the nasopharynx and results in greater deposition in the tracheobronchial tree. Through such a transition, workers performing physical labor may lose the benefit of a major natural defense mechanism (Framkin, 1988). In addition, deep breathing, as during strenuous exercise, increases the amount of inhaled air to the distal airways and promotes alveolar deposition.

Particle deposition is also influenced by its shape and density. As indicated in a classic report by Brain and Valberg (1979), the efficiency of deposition of particles is determined by its size, shape, and density (Fig. 6–5). Deposition of particles with an aerodynamic diameter of several micrometers (μm) is high, diminishes at about 1.0 μm and increases again below 0.5 μm. Those particles with an effective aerodynamic diameter between 0.5 and 5.0 μm (the respirable fraction) can be maintained in the alveoli and bronchioles, setting the stage for pneumoconiosis. Particle filtration in the upper airways and cilial action are important clearance mechanisms. Cilial action may be significantly compromised in smokers or workers who have been continually exposed to some form of toxic material.

Ingestion is the third route of exposure for toxicants. While this route is generally not as significant in the workplace, chemicals can enter the body via contaminated food or water, inhaled particulates collected in the nasopharyngeal region and later swallowed (e.g., lead), or by workers who mouth breath, chew gum or tobacco, or who may place contaminated fingers or materials in their mouths.

Gastric juices can help minimize toxicity through detoxification of the substances; thus, absorption into the bloodsteam may be decreased. However, where substances are metabolized by the liver and the rate of passage is slowed, the length of time during which the compound is available for absorption is increased, such as with mercury or lead (Lewis, 1990).

Factors Influencing Toxicity

In addition to factors related to agent, dose, and route of exposure, several other factors influence toxicity. These include age, gender, ethnicity, nutrition, state of health, individual susceptibility, and previous or concurrent exposures.

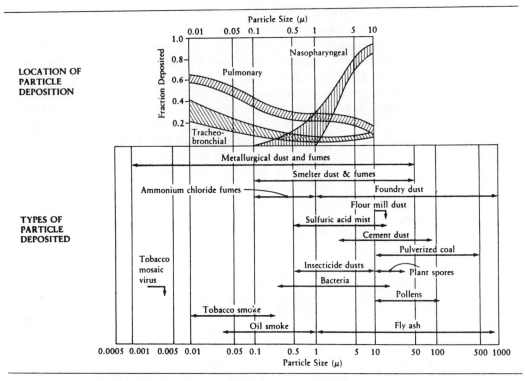

■ **Figure 6–5**   Respiratory deposition of inhaled particles influenced by particle shape and size. (Reprinted from Levy, B & Wegman, D. Occupational health. Boston: Little, Brown and Company, copyright 1988.)

Age

Although data are insufficient, evidence exists that infants and children are at greater risk of toxic insult from chemical exposure than are adults. This is related to a less efficient biotransformation process in infants and because cells divide more rapidly in growing children, making them more vulnerable to attack by chemical carcinogens (Ottoboni, 1991). Although not reported, one might also consider what influence the aging process has on the metabolism of toxic materials. In addition, degenerative changes occurring in organ and immunologic systems may predispose older workers to harmful effects from toxic exposures. Further, the effects of age on healing processes may be an important consideration during the healing phase.

Gender

Gender differences related to toxic effects have been shown in numerous animal studies. However, in humans, differences between the sexes relate primarily to their reproductive roles. While most current knowledge about reproductive toxicity comes from experimental animal studies, epidemiologic studies form the basis for occupational exposure associations in humans related to reproductive toxicity (Buring et al., 1985; Holmberg et al., 1986; Rogers, 1987; Schnorr, 1993; Winder, 1989). NIOSH has included reproductive disorders among their top 10 leading work-related disorders.

Reproductive Toxicity.   It is important that the occupational health professional has a good understanding of the reproductive processes in both the male and female, a thorough knowledge of chemical exposures encountered in the workplace, and how or if these exposures may in any way compromise the reproductive system or outcome. The reproductive process is highly complex and dynamic. Damage by physical or chemical agents to the sperm, ovum, or the fertilized ovum may cause infertility, spontaneous abortion, birth defects, or may result in germ cell mutations that are passed on to future generations. When considering occupational exposures that may damage reproductive processes, the hazard to both men and women must be examined.

In utero, development of the male reproductive system in the fetus begins about seven weeks after conception with development of the male sex organs and testicular descent by seven months gestation. During this process, the phase of spermatogenesis in the male (stem germ cell to mature sperm) takes about 70 to 80 days, during which constant cell division makes the male reproductive system highly susceptible to chemical insult. Chemicals reach the testes by systemic blood distribution through inhalation, ingestion, or transpercutaneously. As shown in Table 6–8, several male reproductive toxins have been occupationally identified, including lead, selected halogenated pesticides, and possibly the organic solvents carbon disulfide (CS_2) and dinitrotoluene.

The term "perinatal toxicology" designates the study of toxic responses to occupational and environmental agents when exposure occurs from the time of conception through the neonatal period (Ottoboni, 1991). It is important to recognize that exposures of the conceptus during specific periods of gestation elicit different responses. Figure 6–6 depicts the stages of gestation and the biological responses associated with exposures to reproductive toxins during specific periods (Williams & Burson, 1985).

Fertilization of the ovum by the sperm occurs in the fallopian tube followed by implantation. During this time the developing embryo is highly susceptible to both genetic abnormalities and toxic insults. Organogenesis occurs between days 20 and 56, followed by a slower development and maturation period including neurological and sexual organ development. During this period of fetal development, toxic exposures can result in neurologic, immunologic, developmental, and endocrine deficits and cancer in the offspring (Fig. 6–6) (Williams & Burson, 1985).

One process whereby some foreign agent, physical or chemical, produces an abnormality in a developing organism during uterine life is called teratogenesis. Teratogens are agents that give rise to malformed or otherwise abnormal fetuses. Some chemicals and certain physical agents, such as natural and man-made radiation, can behave as teratogens. Chemical teratogens may or may not be mutagens and chemical mutagens are not necessarily teratogens. X-rays, in particular, may be both mutagens and teratogens. High doses of a teratogen may result in embryolethality (Gochfeld, 1992b).

In the critical period of embryonic development, cells undergo differentiation and mobilization into tissue groups that differentiate further into major organs and cartilage (preskeleton). The critical stage of organ development for the human is the first three months (first trimester) of pregnancy. The kind of abnormality produced depends on what organ system is undergoing the most rapid development at the time of exposure to the teratogen. For example, exposure to high

■ **TABLE 6–8** Adverse Reproductive Outcomes for Selected Chemicals Used in the Workplace

Chemical Agent	Infertility	Fecundity	Menstrual Disorders	Prematurity, Low Birth Weight	Spontaneous Abortion/ Stillbirth	Birth Defects	Contaminated Breast Milk	Animal Studies
Anesthetic Agents	+				+			+
Anilene			+					+
Antineoplastics					+/+	+		+
Arsenic			+		+	+		+
Benzene			+				+	+
Boron		M						+
Cadmium	+	M		+			+	+
Carbon Disulfide		M	+		+			+
Chloroprene	+	M	+		+			
Chromium				+				
CO				+				+
Copper							+	+
DDT							+	+
Dieldrin							+	
Ethylene Dibrom-ide	+	M						+
Ethylene Oxide					+			+
Formaldehyde			+	+				+
Lead	+	M	+		+/+	+	+	+
Manganese	+	M						+
Mercury		F		+			+	+
Nickel								+
Selenium								+
Toluene		M	+	+				+
Vinyl Chloride					+/+			+
Xylene								+

+ = effect reported; M = male; F = female.
Data from Office of Technology Assessment. Reproductive health hazards in the workplace. Washington, DC: U.S. Government Printing Office, 1985.

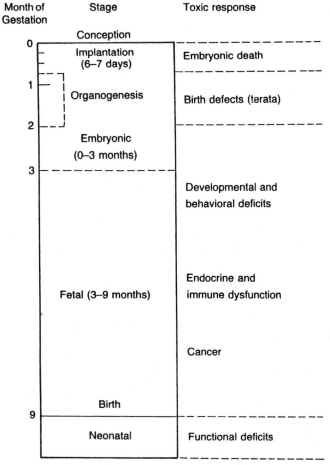

Month of Gestation	Stage	Toxic response

■ **Figure 6–6**   Stages of gestation and potential biological responses related to reproductive toxin exposure. (From Williams, P & Burson, J. Industrial toxicology. New York: Van Nostrand Reinhold, 1985.)

doses of vitamin A on the eighth day of gestation in rats results in skeletal malformations, whereas the same doses on the 12th day result in cleft palate (Williams & Burson, 1985).

For reasons previously stated, the embryo is more susceptible to physical and chemical teratogens than is the mother. Overt toxicity and birth defects are not correlated, and, conversely, a number of chemicals producing toxic effects in the mother do not have an adverse effect on the embryo (Table 6–8). Maternal and placental metabolism of a chemical and the ability of a chemical to move from maternal blood across the placenta into the embryo's blood influence the amount and chemical form of an agent interacting with the rapidly dividing and differentiating cells. Teratogenic effects of a chemical occur within a relatively narrow range of concentration, between intermediate doses that kill the embryo and low doses that have no apparent effect (Ottoboni, 1991).

Mechanisms of teratogenesis are not well understood; however, changes in or inhibition of DNA and RNA, alteration in the structural formation of nucleic acids, or inhibition of enzymatic functions have been implicated. Spontaneous abortions have also been reported as a result of worker exposure to lead, copper, cadmium, anesthetic gases and antineoplastic agents (Paul & Himmelstein, 1988; Rogers, 1987) (Table 6–8). Chemicals can also produce fetal malformations by several mechanisms other than teratogenesis, including preconception parent germ cell mutation and inadequate placental development with resultant disruption in the maternal-fetal nutrient flow and oxygen deficit (Williams & Burson, 1985).

Prevention of reproductive disorders from workplace exposures should be a workplace priority, which the occupational health nurse can facilitate. In order to promote and protect reproductive health, programs for reproductive health surveillance can be instituted in the workplace. The components of the program will be influenced by the nature of the exposures and the workers affected. At the very minimum, a reproductive health questionnaire (Fig. 6–7) should be added to the occupational health history. In addition, periodic examinations, and environmental and biological monitoring can be used to detect exposures (Weeks, Levy, & Wagner, 1991). Education of workers regarding potentially harmful exposures must be an integral component to any reproductive health program.

Nutrition

Nutritional status plays an important role in the ultimate toxic performance of chemicals. A good diet supplies the necessary metals for the biotransformation processes (i.e., those reactions that break down and transform substances into metabolites for excretion from the body), and prevents protein deficiencies that would reduce the ability of the body to supply key enzymes (Williams & Burson, 1985).

Health Status

One's individual responses to a toxic exposure are influenced by one's state of physical and emotional health. For example, individuals with preexisting liver, lung, or immunologic disease may be at greater risk of further injury from a toxic exposure due to already compromised organ systems. The integrity of the body system will have a major determination on how one is able to withstand repeated toxic insults, particularly if previous exposures have occurred.

Individuals may also become predisposed to occupational illness as a result of toxic exposures through lifestyle habits such as smoking, alcohol abuse, or lack of exercise. For example, cigarette smoking has been demonstrated to have important effects on the health of workers exposed to toxic substances. The National Institute for Occupational Safety and Health (NIOSH) has identified six mechanisms by which smoking interacts with occupational exposures. First, certain toxic agents in the workplace, such as carbon monoxide and cadmium, are also present in tobacco or smoke, thereby increasing these exposures. Second, workplace chemicals may be pyrolyzed into more harmful agents, because the temperature of a burning cigarette reaches 1,600 degrees Fahrenheit. Third, tobacco products serve as vectors by becoming contaminated with workplace agents like lead and pesticides, which may enter the body through inhalation, ingestion, or skin absorption. Fourth, there may be additive effects from smoking and exposure to other substances such as chlorine, cotton dust, and coal dust. Fifth, the effects may be synergistic between smoking and asbestos, gold, and

Occupational Health History
for
Reproductive Surveillance in the Workplace

Name _____ Date _____

Duration of Employment _____

Job Title _____

Description of Job Duties _____

_____

_____

_____

Total Work Hours per Week _____ Shift Work? Yes _____ No _____

Do you work overtime? Yes _____ No _____

If yes, how many hours usually per week? _____

1. Physical Requirements of Job. Please indicate and describe if you engage in any of the work activities that are listed below and the approximate number of hours each week you do the activity.

   Bending _____   Sitting _____

   Climbing _____   Standing _____

   Lifting _____   Stooping _____

   Pulling _____   Twisting _____

2. Job Exposures. Please indicate if you have any of the following exposures and describe them giving the amount and duration of the exposure.

   Chemicals (topical) _____   Psychological Stress _____

   _____   _____

   Dusts, fumes, vapors _____   Radiation _____

   _____   _____

   Infectious Agents _____   Sharp Objects _____

   _____   _____

   Metals _____   Temperature Extremes _____

   _____   _____

   Noise _____   Vibration _____

   _____   _____

■ **Figure 6–7** Occupational Health History for Reproductive Surveillance in the Workplace

Illustration continued on following page

Occupational Health History
for
Reproductive Surveillance in the Workplace *Continued*

3. Do you use any of the following protective measures in the workplace?

   Apron/Coat _____   Gloves _____

   Ear Protection _____   Lifting Devices _____

   Eyewear _____   Respirator _____

   Face Mask _____   Ventilation _____

4. Do you have any exposures at home/community (e.g. lead paint)? _____

   _____

   _____

   _____

5. Do you have any hobby exposures? _____

   _____

   _____

6. Cigarette Smoke: Active (No. of packs per day) _____

   Passive _____

7. Alcohol (quantity per day) _____

8. Please answer the following questions related to pregnancy and pregnancy outcomes in the past year.

   A. Have you and your spouse/partner had any problems with fertility or becoming pregnant? Yes _____ No _____

   B. Have you had any miscarriages? Yes _____ No _____

   C. Have you had a baby born to full term? Yes _____ No _____

   D. Have you had a premature or low birth weight baby (born weighing less than 5 lbs. or before the eighth month)? Yes _____ No _____

9. Have you had any child born with a birth defect? Yes _____ No _____

■ **Figure 6–7** *Continued*

rubber industry exposures. Sixth, smoking increases accident rates through loss of attention, preoccupation with the hand, irritation of the eyes, coughing, and fires. Smoking, of course, is associated with the development of lung cancer, increased mortality for workers exposed to asbestos, and increased risk of developing byssinosis in textile workers (Levy & Wegman, 1988). In addition, selected medication intake may pose an interactive effect coupled with exposure to certain toxins, such as a worker exposed to pesticides, who smokes, and is being treated with Isoniazide.

Individual Susceptibility

Individual susceptibility is an important variable with respect to one's response to chemical exposure (Williams & Burson, 1985; Ottoboni, 1991). For example, some individuals respond very differently to the same medications or may have different reactions when exposed to various odorous substances such as perfumes. Other examples related to genetic predisposition include individuals who have red blood cells that are more fragile than usual due to a certain enzyme deficiency, and thus, are more susceptible to chemicals that cause hemolysis. People who have a genetic deficiency of a certain DNA-repair process suffer from xeroderma pigmentosa, a disease that renders them tremendously more susceptible to the carcinogenic effects of ultraviolet radiation on the skin. Albinos, and fair-skinned people in general, are more susceptible to the damaging effects of sunlight.

In addition, individuals may be hypersusceptible, which indicates an unusually high response to some dose of a substance. This may be a genetic predisposition to a toxic effect or a response that is uncharacteristic of the "average" person. Hypersensitivity is a form of hypersusceptibility characterized by an acquired, immunologically mediated sensitization to a substance usually manifested by respiratory or dermatologic responses in the workplace (Framkin, 1988). For example, toluene disocynate (TDI), used in the manufacture of polyurethane, will evoke an asthmatic reaction in a small number of exposed workers even at permissible exposure levels (Wegmen & Christian, 1988).

Occupational History

A worker's prior occupational exposures may have a significant effect on her or his susceptibility to occupational disease based on further occupational exposures. Many forms of occupational cancer are characterized by long latency periods—as long as 35 to 40 years—before the disease is clinically evident. The leading example would be exposure to asbestos. Consequently, an individual with a history of previous toxic exposures may be considered by employers to be a high risk (Lilis, 1992; Travers, 1986).

It is also possible that a prior exposure to a carcinogen may combine with a later exposure (even to a different agent) to produce an effect that neither exposure alone would have produced. For example, the incidence of leukemia among radiation-exposed survivors at Hiroshima and Nagasaki has been shown to be increased where there was occupational exposure to benzene years after the radiation exposure (Upton, 1988).

In addition, exposure to different toxic substances at the same time is common in many industrial settings. The physiological effects of combined exposures may, in some instances, produce a synergistic effect that is greater than simply an additive effect of the single agents alone. For example, it is a well-established fact that smoking potentiates the carcinogenic effects of asbestos resulting in a lung cancer incidence 20 to 30 times greater than in nonsmokers (Selikoff, 1978).

There is still a great deal to be learned about individual reactions to chemicals. Gathering and interpreting data and recognizing important cues indicative of a potential exposure can help reduce associated risks. The occupational health nurse will need to be vigilant for signs and symptoms triggered by seemingly innocuous exposures.

■ SAFETY

Safety in the workplace is everyone's responsibility and awareness of safety and health issues is key to accident prevention. An accident is an unanticipated, sudden event that results in an undesired outcome such as a physical injury or death (Keyserling, 1988). Although the number of fatal occupational injuries has gradually declined in recent years, work-related illnesses and nonfatal injuries appear to be increasing. During 1987 alone, permanent impairments suffered on the job grew from 60,000 to 70,000, total disabling injuries numbered 1.8 million, and combined occupational illnesses and injuries in the manufacturing industries increased by 13.5% (BLS, 1988a). NIOSH estimates that at least 10 million injuries occur on the job each year, about 3 million of which are severe. Every workday more than 10,000 people suffer injuries that result in lost work time. Almost half of all occupational injuries reported in 1986 required either time off from work or restricted job activity. As work-related injuries continue to remain high, prevention of accidents and injuries at the worksite continues to be a major priority in occupational health (BLS, 1988b). The American National Standards Institute (ANSI) classifies work injuries according to accident type, which are briefly summarized in Table 6–9.

Occupational injury causes a major portion of unintentional injury deaths, which are the nation's leading cause of lost productive years of employment. Estimates of combined and specific industry deaths vary widely, with totals for 1987 ranging from 3,400 to 11,000 (NSC, 1987). Approximately 40% of fatal injury victims in 1987 were between 25 and 44 years old. New workers are at special risk in many occupations. More than 20% of fatal occupational injuries in the mid-1980s involved highway vehicle crashes, which were the leading cause of death in seven of eight industry divisions. Although mining (including quarrying and extraction of oil and gas) fatalities fell somewhat during the mid-1980s, they are still among the highest levels of occupational deaths. Beyond the manufacturing and service industries, agricultural work continues to be one of the most hazardous occupations, with death and permanent disability rates that remain consistently high (National Coalition for Agricultural Safety & Health, 1989). The number of fatal injuries in construction (670) and manufacturing (770) were higher than in mining (200) during 1986, but far more people were employed in these nonmining occupations. Agricultural worker deaths may be underestimated because many farm work forces have fewer than 11 workers and are therefore not identified by national data systems. The National Safety Council has estimated a rate as high as 52.1 deaths per 100,000 agricultural workers.

The principal responsibility of the safety professional is to design and implement strategies aimed at preventing and controlling workplace exposures that result in unnecessary injuries and deaths. Training and education of workers about job safety must be emphasized. Heath (1992) reports data obtained from the Bureau of Labor Statistics Work Injury Report Surveys (Table 6–10), which show the percentages of injured workers who reported they did not receive safety education or training for the jobs they were performing when injured. For example, while only 11% of those workers injured during welding and cutting operations indicated they did not receive appropriate job task training, 73% of workers using ladders reported the same! In addition, Heath (1992) states that:

■ **TABLE 6–9** Work Injuries According to Accident Type as Classified by the American National Standards Institute (ANSI)

Work Injury Type	Examples of Preventive Measures
Struck by: Incidents in which the worker is hit by a moving object or particle. Examples include falling or flying object or moving equipment	Use of siderails, toeboards, nets, gratings, safety helmets, and steel-toed shoes
Caught in, under, or between: Incidents involving an injury caused by crushing, squeezing, or pinching of a body part between a moving and stationary object or two moving objects. Examples include operations involving mechanical equipment such as power presses or calenders where tasks place workers' hands near moving parts	Use of barrier guards and equipment enclosures, safety buttons, presence-sensing systems (electric eye), emerging stop buttons, and lockout switches
Fall from elevation: Incidents in which a worker falls to a lower level and is injured on impact against an object on the ground. Examples include falls from ladders and other temporary work surfaces (scaffolds)	Use of guardrails and devices such as safety belts, harnesses, lanyards and lifelines
Falls on same level: Incidents involving workers who lose their footing and fall to surfaces supporting them. Examples include loss of foot traction, walking on wet, oily surfaces or highly polished surfaces (usually from a nonskid surface), trips, and missteps	Use of appropriate tread shoes, good housekeeping, maintenance, and lighting, and placement of warning or caution signs
Overexertion and repetitive trauma: Incidents involving worker injuries caused by excessive physical effort or highly repetitive patterns of localized muscle and joint usage resulting in back injuries, sprains, strains. Examples include manual materials handling, assembly line work, or jobs requiring awkward posture	Use of ergonomically designed equipment, lifting devices, reductions in load weight, and job rotation
Motor vehicle accidents: Incidents involving injury while person is operating a motor vehicle. Examples include internal accidents occurring in the worksite itself (e.g., forklift) and accidents external to the worksite on public roads	Use of training techniques, driver selection processes, vehicle inspection and maintenance programs, and use of seat belts
Other causes of physical trauma: Contact with electric current; struck against; contact with temperature extremes; tissue rubbing or abrading; bodily reaction; contact with radiation, caustics, and toxic and noxious substances; public transportation accident	Use of appropriate measures to reduce the risk of injury such as effective grounding of electrical equipment, insulation of all electric hand tools; use of safety equipment for body protection (helmets); use of robots in extreme temperature situations, and use of appropriate insulating materials; covering sharp objects with padding or handholds

1. Large numbers of injured workers do not receive what little training they do have from their current employers.
2. The training employees received was more than one year prior to their injury-producing event, despite changes in work methods, materials, and equipment.
3. Much of the safety information and instructions the workers do have come

■ **TABLE 6–10**   Percentages of Injured Workers Who Reported Receiving No Safety Training for Task(s) Being Performed at Time of Injury

Type of Injury, Part of Body Injured, or Activity in Which Worker was Engaged at Time of Injury	Size of Injured Worker Population	Percentage of Workers Who Report Never Having Received Training for Job Being Done When Injured
Survey of welding and cutting accidents resulting in injuries	1,364	11
Survey of power saw accidents resulting in injuries	1,746	17
Injuries in oil and gas drilling and services	1,041	21
Injuries to construction workers	3,700	26
Survey of scaffold accidents resulting in injuries	803	27
Injuries in the logging industry	1,086	37
Accidents involving eye injuries	1,053	40
Injuries to warehouse workers	2,700	46
Back injuries associated with lifting	906	51
Accidents involving face injuries	774	59
Survey of injuries to longshore workers	582	59
Work-related upper extremity amputations (arm, hand, or finger)	862	59
Injuries related to servicing equipment	833	61
Work-related hand injuries	944	66
Chemical burn survey	790	67
Accidents involving head injuries	1,033	71
Accidents involving foot injuries	1,251	71
Survey of ladder accidents resulting in injuries	1,419	73

Adapted from Heath, E. Safety and health training quality. In Proceedings of the Occupational Safety and Health Summit. Des Plaines, IL: American Society of Safety Engineers, 1992. Data from the Bureau of Labor Statistics, U.S. Department of Labor, Washington, D.C.

not from their employer or a supervisor, but from a fellow worker. Injured workers, almost uniformly, reported receiving significant amounts of safety education and training from their employee (union) representative, from salesmen for personal protective equipment, and from the printed instructions that came with the protective equipment.

A concerted effort needs to be made on the part of health and safety professionals working together to develop targeted, current, and renewed programs to prevent unnecessary job-related injuries.

Safety Committees and Programs

An effective safety program requires a multidisciplinary effort. The emphasis and commitment on safety starts with top management and extends, by example, throughout the organization to managers and other employees. The establishment of a workplace safety (and health) committee is vital to transforming safety ideas into prevention and protection strategies in terms of policy, procedure, program development, and training and education about safety in the workplace. As a collective group, the safety committee can study and analyze safety and related health problems and recommend policies and programs for the entire organization for an improved safety program. This need can be demonstrated from high or increased illness and injury rates, increased workers' compensation costs, or noted deficits from inspections or regulatory compliance and citations.

The safety committee should include varying levels of members of management, employees, the occupational health nurse, physician, the safety manager, other appropriate health care professionals, and union representatives, if applicable. The safety and health plan with specific goals and objectives should be established within the context of the committee with input from employees and all levels of management. The plan should be reviewed and updated annually and incorporated into the annual budget. Staff safety and health personnel generally know what should be done but often lack the line-management support to get it done. The safety committee can help to establish routine, effective lines of communication within all levels of the organization, from the ranking manager to the employee. This offers an excellent basis for training and informing personnel about safety and health procedures.

Boylston (1990) lists fundamental principles associated with safety and health management, including the following:

1. Safety and health maintenance is a line-management function.
2. Safety and health maintenance is an inherent job responsibility.
3. Minimum acceptable safety and health standards must be established and maintained.
4. Safety responsibility and accountability must be achieved in the same manner as are responsibilities for production, quality, cost control, and personnel relations.

Keyserling (1988) identifies the following basic policy components that govern an effective safety program at the worksite:

1. A commitment to provide the greatest possible safety to all employees and to ensure that all facilities and processes will be designed with this objective. Similarly, purchasing policies must provide that all equipment, machines, and tools meet the highest safety standards.
2. A requirement that all occupational injuries and accidents be reported and corrective action taken to ensure that similar incidents do not occur.
3. Clear explanations to all employees of the safety and health hazards to which they are exposed and the establishment of training progams to inform employees of how to minimize their risk of being affected.
4. Regularly scheduled systems safety analyses of all processes and work stations to identify potential safety hazards so that corrective actions can be taken before accidents occur.
5. Disciplinary procedures for employees who engage in unsafe behavior and for supervisors who encourage or permit unsafe activities.

While the chief executive officer is charged with the ultimate responsibility for the safety of all employees, this responsibility should be delegated and shared throughout the organization.

Larger companies may employ a full-time safety director to manage the safety program. Ideally, this person should be a Certified Safety Professional. The safety director works with all departments to ensure that related safety principles are being observed and monitored.

Line supervisors are responsible to ensure that appropriate and safe equipment are available for employee use, that employees adhere to safety standards, regulations, and safe work practices, and that injuries are promptly reported and treated. Safety contests have been used to promote and encourage worksite safety practices; however, caution should be taken that these competitions do not undermine the safety effort through inaccurate or underreporting of injuries.

Occupational health personnel, including nurses and physicians, are integral to the safety program through identification of workplace hazards from observations and worker complaints, and through the provision of primary treatment of injured employees. Health personnel must work closely with the line supervisors to help prevent repeated accidents and injuries by providing data related to the causes of workplace injuries and ensuring prompt injury reporting.

Employee participation in the safety program is critical to its success. This includes participation in safety education and training about specific job related hazards, design and discussion of safer methods to perform the job, maintenance of a safe work area and practices, and appropriate use and maintenance of work equipment and personal protective equipment, when needed.

Boylston (1990) suggests that the safety and health committee be divided into eight task groups including the following:

- Safety activities
- Rules and procedures
- Inspections and audits
- Fire and emergency
- Education and training
- Health and environmental
- Accident and investigation
- Housekeeping

However, the division of tasks and groups may be dependent on the size of the company. Thus, in a smaller company, task groups may be combined or composed of smaller numbers. Each task group must develop its goals and objectives annually, which then become part of the overall safety and health plan. The purpose and activities of each task area is briefly summarized below.

Safety activities involve overseeing the entire safety program to ensure program effectiveness in reducing illness and injury and include the following:

- review annually safety program activities
- determine strategies to obtain employee input regarding program activities
- recommend special safety emphasis programs
- analyze workplace injuries to determine strategies for corrective actions
- publicize safety programs (e.g., bulletin boards, pamphlets, brochures)
- disseminate safety information to employees
- coordinate safety awards/conferences/contests

Rules and procedures communicate to all managers, supervisors, and employees safe ways to perform every job. Specific activities include the following:

- recommend compliance procedures that can be followed
- audit the workplace for compliance with procedures and recommend corrective actions
- develop and review the safety manual and make it accessible in each department (Fig. 6–8)

Text continued on p. 134

SAFETY MANUAL CHECKLIST		Date:
		Page 1 of 5
Employer	**Facility**	**Unit**
Address		

General Information

Every employer should have a safety and health policies and procedures manual. A written manual is important to:

- Document company/governmental safety and health policies

- Train and educate employees as to safety and health policies

- Establish a safety and health management program that includes both management and hourly employees

- Enforce safety policies fairly and consistently

- Organize and address all safety and health issues

This manual should be developed with input from all levels of the organization. Every policy should be written and feasible, employees trained, and the policies enforced. A number of resources are available to obtain prepared policies that can be adapted to a worksite. Those resources include:

- Governmental Regulatory Agencies

- Industry Associations

- Safety and Industrial Hygiene Associations

- National Safety Council's *Accident Prevention Manual*

- OSHA, ANSI, NFPA, etc., Standards

■ **Figure 6–8**   Sample checklist form for safety and health manual. (From Boylston, R. Managing safety and health programs. New York: Van Nostrand Reinhold, 1990.)

Illustration continued on following page

SAFETY MANUAL CHECKLIST		Date:		
		Page 2 of 5		
Check When Complete	**Subject**	**To Be Developed By**	**Dates**	
			Target	**Completed**

	I. Safety and Health Program/ Organization
	
	A. Policy Statement
	B. Central Safety Committee/Task Groups
	     1. Safety Activities Task Group
	     2. Rules and Procedures Task Group
	     3. Inspections and Audits Task Group
	     4. Fire and Emergency Task Group
	     5. Education and Training Task Group
	     6. Health and Environmental Task Group
	     7. Accident Investigation Task Group
	     8. Housekeeping Task Group
	C. Plant Safety and Health Committee
	
	II. Safety and Health Rules
	
	A. General Plant Safety and Health Rules
	B. Specific Division/Department Rules
	
	III. Duties and Responsibilities
	
	A. Chief Executive Officer, Ranking Official
	B. Directors, Managers, and Supervisors
	C. Employees
	D. Plant Safety and Health Coordinator
	E. Employee and Supervisory Performance Appraisals
	F. Central Safety Committee and Task Group Responsibilities			

■ **Figure 6–8** *Continued*

SAFETY MANUAL CHECKLIST		Date:		
		Page 3 of 5		
Check When Complete	Subject	To Be Developed By	Dates	
			Target	Completed
	IV. Safety and Health Training			
	A. Employee Selection and Placement			
	B. Safety Orientation and Training			
	C. Supervisory Safety Training			
	D. Employee Safety Meetings and Contacts			
	E. Special Safety and Health Training			
	1. Transfers			
	2. New Assignments			
	V. Accident/Incident Response			
	A. Accident Reporting			
	B. Accident Investigation			
	C. Injury and Illness Recordkeeping			
	D. Transportation of Injured/Ill Employees			
	E. Notification of Injured's Family			
	VI. Inspection and Audit Programs			
	A. Safety Audit and Inspection Procedure			
	B. Safety Inspection Checklists			
	C. Safety Audits of New or Modified Equipment and Facilities			
	D. Capital Project Insurance Review Procedure			
	E. Monitoring for Air Contaminants			
	F. Monitoring for Physical Health Hazards			
	VII. Effective Management Action			
	A. Corrective Action Procedures			
	B. Follow-Up Assessments			
	C. Safety Work Orders			

■ **Figure 6–8** *Continued*

Illustration continued on following page

Check When Complete	SAFETY MANUAL CHECKLIST		Date:		
			Page 4 of 5		
Check When Complete	Subject	To Be Developed By	Dates		
			Target	Completed	

Check When Complete	Subject	To Be Developed By	Target	Completed
	VIII. Safety Permits			
	A. Permit Systems			
	B. Confined Space Entry			
	C. Hot Work Permit			
	D. Electrical Hot Work Permit			
	E. Temporary Wiring Permit			
	IX. Electrical Safety			
	A. Hazardous Locations			
	B. Temporary Electrical Wiring			
	C. Electrical Safety for Employees			
	X. OSHA Inspections			
	XI. Contractor and Visitor Safety and Health			
	XII. Safety and Health Procedures			
	A. Emergency Action Plan			
	1. Fire and Explosions			
	2. Chemical Leaks and Spills			
	3. Meteorological Occurrences			
	4. Bomb Threats/Public Disorders			
	B. Hazard Communication Program			
	C. Locking and Tagging Procedure			
	D. Respiratory Protection Program			
	E. Job Safety and Health Analysis			
	F. Hearing Conservation Program			
	G. Medical Surveillance Program			
	H. Employee Exposure and Medical Records Policy			
	I. Confined Space Entry			
	J. Hot Work Procedures			
	K. Personal Protective Equipment			
	L. Barricade Procedures			
	M. Ladders, Scaffolds, Platforms, Manlifts			

■ **Figure 6–8** *Continued*

SAFETY MANUAL CHECKLIST			Date:		
			Page 5 of 5		
Check When Complete	Subject	To Be Developed By	Dates		
			Target	Completed	
	N. Office Safety				
	O. Walking and Working Surfaces				
	P. Manual Material Handling				
	Q. Machinery and Equipment				
	R. Compressed Gas Storage and Handling				
	S. Housekeeping				
	T. Railroad Safety				
	U. Forklifts, Industrial Trucks				
	V. Cranes and Hoists				
	W. Tools				
	X. Fall Protection				
	Y. Color Coding				
	Z. Excavating				
	AA. Traffic Rules				
	BB. Flammable and Combustible Liquids				
	CC. Open Flames and Sparks				
	DD. Fire Protection				
	EE. Compressed Air				
	FF. Process Hazards				
	GG. Fleet Safety and Vehicle Maintenance				
	HH. Asbestos Maintenance and Removal				

■ **Figure 6–8** *Continued*

- recommend necessary training and enforcement procedures
- review rules/procedures annually and update them with input from other groups
- review, evaluate, and recommend improvements in recordkeeping
- establish minimum safety rules (Table 6–11)

Inspection and audit involves identifying workplace hazards through systematic inspection and recommending corrective actions for defects and to prevent occurrences (Fig. 6–9). Specific activities include the following:

- determine what is to be inspected and by whom
- develop audit/inspection checklist and determine inspection frequency (i.e., periodic, special, continuous)
- establish and participate in inspection procedures
- compile statistics on injury events
- highlight repeated injury events and problem areas and recommend control strategies
- ensure equipment maintenance
- monitor inspection outcomes for timely deficit correction

Accident investigation involves determining cause for accident occurrence and formulating methods to prevent recurrence. Specific activities include the following:

- investigate accident events promptly and document them
- review all accident reports to identify potential and actual causes and determine best control strategies
- discuss accident occurrence with employees and methods to reduce risk of recurrence
- observe work areas for contributing factors
- follow up to determine compliance with directives and abatement of hazard
- compile statistics for analysis
- maintain records

Education and training involve assisting employees to recognize safety hazards and how to control them. Specific activities include the following:

- manage and coordinate the safety education and training program related to, for example, new employees, new regulations, new work processes, new procedures, employee transfers, and national standards (e.g., ANSI) (A sample checklist for new employee orientation is shown in Figure 6–10.)
- establish a training schedule and assign administrative responsibilities
- maintain and store training records
- evaluate training effectiveness for content and instruction

Health and environment involve coordinating all health and environment activities in the organization and recommending measures for health promotion and protection, environment protection, and hazard reduction or elimination. Specific activities include the following:

- review safety program to ensure adequate health emphasis
- conduct on-site inspections with safety personnel to identify potential/actual exposures
- recommend control strategies to reduce health hazard exposures

■ **TABLE 6–11** Minimum Safety Rules

1. All plant injuries must be reported immediately to supervision and medical staff.
2. Horseplay, scuffling, and fighting are prohibited.
3. Unauthorized operation or maintenance of equipment is prohibited.
4. Rings, bracelets, wristwatches, loose adornments, long hair (at or below shoulder), and loose clothing must not be worn within 3 feet of operating machinery or moving products.
5. All guards and safety devices must be in place before equipment is operated, except as provided in written approved procedures.
6. "Lock, tag, and try" procedures described in written company safety procedures must be followed by all employees to avoid injury while repairing, adjusting, or cleaning machinery or processes.
7. Roped-off or barricaded areas may be entered only by permission of personnel working in the en-closed area or of the supervisor responsible for the work.
8. Safety spectacles must be worn as minimum eye protection for protection against flying objects, glare, and radiation, as specified by job safety procedures. Goggles are required for employees using air hoses to blow off equipment and for liquid splash protection.
9. Strike-anywhere matches, firearms, explosives, and ammunition are prohibited unless authorized.
10. Smoking is permitted only in designated areas. Cigarettes, cigars, and matches must be discarded only in ashtrays and specifically identified containers.
11. Posted speed limits for in-plant and outside vehicles must be observed.
12. Intoxicants, narcotics, and persons under the influence of these are prohibited in the plant, except as authorized by medical staff.
13. Emergency exits, evacuation routes, and emergency equipment must not be obstructed.
14. Running in the plant is prohibited, except to prevent loss of life or serious injury.
15. All chemicals used in the plant must be approved through the Central Safety and Health Committee, and chemical containers must be identified.
16. All scissors, knives, razor blades, and sharp-pointed tools used by employees must be specifically approved by management for their intended use.

From Boylston, R. Managing safety and health programs. New York: Van Nostrand Reinhold, 1990.

Fire and emergency include developing and implementing effective emergency management procedures to protect people, property, and the environment. Specific activities include the following:

- develop written emergency plan and organize an emergency response program (e.g., safety, security, fire brigade) including damage control, follow-up, and operation resumption
- develop proper training program
- conduct mock emergency preparedness situations
- disseminate emergency plan to all employees (department contact person, report mechanisms, escape procedures, employee accountability, rescue/medical duties, training, evaluation)
- evaluate new facilities, equipment, and work processes to identify potential emergency situations and controls
- evaluate procedures for emergency preparedness

Housekeeping involves maintaining proper mechanisms for workplace cleanliness and orderliness to help enhance safety, productivity, and morale. Specific activities include the following:

- observe workplace for safe and clean work surfaces
- ensure clutter-free stairways, corridors

Text continued on page 140

SAFETY AND HEALTH INSPECTION	Date		Page 1 of 3		
Organization		Location			Unit
Inspection Time—From To		Inspectors			
General—This safety and health inspection checklist is intended as a reminder for inspectors. It does not and cannot cover all safety and health items. Refer to specific standards, codes, and regulations for more details concerning safety and health inspection requirements.					
No.	**Item**	**Reference**	**Yes**	**No**	**Comments**
	Rules and Procedures				
1.	Are rules and procedures known, under-stood, and followed?				
2.	Are assignments performed right—the safe way?				
	Housekeeping				
3.	Is the work area clean and orderly?				
4.	Are floors free from protruding nails, splinters, holes, and loose boards?				
5.	Are aisles and passageways kept clear of obstructions?				
6.	Are permanent aisles and passageways clearly marked?				
7.	Are covers or guardrails in place around open pits, tanks, and ditches?				
	Floor and Wall Openings				
8.	Are ladderways and door openings guarded by a railing?				
9.	Do skylights have screens or fixed railings to prevent someone from falling through?				
10.	Do temporary floor openings have standard railings or someone constantly on guard?				
11.	Are wall openings with a drop of more than 4 feet guarded by a standard railing?				
12.	Are open-sided floors, platforms, and run-ways with a drop of more than 4 feet guarded by a standard railing and toeboard?				
13.	Do all stairways with 4 or more risers have a handrail?				
14.	Are stairways strong enough? too steep? adequately illuminated? slip resistant?				

■ **Figure 6–9**   Sample checklist for safety and health inspection. (From Boylston, R. Managing safety and health programs. New York: Van Nostrand Reinhold, 1990.)

No.	Item	Reference	Yes	No	Comments
	SAFETY AND HEALTH INSPECTION CHECK SHEET	No: Page 2 of 3			
	Means of Exit				
15.	Are there enough exits to allow prompt escape?				
16.	Do employees have easy access to exits?				
17.	Are exits unlocked to allow egress?				
18.	Are exits clearly marked?				
19.	Are exits and exit routes equipped with emergency lighting?				
	Personal Protective Equipment				
20.	Is required equipment provided, maintained, and used?				
21.	Does equipment meet safety requirements? Is it reliable?				
	Employee Facilities				
22.	Are facilities kept clean and sanitary?				
23.	Are toilets kept clean and in good repair?				
24.	Are cafeteria facilities provided where toxic chemicals are used? Do employees use them?				
	Medical and First Aid				
25.	Is there a hospital, clinic, or infirmary nearby?				
26.	Are employees trained as first-aid practitioners present on each shift worked?				
27.	Are physician-approved first-aid supplies available?				
28.	Are first-aid supplies replenished as they are used?				
	Fire Protection				
29.	Are fire extinguishers suitable for the type of fire most likely in that area?				
30.	Are enough extinguishers present to do the job?				
31.	Are extinguisher locations conspicuously marked?				
32.	Are extinguishers properly mounted and easily accessible?				
33.	Are all extinguishers fully charged and operable?				
34.	Are special-purpose extinguishers clearly marked?				

■ **Figure 6–9** *Continued*

Illustration continued on following page

SAFETY AND HEALTH INSPECTION CHECK SHEET		No:			
		Page 3 of 3			
No.	**Item**	**Reference**	**Yes**	**No**	**Comments**
	Materials Handling and Storage				
35.	Is adequate clearance allowed in aisles where materials must be moved?				
36.	Are tiered materials stacked, interblocked, locked and limited in height to maintain stability?				
37.	Are storage areas kept free of tripping, fire, explosion, and pest hazards?				
38.	Is proper drainage provided?				
39.	Are signs warning of clearance limits posted?				
40.	Are powered industrial truck operators adequately trained?				
	Machine Guarding				
41.	Are point-of-operation guards in place and working on all operating equipment?				
42.	Are all belts and pulleys that are less than 7 feet from the floor (and within reach of workers) guarded?				
43.	Are spinning parts guarded?				
	Electrical				
44.	Are all machines properly grounded?				
45.	Are portable hand tools grounded or double insulated?				
46.	Are junction boxes closed?				
47.	Are extension cords out of the aisles (where they might be abused by heavy traffic)?				
48.	Are extension cords being used as permanent wiring? (It's a dangerous thing to do.)				

■ **Figure 6–9** *Continued*

SUBJECT: NEW EMPLOYEE ORIENTATION AND TRAINING CHECKLIST

Name:_____ S.S.# _____

Job Assignment: _____ Supervisor: _____

Employment Date: _____

1. By Personnel Department on the First Day of Employment:

   ☐ Management's safety and health philosophy

   ☐ Management's, supervisor's, and employees' safety and health responsibilities

   ☐ General plant safety and health rules

   ☐ Hazard communication audiovisual presentation

   ☐ Location and availability of the hazard communication program

   ☐ Access to employee exposure and medical records

Completed by: _____ Date: _____

2. By New Employee's Immediate Supervisor

   A. First Day in Work Area   Date: _____

   ☐ Introduction to operations where chemical and physical hazards are present
      —types of hazards encountered

   ☐ Required work practices

   ☐ Personal protective equipment

   ☐ Emergency procedures

   ☐ Detection of chemical hazards

   ☐ Location and availability of Material Safety Data Sheets

   ☐ Labeling systems

   B. One Week Follow-up   Date: _____

   ☐ Review work practices and procedures with employee

   ☐ Answer employee questions

   ☐ Return completed checklist to Personnel Department for filing in employee
      personnel folder.

Completed by: _____ Date: _____

Employee's Signature: _____ Date: _____

■ **Figure 6–10**   New employee orientation and training checklist. (From Boylston, R. Managing safety and health programs. New York: Van Nostrand Reinhold, 1990.)

- manage waste and spill refuse
- report noted deficits affecting worksite safety

Within the context of a multidisciplinary effort, the occupational health nurse has an important role contributing to the overall management of the safety program. Training and education of workers about safety issues, initiation of effective prevention strategies, and full participation on health and safety committees are part of the effort. The occupational health nurse will need to work with management to secure a commitment to an active safety program.

■ ERGONOMICS

Historical evidence exists in the writings of Ramazzini (1713), in what we now refer to or think of as ergonomic factors, regarding the effects of work on the worker, wherein he writes:

> The maladies that affect the clerks (aforesaid) arise from three causes: first, constant sitting, secondly, the incessant movement of the hand and always in the same direction, thirdly, the strain on the mind from the effort not to disfigure the books by errors or cause loss to their employers when they add, subtract, or do other sums in arithmetics.

This historical perspective provides some insight into the long-standing problem of matching the worker to the job and work environment, within the context of effective, healthy, and safe human capabilities. Ergonomics-related injuries are a rapidly growing concern in today's workplace. For example, the Bureau of National Affairs reports the following:

- In 1990, $27 billion was spent on cumulative trauma disorders (CTDs). This includes medical care and lost income.
- U.S. corporations face more than 16 million lost workdays each year as a result of CTDs.
- In 1988, more than $10 billion (about a third of workers' compensation) was paid for repetitive motion injuries.
- The number of reported cases of repetitive motion has increased eight-fold since 1981 from slightly more than 20,000 to nearly 160,000.
- More than half of the recordable injuries in 1989 and 1990 were ergonomic-related.
- In 1989, the Bureau of Labor Statistics reported that 52% of all occupational illnesses result from cumulative trauma disorders (CTDs). The CTD incidence rate has increased more than 3,000% among certain clothing industry sectors and more than 2,500% among automobile workers.
- 40 million people who work with visual display terminals have suffered an unprecedented increase in CTDs.
- Postal service workers who are 27% of the federal work force filed 60% of the federal workers' compensation on carpal tunnel syndrome in 1990. The number of reported CTD cases among postal workers nearly doubled between 1989 and 1990 resulting in $3.8 million in benefits being paid to injured postal workers.

In addition to increased awareness by industry, employees, and government in reporting ergonomic-related disorders, the frequency of these injuries are due to changes in work processes and technology that expose employees to increased repetitive motion risk factors, resulting in increased costs (USDOL, 1991). This has brought about the need for finding effective solutions to manage ergonomic hazards and problems in the workplace.

The term ergonomics is derived from two Greek words, "ergos" meaning work and "nomos" meaning laws; thus the laws of work. Ergonomics has been defined by several authors; however, Keyserling and Armstrong (1992) define ergonomics as "the study of humans at work and the evaluation of the stresses that occur in the work environment and the ability of people to cope with these stresses. The goal of ergonomics is to design facilities (e.g., factories and offices), furniture, equipment, tools, and job demands to be compatible with human dimensions, capabilities, and expectations, and thus reduce stress. All work, regardless of its nature, places both physical and mental stresses on the worker." The National Safety Council offers a simple but consistent definition: "Ergonomics is the science of designing the job and the workplace to fit the worker. The goal of ergonomics is to allow work to be done without undue stress." Within the framework of these definitions the goal remains the same, that is, to match job demands and requirements to the abilities and capabilities of the worker (Sluchak, 1992).

Keyserling and Armstrong (1992) state that ergonomics is a multidisciplinary science with four major areas of specialization:

1. Human factors engineering (sometimes called engineering psychology) is concerned wtih the information processing requirement of work. Major applications include designing displays (e.g., gauges, warning buzzers, signs, instructions) and controls to enhance performance and minimize the likelihood of error.
2. Anthropometry is concerned with the measurement and statistical characterization of body size. Anthropometric data provide important information to the designers of clothing, furniture, machines, and tools.
3. Occupational biomechanics is concerned with the mechanical properties of human tissue, particularly the response of tissue to mechanical stress. A major focus of occupational biomechanics is the prevention of over-exertion disorders of the low back and upper extremities.
4. Work physiology is concerned with the responses of the cardiovascular system, pulmonary system, and skeletal muscles to the metabolic demands of work. This discipline is concerned with the prevention of whole body and localized fatigue.

Although ergonomics is concerned with matching work and job design to fit the capabilities of most people by adapting the product to fit the user rather than vice versa, Pheasant (1991) and Rodgers (1992) state that the design of the work environment should be flexible enough to consider the need for individual variation (Sluchak, 1992). For example, two people with the same height and weight may have a different arm reach or strength, and accommodations for those differences should be available. In order to make these changes, anthropometric analysis, that is, determining the relationship of the physical features of the human body (e.g., weight, size, range of motion) to the work and environment, may need to be taken into account.

Several studies have been done citing numerous health problems, such as back injuries (Bigos et al., 1986; Jensen, 1987), carpal tunnel disorders (Moore & Garg, 1991; Nathan et al., 1988; Osorio, 1993), and neurologic problems

(Mandel, 1987) as a result of ergonomic hazards. In addition, OSHA has written guidelines, *Ergonomics Program Management Guidelines for Meatpacking Plants,* to address growing concern regarding CTDs and other work-related ergonomic problems in the meatpacking industry (USDOL, 1991). However, these guidelines can be adapted for use in other settings. The OSHA ergonomic guidelines are intended to provide information to help employers:

- determine if they have ergonomic-related problems in their workplaces
- identify the nature and location of these problems
- implement measures to reduce or eliminate the problems

While the scope of these guidelines will not be fully described, the major elements will be reviewed. Hales and Bertsche (1992), however, provide an extensive discussion of the application of the guidelines.

Critical to the development of any program is management commitment and employee involvement. This is outlined by OSHA as follows:

1. Obtain management commitment to reduce ergonomic hazards through active participation, policy development, resource allocation, and accountability for program implementation at all levels in the organization.
2. Develop a goal-directed written program for job safety, health, and ergonomics that is communicated to all employees.
3. Encourage employee involvement in the ergonomics program and decision making through mechanisms that bring their concerns to management, and procedures that support the reporting, analysis, resolution and monitoring of ergonomic problems.
4. Develop mechanisms to evaluate program progress including analysis of trends in illness/injury rates, employee surveys, and management's evaluation of job/worksite changes (USDOL, 1991).

In keeping with OSHA's emphasis on management commitment and employee involvement, Travers (1992) points out that successful program implementation is most often seen in the gradual steps of continuous improvement that focus on implementation of employee education programs on ergonomics; customizing work areas with relatively inexpensive assistive devices or accommodations; increasing awareness so that new office or production designs incorporate ergonomic principles before a new facility is built or a process becomes operational; identifying health patterns or trends so that intervention strategies can be prioritized; and reporting to upper management the return on investment so that ergonomic strategies are viewed as cost effective.

The OSHA ergonomic guidelines (USDOL, 1991) describe four major program elements including worksite analysis, hazard prevention and control, medical management, and training and education. Worksite analysis identifies existing hazards and conditions, operations that create hazards, and areas where hazards develop. This should include the following:

1. An analysis of all illness and injury records for evidence of ergonomic problems and trends related to specific departments, jobs, titles
2. Identification of jobs, operations, processes, and work stations or methods that contribute to ergonomic risk factors. For example, some of the risk factors for CTDs include the following:
   - repetitive and/or prolonged activities

- forceful exertions, usually with the hands (including pinch grips)
- prolonged static postures
- awkward postures of the upper body, including reaching above the shoulders or behind the back, and twisting the wrists and other joints to perform tasks
- continued physical contact with work surfaces (e.g., contact with edges)
- excessive vibration from power tools
- cold temperatures
- inappropriate or inadequate hand tools

2. Risk factors for back disorders include items such as the following:
   - bad body mechanics including (1) continued bending over at the waist; (2) continued lifting from below the knuckles or above the shoulders; and (3) twisting at the waist, especially while lifting
   - lifting or moving objects of excessive weight or asymmetric size
   - prolonged sitting, especially with poor posture
   - lack of adjustable chairs, footrests, body supports, and work surfaces at work stations
   - poor grips on handles
   - slippery footing

3. Performance of initial and periodic job hazard analysis in order to detect situations that place workers at risk of ergonomic hazards. This would include an analysis of the work environment, work station, and manual materials lifting. Use of a videotape analysis method is recommended, if feasible.

An ergonomic workplace analysis can be facilitated through use of a workplace checklist specific for ergonomic concerns. This will help to provide for a systematic analysis approach, and obtain objective, quantifiable data. An example can be found in Table 6–12.

As described in the OSHA guidelines, hazard prevention and control of ergonomic risks is accommodated primarily through effective design of the work station, tools, and jobs through engineering, work practice, personal protective equipment, and administrative controls. Engineering techniques, where feasible, are the preferred method of control. The focus of an ergonomics program is to make the job fit the person, not to force the person to fit the job. This can be accomplished by designing or modifying the work station, work methods, and tools to eliminate excessive exertion and awkward postures and to reduce repetitive motion. Work stations should be easily adjustable and either designed or selected to fit a specific task so they are comfortable for the workers using them. Work methods should be designed to reduce static, extreme, and awkward postures, repetitive motion, and excessive force. Work method design addresses the content of tasks performed by the workers.

The appropriate tool should be used to do a specific job. Tools and handles should be selected to eliminate or minimize the following stressors:

- chronic muscle contraction or steady force
- extreme or awkward finger/hand/arm positions
- repetitive forceful motions
- tool vibration
- excessive gripping, pinching, or pressing with the hand and fingers

■ **TABLE 6-12** A Sample Ergonomic Checklist to Identify Potential Hazards in the Workplace

General Work Environment
    Workforce characteristics
        Age, sex, anthropometrics (body size and proportions)
        Strength, endurance, fitness
        Disabilities
        Diminished senses
        Communication/language problems (e.g., non-English-speaking or illiterate workers)
    Lighting
    Climate
    Noise level
    Health and safety safeguards
Job and Workstation Design
    Location of controls, displays, equipment, stock
        Accessibility
        Visibility
        Legibility
        Efficiency of sequence of movements during operation or use
        Use of pedals
        Posture of workers
           Sitting, standing, combination
           Possibility for variation
           Stooping, twisting, or bending of the spine
        Chair availability, adjustments
        Room to move about
        Work surface height
    Predominantly dynamic or static work
        Alternation possible
        Use of devices such as clamps or jigs to avoid static work
        Availability of supports for arms, elbows, hands, back, feet
Muscle-Work-Load Task Demands
    Repetitiveness
        Frequency
        Force
        Availability of rest pauses
        Possibility for alternative work
        Skill, vigilance, perception demands
        Efficiency of organization (supplies, equipment)
    Use of hand tools
        Hand and wrist posture during use
        Work surface height
        Size and weight of tool
        Necessity, availability of supports
        Shape, dimensions, and surface of hand grip
        Vibratory or nonvibratory
Physical strength requirements
    Strength capabilities
    Working pulses/respiratory rate
    Loads lifted, carried, pushed, or pulled
        Manner in which handled
        Weight and dimensions of objects handled

Reprinted by permission of the American Association of Occupational Health Nurses from Frederick, L, Habes, D, Schloemer, J. AAOHN Journal, *32*(12): 643–645, 1984.

Key elements of a good work practice program for ergonomics include proper work techniques, employee conditioning, regular monitoring, feedback, maintenance, adjustments and modifications, and enforcement. A program for proper work techniques, such as the following, includes appropriate training and practice time for employees:

- proper maneuvering techniques, including work methods that improve posture and reduce stress and strain on extremities
- correct lifting techniques (proper body mechanics)
- proper use and maintenance of tools and equipment
- correct use of ergonomically designed work stations and fixtures

Personal protective equipment (PPE) should be selected with ergonomic stressors in mind. Appropriate PPE should be provided in a variety of sizes, should accommodate the physical requirements of workers and the job, and should not contribute to extreme postures and excessive forces.

A sound overall ergonomics program includes administrative controls that reduce the duration, frequency, and severity of exposures to ergonomic stressors. Examples of administrative methods include the following:

- reducing the total number of repetitions per employee by such means as decreasing production rates and limiting overtime work
- providing rest pauses to relieve fatigued muscle-tendon groups. The length of time needed depends on the task's overall effort and total cycle time
- increasing the number of employees assigned to a task to alleviate severe conditions, especially in lifting heavy objects
- using job rotation with caution and as a preventive measure not as a response to symptoms
- effective housekeeping programs to minimize slippery work surfaces and related hazards such as slips and falls

Travers (1992) identifies several common ergonomic concerns and associated corrective measures in the office environment (Table 6–13, p. 148).

An effective ergonomic health and medical program should encompass a multidisciplinary approach and include early identification, evaluation, treatment, follow-up, rehabilitation, and recording of signs and symptoms by health care providers knowledgeable in these areas and with respect to the company's operations, work practices, and light duty jobs. A survey of employees can be conducted to measure employee awareness of work-related disorders, and to report the location, frequency and duration, of discomfort (Fig. 6–11) (Silverstein & Fine, 1984). Body diagrams can be used to facilitate and clarify information gathering. A physician or occupational health nurse with appropriate ergonomics prevention/management training should oversee the program. The health/medical management program as identified by OSHA (USDOL, 1991) should include:

- injury and illness recordkeeping
- early recognition and reporting
- systematic evaluation and referral
- conservative treatment
- conservative return to work

Symptoms Survey: *Ergonomics Program*

DATE_____/_____/_____

_____   _____   _____   _____
Plant   Dept #   Job #   Job Name

_____   _____   _____   _____years_____months
Shift   Supervisor   Hours worked/week   Time on THIS job

Other jobs you have done in the last year (for more than 2 weeks)

_____   _____   _____   _____   _____months_____weeks
Plant   Dept #   Job #   Job Name   Time on THIS job

_____   _____   _____   _____   _____months_____weeks
Plant   Dept #   Job #   Job Name   Time on THIS job

(If more than 2 jobs, include those you worked on the most)

Have you had any pain or discomfort during the last year?
❑ Yes   ❑ No   (If NO, stop here)

If YES, carefully shade in the area of the drawing which bothers you the MOST.

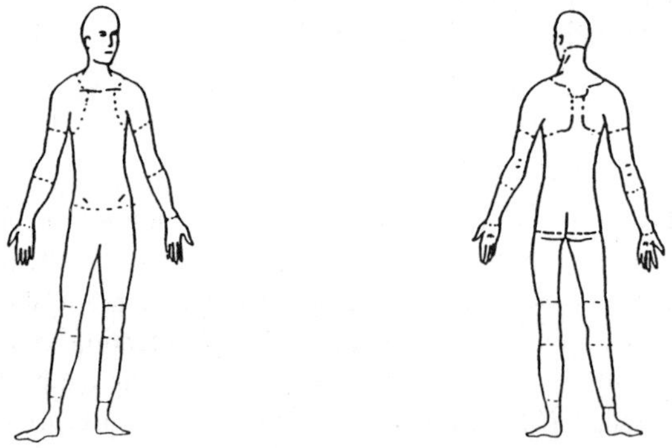

Front   Back

(Continued)

■ **Figure 6–11** Symptoms survey: ergonomics program. (From Silverstein, BA & Fine, L. Evaluation of upper extremity and low back cumulative trauma disorders. A screening manual. Ann Arbor, MI: University of Michigan, School of Public Health, 1984.)

- systematic monitoring
- adequate staffing and facilities.

In an effective program, health care providers should conduct periodic, systematic, workplace walkthroughs to remain knowledgeable about operations and work practices, to identify potential light duty jobs, and to maintain close contact

(Complete a separate page for each area that bothers you)

Check Area: ☐ Neck   ☐ Shoulder   ☐ Elbow/Forearm   ☐ Hand/Wrist   ☐ Fingers
　　　　　　 ☐ Upper Back   ☐ Low Back   ☐ Thigh/Knee   ☐ Low Leg   ☐ Ankle/Foot

1. Please put a check by the word(s) that best describe your problem
　　　☐ Aching
　　　☐ Burning
　　　☐ Cramping　　　　☐ Numbness (asleep)　　　☐ Tingling
　　　☐ Loss of Color　　☐ Pain　　　　　　　　　☐ Weakness
　　　　　　　　　　　　☐ Swelling　　　　　　　　☐ Other
　　　　　　　　　　　　☐ Stiffness

2. When did you first notice the problem? _____(month) _____(year)

3. How long does each episode last? (Mark an X along the line)

　　　_____/_____/_____/_____/_____
　　　　1 hour　　 1 day　　 1 week　　 1 month　　 6 months

4. How many separate episodes have you had in the last year?_____

5. What do you think caused the problem?_____
_____

6. Have you had this problem in the last 7 days?　　☐ Yes　　☐ No

7. How would you rate this problem (mark an X on the line)
　NOW

　None　　　　　　　　　　　　　　　　　　　　　　　　　　Unbearable

　When it was the WORST

　None　　　　　　　　　　　　　　　　　　　　　　　　　　Unbearable

8. Have you had medical treatment for this problem?　　☐ Yes　　☐ No
　　8a. If NO, why not_____

　　8b. If YES, where did you receive treament?_____
　　　　1. Company Medical ☐　　Times in past year_____
　　　　2. Personal doctor ☐　　Times in past year_____
　　　　3. Other ☐　　　　　　　Times in past year_____
　　8c. If YES, did the treatment help?　　☐ Yes　　☐ No

9. How much time have you lost in the last year because of this problem?_____days

10. How many days in the last year were you on restricted or light duty because of this problem?
　　_____days

11. Please comment on what you think would improve your symptoms
_____
_____
_____
_____

■ **Figure 6–11** *Continued*

with employees. Health care providers also should be involved in identifying risk factors for CTDs in the workplace as part of the ergonomic team. The ergonomist or other qualified person should analyze the physical procedures used in the performance of each job, including lifting requirements, postures, hand grips, and frequency of repetitive motion. The ergonomist and health care providers should develop a list of jobs with the lowest ergonomic risk. For such

■ **TABLE 6–13** Common Ergonomic Concerns and Corrective Measures*

Problems	Recommendations
Chair not adjusted; feet not flat on the floor; inadequate lumbar support.	**ENGINEERING CONTROLS** 1. Adjust height and position of chair so that feet are flat on floor, arms are close to the body. 2. Adequate lumbar support by using a rolled towel, pillow, cushion, or lumbar support. 3. Footrest. **ADMINISTRATIVE CONTROLS** 1. Employee education on adjusting chair and the importance of assuming varied postures throughout the course of any day.
Keyboard too high, causing wrists and elbows to be in non-neutral positions; reaching motions.	**ENGINEERING CONTROLS** 1. Lower keyboard by using desk drawer, articulating shelf, or lowering desk or table; or raise chair and use a footrest. 2. Position keyboard and other input devices to avoid reaching motions. **ADMINISTRATIVE CONTROLS** 1. Employee education on reasons for setting up areas to foster neutral body positions. 2. Work practice changes so that no one position is assumed for long periods of time.
Glare on terminal screen from overhead lighting or reflections from direct sunlight.	**ENGINEERING CONTROLS** 1. Place screen perpendicular to the light source. 2. Close blinds on windows or rearrange office setup to decrease glare from sunlight. **ADMINISTRATIVE CONTROLS** 1. Regularly clean screen so vision is not hampered by smudge marks or an accumulation of dust. 2. Have vision checked for viewing distance to screen. If needed, obtain glasses for specific viewing distance.
Terminal screen too low.	**ENGINEERING CONTROLS** 1. Raise terminal by using terminal stand, wooden box, or two-leveled stand.
Contact with sharp edges.	**ENGINEERING CONTROLS** 1. Pad edge of table or desk with foam rubber, cushion, towel, or wrist support. **ADMINISTRATIVE CONTROLS** 1. Employee education on how to set up work area, symptoms, reasons for symptoms, and ways to avoid discomfort.

*These are examples of some of the solutions that can be implemented.
Reprinted by permission of the American Association of Occupational Health Nurses from Travers, PH. AAOHN Journal, *40*(3): 129–137, 1992.

jobs, the ergonomic risk should be described. This information will assist health care providers in recommending assignments to light or restricted-duty jobs. The light-duty job should therefore not increase ergonomic stress on the same muscle-tendon groups. Prior to assignment, all new and transferred workers who are to be assigned to positions involving exposure of a particular body part to ergonomic stress should receive baseline health surveillance.

Baseline and periodic health surveillance should be performed on all workers who are assigned to positions involving exposure to a particular body part to an ergonomic stressor. Employees should be encouraged to report systems so that adequate evaluation, treatment, and follow-up of the specific condition can be received to prevent irreversible tissue damage and functional impairment.

In the work setting the health care professional must be knowledgeable and skilled to recognize symptoms and make appropriate decisions regarding etiology, and on-site treatment versus referral. The OSHA Ergonomics Guidelines Medical Management Section (USDOL, 1991) outlines specifics related to management of CTDs and provides a useful algorithm for management of upper extremity cumulative trauma disorders. A similar algorithm (Fig. 6–12) is provided by Hales and Bertsche (1992).

Training and education are critical components of an ergonomics program for employees potentially exposed to ergonomic hazards. Training allows managers, supervisors, and employees to understand ergonomic and other hazards associated with a job or production process, their prevention and control, and their health/medical consequences. Employees who are potentially exposed to ergonomic hazards should be given formal instruction on the hazards associated with their jobs and related equipment. New employees and reassigned workers should receive an initial orientation and hands-on training prior to being placed in a full-production job. On-the-job training should emphasize employee development and use of safe and efficient techniques.

Supervisors are responsible for ensuring that employees follow safe work practices and receive appropriate training to enable workers to follow through. Supervisors, therefore, should undergo training comparable to that of the employees, and such additional training as will enable them to recognize early signs and symptoms of CTDs, to recognize hazardous work practices, to correct such practices, and to reinforce the employer's ergonomic program, especially through the ergonomic training of employees as may be needed. Resolution of ergonomic problems is best accomplished through a team problem-solving approach. Rodgers (1992) provides several examples of aproaches to ergonomic problems utilizing a team oriented framework (Table 6–14).

■ OCCUPATIONAL MEDICINE

Occupational medicine is a subspecialty of preventive medicine as designated by the American Board of Preventive Medicine. While some medical schools offer some academic coursework in occupational medicine, post-graduate training in occupational medicine can be obtained through NIOSH Educational Resource Centers.

Felton (1990) offers a definition of occupational medicine as concerned with (1) the assessment, maintenance, restoration, and improvement of the health of the worker through the application of the principles of preventive medicine, emergency medical care, rehabilitation, and environmental medicine; (2) the

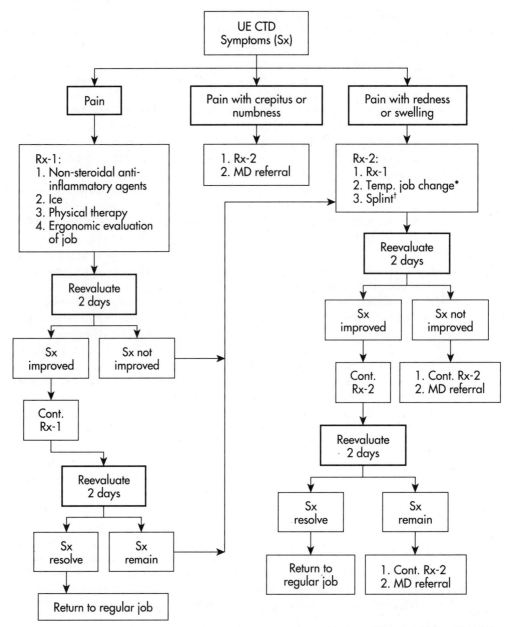

■ **Figure 6–12** Upper extremity cumulative trauma disorders algorithm. (Reprinted by permission of the American Association of Occupational Health Nurses from Hales, TR & Bertsche PK. AAOHN Journal, *40*(3): 118–128, 1992.)

promotion of a productive and fulfilling interaction of workers with their work, through the application of the principles of human behavior; and (3) the active appreciation of the social, enconomic, and administrative needs and responsibilities of both the worker and the work community.

Levy and Wegman (1988) state that physicians employed by companies have responsibilites in three general areas:

■ **TABLE 6–14** Examples of Approaches to Find Ergonomic Solutions

WORKPLACE DESIGN

1. Work height adjustments
   a. Adjust the work surface height
      (1) Adjustable height surface
      (2) Cut off or add blocks to work surface to change present height or use platform under supply bins
   b. Adjust height of person relative to work surface
      (1) Platforms
      (2) Chair adjustability
   c. Change the location of the operation to another part of the line where the height is more appropriate
2. Reach improvements
   a. Work height adjustments
      (1) Adjust work surface
      (2) Adjust person
   b. Reduce forward reach requirements
      (1) Work surface design changes (e.g., cut-outs)
      (2) Provision of reach extenders
3. Orientation of workplace and location of supplies
   a. Redesign line supply systems
      (1) Conveyors
      (2) Location relative to line
   b. Provide for resupply of parts from existing storage
      (1) Hoists
      (2) Roller conveyor sections
      (3) Hoppers

ENVIRONMENTAL DESIGN

1. Lighting
   a. Improve quality of lighting
      (1) Task lighting
      (2) Type of lighting
      (3) Glare reduction
   b. Use specialized lighting for inspection
      (1) Lighting angle adjustment
      (2) Special light sources (e.g., polarized light, projected stripes)
2. Temperature and humidity
   a. Modify ventilation systems
      (1) Two-speed fans
      (2) Alter duct or thermostat locations
   b. Provide localized cooled or heated areas
      (1) Break areas
      (2) Spot cooling or heating
   c. Vary workload requirements during hotter weather
      (1) Alternate tasks for recovery from heat exposure
      (2) Implement work practices to reduce heat illness

EQUIPMENT DESIGN AND SELECTION

1. Tools
   a. Choose best tool for task
      (1) Specialized tools—bend tool not wrist
      (2) Computer torque tools
      (3) Triggering versus push-to-start tools

Table continued on following page

■ **TABLE 6–14** Examples of Approaches to Find Ergonomic Solutions *Continued*

  b. Maintain tools
    (1) Vibration reduction
    (2) Keep torque capabilities
2. Provide protective equipment
  a. Vibration protection—Sorbothane/Viscolas
  b. Stall bars on tools
  c. Choice of gloves
  d. Choice of eye wear
3. Reduce complexity of information
  a. Use understandable, action-oriented language
  b. Provide troubleshooting aids
  c. Use legible presentation
    (1) Character size versus distance
    (2) Code use—shape, color, size, alphanumeric
    (3) Color contrast
    (4) Proper lighting
    (5) Reduce numbers of unnecessary quantitative displays

JOB DESIGN
1. Provide worker control
  a. Reduce tight external pacing
    (1) Incorporate in-process inventory or off-line areas in highly paced operations
    (2) Provide easy access to parts, close to line
    (3) Allow for some working ahead of or behind line speed
    (4) Provide a "floater" to help reduce pressure on line workers
  b. Provide training for new or transferred employees
    (1) Provide some off-line training initially
    (2) When a job, equipment, or methods change, provide some time for learning during its implementation
2. Reduce manual lifting demands
  a. Find ways to slide the load rather than lift it
    (1) Design to minimize handling
    (2) Adjust heights to permit horizontal transfer at about 75-100 cm (30-40 in.) above the floor
    (3) Use ball-bearing tables or roller conveyor sections to move parts between locations
  b. Use bulk transfer devices to handle parts
    (1) Hoppers, super sacks
    (2) Lowerators
    (3) Hoists, magnets
3. Train workers to increase their work capacities
  a. Provide on-the-job work-related fitness programs
  b. Identify skills and strengths/endurances for jobs that are difficult to redesign. Determine what capabilities are needed and look for people with those capabilities.

From Rodgers, S. Occupational Medicine: State of the Art Reviews, *7*(4): 679–712, 1992.

1. prevention and early detection of occupational disease and injury
2. diagnosis and treatment of occupational disease and injury (emphasizing return of workers to their job)
3. diagnosis and treatment of nonoccupational disease or injury in emerging situations or when community resources are unavailable

Some of what is described in these definitions represents overlapping or shared functions with nursing and/or other disciplines within the parameters of state practice acts; thus, the need for close collaboration between the occupational health nurse and physician is imperative. Felton (1990) points out that occupational health includes activities of all members of the occupational health team, and implies cooperative functioning of all members of the group charged with operation of a program in occupational health. There is much work to be done, and promoting and protecting worker health and this philosophy of collaboration is facilitative of this effort.

The occupational health nurse practicing in the clinical setting will need to be familiar with occupational diseases and injuries within the context of nursing practice and process. The occupational health nurse will find the addition of reference sources to her/his library in a variety of fields, such as textbooks in occupational medicine, safety, epidemiology, and toxicology very valuable.

■ SUMMARY

Effective assessment and management of workplace hazards and related health effects requires collaboration among multidisciplines. The occupational health nurse is often the primary health care professional at the worksite who is engaged in identifying work-related health hazards. As foundational to the knowledge base in occupational health nursing, the nurse must be familiar with key concepts and principles of related disciplinary knowledge. This will help to enhance skills and expertise in hazard recognition and control, and risk reduction. Collaborative efforts in providing health care at the worksite is essential in preventing unnecessary harm and risk, and protecting and promoting worker health and a safe and healthful work environment.

References

American Conference of Governmental Industrial Hygienists. Threshold limit values and biological exposure indices 1990–1991. Cincinnati: Author, 1990.

American Industrial Hygiene Association: Definition, scope, function and organization. American Industrial Hygiene Association Journal, *20:* 428, 1959.

Armitage, P. Multistage models of carcinogenesis. Environmental Health Perspectives, *63:* 195–201, 1985.

Becker, C. Gases. In J. LaDow (Ed.), Occupational medicine (pp. 432–442). Norwalk, CT: Appleton Lange, 1990.

Bigos S, Spengler, DM, Martin, NA, et al. Back injuries in industry: A retrospective study: II. Injury factors. Spine, *11:* 246–251, 1986.

Boylston, R. Managing safety and health programs. New York: Van Nostrand Reinhold, 1990.

Brain, JD & Valberg, PA. Aerosol deposition in the respiratory tract. American Reviews of Respiratory Diseases, *120:* 1325–1373, 1979.

Bureau of Labor Statistics. Annual survey of occupational injuries and illnesses. Washington, DC: Department of Labor, 1988a.

Bureau of Labor Statistics. Occupational injuries and illnesses in the U.S., by industry, 1986 Bulletin 2308. Washington, DC: Department of Labor, 1988b.

Buring, JE, Hennekens, CH, Mayrent, SL. Health experiences of operating room personnel. Anesthesiology, *62:* 325–330, 1985.

Danse, IR. Common sense toxics in the workplace. New York: Van Nostrand Reinhold, 1991.

Felton, J. Occupational medical management. Boston: Little, Brown & Company, 1990.

Fowler, D. Industrial hygiene. In J. Ladow (Ed), Occupational medicine (pp. 499–513). Norwalk, CT: Appleton Lange, 1990.

Framkin, H. Toxins and their effects. In B. Levy & D. Wegman (Eds.), Occupational health (2nd ed.) (pp. 193–214). Boston: Little, Brown & Company, 1988.

Frederick, L, Habes, D, & Schloemer, J. An introduction to the principles of ergonomics. AAOHN Journal, *32*(12): 643–645, 1984.

Gibaldi, M & Perrier, D. Pharmakokinetics. New York: Marcel Decker, 1982.

Gochfeld, M. Toxicology. In J. Last & R. Wallace (Eds.), Public health and preventive medicine (13th ed.) (p. 315–324). Norwalk, CT: Appleton & Lange, 1992a.

Gochfeld, M. Environmental risk assessment. In J. Last & R. Wallace (Eds.), Public health and preventive medicine (13th ed.) (p. 332–342). Norwalk, CT: Appleton & Lange, 1992b.

Hales, TR & Bertsche, PK. Managing of upper extremity cumulative trauma disorders. AAOHN Journal, 40(3): 118–128, 1992.

Hansen, D. The work environment: Occupational health fundamentals. Chelsea, MI: Lewis Publishers, 1991.

Hathaway, B. Toxicology: An overview. AAOHN Journal, 34(11): 518–523, 1986.

Heath, E. Safety and health training quality. In Proceedings of The Occupational Safety and Health Summit (pp. 59–88). Des Plaines, IL: American Society of Safety Engineers, 1992.

Holmberg, PC, Kurppa, K, Riala, R. Solvent exposures and birth defects: An epidemiologic survey. Progress in Clinical Biological Research, 220: 179–184, 1986.

Horstman, S. Industrial hygiene. In J. Last & R. Wallace (Eds.), Public health and preventive medicine (13th ed.) (pp. 547–550). Norwalk, CT: Appleton & Lange, 1992.

Jensen, RC. Disabling back injuries among nursing personnel: Research needs and justification. Research in Nursing and Health, 10: 29–38, 1987.

Jones, SE, Hosein HR, Swain, GR, & Yablonsky, SF. Occupational hygiene management guide. Chelsea, MI: Lewis Publishers, 1990.

Kayafas, N. Employee health and industrial hygiene. Independence, MS: TIV Press, 1989.

Keyserling, WM & Armstrong, TJ. Ergonomics. In J. Last & R. Wallace (Eds.), Public health and preventive medicine (13th ed.) (pp. 533–546). Norwalk, CT: Appleton & Lange, 1992.

Keyserling, WM. Occupational safety: Preventing accidents and overt trauma. In B. Levy & D. Wegman (Eds.), Occupational health (2nd ed.) (pp. 105–120). Boston: Little, Brown & Company, 1988.

Levy, B. & Wegman, D. Occupational health. Boston: Little, Brown & Company, 1988.

Lewis, R. Metals. In J. Ladou (Ed.), Occupational medicine (pp. 297–326). Norwalk, CT: Appleton & Lange, 1990.

Lilis, R. Diseases associated with exposure to chemical substances. In J. Last & R. Wallace (Eds.), Public health and preventive medicine, (13th ed.) (pp. 403–432). Norwalk, CT: Appleton & Lange, 1992.

Lioy, PJ. Assessing total human exposure to contaminants. Environmental Science Technology, 24(7): 938–945, 1990.

Mandel, S. Neurologic syndrome from repetitive trauma at work. Postgraduate Medicine, 82(6): 87–92, 1987.

Moore JS & Garg, A. Determination of the operational characteristics of ergonomic exposure assessments for prediction of disorders of the upper extremities and back. In Proceedings of the 11th Congress of the International Ergonomics Association. London, Taylor & Francis, pp. 144–146, 1991.

Nathan PA, Meadows, KD, & Doyle, LS. Occupation as a risk factor for impaired sensory conduction of the median nerve at the carpal tunnel. Journal of Hand Surgery, 13B, 167–170, 1988.

National Coalition of Agricultural Safety and Health. A Report to the nation: Agriculture at risk. Iowa City: The University of Iowa, 1989.

National Safety Council. Ergonomics: A practical guide. 1988.

National Safety Council. Work injury and illness rates. Chicago: Author, 1987.

Needleman, H, Gunnoe, C, Leviton, A, Reed, R, Peresie, H, Maher, C, & Berrett, P. Deficits in psychologic and classroom performance in children with elevated lead levels. New England Journal of Medicine, 300, 689–695, 1979.

Neuberger, JS, Harris, J, Kundin, ND, Bishone, A, & Chin, T. Incidence of needlestick injuries in hospital personnel: Implications for prevention. American Journal of Infection Control, 12(3): 171–176, 1984.

Osorio, A. Carpal tunnel syndrome among grocery store workers. In K. Steenland. Case studies in occupational epidemiology, (pp. 127–141). New York: Oxford University Press, 1993.

Ottoboni, MA. The dose makes the poison. New York: Van Nostrand Reinhold, 1991.

Paul, ME & Himmelstein, J. Reproductive hazards in the workplace: What the practitioner needs to know about chemical exposures. Obstetrics & Gynecology, 7: 921–926, 1988.

Pheasant, S. Ergonomics, work and health. Gaithersburg, MD: Aspen, 1991.

Plog, BA. Fundamentals of industrial hygiene. Chicago: National Safety Council, 1989.

Ramazzini, B. DeMorbis Artificum (1713). Trans. W.C. Wright. Diseases of Workers. Chicago: University of Chicago, 1940.

Rodgers, S. A functional job analysis technique.

Occupational Medicine: State of the Art Reviews, *7*(4): 679–712, 1992.

Rogers, B & Emmett, E. Handling antineoplastics agents: Urine mutagenicity in nursing personnel. Image, *19*(3): 108–113, 1987.

Schnorr, T. Video display terminals and adverse pregnancy outcomes. In K. Steenland. Case studies in occupational epidemiology (pp. 7–20). New York: Oxford University Press, 1993.

Selikoff, IJ & Lee, DH. Asbestos and disease. New York: Academic Press, 1978.

Silverstein, M. Labor unions and occupational health. In B. Levy & D. Wegman (Eds.), Occupational health (2nd ed.) (pp. 537–551). Boston: Little, Brown & Company, 1988.

Silverstein, BA & Fine, L. Evaluation of upper extremity and low back cumulative trauma disorders. A screening manual. Ann Arbor, MI: University of Michigan, School of Public Health, 1984.

Sluchak, TJ. Ergonomics: Origins, focus, and implementation considerations. AAOHN Journal, *40*(3): 105–112, 1992.

Smith, T. Industrial hygiene. In B. Levy & D. Wegman (Eds.), Occupational Health (2nd ed.) (pp. 87–104). Boston: Little, Brown & Company, 1988.

Travers, P. Application of toxicological concepts to the occupational history. AAOHN Journal, *34*(11): 524–529, 1986.

Travers, PH. Implementing ergonomic strategies in the workplace: An occupational health nursing perspective. AAOHN Journal, *40*(3): 129–137, 1992.

Upton, A. Ionizing radiation. In B. Levy & D. Wegman (Eds.), Occupational health (2nd ed.) (pp. 231–245). Boston: Little, Brown & Company, 1988.

U.S. Department of Agriculture. Hazard communication: A program guide for federal agencies. Washington, DC: U.S. Government Printing Office, 1987.

U.S. Department of Health and Human Services. National Institute for Occupational Safety & Health. Pocket guide to chemical hazards. NIOSH Pub # 90–117. Cincinnati: Author, 1990.

U.S. Department of Labor, Occupational Safety & Health Administration. Ergonomics program management guidelines for meatpacking plants. Publication # 3123. Washington, DC: Author, 1991.

Verma, D & Vernall, B. Principles of industrial hygiene. AAOHN Update Series, *2*(26): 2–11, 1985.

Weeks, J, Levy, B, & Wagner, G. Preventing occupational disease and injury. Washington, DC: American Public Health Association, 1991.

Wegman, D & Christian, D. Respiratory disorders. In B. Levy & D. Wegman (Eds.), Occupational health (2nd ed.) (pp. 319–344). Boston: Little, Brown & Company, 1988.

Williams, P & Burson, J. Industrial toxicology. New York: Van Nostrand Reinhold, 1985.

Wills, JH. Nasal carcinoma in woodworkers: A review. Journal of Occupational Medicine, *24:* 526–533, 1982.

Winder, C. Reproductive and chromosomal effects of occupational exposure to lead in the male. Reproductive Toxicology, *3:* 221–226, 1989.

AN OSHA Material Safety Data Sheet

Material Safety Data Sheet May be used to comply with OSHA's Hazard Communication Standard, 29 CFR 1910.1200. Standard must be consulted for specific requirements.	**U.S. Department of Labor** Occupational Safety and Health Administration (Non-Mandatory Form) Form Approved OMB No. 1218-0072
IDENTITY *(As Used on Label and List)*	Note: *Blank spaces are not permitted. If any item is not applicable, or no information is available, the space must be marked to indicate that.*

Section I

Manufacturer's Name	Emergency Telephone Number
Address *(Number, Street, City, State, and ZIP Code)*	Telephone Number for Information
	Date Prepared
	Signature of Preparer *(optional)*

Section II — Hazardous Ingredients/Identity Information

Hazardous Components (Specific Chemical Identity; Common Name(s))	OSHA PEL	ACGIH TLV	Other Limits Recommended	% *(optional)*

Section III — Physical/Chemical Characteristics

Boiling Point		Specific Gravity (H$_2$O = 1)	
Vapor Pressure (mm Hg.)		Melting Point	
Vapor Density (AIR = 1)		Evaporation Rate (Butyl Acetate = 1)	
Solubility in Water			
Appearance and Odor			

Section IV — Fire and Explosion Hazard Data

Flash Point (Method Used)	Flammable Limits	LEL	UEL
Extinguishing Media			
Special Fire Fighting Procedures			
Unusual Fire and Explosion Hazards			

Section V — Reactivity Data

Stability	Unstable		Conditions to Avoid
	Stable		

Incompatibility (*Materials to Avoid*)

Hazardous Decomposition or Byproducts

Hazardous Polymerization	May Occur		Conditions to Avoid
	Will Not Occur		

Section VI — Health Hazard Data

Route(s) of Entry:	Inhalation?	Skin?	Ingestion?

Health Hazards (*Acute and Chronic*)

Carcinogenicity:	NTP?	IARC Monographs?	OSHA Regulated?

Signs and Symptoms of Exposure

Medical Conditions
Generally Aggravated by Exposure

Emergency and First Aid Procedures

Section VII — Precautions for Safe Handling and Use

Steps to Be Taken in Case Material Is Released or Spilled

Waste Disposal Method

Precautions to Be Taken in Handling and Storing

Other Precautions

Section VIII — Control Measures

Respiratory Protection (*Specify Type*)

Ventilation	Local Exhaust	Special	
	Mechanical (*General*)	Other	

Protective Gloves	Eye Protection

Other Protective Clothing or Equipment

Work/Hygienic Practices

APPENDIX

6–2

A Manufacturer's Material Safety Data Sheet

Vinyl Chloride
CAS #75-01-4

Manufacturer's Name & Address
XYZ Chemical, Inc.
440-01 Carcin Alley
Elizabeth, New Jersey 07231

Emergency Contact
John H. Doe (615) 211-2233

Information Contact
Susan S. Smith (615) 211-2234

Prepared By
Susan S. Smith

Date Prepared
2/18/94

Chemical Identity
Vinyl Chloride Monomer
CAS #75-01-4
$CH_2 = CHCl$

Synonyms, Trade, and Common Names
VCM; Vinyl Chloride, inhibited; Chloroethylene; Chloroethene; Monochloroethylene; Ethylene monochloride

OSHA PEL
1 ppm (8 hr. TWA); 0.5 ppm (8 hr. TWA) action level; 5 ppm ceiling concentration

ACGIH TLV
5 ppm (8 hr. TWA); Human carcinogen

Other Limits Recommended
NIOSH - Lowest detectable (NIOSH Recommended Exposure Level, REL)

Hazardous Components/Ingredients
Vinyl chloride monomer 99.9%
Contaminants may include acetaldehyde, acetylene, iron, hydrogen chloride.
An inhibitor (e.g., approx. 50 ppm phenol) may be added to prevent polymerization during storage.

Physical/Chemical Characteristics

Boiling Point:	7°F (-14°C)
Specific Gravity ($H_2O = 1$):	0.91
Vapor Pressure:	230 mm Hg at 20°C
Solubility in Water:	Negligible (0.1% at 25°C)
Appearance and Odor:	Colorless, sweet-smelling gas at room temperature. Readily liquefies below -14°C or at increased pressures.
Vapor Density (Air = 1):	2.2
Melting Point:	-245°F (-160°C)
Evaporation Rate: (Butyl Acetate = 1)	Information not available

Fire and Explosion Information
Flash Point (Method Used): 108°F/ -77°C (COC)
Flammable Limits in Air (% by volume):
  Lower (LEL) 3.6%
  Upper (UEL) 33%

Extinguishing Media: Dry chemical or carbon dioxide for small fires. Heavy water spray, fog or alcohol foam for larger fires to cool containers and protect response workers (ineffective extinguishing material).

Special Fire Fighting Recommendations: Stop flow of gas if possible; if flow cannot be stopped, fight fires from a distance or allow to burn. If possible, remove container from fire area and/or isolate from other flammable materials.

Unusual Fire and Explosion Hazards: Heavier than air - can flow along surfaces to distant sources of ignition and flash back. VCM is highly flammable and can form explosive mixtures in air. If heated or exposed to light, air or catalyst, it can undergo violent exothermic reaction.

Reactivity Data

Stability: Inhibited VCM is stable at room temperature.

Conditions to Avoid: Heat, sparks, or other sources of ignition can result in a flashback fire and/or explosion. Exposure to heat, light, air, oxidizing agents, copper, or aluminum can result in vigorous reaction.

Hazardous Polymerization: X̲ may occur _____ does not occur

Hazardous Decomposition Products: Hydrogen chloride, carbon monoxide, phosgene.

Health Hazard Data

Main Route(s) of Exposure: Inhalation, Skin, Eye contact

Signs and Symptoms of Overexposure:

Acute: Central Nervous System (CNS) disturbances (e.g., headache, nausea, drunkenness, drowsiness, narcolepsy, unconsciousness, respiratory paralysis, euphoria, cardiac arrest); Asphyxia, Pulmonary damage; Liver and Kidney damage; Dimmed vision; Skin irritation, redness, frostbite and pain; Nonpermanent corneal injury with eye contact.

Chronic: Cancer; CNS and autonomic nervous system effects; Peripheral circulation disturbances (Raynaud's phenomenon), skeletal and skin changes, immunosuppression.

Carcinogenicity: NTP-Yes	IARC-Human Yes	OSHA-Yes
	-Animal Yes	(29 CFR 1910.1017)

Medical Conditions Aggravated by Exposure: No information available

Emergency and First-Aid Procedures

Inhalation: Promptly take victim to uncontaminated, well-ventilated area. Resuscitate if necessary (oxygen may be necessary). GET MEDICAL ATTENTION IMMEDIATELY.

Skin Contact: Promptly remove contaminated shoes and clothing and thoroughly wash affected areas with large amounts of warm water. If frostbite occurs, warm affected parts by wrapping. Gently exercise affected parts to restore circulation.

Eye Contact: Immediately flush eyes with large amounts of water with lids lifted, for no less than 15-20 minutes. GET IMMEDIATE MEDICAL ATTENTION.

Precautions for Safe Handling and Use

Storage and Handling Precautions: Store in a cool, well-ventilated area isolated from ignition sources or oxidizing agents. Cylinders must be protected from physical damage.

Other Precautions: VCM is a cancer hazard and must be stored in a designated regulated area with con-

Precautions for Safe Handling and Use *Continued*

trolled and limited access. Where workers may be exposed, storage and other areas must be monitored periodically for levels above the 0.5 ppm action level.

Spill and Leak Procedures: Immediately remove and/or turn off all sources of ignition. Evacuate and isolate area until leak has been stopped and area well-ventilated. Stop leak if possible and spray area with large amounts of water to suppress vapors and reduce temperatures. Response personnel must use appropriate personal protective clothing and equipment to prevent breathing contaminated air or coming into contact with liquid VCM.

Waste Disposal Method: High-temperature incineration in accordance with EPA guidelines.

Control Measures

Ventilation: Local exhaust, explosion-proof. Process enclosure, if possible.

General ventilation must also be explosion-proof.

Respiratory Protection (Specific Type):

Up to 10 ppm: 1. Combination Type C supplied air respirator (SAR), demand type with half-mask facepiece and auxiliary self-contained air supply; or

2. Type C SAR, demand type with half-mask facepiece; or

3. Any chemical cartridge respirator with an organic vapor cartridge that has at least a one-hour service life in concentrations of vinyl chloride up to 10 ppm.

(See 29 CFR 1910.1017(g) (4) for the required selection of respirators at higher concentrations.)

Protective Gloves: Neoprene or other VCM-impermeable material.

Eye Protection: Chemical-protective goggles or faceshield, as needed. Eyewash station must be in working order and readily accessible for emergency use.

Other Protective Clothing/Equipment: Chemical-protective clothing and boot covers.

Work/Hygienic Practices: Safety showers and eyewash stations must be in working order and readily accessible in the work areas.

From U.S. Department of Agriculture. Hazard communication: A program guide for federal agencies. Washington, DC: U.S. Government Printing Office.

7

DEVELOPING OCCUPATIONAL HEALTH SERVICES AND PROGRAMS: A CONCEPTUAL MODEL

Occupational health nursing practice is committed to the promotion, maintenance, and restoration of worker health within the context of health promotion and preventive strategies to improve health and reduce work-related health risks. To achieve this commitment, occupational health nurses develop and provide numerous occupational health and safety programs and services and are challenged to do so with emphasis on quality and cost containment. This chapter presents a conceptual framework or model, which can serve as a guide for a systematic approach to program development in occupational health in the work setting. As an extension of the occupational health nursing practice model described in Chapter 3, this model is predicated on the general systems theory and approach developed by von Bertalanfly (1968). However, before discussing the application of this model in the occupational health setting, it is necessary and important to describe basic systems theory definitions and conceptual linkages to clarify the essential model elements in order to fully explicate its meaning and value.

The systems theory provides an approach to examine organizational interactions and how they can be integrated to achieve outcomes or goals. Systems are arranged in a hierarchical order and thus all systems or entities are simultaneously parts of larger entities (suprasystems). For example, Putt (1978) describes that an individual can be conceptualized as being composed of a number of body systems, or subsystems, such as the circulatory system or respiratory system. At the same time, an individual is part of a number of larger systems, such as family, a work or school group, community, and society. In like manner, the occupational health unit can be considered a subsystem within the business, industry, or institutional system, which may also be part of a complex organizational or corporate structure, or suprasystem, and is influenced by the external environment. Changes in one system are likely to affect another system. Hall and Weaver (1985) point out that all systems, because of their interrelated hierarchical arrangement, may also be viewed as subsystems or suprasystems, depending on one's focus or location within the hierarchy. Thus, it is important to specify which system is the system of analysis or focus, that is, the *target* system.

■ SYSTEMS APPROACH AND COMPONENTS

Figure 7–1 displays the basic elements of a system that can be applied to any organizational setting. In general systems theory, a system is defined as a set of components or units interacting with each other (Hazard, 1978; von Bertalanfly, 1968). All living systems are open systems and as depicted in Figure 7–1, there is a continual exchange of information and energy from the interactions of the system with the environment through a semi-permeable boundary (dotted line). This boundary allows for the filtering of information into and out of the system (Griffith-Kenney & Christensen, 1986). For example, many occupational health and safety activities are impacted by regulatory agencies such as the Occupational Safety and Health Administration (OSHA). Thus, the employer needs to develop mechanisms to meet regulatory requirements and provide data through accurate recordkeeping to assure compliance with these requirements.

Components of all systems have inputs, throughput processes, outputs, and feedback mechanisms and function within the context of the environment. The environment of the system includes all factors that affect the system and also all factors that are affected by the system, such as economic and legislative influences. In order for a system to survive, it must have adaptation with the environment, integration of system or subsystem components, and effective decision making about the allocation of resources to achieve organizational and system goals.

From a systems perspective, inputs are supports, demands, or some form of energy or information taken into the system that is then processed through into the system's outputs (Hazard, 1978). For example, in the simplest form, the employee enters the company system and processes work to achieve the desired output, that is, the product or service of the industry or organization. From the

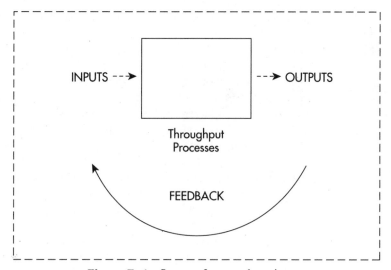

■ **Figure 7–1** Systems framework environment.

occupational health perspective, the occupational health unit as a subsystem influenced by external entities such as OSHA (environment) obtains and uses resources or energy in the form of workers, work processes, health care, budget, and so forth (input) that interact together, and are then processed (throughput) and returned in an altered or changed form such as a reduction in work-related injuries or improved work practices (output). The feedback mechanism allows the system to use output information as a measure of the effectiveness of system functioning. Feedback may be positive, negative, or neutral and is reintroduced into the system as input data in order to improve, adjust, modify, or make corrections as needed. For example, if an occupational health goal is thwarted because employees are unable to participate in occupational health programs on company time (e.g., smoking cessation program), the occupational health professional will need to reexamine and renegotiate approaches and strategies with management to achieve the desired goal.

■ CONCEPTUAL APPROACH TO OCCUPATIONAL HEALTH PROGRAMMING

The conceptual model shown in Figure 7–2 can serve as a guide for the application of the systems approach for developing and analyzing occupational health and safety services and programs. The framework illustrates the relationship between the system as a whole, its external environment, and the internal functioning of the system through the flow of inputs, throughput processes, related interventions, and outputs to achieve the goals or outcomes desired. The feedback mechanism represents a control function to improve the overall functioning of the system. In systems theory, as previously mentioned, all systems are arranged within a hierarchical order; however, each subsystem, system, or suprasystem retains the functioning properties and elements of a system (i.e., contextual environment, system inputs, throughputs, outputs, and feedback). Thus, this model is an application of the systems approach to the occupational health unit viewed as the target system, albeit a subsystem of the business or organization in which it functions. The description of some elements of this model (e.g., external influences, scope of practice) have been previously mentioned within the context of the occupational health nursing practice model in Chapter 3, but will be reviewed here for purposes of continuity.

Environmental Influences

An examination of the model shows that the business and ultimately the occupational health unit are affected or influenced by external contextual factors including population and health care trends, legislation/politics, the economy, and technology. This relationship is depicted through environmental-system interaction via the dashed interface line (Fig. 7–2). Examples of external contextual factors are shown in Table 7–1.

Population and health trends are important factors affecting the business and occupational health unit as these same indices are often reflected in the workforce. Typically, workers are hired from the community wherein the business resides; thus, knowledge of the community culture and demographics of the population can provide anticipatory information about the potential workforce. For example, population data clearly indicate a continued increase in the aging of the population with concomitant chronic illnesses, which may indicate a need for different types of programs offered at the worksite as well as an increase in health care costs

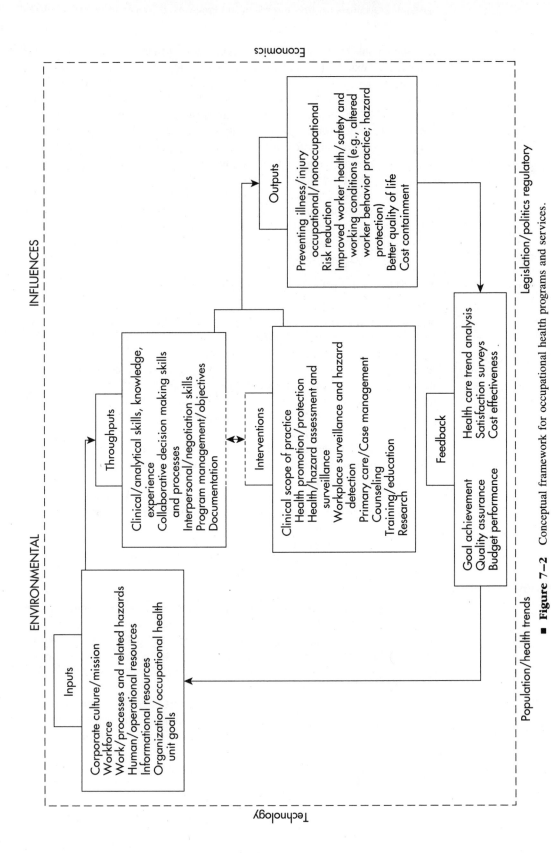

■ **Figure 7–2** Conceptual framework for occupational health programs and services.

■ **TABLE 7–1**   Examples of External Environmental Influences

Population/Health Trends	Legislation/Politics Regulatory	Technology	Economy

Population Demographics
  Aging workforce
  More women workers
  Ethnic diversity
  Bipolar aged work-
    force
Increased chronic illness
Prenatal/child health
  care issues
	OSH Act
	Regulatory
	  Hazard Communi-
	    cation Standard
	  Americans with
	    Disabilities Act
	  Recordkeeping
	  Nurse Practice Acts
	  Lobbying
		New/redesigned
		  work processes
		New chemicals
		Computerization
		Robotics/worker dis-
		  placement
			Increased health care
			  costs
			  Worker's compensation
			  Health insurance
			Cost containment
			Managed care

via insurance premiums. In addition, some job redesign may be in order to continue to match job demands with older workers' needs and with the needs of disabled workers. Increased ethnic diversity in the population and workforce will also require a better understanding of variations in ethnic culture. The latter may provide more insight into how workers perceive or value health and/or how and under what circumstances health care delivery is received by targeted populations.

With the continued increase of women in the workforce, who may also be single heads of households, more flexibility in work schedules, flex-time, job sharing, and accommodations for child care must be considered. Evidence exists that employee concern regarding child-care arrangements may increase worker anxiety, stress, and illness, and reduce productivity (Mastroianni, 1992). Depending on how the population grows, a bipolar aged workforce, that is, the very old and very young, may be apparent and will require a diversity in health care programs provided for these groups. Other examples of societal health issues needing attention include substance abuse problems, violence, the need for better access to health care including prenatal care, and control of communicable diseases for which programs can be designed and delivered at the worksite.

It is important that the occupational health nurse have a good understanding of another major group of contextual factors that include the laws and regulations affecting industry and occupational health as well as the political influences affecting the processes of legislation and regulation. For example, over the past several decades, several pieces of legislation have been enacted including the Federal Coal Mine Safety and Health Act (1969); the Occupational Safety and Health Act (1970); the Noise Control Act (1972); the Toxic Substances Control Act (1976); the Hazard Communication Standard (1983); the Americans With Disabilities Act (1990); and the Bloodborne Pathogens Standard (1991). Laws such as these and resultant regulations impact the workplace and workforce in terms of mandated programs and the requirement for occupational health and safety program initiatives and expansion, program administration, the institution of control strategies to meet regulatory mandates and reduce worker exposures, and the acquisition of necessary resources to achieve occupational health requirements and goals. The occupational health nurse is in a key position to help interpret the meaning of regulations with respect to appropriate and necessary health-related programs, strategies, and interventions, and to help the company comply with regulatory requirements. As one can imagine, the implementation of strategies to effect compliance with regulations may pose a significant economic burden on business and industry. Thus, effective programs to reduce work-related injuries and illnesses and resulting costs are critical.

Political influences, such as special interest groups, can affect the passage of legislative acts and the occupational health nurse will want to recognize these influences and their impact, and individually or collectively be involved in the political process to improve worker and workforce health and safety. For example, the American Asssociation of Occupational Health Nurses (AAOHN), through its governmental affairs program, monitors proposed legislation affecting occupational health and safety and provides testimony before congressional committes to influence passage, modification, or nonpassage of related legislative acts such as the Bloodborne Pathogens Standard or OSHA Reform Act. The occupational health nurse will want to keep abreast of these issues in order to effectively monitor and communicate the potential impact at the worksite.

Technological advances add to industries' capacity to develop and implement new or improved work processes, systems for more effective monitoring and analysis of work-related illness and injuries trends, and enhanced computer applications for more efficient recordkeeping. It is important that new or redesigned work processes be examined prior to implementation and continually monitored to determine the potential for work-related hazardous exposures. In addition, in the face of new or computerized manufacturing work processes, workers may be displaced, requiring job retraining and the acquisition of new skills; or workers may be terminated, with the loss not only of income but also of health insurance benefits, creating uncertainty and anxiety for workers (and families) and business.

Computerized record systems can serve to enhance the tracking of work-related illness and injury trends, resulting in more effective evaluation of occupational health data and targeted programs to address high risk situations. These systems can be carried over into employee health recordkeeping to provide for more systematic data collection that will improve health care service delivery and more consistent data for research analysis. However, care needs to be taken with respect to appropriate controls regarding confidentiality mechanisms.

Economic variables are of major contextual importance as they affect the overall health of the company in terms of profitability, growth, and expansion. This in turn affects the stability, morale, and productivity of a workforce. Costs associated with work-related injuries have increased dramatically in workers' compensation claims, health care and health insurance costs, and related indirect costs. This is described in Chapter 1. As injury rates increase, workers' compensation insurance premiums also rise adding to employer economic liabilities. Employers must consider the value of the implementation of occupational health and safety programs and the potential savings derived even in the face of associated direct costs, whether they are mandated regulatory programs or health promotion programs. However, occupational health professionals bear the responsibility for developing programs and services that are cost-effective. In addition, providing primary care services at the worksite can potentially decrease the utilization of external health care services, which can be very costly. Evidence exists to support the use of nurse practitioners at the worksite as cost-effective and cost-containment strategies; thus, primary care services could be increased through utilization of these practitioners (Touger & Butts, 1989).

System Inputs

The inputs into the occupational health unit system are determined by the business or organization and include the corporate culture, mission, and philosophy; the workforce; the work, work processes, and related hazards; available human and operational resources; and the organizational and occupational health unit goals. The interaction and flow of these inputs into the system are ultimately transformed into system outputs (Fig. 7–2).

The importance of understanding the corporate or company mission, philosophy, and culture cannot be overstated. The occupational health nurse will want to gather information about management's commitment to providing health care programs at the worksite, including occupational and nonoccupational health services. Management's commitment to occupational health is usually demonstrated through the establishment of and participation on health and safety committees; resource allocation for occupational health and safety programs; the inclusion of employees in decision-making processes regarding health; the promotion of health, wellness, and risk reduction through company-sponsored health programs on company time; and the incorporation of a concept of health which may extend beyond the workplace to include family participation in worksite health activities and industry-sponsored occupational health events such as health fairs or support for educational activities.

Management's philosophy about work and health and the interrelationships as it affects workers productivity, morale, and well-being will provide the underpinning for the success of the occupational health service. If management has a lukewarm attitude toward worker health, then occupational health services and programs are not likely to be viewed as a priority except for meeting mandated programs as required. The occupational health nurse will want to influence management's perception about the value of occupational health and safety programs by demonstrating that these programs can be cost-effective, can increase employee morale and productivity, and can improve the company's image among the workforce and community.

The company culture is concerned not only with management attitudes, values, and beliefs about work and health, but also that of the workers. This may be witnessed in workers' participation in health and wellness programs, compliance with regulatory mandates, and overall observation of safe and healthful work practices. The occupational health nurse needs to understand the value of company culture as this can have a major impact on the success of any program. Organizational culture exerts considerable influence on types of changes made and behavior expressed. These points are described more fully in Chapters 8 and 13.

Workforce inputs are important to be examined so that the occupational health nurse can plan and implement effective occupational health and safety programs relative to the needs of the workers. The aggregate workforce should be viewed in terms of the size and distribution of the workforce, demographic characteristics, and health status indicators including morbidity and mortality trends and patterns. It is also important to assess worker perceptions about health, accident prevention, work and risk acceptance, and related work practice behaviors. The health status and occupational history of workers also need to be assessed so that workers are appropriately matched to their respective jobs. This is discussed in more detail in Chapter 10.

Workers are employed to produce a certain product or service. Depending on the type of work and related work processes, workers may potentially be exposed to various workplace hazards from biological, chemical, environmental/ergonomic, physical, or psychosocial agents. The occupational health professional will need to have a thorough understanding of the industry's work processes, workers' job tasks and demands, and working conditions in order to recognize potential and actual hazards and be able to design, implement, and monitor strategies to prevent potential hazard exposure or alter existing hazardous conditions. This can be accomplished through reviewing company information related to work processes, associated technical reports and health hazard evaluations, and through conducting workplace walk-throughs. Depending on potential or actual exposures involved, the interaction of the worker with the work and its processes can clearly affect the health end points of the individual worker and the collective workforce. Hazard identification and evaluation are described more in-depth in Chapters 6 and 9.

In order to have an effective occupational health and safety program, it is essential to have adequate human and operational resources. With respect to human resources, the best approach to comprehensive occupational health and safety programming is through a multidisciplinary effort. The core disciplines of the occupational health and safety team include the occupational health nurse, physician, industrial hygienist, and safety specialist. Other team members may also include an ergonomist, toxicologist, and psychologist/EAP counselor. While the interdisciplinary approach to occupational health and safety management is the most effective, most businesses who employ occupational health and safety professionals primarily employ occupational health nurses. From surveys conducted by the AAOHN of its membership, approximately 50% of occupational health nurses employed are sole health care providers at the worksite (AAOHN, 1992). Thus, the occupational health nurse is central to the management and coordination of occupational health unit activities. The occupational health nurse must have adequate and appropriate education, knowledge, and skills in the nursing, public health, occupational health, and behavioral sciences, management concepts and principles, and be knowledgeable about laws and regulations specific to occupational health. The knowledge and skills acquired are applied through the roles the nurse assumes in the occupational health setting, including clinician, manager, education, researcher, or consultant, described in more detail in Chapter 4.

As part of the interdisciplinary team, occupational health physicians may be employed full-time or part-time by the company to provide direct care services in evaluating employee work-related illnesses and injuries. More often, companies will have contractual relationships with community physicians or providers at health maintenance organizations to provide the services needed (Felton, 1990). Industrial hygienists engage in recognizing, evaluating, and controlling workplace hazards through walk-through observation of the workplace, measurement of workplace exposures, and through recommending and instituting control strategies to prevent unnecessary exposures. Safety specialists conduct safety audits to identify hazardous and unsafe situations in the work environment, investigate accidents and work-related injuries, and institute worker training and education programs related to safety in the workplace. Even if the company does not employ these types of health care professionals, appropriate and specific services can be obtained from private consultants or through state-level health agencies.

It is important to emphasize that the worker must be included as a member of the occupational health team if appropriate and realistic strategies for risk reduction are to be developed and implemented. The team approach in assessing and evaluating work-related problems will lend itself to a broader perspective and interpretation of factors that impact worker health, and also to a wider array of alternative control strategies.

Collaboration between professional disciplines and management is essential to effective, efficient programs and resource management. In addition to professional personnel, support personnel should be employed to handle the clerical and nonprofessional tasks. This will ensure better use of professional skills and more efficient use of scarce resource dollars. Further information on occupational health and safety specialty areas can be found in Chapters 6 and 11.

Operational resources include an adequate budget, facilities, equipment, supplies, and so forth necessary to operate the occupational health and safety program. The occupational health unit budget should be developed based on established goals and objectives reflective of the needs for promoting and protecting worker health. It is important that the occupational health nurse manager develop or have input into the budget process as she/he is the person most familiar with the program unit goals and can most effectively manage the occupational health unit budget. In other words, the individual who controls the budget in essence controls the program.

Management should commit sufficient space for the occupational health unit. Facilities need to be designed that are adequate to meet the space needs for the staff and employee population, and should also be comfortable and attractive. The size of the occupational health unit will vary and is often governed by space available. Other factors to consider include the number of employees, work shifts, and scope and type of services to be provided. Felton (1990) estimates approximately 175 square feet per employee up to 1,000 employees. Guidotti et al. (1989) suggests that a more modern facility should provide 1.5 square feet per employee above 200 employees.

Access to the occupational health unit is critical and the unit should be located as central as possible to the majority of the workers. It should be barrier-free and equipped for handicapped individuals. The floor plan should be simple in design to facilitate the flow of work. Component areas include reception, record storage, diagnostic and treatment services, employee function areas (hygiene facilities, dressing rooms), and conference space. Additional space for special program areas may be desirable depending on the types of services offered (e.g., physical therapy, fitness, library).

Equipment needed in the occupational health unit can be expensive, so its purchase should be based on need and volume of use (i.e., occupational, nonoccupational, and health promotion activities). Extensive laboratory equipment is generally unnecessary where contractual laboratory services are more cost-effective and when the health care professional does not possess the skills appropriate to conduct the test. As with any clinical setting, current, up-to-date equipment should be provided. The occupational health nurse should develop and maintain an inventory of supplies and equipment necessary for the occupational health services. An example of an inventory list of equipment/supplies can be found in Appendix 7–1.

Information resources are needed to assist the occupational health professional in making decisions in occupational health programming. This includes, for example, data on health and illness trends of the workforce, health needs of the workforce for services and programs, health insurance and claims data, and costs of goods and services. In addition, informational resources such as library/journal references, health- and management-related materials, and computer linkages for data access and analysis and networking are valuable tools.

The last major system input is the establishment of occupational health unit goals. These goals must be congruent with the overall business or industry goals and should address such areas as high risk situations in terms of work-related illness/injury episodes and trends, worker needs, working conditions, and health promotion. The goals set the blueprint or direction for occupational health unit activities from which objectives will be derived (throughput process), the achievement of which will be measured as a system output. A more in-depth discussion of goals and objectives is addressed in Chapters 12 and 13.

System Throughput Processes and Interventions

System inputs interact together and, as depicted in Figure 7–2, are transformed through a complex set of dynamic processes or throughputs to achieve the desired system output or outcome through organized interventions. System processes or throughputs and interventions are variable and numerous depending on the system and its needs. When considering the occupational health unit system inputs described, the following are examples of major throughput processes and interventions.

In the throughput process, the occupational health professional effectively utilizes knowledge and skills to achieve the specified goals reflected in outputs. This includes the ability to analyze with other team members the interaction of system inputs; prioritize program interventions; employ effective interpersonal skills to communicate to management and the workforce the value of and need for health programs; develop achievable objectives; negotiate for additional or strategic resources; and make collaborative decisions with interdisciplinary team members, management, and workers regarding the development and implementation of effective strategies to improve worker health and safety. Appropriate documentation including record keeping and administrative and legal reports is essential.

Interventions are tied to the throughput processes as products of the processes described above. Occupational health nurses practice within the legal framework of state nurse practice acts (Chapter 15), the occupational health nursing scope of practice (Table 7–2) (described in detail in Chapter 3), the nursing process, clinical nursing guidelines as appropriate (Chapter 11), and ethical parameters for practice derived from the code of ethics (Chapter 16). Interventions are derived from the scope of practice, are designed to meet the needs identified through throughput processes, and lead to system outputs. Examples might include developing health promotion and health protection programs such as health appraisals, smoking cessation, wellness, hearing conservation, and employee

■ **TABLE 7–2**   Scope of Practice in Occupational Health Nursing

Health promotion/protection
Worker health/hazard assessment and surveillance
Workplace surveillance and hazard detection
Primary care/case management
Counseling
Management/administration
Research
Legal/ethical monitoring
Community orientation

assistance programs; health teaching and counseling regarding appropriate work practice measures; and the delivery of appropriate primary care services for occupational and nonoccupational health services. Training and education related to mandatory programs such as the Hazard Communication Standard or Bloodborne Pathogens Standard and return-to-work programs are designed to improve the health and safety of the worker as well as the quality of life. Participating in and/or conducting research is essential to improving practice.

System Outputs

Through utilization of knowledge and skills in analysis, communication and negotiation techniques, decision making, interpersonal relationships, and collaboration, the occupational health nurse is able to better understand the interaction of the inputs and design interventions that result in system outputs. These outputs reflect the product or service of the occupational health unit, that is, a healthy worker population, and achievement of this desired end state. The major products produced are related to the following factors:

1. prevention of work-related illness and injury episodes:
   • decreased incidence and prevalence of work-related injuries, illnesses, and disabilities
   • reduction in premature morbidity
   • decreased workers' compensation claims
2. improvement in the health and safety of the workforce and work environment:
   • enhanced managerial commitment to a health/safety supportive environment
   • improved population health and quality of life
   • increased health promotion-oriented programs
   • improved occupational health and safety risk reduction programs
   • increased or altered work behavior practices to support safe and healthful working conditions
   • increased compliance with health and safety strategies (mandated, recommended)
3. improved cost-effective programs:
   • decreased health care costs (i.e., workers' compensation and health insurance premiums)

- decreased absenteeism and lost work time
- increased productivity

The occupational health nurse will want to determine if and to what extent outputs or outcomes have been achieved. This is best accomplished through determining if occupational health services and programs were effective in meeting objectives, altering risk, improving health parameter measurements (e.g., morbidity and mortality trends), and reducing costs.

In the process of transforming inputs and throughputs into outputs, objectives are determined in the throughput phase for meeting occupational health and safety program goals. These objectives should be explicit and quantifiably measurable so one can determine their achievement. For example, if the occupational health nurse identified from system inputs that employees were potentially exposed to blood and were not using personal protection equipment, or that there were increased complaints regarding cumulative trauma disorders, later validated through examinations, objectives would have been developed related to increasing the use of protective equipment and reducing the incidence of cumulative disorders, respectively, and measured as an output.

System Feedback

The occupational health unit system is dependent on larger systems and influences, that is, the company and environment for its inputs and also for acceptance of its outputs (Gibson et al., 1985). The feedback mechanism is designed so that the system can make adjustments that are more responsive to worker needs, organizational and occupational health goals, and environmental demands. Feedback is concerned not only with identifying goal achievement or lack thereof but also with what needs to be altered or improved to correct the deviation or with what successful endeavors need to be enhanced or promoted. For example, if a hypertension screening program was implemented but was poorly attended, one might find that the lack of participation was due to a scheduling problem which could be altered.

Another important feedback mechanism with respect to the value of occupational health services is the use of satisfaction surveys of workers and management (Rogers et al., 1993). Based on data obtained regarding how individuals feel about the delivery and quality of occupational health services, modifications or adjustments can be made to improve or enhance the program. Measurement of illness/injury trend data over time can also provide information about the effectiveness of program strategies. For example, one can examine and analyze data collected from the OSHA log from one year to the next and use these as a basis for comparison related to the effectiveness of interventions/programs. Development and measurement of objectives and analysis of epidemiologic trends are described in more detail in Chapters 13 and 5 respectively.

■ SUMMARY

The use of a conceptual approach to develop occupational health and safety programs and services provides a systematic method to examine and analyze the occupational health system within the context of the company and external environment. This will help to focus on system and environmental demands that are directed toward improving worker health and reducing work-related risks.

The occupational health nurse will want to thoroughly examine system inputs in order to determine what skills (i.e., analysis, negotiation) need to be employed to achieve the outputs and outcomes desired. This approach will allow for a better understanding of how systems function and interact to achieve organizational and occupational unit goals.

Budget analysis should be performed to measure the budget match with goals and objectives. In addition, examining the cost effectiveness of occupational health with programming should be an integral component of occupational health objectives.

References

American Association of Occupational Health Nurses. Membership Statistics, 1992.

Felton, JS. Occupational medical management. Boston: Little, Brown & Company, 1990.

Gibson, JL, Ivancevich, JM, Donnelly, JH. Organizations. Piano, TX: Business Publications, 1985, pp. 5–21.

Griffith-Kenney, JW & Christensen, PJ. Nursing process: Application of theories, frameworks, and models. St. Louis: The C.V. Mosby Co., 1986.

Guidotti, T, Cowell, J, Jamieson, G & Engleberg, AL. Occupational health services: A practical approach. Chicago: American Medical Association, 1989.

Hall, J & Weaver B. Distributive nursing practice: A systems approach to community health. Philadelphia: J.B. Lippincott, 1985.

Hazard, ME. An overview of systems theory. Nursing Clinics of Nursing America, 6(3): 385–393, 1978.

Mastroianni, K. Child day care arrangements and employee health. AAOHN Journal, 40(2): 78–83, 1992.

Putt, A. General systems theory applied to nursing. Boston: Little, Brown & Co., 1978.

Rogers, B, Winslow, B & Higgins, S. Employee satisfaction with occupational health services. AAOHN Journal, 41(2): 58–65, 1993.

Touger, GN & Butts, J. The workplace: An innovative and cost-effective practice site. The Nurse Practitioner, 14(1): 35–42, 1989.

von Bertalanfly, L. General systems theory. New York: George Braziller, 1968.

APPENDIX

7–1

Equipment and Supplies for an Occupational Health Unit

FURNISHINGS
Office
Desks
Chairs
Bookcases
Filing cabinets with locks
Storage cabinets with locks
Wall clocks

FURNISHINGS *Continued*

Office

Word processor, typewriters, computer
Tables
Wastebaskets
In/Out baskets
Desk lamps
Bulletin boards
Calculators

Clinic

Stools, height appropriate to counter, with adjustable backs
Chart-holders, with priority and occupancy indicators
Stretcher, wheelchairs, beds
Sinks with surgical handles on faucets, towel racks
Examination tables
Chairs
Medication cabinet with locks
Pedal-operated wastebaskets with lid and liners
Health records filing cabinets
Instrument trays
Autoclave (optional)
Refrigerator
Oxygen unit

EQUIPMENT

Major instruments

Wall-mounted oto-/ophthalmoscope
Wall-mounted sphygmomanometer (blood pressure cuff)
Crash cart (cardiopulmonary resuscitation) must be fully equipped and provided with a
    seal to ensure that it is not opened and drugs and equipment are not used except in
    a true emergency
Scales
Electrocardiograph
Audiometer (optional)
Vision screening apparatus
Recording spirometry (optional)
Suction apparatus

Hand-held instruments

Irrigating syringe, suitable for removal of cerumen from ear
Assorted clamps
Dental mirror
Dynamometer (for measuring grip strength)
Flashlights
Laryngoscope (in crash cart)
Sphygmomanometer with varying cuffs (small, medium, large, i.e., thigh)–hand held
Magnifying lens
Percussion hammer
Scalpels
Surgical scissors
Ear specula
Nasal specula
Vaginal specula
Stethescope
Tape measures
Thermometer

Tuning forks
Color vision chart (Ishihara plates)
SUPPLIES
Syringes
Needles
Gloves
Vacutainers and assorted blood-drawing apparatus
Tongue depressors
Cotton swabs
Gauze pads
Assorted dressings
Suture material and needles/suture removal materials
Specimen containers
Elastic bandages, in assorted sizes
Self-adhering gauze bandage rolls
Large compresses
Butterfly closures (steri-strips)
Adhesive tape
Ace bandages
Portable emergency list
Stockinette bandage
Telfa pads of different sizes
Sling
Pressure bandages (2-3-4-6 inches in width)
Triangular bandages
Cold packs
Cervical collars
Surgical masks and hoods
Eye patches and pads
Cotton, in various forms
Inflatable splints
Various types of splints, such as wrist and leg
First aid boxes, first aid manual
First aid scissors, bandage scissors, straight scissors
First aid tweezers, splinter forceps, nail clippers
Basins of various sizes and capacity
Crutches
Instrument trays with covers
Heating pad set-up, hydroculator and pads
Finger cots
Antiseptics
Blankets
Examination gowns and paper sheets
Eye irrigating solutions
Facial tissue
Pillows with pillow cases
Safety pins
Sheets (including sterile burn sheet)
Towels (varying sizes)

MEDICATIONS COMMONLY USED IN AN OCCUPATIONAL HEALTH SERVICE
Acetylsalicylic acid 325 mg tablets (Aspirin)
Acetaminophen 325 mg tablets (Tylenol)
Actifed tablets

MEDICATIONS COMMONLY USED IN AN OCCUPATIONAL HEALTH SERVICE—cont'd

Chlorpheniramine maleate tablets (Chlor-Trimeton)

Dimenhydrinate tablets and suppositories (Dramamine)

Diphenhydramine hydrochloride 25 mg (Benadryl Caps); cream and injections 50 mg/ml

Epinephrine (Adrenalin)

Magnesia & alumina suspension (Maalox)

Kaopectate

Guaifenesin syrup 100 mg/5 ml (Robitussin)

Bacitracin 500 unit/g ointment (Baciguent)

8

ASSESSING THE ORGANIZATION

■ ORGANIZATIONAL CULTURE

An organization is defined as a group or groups interacting to achieve some common goal. Groups interact and articulate together in such a way that the behavior of one member or group influences the behavior of another. The work of groups is to share common goals and values to facilitate goal achievement (Katz & Kahn, 1978). Every organization has cultural norms and values that hold the organization together.

Organizational culture has been defined as the learned values, assumptions, and behaviors that knit a community together (McNeil & Garcia, 1991; Schein, 1985; Turnipseed, 1990). It preserves and unifies the social structure through a system of norms, expectations, and assumptions about the way individuals feel or behave within a group. For example, if a healthy workforce and healthful workplace are considered important and valued within the context of the organization, then organizational goals must be reflected in the actual implementation of programs and role modeling organizational behaviors that support, promote, and protect health (e.g., hazard exposure control, nutrition awareness, stress management). "Culture, conceived as shared key values and beliefs, fulfills several important functions. First, it conveys a sense of identity for organization members. Second, it facilitates the generation of commitment to something larger than self. Third, it enhances social system stability, and fourth, it serves as a sense-making device that guides and shapes behavior" (Smircich, 1983, p. 346).

Culture within organizations exerts a powerful influence on the types of decisions that are made, the kinds of information that are shared, when and in what manner information is disseminated, who is considered powerful, and what employee behaviors are deemed acceptable. Goodstein et al. (1992) term some members in the organization as heretics, that is, those who challenge the basic assumptions and beliefs of the system and the established order. Members who violate organizational norms are initially pressured to conform. If pressure does not produce the desired conformity, then severe sanctions may be imposed. However, it should be pointed out that large-scale cultural change requires heretical challenges that can precipitate the emergence of a new order.

Harrison and Stokes (1990) describe a typology of organizational cultures that involves four generic types: the power culture, the role culture, the achievement

■ **TABLE 8–1**   Typology of Organizational Cultures

1. Power Culture. This culture is based on an assumption that an inequality of resources such as money, privileges, security, and overall quality of life is natural. Hierarchical structure of the organization is accepted. Strong leaders are needed to manage these inequalities and provide balance to the system. These leaders are firm but fair in power cultures that work well. Poorly managed power cultures are ruled by fear with power abused by the leaders and their followers for personal gain. Playing "politics," manipulation, and infighting is common. Power cultures are best suited for start-up organizations in need of direction; however, as the organization expands, the need for delegation and functional systems is needed for efficiency and continued growth.
2. Role Culture. The basis of this culture is that work is best accomplished through rules and procedures. Roles are identified that clearly delineate each person's responsibilities and rewards. The system is managed through task delegation rather than arbitrary (power) control from the top. Role cultures provide stability, justice, and efficiency. Bureaucracies are typical role-oriented cultures that are generally efficient because work is routine and can be managed by rules, regulations, and procedures. However, they tend to be rigid and inflexible, thwarting creativity and innovation, which can hamper organizational growth and dynamism.
3. Achievement Culture. Within the organizational context, this culture supports the notion that people want to make significant contributions to work and society, and derive satisfaction from a job well done and meaningful interactions with others in the work environment. The role of management in this culture is to support workers in achieving the organizational mission and to empower workers to achieve both organizational and professional goals. Sustaining a high level of energy and enthusiasm and dealing with a lack of attention to organizational structures and systems may be difficult.
4. Support Culture. This culture's primary motivation is to develop mutual trust and support between the organization and individual. The valuing and nurturing of the human being is critical in this type of organization with harmony, warmth, and caring deeply valued, and confrontation avoided. This support culture meets important human needs often ignored in organizations; however, commitment to goal/task achievement may be compromised.

culture, and the support culture (Table 8–1). This model does not presume to categorize organizations by type but rather to assess the degree to which each of these four cultures are represented in an organization. While models will never fit any organization exactly, they are useful in understanding the focus and parameters of cultural norms.

The challenge for successful managers is to understand the organizational culture well enough to be able to tailor their behavior and strategies to comply with existing norms and values (del Bueno & Freund, 1986). How successful the occupational health nurse manager is will depend in part on successful interrelationships and interactions both vertically and horizontally within the organization and with external groups and constituents and recognizing and understanding the dynamics of the organizational culture.

Most nurses work in traditional health care settings such as hospitals, nursing homes, and public health agencies where health care is the primary service. In contrast, the occupational health nurse practices in a business setting, where the provision of health care is not the primary product, rather a support service to the primary mission (McNeil & Garcia, 1991). Occupational health services and programs are aimed at ensuring a healthy workforce and a safe, healthful work environment in order to reduce or eliminate work-related illnesses and injuries and promote worker health and productivity. From this perspective it is important to recognize the value and relationship of the occupational health unit to the other organizational units. Understanding how the occupational health unit is perceived and fits into the total organization can help the occupational health nurse determine the value and effectiveness of occupational health contributions.

■ ORGANIZATIONAL ASSESSMENT

A concept closely related to organizational culture is that of the social climate of the environment or organization. Moos (1987) defines social climate as the "personality" of a work setting or organization that impacts the work environment, work outcomes, and job satisfaction. Moos and colleagues (1986) have developed a 90-item Work Environment Scale (WES) that comprises 10 subscales that measure the social environment of the work setting. The subscales assess three major dimensions: Relationships, Personal Growth, and System Maintenance and Change. The Relationship dimensions are measured by the Involvement, Peer Cohesion, and Supervisor Support subscales; the Personal Growth dimensions are measured by Autonomy, Task Orientation, and Work Pressure subscales; the System Maintenance and Change dimensions are measured by the Clarity, Control, Innovation, and Physical Comfort subscales. The WES can also be used to compare employee and manager perceptions and actual and preferred work environments, enhance organizational development, and identify interventions to foster job satisfaction and productivity, including evaluating organizational dynamics, planning for organizational change, encouraging teamwork and cohesiveness, facilitating organizational management, and planning for physical environmental change (Flarey, 1991). Sample items for the WES as related to each subscale are shown in Table 8–2. The complete instrument can be obtained from Consulting Psychologists Press.

Within the context of organizational culture and social climate, it is important to examine organizational politics and several other factors, such as the formal structure, formal and informal communication patterns, leadership styles/behaviors, the work environment, projected/perceived image, status symbols, rituals and stories, and evidence of strategic planning (Beyers, 1984; Dieneman, 1989; Hein & Nicholson, 1986; McNeil & Garcia, 1991). A brief discussion of each of these factors follows. In addition, the concept of power is important as power sources clearly exert a major impact on the organization; these will be discussed in more detail. A detailed checklist for organizational assessment can be found in Appendix 8–1.

Assessment of organizational politics is a critical element and can reveal much information about power relationships, decision-making roles and alliances, and who influences resource allocation. A certain amount of politics is inevitable in every organization, and the occupational health nurse must be able to recognize the power/politics game and players, and develop political skills and savvy while maintaining integrity. Del Bueno & Freund (1986, pp. 12–14) identify several strategies for dealing with organizational politics (see Table 8–3).

While acquisition of resources may realistically be tied to political tactics and strategies, it is clearly important to assess the organization's values and beliefs with respect to political harnessing. Politicizing can breed contempt and distrust or one can quickly become politically vulnerable, scapegoated, or expendable. The manager must be astutely aware of political interrelationships and agendas and use caution and assertiveness as appropriate and necessary.

Assessment of the organization's formal structure is an obvious and key

■ **TABLE 8–2**   Items from Work Environment Scale—Real Form (90 Items Total)

Directions: These statements are about the place in which you work. The statements are intended to apply to all work environments. However, some words may not be quite suitable for your work environment. For example, the term "supervisor" is meant to refer to the boss, manager, department head, or the person or persons to whom an employee reports. You are to decide which statements are true of your work environment and which are false.

Involvement Scale
1. The work is really challenging.
Peer Cohesion
2. People go out of their way to help a new employee feel comfortable.
Task Orientation
5. People pay a lot of attention to getting work done.
Work Pressure
6. There is a constant pressure to keep working.
Control
8. There's a strict emphasis on following policies and regulations.
Innovation
9. Doing things in a different way is valued.
Supervisor Support
13. Supervisors usually compliment an employee who does something well.
Autonomy
14. Employees have a great deal of freedom to do as they like.
Clarity
17. Activities are well-planned.
Physical Comfort
20. The lighting is extremely good.

NOTE: The numbers represent the numbered items within the WES.
From Work Environment Scale by Paul M. Insel and Rudolf H. Moos. Copyright 1974 by Consulting Psychologists Press, Inc., Palo Alto, CA. All rights reserved. Further reproduction is prohibited without the Publisher's written consent.

element that can help the occupational health nurse understand the design, management, and visionary force supporting the organization, the decision-making authority centers, and where and at what level the occupational health unit fits within the formal and policy making structure. Examples of key formal structure assessment elements include: mission/philosophy statements and organizational goals, the organizational chart, key policy and procedure documents, and job descriptions.

Assessment of both formal and informal communication structures and patterns is critical to understanding how information is disseminated, received, and interpreted. In all organizations, the potential for communication breakdown and distortion always exists and information may be directed without clarity. How vertical (upward and downward) information flows between managers and workers establishes the limits, accessibility, and flexibility with respect to organizational communications. Horizontal communication between workers reflects a degree of teamwork within and across groups. How individuals communicate with each other irrespective of the type of communication is a measure of the level of personal and professional respect encouraged and supported within the organization. Examples of key formal communication assessment elements in-

■ **TABLE 8–3**   Strategies For Dealing With Organizational Politics

---

• Establish alliances with superiors and peers but choose your friends and confidants carefully.
• Use all possible channels of communication including formal, informal, and the grapevine.
• Know when to be fair to subordinates but recognize aggressive and manipulative individuals who may want to take over.
• Know how decisions are made, including the influence of powerful people and their biases (not necessarily based on ideas of merit).
• Be courteous, as this is a very powerful tool that increases others' self-esteem.
• Maintain a flexible/adaptable position and do not be uncompromising except on positions or issues that are morally or ethically essential.
• Use passive resistance or delay action when you are under pressure from demands that you cannot openly challenge.
• Project an image of status and power as too much modesty may be perceived or mistaken as lack of power.

Adapted from del Bueno, D & Freund, C. Power and politics in nursing administration: A casebook. Owings Mills, MD: National Health Publishing, 1986.

clude: memos, performance appraisal techniques and documents, one-to-one discussions, and meeting structures and frequency.

Informal communication structures are equally important as these represent the grapevine exchange of information and key data references for the manager to be able to determine how information is received, filtered, and interpreted. Informal communication channels can be skillfully manipulated to achieve hidden agendas. How workers and managers use the informal structure to pass along and collect information is important to assess. Examples of informal communication assessment elements include: observations of social relationships on and off the job between and among coworkers and managers, who avoids whom, who criticizes and supports ideas, and who speaks out.

Leadership styles and behaviors ebb from the context of the organization. The organization itself is steeped in history and tradition and is characterized by certain modes of leadership behaviors that are often considered institutionalized. As described previously, the organization has a style and value system with which the leaders articulate, and leaders are often selected to match this style and behavior. Thus, it is important that the occupational health nurse recognize and understand organizational leadership behaviors and their impact on workers' behaviors and performance. Examples of leadership assessment elements include: types of leadership, perception of leadership style used, intimidation tactics, value the leaders place on worker health and safety, and role modeling behaviors.

Assessment of the work environment is particularly important as this can greatly affect the physical and mental well-being of the workplace inhabitants. The physical condition and hygiene of the environment may be perceived, to some extent, as how management and the workers feel about the workplace. Employee satisfaction with the organizational culture is important to consider as it impacts the productivity and cohesiveness of the organization (Blancett, 1992). Issues related to workplace safety, working conditions, stress production and management, and how people are treated are important to assess. Examples of environmental assessment elements include: design and structure of existing buildings, adequacy of equipment and supplies, health and safety awareness, eating and comfort facilities, and location and adequacy of the occupational health unit.

Assessment of the image the organization portrays or strives to portray is important in order to determine how the organization desires to be perceived by the external community and environment. In addition, the relationship of the organization to the external community is vital to assess as the organization is affected by the population characteristics and makeup of the community (e.g., age of residents, ethnic makeup, and values). Examples of key image assessment elements include: slogans or phrases describing the organization, public relations activities, employee dress, organizational health consciousness (e.g., smoking, exercise), publications, and involvement in community activities.

Assessment of status symbols can provide information about who has power, who is considered successful, and the degree of corporate elitism. Examples of key status symbol assessment elements include: allocation and location of parking spaces, the size, appearance and location of office space, and the ability to determine one's working hours.

While assessing the organizational culture, it is important to consider rituals and stories. Rituals are time-honored customs that enable individuals to understand social relationships, reduce uncertainty and anxiety, and exert control (e.g., committee meetings that are routinely held without reason and/or productivity) (del Bueno & Freund, 1986). Stories help describe conflicts, events, and relationships, reinforce the history of decision making, and facilitate the cultural linkages. As stated by del Bueno and Freund (p. 20),

It is not sufficient to have knowledge of the formal structure, the written rules and policies. These only represent the surface or the conscious life of the organization. Penetration beneath the surface level is neccesary to understand the true reality of the organization, which consists of both the overt and the covert or the conscious and the unconscious. Linkage among values, beliefs, and actions are often explained by the organization's rituals, myths, and stories. A diverse sample of these and other indicators are necessary to form a true picture of an organization's culture.

Examples of organizational rituals include holiday parties, company picnics, and sports events participation.

For many organizations it is important to know if there is a strategic management plan, as this implies a future-oriented organization. Strategic planning allows for an integration of a shared vision regarding the organization's future direction. The strategic planning process should provide the criteria for making organizational decisions and should provide a template against which all such decisions can be evaluated.

Simyar and Lloyd-Jones (1988) describe strategic planning as the process of defining an organization, its mission, and the set of goals and objectives it is to pursue given certain environmental factors. Goodstein et al. (1992, p. 3) define strategic planning as "the process by which the guiding members of an organization envision its future and develop the necessary procedures and operations to achieve that future." Strategic management is defined as the day-to-day implementation of the strategic plan and involves formalizing the plans, policies, structure, standards of conduct, courses of action, allocation of resources, and tasks that are to be included in an organization's planning cycle. Several questions

■ **TABLE 8–4** Assessing Strategic Status

• Where is the enterprise currently?
• Where does the organization wish to be in the future?
• What steps are needed to achieve the desirable state?
• What is the environmental context?
• How do the internal strengths and weaknesses relate to the external opportunities and threats?

to consider when assessing the organization's strategic status are shown in Table 8–4.

Changes in the external environment make it critical for organizations to develop a strategic vision, as this helps to define the organization for the future and shape services and ventures. Critical factors to consider and predict are information technology, regulations, and competitors. The strategic planning process does more than plan for the future; it helps an organization to create its future.

■ **POWER CONCEPTS AND RELATIONSHIPS**

Power and influence are concepts that are interrelated. Influence is considered the effect one party has on another. Even though simply stated, the process of influence may take different forms and result in different outcomes. For example, when one party (agent) is attempting to get another party (target) to accept an idea, proposal, or decision, the result may include a commitment to the decision or request with an enthusiasm to implement the decision; compliance with the decision but apathy or minimal effort toward decision implementation; or resistance to the proposal or decision through active opposition to implementation, such as making excuses, trying to influence withdrawal of the request, sabotaging the implementation plan, and outright refusing to carry out the request (Yukl, 1989).

Power generally refers to the capacity or ability of an individual or group to influence, modify, or control the behavior of another individual or group in such a way that desired results are achieved (Janik, 1986). In organizations, power can be derived from several sources, which are displayed in Table 8–5 (French & Raven, 1959; Hersey & Blanchard, 1988; Yukl, 1989).

Formal authority or legitimate power is based on the leadership position one holds in the organization and associated rights and responsibilities inherent in that position. The manager has the right to make requests, such as certain work assignments, and workers have an obligation to comply. Tied to formal authority is the manager's authority to make decisions regarding allocation of resources. The higher one's authority position in the organization, the more control she or he has over resources.

Power related to reward and punishment is based on the perceived credibility of the manager to effect the reward or punishment as promised. The capacity to provide compensation, promotions, more responsibility, or status symbols such as larger office space or reserved parking are examples of reward power. The organization also uses formal authority in the form of punishment or coercive power to influence workers, although this method of power is not very effective

■ **TABLE 8–5**   Sources of Power

Legitimate Power is based on the position held by the leader. Normally, the higher the position, the higher the legitimate power tends to be. Leaders high in legitimate power induce compliance or influence others because they feel they have the right, by virtue of position in the organization, to expect that suggestions will be followed.

Reward Power is based on the leader's ability to provide rewards for other people who believe that compliance will lead to positive incentives such as pay, promotion, or recognition.

Coercive/Punitive Power is based on fear. A leader high in coercive power is seen as inducing compliance because failure to comply will lead to punishment such as undesirable work assignments, reprimands, or dismissal.

Information Power is based on the leader's possession of or access to information that is perceived as valuable by others. This power base influences others because they need this information or want to be in on things.

Expert Power is based on the leader's possession of expertise, skill, and knowledge, which, through respect, influences others and leads to compliance with the leader's wishes. A leader high in expert power is seen as possessing the expertise to facilitate the work behavior of others.

Referent Power is based on the leader's personal traits. A leader high in referent power is generally liked and admired by others because of personality, which allows for personal influence.

Connection Power is based on the leader's "connections" with influential or important persons inside or outside the organization. A leader high in connection power induces compliance from others because they aim at gaining the favor or avoiding the disfavor of the powerful connection.

and is used infrequently (Katz & Kahn, 1978). Punitive power such as job dismissal for arbitrary reasons is usually prohibited; however, in situations where workers do not perform their duties or thwart the organizational goals, some form of disciplinary or punitive action may be expected. A leader with substantive reward and punishment power is more likely to obtain worker compliance with requests and demands even when no explicit promises or threats have been made. However, workers are more likely to acknowledge being influenced by referent or expert power than to admit to succumbing to change based on compensation or fear of reprisal (Yukl, 1989).

One's access to and control over the distribution of vital information to others is an important source of power. Control of information downward can involve selective interpretation and filtering and may also involve distortion of information in an attempt to dictate a certain course of action. In addition, withholding information from workers may also serve to increase worker dependence on the leader for decision making and, in effect, decrease worker autonomy.

Types of personal power, which are viewed as facilitating the work, include expert and referent power. Expert power is based on one's possession of expertise, knowledge, and skills in problem solving and task performance. Perceived expertise can be as influential as actual expertise; however, in the long term actual expertise will need to be demonstrated and certainly expertise must be maintained. Specialized knowledge and skill will remain a source of power as long as there is continued dependence on the person who possesses these characteristics.

Referent power is based on one's personal traits wherein the leader is liked and admired by others. This type of power is often dependent upon feelings of friendship and loyalty, and often the worker identifies with a likeable leader, perceiving some of the same qualities in herself or himself. Referent power is an important source of upward, horizontal, and downward power in organizations; that is, praise, flattery, and loyalty given sincerely can be very influential at all levels (Dubin, 1978; Kaplan, 1984).

The power of politics is pervasive in organizations and includes such strategies as co-optation, connection, and coalitions. Co-optation is a form of political action wherein the objective is to overcome the opposing party by encouraging the group or a member of the group to become a part of the project, committee, or function responsible for the decision making. The result then usually favors the proposed action through individual or group attitude change and ownership, and thus the member and / or group are co-opted to carry out the decision (Pfeiffer, 1981).

Connection power refers to the leader's connection to or relationship with other influential individuals who have the capacity to reward or disfavor, either within or external to the organization. The leader is thus viewed as powerful "by association" and workers, peers, or colleagues may feel they can gain by the association with the leader.

Coalitions represent a political force that acts together to get what it wants either in supporting or opposing a particular change or program (Stevenson et al., 1985). In a coalition, two or more groups (e.g., departments) unite, generally to achieve a common goal, such as better or increased human and physical resources. Another common example is the use of collective bargaining strategies to acquire more benefits such as increased compensation or better working conditions.

In organizations, the use of power varies greatly, depending on individual relationships (i.e., upward, downward, lateral) and the situational context. Effective leaders are likely to use a mix of power tactics to effect change. Over time, leaders gain and lose power in organizations depending on such factors as loyalty, competence, and success. Political processes and other types of power are used to protect and increase one's power in organizations, and it is important to recognize and understand how these processes are used and the consequences of the action.

It is also important to recognize that conflict in organizations exists and that potential or probable reasons for the conflict often occur between individuals or groups because of power struggles related to philosophical differences and competing values and in the heat of competing for scarce resources. In working with people and organizations, the occupational health nurse manager can utilize skills and tactics to help prevent or resolve power struggles and conflicts as previously described.

■ SUMMARY

There is no doubt that organizational culture is an important force in determining the direction, support, and influence with respect to the health of the work environment. While health care managers and administrators spend a lot of time attending to management and delivery of workplace health services, it is imperative that they carefully assess organizational culture, politics, and variables such as formal and informal structures and power relationships in order to effectively understand decision-making tactics, the role they play, and their influence on the decision-making process.

References

Beyers, M. Getting on top of organizational change. Journal of Nursing Administration, *14:* 32–37, 1984.

Blancett, S. Satisfaction: It's more than effectiveness and efficiency. Journal of Nursing Administration, *22:* 5, 1992.

del Bueno, D & Freund, C. Power and politics in nursing administration: A casebook. Owings Mills, MD: National Health Publishing, 1986.

Dieneman, J. Theoretical perspectives in organization science for nursing administration. In: Henry, B, Arndt, C, Divincetti, M & Marriner-Torney, A (Eds.), Dimensions of nursing administration. Boston: Blackwell Scientific Publications, 1989.

Dubin, AJ. Human relations: A job oriented approach. Reston, VA: Reston, 1978.

French, J & Raven, B. The bases of social power. In: Cartwright, D (Ed.), Studies of social power. Ann Arbor, MI: Institute for Social Research, 1959.

Flarey, D. The social climate: A tool for organizational change and development. Journal of Nursing Administration, *21:* 37–44, 1991.

Goodstein, LD, Nolan, TM, & Pfeiffer, JW. Applied strategic planning. San Diego: Pfeiffer & Company, 1992.

Harrison, R & Stokes, H. Diagnosing organizational culture. Mountain View, CA: Harrison Associates, 1990.

Hein, E & Nicholson, J. Assessing organizational structure. In: Hein E & Nicholson, J, Contemporary leadership behavior: Selected readings. Boston: Little, Brown & Company, pp. 353–362, 1986.

Hersey, P & Blanchard, K. Management of organizational behavior. Englewood Cliffs, NJ: Prentice Hall, 1988.

Janik, A. Power base of nursing in bargaining relationships. In: Hein, E & Nicholson, J. Contemporary leadership behavior: Selected readings. Boston: Little, Brown & Company, pp. 179–185, 1986.

Kaplan, RE. Trade routes: The manager's network of relationships. Organizatinal Dynamics, Spring: 37–52, 1984.

Katz, D & Kahn, RL. The social psychology of organizations. New York: John Wiley, 1978.

Moos, R. Work environment scale manual (2nd ed.). Palo Alto, CA: Consulting Psychologists Press, 1986.

Moos, R. The social climate scale: A user's guide. Palo Alto, CA: Consulting Psychologists Press, 1987.

McNeil, V & Garcia, MA. Enhancing program management through cultural organizational assessment. AAOHN Update Series, *4*(6): 1–8. Skillman, NJ: Continuing Professional Education Center, 1991.

Pfeiffer, J. Power in organizations. Marshfield, PA: Pittman, 1981.

Schein, E. Organizational culture and leadership. San Francisco: Jossey-Bass, 1985.

Simyar, F & Lloyd-Jones, J. Strategic management in the health care sector: Toward the year 2000. Englewood Cliffs, NJ: Prentice Hall, 1988.

Smircich, L. Concepts of culture and organizational analysis. Administrative Science Quarterly, *28:* 339–358, 1983.

Stevenson, W, Pearce, J, & Porter, L. The concept of coalitions in organization and theory and research. Academy of Management Review, *10:* 256–268, 1985.

Turnipseed, D. Evaluation of health care work environments via a social climate scale: Results of a field study. Hospital Health Services Administration, *35:* 245–262, 1990.

Yukl, L. Leadership in organizations. Englewood Cliffs, NJ: Prentice Hall, 1989.

--- APPENDIX ---

8–1

An Organizational Culture Checklist

What beliefs and norms organize and influence rules, policies, and behavior in your organization? What is the desired image? What is explicit and what is implicit? The following checklist is neither all-inclusive nor universally applicable. It may be helpful, however, for learning about and understanding your organization's culture and subcultures.

IMAGE

- How does the organization wish to be perceived? What word, slogans, or phrases are used in describing the organization? Examples: friendly, caring, innovative, safe, up-and-coming, biggest, oldest, dependable.
- Is money obviously being spent on creating this image with respect to decor, landscaping, equipment, signage, public relation activities, annual reports, or community activities?
- How does the public get access to the organization? Through a lobby, parking garage, clinic, or reception area? How comfortable, attractive, and secure is this access?
- How are visitors treated? Does the treatment depend on socioeconomic status?
- Is community involvement expected of employees? If so, does it depend on position or status in the organization?

DEPORTMENT

- Is there a dress code? How strictly is it enforced? Is it different for men and women? Do people dress formally/informally? Does this depend on status in the hierarchy?
- Is facial hair tolerated on men? Is hair length or style an issue? How much makeup and jewelry can women wear?
- Is touching acceptable or desirable? Only between same-sex employees or between opposite sexes? How much, if any, affection is acceptable?
- What kind of relationships are acceptable off the job between different sexes, at different job or position levels?
- Can people "let themselves go" at parties or social events?
- Is social drinking or smoking acceptable on the job?
- Are there off-limits places for employees?
- Does it matter whom you hang around with or does it depend on your position?
- Are there social stratifications? If so, what is the basis of this stratification: title, department, personal relationship?
- Is swearing or use of four-letter words acceptable? Can employees tell off-color or ethnic jokes?
- Do employees use first names or last names with each other? Does it depend on job position or gender? Does it depend on the setting (e.g., social gatherings versus work)?
- Are sexist behaviors tolerated? Does it depend on title or status?

STATUS SYMBOLS AND REWARD SYSTEMS

- Are there any acknowledged symbols of status such as space, titles, or special privileges?
- On what basis are promotions given: performance, longevity, loyalty? Are upper-level positions given to outsiders or only to those who have "earned their stripes?"
- Are there restricted areas or areas that are off-limits except for special groups, such as meeting rooms or lounge spaces?
- Do only specific individuals or positions warrant reserved parking or personal bathrooms or closets?
- What are the elitist committees, societies, projects, or events?
- Do certain people receive special perquisites such as a company car, country club membership, or professional association dues? Who are those individuals?
- What badges or physical indicators such as beepers, personal desktop computers, different uniforms, or clipboards set people apart as being special?
- Who gets sent to the fun cities for conventions and meetings?
- Do titles truly reflect status and authority in the organization?

ENVIRONMENT AND AMBIANCE

* Are there lounges or places for employees to relax? Where are they located? How attractive and comfortable are they?
* Are eating and drinking allowed in the work area?
* Are there public eating areas? Who has access? What is the appearance and ambiance?
* Can employees have plants, photographs, posters, or other individual touches in their work area or offices?
* Is there a company color scheme? If so, is it subdued, bright, sterile?
* Is music provided or acceptable in work areas or offices?
* What are the norms in regard to starting time, quitting time, and "goof-off" time?
* Who eats with whom? Are there separate eating areas for special groups?
* How is office furniture arranged? Is open seating at tables or in a circle encouraged?

COMMUNICATION

* Is the norm for important communication verbal or written?
* Are written communications formal or informal? Is the preferred style narrative or memo? Is language to the point or circuitous?
* Is jargon acceptable or desirable? In the organization? with clients or outsiders?
* Are minutes of meetings kept? Are they circulated? If so, to whom? What kind of reports are important and what kind are filed in the wastebasket?
* Is rumor the usual method of information distribution?
* Are there bulletin boards, company newsletters, or house organs? How important or meaningful are these means of communication? What is their purpose: recognition, information, or both?
* Does important information flow from the top down or from the bottom up? Can the chain of command be circumvented without punishment?
* Where does important communication take place: in meetings, in the hall, at social functions, away from the place of business, in the men's room?

MEETINGS

* Are there unwritten rules about who speaks first and last at meetings?
* What meetings can you skip without being punished or missing anything important?
* Is it permissible to come late or leave early, or does it depend on whose meeting it is?
* Where are people seated? Are there territorial rights? Are there established arrangements based on status or hierarchy?
* Is discussion allowed? Is the agenda predetermined and no adjustments permissible?
* Are refreshments provided? Who pours or serves the refreshments? Does everyone help himself?
* Are time limits strictly enforced?

RITES, RITUALS, AND CEREMONIES

* Are there established rituals that must be attended, such as Monday morning executive breakfast meetings, Friday afternoon drinks or beer bashes, Christmas parties, the annual picnic?
* Is orientation to the organization special? Who greets new employees? Is orientation different for different position levels?
* What does the organization do to recognize length of service? birth of employees' children? retirement? marriage? death in employees' families?
* Are there sports teams? How important is membership or participation?
* Are there rules or assumptions about how long you have to be employed before you are considered an insider?

SACRED COWS

- (A sacred cow is a person, place, thing, or belief that cannot be discussed, attacked, or ignored. Sacred cows are revered and protected. Denial of the existence of sacred cows or failure to give fealty to them is fraught with risk.)
- Are there heroes, living or dead, in the organization who are revered and honored? How did these individuals get to be heroes?
- Are there any myths about the organization that must be perpetuated, such as, "We have a mission to the poor and needy"?
- Are there any subjects or ideas that are taboo, such as unionization or merit systems?
- Are there rules or policies that are sacrosanct and cannot be changed even if outdated, ineffective, or illogical?
- Are there relationships between departments, individuals, or groups that cannot be threatened, challenged, or questioned, such as between physicians and nurses or between lay members and professional or religious members of the board?
- If there is a difference between what we do and what we say, is it acceptable to acknowledge this inconsistency or is it taboo to suggest that such a situation even exists?
- Can employees speak freely to the media or are all public relations and statements carefully controlled?

SUBCULTURES

- Are there any? If so, what purpose do they serve? Is the purpose deliberate?
- If there are subcultures are they subrosa or overt? Are they tolerated or pointed to with pride as our unique group, department, or unit?

From del Bueno, D & Freund C. Power and politics in nursing administration: A casebook. Owings Mills, MD: National Health Publishing, 1986.

9

ASSESSING WORK AND THE WORK ENVIRONMENT

The primary goal of a comprehensive occupational health program is the preservation, protection, and improvement of the health of the workforce. The Occupational Health and Safety Administration (OSHA) has published Guidelines for General Safety and Health Programs (USDOL, 1989), which describes an effective program as one that looks beyond the specific requirements of the law in addressing general and specific workplace hazards. An essential component of the program is a thorough assessment of the work and work environment to determine potential and actual work-related hazards to which workers may be exposed. In addition, factors that influence a healthy workforce/workplace orientation, such as adequate resources and management commitment, are considered.

In order to relate any human response to a work-related exposure or within an occupational context, the occupational health nurse needs to be familiar with worker jobs and demands, steps in the work processes, and all aspects of the work environment. With virtually thousands of new chemicals and processes active in the occupational environment (Love & Upton, 1987), it is incumbent upon all health care professionals to delineate new occupational hazards, detect existing problems, and develop and implement preventive strategies before human harm occurs.

The occupational health nurse is often the only health and safety professional at the worksite and thus plays a critical role in worksite assessment. However, using a team approach to worksite assessment whenever possible, which may involve management, workers, union representatives, and other health care professionals, will add to the breadth and depth of the investigation. In addition, collaborative efforts will foster the understanding of human consequences from hazardous workplace exposures, as well as add input for remedies regarding hazard abatement. Further, worksite assessments can help to link employee health complaints and data regarding illness and injury trends to workplace hazards.

The purpose of a worksite assessment is to ensure a safe and healthful work environment and thereby protect and promote the physical and mental well-being

■ **TABLE 9–1**   Elements of a Comprehensive Worksite Assessment

- Determination of management philosophy and commitment
- Familiarization with and/or review of the work, work processes, and products
- Knowledge of the composition, demographic characteristics, and health status of the workforce
- Review of existing occupational health and safety programs
- Conduct of the worksite walk-through
- Observation and review of control strategies
- Report of the assessment, in writing, including recommendations for abatement

of the worker. In order to do this it is necessary to identify high-risk personnel and work areas, materials, and processes; determine the effectiveness of existing health and safety programs and control measures; and recommend target areas for worksite and work process modification and/or training and education needs (Camp & Tanberg, 1985; Rogers, 1990). Although a walk-through survey is a key component of the assessment, several elements comprise a comprehensive worksite assessment (Table 9–1). The occupational health nurse may want to develop a guide or tool to use when assessing the worksite. An example of a Worksite Assessment Guide can be found in Appendix 9–1.

■ MANAGEMENT PHILOSOPHY AND COMMITMENT

Management plays an important role in the overall company health program and must be fully cognizant that the occupational health program is preventive in nature and not simply a tool to reduce compensation costs or improve the company safety record (USDHHS, 1983). It is important that the occupational health nurse understand the philosophy of corporate management with respect to health and safety.

Although the mission of business and industry encompasses a profit motive, ideally, management philosophy will embody a commitment to worker health promotion and protection. This will be reflected in policies and programs for a healthful work environment, resources to support program activities, including adequate levels and types of health care professionals, promotion of education and research to improve worker health and safety, and a mechanism for quality assurance, all of which should be specified in clear goals and measurable objectives. The support for establishment of a Health and Safety Committee should also be evident as this committee is critical in assisting management to ensure a safe and healthful environment. The committee should review accidents and data related to health and safety issues at work and make recommendations for corrective action and policy. In addition, management must be willing to delegate authority and responsibility for program management to the appropriate health care professionals, if the program is to be successful (Felton, 1990).

Management's commitment can be demonstrated by active involvement in the health and safety program such as through participation in health and safety meetings, walk-through surveys, and through appropriate allocation of capital equipment, materials, and human resources to provide quality services and control measures for hazard abatement and risk reduction. If management displays a lukewarm attitude toward a comprehensive occupational health program, the occupational health nurse will need to help educate management as to the benefits of the program, such as a decrease in work-related illnesses, injuries, and associated health care costs, and an increase in employee morale and productivity (AAOHN, 1987). In addition, obtaining background information on the industry may provide a historical context about the evolution of the organizational culture and perspective on how health and safety has been viewed, which the occupational health nurse may find helpful in terms of negotiating for program expansion. Sometimes information may be difficult to obtain because management may be uncertain as to how the data will be used. A meeting with management can facilitate an understanding of the assessment process (Sutherland & Ameen, 1991).

Management's commitment should extend to encouraging employee involvement in the program operation and participation in health and safety program decision making. Employees' input regarding knowledge of their jobs can provide firsthand information about work procedures and associated hazards (Patty, 1981). In addition, employee involvement should be sought for worksite inspections, and recommendations regarding work modification, hazard control measures, and development of training programs for job safety.

■ WORK AND WORK PROCESSES

Health care professionals need to have a certain degree of suspicion about the work environment in order to identify potential or actual workplace hazards (Burgess, 1981; Froines et al., 1986). This can be accomplished in part through a prior review of the work processes, materials, and products. Resource books and technical publications are helpful in describing the manufacturing or work processes and providing information about health hazards, acute and chronic symptoms related to selected exposures, and adverse health outcomes. NIOSH criteria documents and a review of Material Safety Data Sheets (MSDS) will also provide useful information about the composition, physical, and chemical properties of materials used in the work processes. An inventory of chemicals used and produced in the manufacturing process should be developed, maintained, and updated regularly.

To recognize certain workplace hazards it is necessary to know about the raw materials. Although hazards from raw materials may be predicted from animal toxicity data, many materials used in industry may not have been adequately evaluated for possible harmful effects. By-products, intermediates, and final products formed by the raw materials may be difficult to determine.

Each step from raw materials to finished product must be evaluated. It is important to understand the processes well enough to determine where contaminants are released, who is exposed, and to what degree. This may be dependent on or affected by such variables as room air currents, work practices/patterns (e.g., shiftwork, overtime), temperature, and environmental hygiene factors.

It should be emphasized that the toxicity of a substance is not necessarily the most important factor in determining the extent of a health hazard associated with the use of that material. The nature of the process in which that material is used or generated, the possibility of reaction with other agents (biological, physical, or chemical), the extent and duration of exposure, and the degree of effective ventilation and other control measures all relate to the potential hazard associated with the use of that material. Consideration should also be given to the type and degree of toxic response the material may elicit in both the average and the hypersusceptible worker (Danse, 1991; Olishifski, 1983).

Knowledge of the work processes and materials will aid in preparation and preplanning for the worksite survey as well as assist in the organization and efficiency in the conduct of the survey. A map or layout of the work environment usually will provide a good description of the general operations involved, and work areas that are high risk. This information will help the occupational health nurse to avoid missing critical functions in the operations of the "plant" and pinpoint potentially dangerous or hazardous conditions such as repetitive operations on assembly lines, or exposure to chemical or physical agents associated with a specific process such as crushing, grinding, heating, and electrolysis (Olishifski, 1983; Camp & Tanberg, 1985).

A flow sheet that identifies each step of the work process from start to finish should be obtained and reviewed prior to the survey. The flow sheet should indicate the fate of raw materials from the time they enter the worksite; how they are used and transformed in the process; the various pieces of equipment involved; and by-products produced at any step in the process (Verma & Verrall, 1985). An example of a flow process for pulp and paper is shown in Figure 9-1.

In addition to examining the flow process of raw materials, an analysis of each job and its related hazards provides valuable information. The job hazard analysis is a tool that provides a blueprint about how to do a critical job in a safe, productive manner, identifies actual or potential sources of occupational health problems/hazards, and specifies recommendations for prevention and control measures. A job hazard analysis is best completed by the occupational health team or occupational health and safety committee so that employees can be involved in the process. Direct observation of the worker(s) performing the job or videotaping of job activities, which allows for a careful step-by-step review of the tasks performed, is essential for an accurate analysis. An example of a job hazard analysis tool is shown in Table 9-2. Analysis of jobs performed at the worksite prior to the walk-through survey will assist in anticipating the physical and psychosocial demands placed on workers and detecting potential sources of injury and exposure.

Of interest in categorizing specific types of industries is the *Standard Industrial Classification* system (USOMB, 1987). The *Standard Industrial Classification* (SIC) was developed for use in the classification of establishments by type of activity in which they are engaged; for purposes of facilitating the collection, tabulation, presentation, and analysis of data relating to establishments; and for promoting uniformity and comparability in the presentation of statistical data collected by various agencies of the United States government, state agencies, trade associations, and private research organizations.

The SIC is intended to cover the entire field of economic activities: agriculture, forestry, fishing, hunting, and trapping; mining; construction; manufacturing; transportation, communications, electric, gas, and sanitation; wholesale trade; retail trade; finance, insurance, and real estate; personal, business professional, repair, recreation, and other services; and public administration. Each operating establishment is assigned an industry code on the basis of its primary activity, which is determined by its principal product or group of products produced or distributed, or services rendered. The structure of the classification makes it

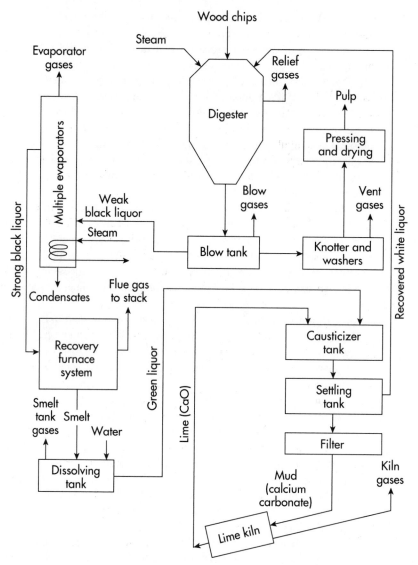

■ **Figure 9–1** Flow process for pulp and paper operation. (From Burgess, WA. Recognition of health hazards in industry. New York: John Wiley & Sons, 1981.)

possible to tabulate, analyze, and publish establishment data on a divison, and within that divison, a two-digit major group, a three-digit industry group, or a four-digit industry code basis, according to the level of industrial detail considered most appropriate.

The 10 major establishment divisions and one division identified as nonclassifiable establishments (A-K) are shown in Table 9–3. Within each division as a whole are major groups, each specified by two-digit numbers that further narrow or define the industry division. For example, division E, "transportation, communications, electric, gas, and sanitation," is identified by *SIC* numbers 40 through 49. These major groups are then subdivided into industry groups as specified by the addition of a third digit and then further subdivided according

■ **TABLE 9–2** Sample Job Hazard Analysis: Cleaning Inside Surface of Chemical Tank—Top Manhole Entry

Step	Hazard	New Procedure or Protection
1. Select and train operators.	Operator with respiratory or heart problem; other physical limitation.	• Examination by industrial physician for suitability to work.
	Untrained operator—failure to perform task.	• Train operators. • Dry run. [Reference: National Institute for Occupational Safety and Health (NIOSH) Doc. #80-406]

2. Determine what is in the tank, what process is going on in the tank, and what hazards this can pose.	Explosive gas.
	
	Improper oxygen level.
	Chemical exposure—
	Gas, dust, vapor:
	  irritant
	  toxic
	Liquid:
	  irritant
	  toxic
	  corrosive:
	Solid:
	  irritant
	  corrosive
		• Obtain work permit signed by safety, maintenance and supervisors.
		• Test air by qualified person.
		• Ventilate to 19.5%-23.5% oxygen and less than 10% LEL of any flammable gas. Steaming inside of tank, flushing and draining, then ventilating, as previously described, may be required.
		• Provide appropriate respiratory equipment—SCBA or air line respirator.
		• Provide protective clothing for head, eyes, body and feet.
		• Provide parachute harness and lifeline. [Reference: OSHA standards 1910.106, 1926.100, 1926.21(b)(6); NIOSH Doc. #80-406]
		• Tanks should be cleaned from outside, if possible.

3. Set up equipment.	Hoses, cord, equipment—tripping hazards. Electrical—voltage too high, exposed conductors. Motors not locked out and tagged.	• Arrange hoses, cords, lines and equipment in orderly fashion, with room to maneuver safely. • Use ground-fault circuit interrupter. • Lockout and tag mixing motor, if present.
4. Install ladder in tank.	Ladder slipping.	• Secure to manhole top or rigid structure.
5. Prepare to enter tank.	Gas or liquid in tank.	• Empty tank through existing piping. • Review emergency procedures. • Open tank. • Check of job site by industrial hygienist or safety professional. • Install blanks in flanges in piping to tank. (Isolate tank.) • Test atmosphere in tank by qualified person (long probe).
6. Place equipment at tank-entry position.	Trip or fall.	• Use mechanical-handling equipment. • Provide guardrails around work positions at tank top.

Table continued on following page

■ **TABLE 9–2**   Sample Job Hazard Analysis: Cleaning Inside Surface of Chemical Tank—Top Manhole Entry *Continued*

Step	Hazard	New Procedure or Protection
7. Enter tank.	Ladder—tripping hazard.	• Provide personal protective equipment for conditions found. [Reference: NIOSH Doc. #80-406; OSHA CFR 1910.134]
	Exposure to hazardous atmosphere.	• Provide outside helper to watch, instruct, and guide operator entering tank, with capability to lift operator from tank in emergency.
8. Cleaning tank.	Reaction of chemicals, causing mist or expulsion of air contaminant.	• Provide protective clothing and equipment for all operators and helpers. • Provide lighting for tank (Class I, Div. 1). • Provide exhaust ventilation. • Provide air supply to interior of tank. • Frequent monitoring of air in tank. • Replace operator or provide rest periods. • Provide means of communication to get help, if needed. • Provide two-man standby for any emergency.
9. Cleaning up.	Handling of equipment, causing injury.	• Dry run. • Use material-handling equipment.

From U.S. Department of Labor, Occupational Safety and Health Administration, 1988.

to the primary products of the industry, hence a fourth digit. In this classification scheme then, the SIC number 47 specifies the major group "transportation services," the SIC number 472 designates the industry group "arrangement of passenger transportation," and SIC number 4724 indicates "travel agencies." The SIC is used to promote the comparability of established data relative to the U.S. economy. In addition, data can be categorized according to work-related illnesses

■ **TABLE 9–3**   Major Industrial Divisions Within the Standard Industrial Classification Systems

Division	Industry Description
A	Agriculture, forestry, and fishing
B	Mining
C	Construction
D	Manufacturing
E	Transportation, communications, electric, gas, and sanitation
F	Wholesale trade
G	Retail trade
H	Finance, insurance, and real estate
I	Services
J	Public administration
K	Nonclassifiable establishments

and injuries; thus, a high estimation of hazard/risk can be determined through analysis of SIC codes.

■ WORKFORCE CHARACTERISTICS

Information about the demographic characteristics of the workforce such as the number and distribution of employees by age, sex, ethnicity, and by department, job title/responsibilities, and shift of work is an essential component of the worksite assessment. Knowledge of these characteristics will help to determine if there are patterns or trends in illnesses and injuries that may be associated with selected personal variables, certain jobs or departments, or rotation of work schedules and areas (Rogers & Travers, 1991). For example, a workforce comprised primarily of women will present different problems contrasted with a workforce made up of mostly men (e.g., certain reproductive toxicities).

Additional information about the worker and her or his job may be obtained from the *Dictionary of Occupational Titles* (DOT). This dictionary provides standardized occupational information based on on-site job analyses to provide definitions of approximately 20,000 jobs (USDOL, 1990). This information can be useful not only in enumerating and categorizing the types of jobs specific to a particular industry, but can also be helpful in furthering the understanding of job tasks and functions for job hazard analyses.

The DOT groups jobs into occupations based on similarities of job performance, thus defining the structure and content of all listed occupations. Each occupation is given a nine-digit code number, for example, 652.382-010. These digits specify a particular occupational category, division, and group within the category (first three digits); worker functions as related to data, people, and things (middle three digits); and the job title (last three digits). Thus, the code number indicated above specifies a "machine trades occupation" in a "printing occupation" involving "printing machine occupations" (652), with work functions of "compiling" data, "taking instructions helping" people, and "operating/controlling" things (382). The final three digits (010) specify a code applicable to only one occupational title, "cloth printer." Each designated job specifies duties and tasks of, and machine equipment and materials used by, the worker. Thus, the DOT provides a unique code/description of each occupation within a designated industry. The reader is referred to this source for more specific information.

■ OCCUPATIONAL HEALTH PROGRAMS

Within the scope of the workplace assessment is a review of the types of programs and services offered to determine if they are appropriate and responsive to the health promotion and protection needs of the workers. Health promotion programs such as exercise and nutrition may improve the overall health and fitness of workers, thus decreasing vulnerability to exposure and injury, while health protection programs such as use of universal precautions and protective equipment may significantly reduce exposure levels. Observation of workers with respect to work practices or behaviors, which may contribute to health damage, should be assessed within the context of the overall health program. For example, if the occupational health nurse observes poor lifting techniques that may contribute to back injuries, or witnesses unsafe handling of laboratory specimens, health education programs on appropriate lifting and handling techniques may be in order. Some common specific health hazard control programs include hearing conservation against noise; eye protection against flying particulates and chemical exposures; and respiratory protection against such airborne agents as lead, silica, asbestos, cotton, and solvent vapor.

An examination of written reports, logs, sampling data, health and exposure records, and insurance data can aid the occupational health nurse to better target specific areas for observation, investigation, or follow-up (Cahall, 1984). This type of review prior to any walk-through survey may provide information on specific work-related illnesses and injuries prevalent at the worksite, and help identify trends in occupational health unit visits or exposures for which specific programs are in place (e.g., noise and hearing protection) but require monitoring for compliance and improvement.

■ WORKSITE WALK-THROUGH SURVEY

The actual walk-through survey is conducted to identify potential and actual hazards in the workplace, to observe workers and their work practices and activities, to determine if the health and safety policies and programs have been successfully implemented, and to monitor compliance with such policies (Camp & Tanberg, 1985). The walk-through may also help to clarify a relationship between what may be presumed to be a nonoccupational complaint and a work-related exposure.

The walk-through survey may be a baseline, periodic, or specific complaint investigation (Verma & Verrall, 1985). The baseline survey is done to initially assess the complete operation of the worksite. The periodic survey is done to monitor worksite operations and processes, update existing data, and examine new processes added. A specific complaint survey is done to investigate a specific area of the work environment or particular operation, based on worker complaints such as headaches, odors, skin irritations, or back problems. In all instances observation of the workers performing their jobs should be conducted.

As previously described, once preparation and planning for the survey has been completed, the walk-through can begin and should start at the beginning where the raw products, materials, supplies, and so forth enter the worksite to initiate the production process. Information about work processes obtained from resource materials, flow diagrams, and inventory lists will be helpful in identifying potential problems. It is best if walk-through surveys can be conducted with team members, particularly the industrial hygienist and/or technical production personnel, especially when new processes are introduced or if a better understanding of existing processes and controls is needed (USDHHS, 1983). With the aid of the floor plan, which can identify areas of high risk, and the process flow sheet, a planned, systematic examination of the workplace, including area sampling, can be conducted to locate critical functions of the operation and potential sources of contaminants. Potential for worker exposure should be carefully noted as to whom and how many workers are exposed, and the types of job categories involved. In addition, discussions with workers regarding potential and actual exposures will provide invaluable information (Verma and Verrall, 1985).

An industry worksite checklist can be developed in advance to provide a more systematic method for and improved efficiency in data collection. (See Figure

6–1.) However, a more specific guide may be needed for the worksite being surveyed. In addition, the occupational health nurse and/or team conducting the walk-through may need to look beyond the items identified in the checklist for conditions or processes that have changed since the last inspection (Stanevich & Stanevich, 1989). As previously discussed, job hazard analyses can aid in determining specific tasks or areas to inspect, and job observation can also be utilized to:

* improve job procedures and safe work behaviors;
* determine compliance with safety rules and standards;
* monitor work practices and use of personal protective equipment;
* monitor effectiveness of training procedures and identify a need for retraining;
* increase worker and management understanding of work-related hazards; and
* reinforce positive work behaviors (Rogers, 1990; Stanevich & Stanevich, 1989).

As mentioned previously, employee and management participation in the walk-through survey is especially important. Employee interest in helping to identify problems needing correction will be increased if their participation is not only requested but valued. This can be demonstrated by management's like commitment to improving workplace health and safety. In addition, any changes or modifications recommended by the team or program manager should be implemented as soon as feasible. Otherwise, employees and the health care team may view this as an intellectual exercise only, and without applied merit and sincere interest on the part of management. A system for monitoring and evaluating the effectiveness of the changes should also be implemented.

The walk-through survey should be conducted at a time when the operation is in progress in order to fully observe the processes, workers, and potential exposure points. Processes and job operations that are run only intermittently may present some of the greatest potential health hazards. Assessment of all shifts should be conducted. If work is done on the night shift or on weekends, a survey should also be made at these times to see if there are any differences in air contaminant concentrations at night as compared to regular daytime operations. Because the production rate may be significantly different on the night shift, conditions could be better or worse (Jones et al., 1990; Hansen, 1991).

Of particular concern during the walk-through survey are all the work areas that have excessive exposures or poor work conditions such as excessive noise, excessive heat, inadequate ventilation, awkward operation positions, radiation exposure (ionizing and nonionizing), excessive air contaminants, and man/machine interface. Exposure characteristics and patterns, and working conditions including the following should be assessed:

* types of agents in the work environment (biological; chemical; ergonomic/environmental/mechanical; physical; psychosocial);
* potential hazards associated with each agent and unique work process including work station design;
* types and numbers of workers exposed either directly or indirectly;

- concentration, frequency, occurrence (shift patterns), and location of exposure (microenvironmental and macroenvironmental);
- routes of entry (inhalation, transdermal, ingestion);
- factors contributing to the exposure such as performance of the job task, personal protective equipment, control mechanisms, individual susceptibility, and work practices;
- cleanliness of the work environment;
- equipment functioning and maintenance;
- general environmental milieu; and
- surveillance and monitoring activities.

Sensory perception also provides valuable information for walk-through assessment purposes. For example, dusty operations can easily be seen; noise that exceeds the OSHA permissible exposure level (PEL) can be audibly detected; and vapors and gases exceeding the OSHA PEL are often odorous. Obvious exposures should provide direction for future exploration and investigation including measurements of potential hazards with the aid of an industrial hygienist and/or safety specialist (Williams & Burson, 1985). Once a hazard has been identified, a more detailed analysis of the worksite, work processes, and practices can be conducted to determine the scope of the problem and potential strategies for abatement.

■ CONTROL STRATEGIES

Control strategies are designed to minimize worker exposure from hazardous substances, and determination of the effectiveness of these strategies is important to assess. Where possible, the hazard should be eliminated; however, the following control strategies may be utilized:

- substitution: replacement of a toxic substance with a less toxic or nontoxic substance (e.g., use of xylene rather than benzene), or change or replacement of an operational process, such as quiet for noisy machinery;
- engineering: removal or elimination of the hazard, such as, using local exhaust ventilation to remove air contaminants before they are released into the worker's breathing zone;
- work practice: use of careful work practices and good hygiene measures, and the provision of adequate and well-maintained equipment to reduce exposure;
- administrative: removal of employees from the hazard totally or partially such as through job rotation; enforcement of health and safety policies, housekeeping strategies, and training procedures;
- personal protection: use of devices designed to reduce point exposure such as through eye and respiratory protection, earplugs, and protective clothing.

The use of control strategies is presented here in a hierarchical order of effectiveness. Personal protective equipment is considered the least effective because it can only be effective if appropriate and reliable equipment is provided and if employees consistently use it (COH, 1985; Levy & Wegman, 1988).

Four important considerations deserve special attention when the decision has been made that a need exists for personal protective equipment:

1. selection of the proper type of protective device;
2. employee fit with the equipment and instruction on its proper use;
3. enforcement of standards created; and
4. an effective system of equipment sanitation and maintenance.

To assure proper use, one should make sure that workers understand why protection is necessary, so they will want to use it. In addition, special attention should be given to the ease and comfort with which it can be used, so that it will be used. Personal protective equipment can be misused or disused to varying degrees depending on a variety of program factors. Therefore, it behooves the occupational health nurse and other health professionals to constantly recognize that this approach to hazard control should always be secondary to a sincere effort to eliminate the exposure.

The frequency of worksite walk-through surveys should be determined by the nature of the work and major changes in procedures or materials; however, even a brief walk-through should be regularly conducted by the occupational health nurse. Worksite surveys serve to demonstrate to workers that health and safety at the worksite are important to management as well as to the workers.

▪ ABATEMENT/PROGRAM STRATEGIES AND REPORTS

Once work-related problems/hazards are identified, steps can be taken for hazard abatement and risk reduction, including the institution of control measures previously mentioned, modification of existing or development of new health and safety programs, and the improvement or implementation of worker and management training and education programs.

Jensen (1988) states that the importance of education and training in occupational health is reflected in the disproportionately high injury rates among workers newly assigned to work tasks, much of which is related to inadequate knowledge of job hazards and safe work practices. Workers need training and education about general and specific hazards of the worksite and work processes, safety rules and procedures related to the particular work assignment, and prevention and control strategies including work practice behaviors.

Supervisors and managers also have a responsibility to understand the work processes and related hazards and provide for health protection of the workforce through job training or retraining, formal health education sessions, and job hazard analyses. Occupational health nurses have the necessary skills to help develop and implement an effective occupational health and hazard control education program.

Once the walk-through survey is completed and all background data are collected and reviewed, results and recommendations should be described in a written report with a copy maintained in the occupational health unit. The report should have input of and discussion by all team members with recommendations for hazard abatement and improvement or modification of the occupational health and safety plan. A summary report should accompany the full report to management, and should include costs and benefits associated with the recommendations.

Based on this comprehensive worksite assessment, the occupational health nurse should be in a better position to evaluate the occupational health and safety program and address the need for change including:

- development of new programs for health promotion, protection, and hazard control, such as disability management, prenatal care, disaster preparedness, substance abuse, waste management;
- revision of policies and procedures for health and safety programming;
- procurement of additional resources for program management and expansion, including upgrading and maintenance;
- improvement and expansion of health and safety training and education programs; and
- establishment of quality assurance and research programs to evaluate health program effectiveness and improve worker health.

■ CONCLUSION

The occupational health nurse is a critical member of the occupational health and safety team and is the key figure for interpreting the health aspects of the safety program to employees. In the occupational setting both the workforce and worksite are the clients. The occupational health nurse provides valuable skills in observing the workforce for changes in health status and the worksite for hazardous conditions. Worksite assessment and analysis involves all workers and management in determining the most effective and efficient methods for health promotion and hazard reduction.

References

American Association of Occupational Health Nurses. A comprehensive guide for establishing an occupational health service. Atlanta: Author, 1987.

Burgess, WA. Recognition of health hazards in industry. New York: John Wiley & Sons, 1981.

Cahall, J. Surveying the work environment to maintain the health of the worker. AAOHN Update Series, *1* (23): 1–7, 1984.

Camp, J & Tanberg, S. Assessment of the worksite: A guide for the occupational health nurse. AAOHN Update Series, *2*(4): 2–7, 1985.

Council on Occupational Health. Surveying hazards in the occupational environment. Archives of Environmental Health, *10:* 115–130, 1985.

Danse, I. Common sense toxics in the workplace. New York: Van Nostrand Company, 1991.

Felton, J. Occupational medical management. Boston: Little, Brown & Co., 1990.

Froines, JR, Dellenbaugh, CA & Wegman, DH. Occupational health surveillance: A means to identify work-related risks. American Journal of Public Health, *76:* 1089–1096, 1986.

Hansen, D. The work environment: Occupational health fundamentals. Chelsea, MI: Lewis Publishers, 1991.

Jensen, R & Sinkule, E. Safety and education

in the workplace. Journal of Safety Research, *19:* 125–133, 1988.

Jones, S, Hosein, HR, Swalm, G, & Yablonsky, J. Occupational hygiene management guide. Chelsea, MI: Lewis Publishers, 1990.

Levy, B & Wegman, D. Occupational health: Recognizing and preventing work-related diseases. Boston: Little, Brown & Company, 1988.

Love, L & Upton, A. Toxic chemicals, health and the environment. Baltimore: Johns Hopkins University Press, 1987.

Olishifski, J. Fundamentals of industrial hygiene. Chicago: National Safety Council, 1983.

Patty's Industrial Hygiene and Toxicology. General Principles, Vol. 1. New York: John Wiley & Sons, 1981.

Rogers, B. Occupational nursing practice, education & research: Challenges for the future. AAOHN Journal, *38:* 581–585, 1990.

Rogers, B & Travers, P. An overview of work-related hazards in nursing: Health & safety issues. Heart & Lung, *20:* 486–497, 1991.

Stanevich, R & Stanevich, R. Guidelines for an occupational safety and health program. AAOHN Journal, *37:* 205–214, 1989.

Sutherland, J & Ameen, D. The first step to managing costs-assessment. AAOHN Update Series, *4*(5): 1–8, 1991.

U.S. Department of Health and Human Services,

National Institute for Occupational Health & Safety. The industrial environment—its evaluation and control. Washington, DC: Government Printing Office, 1983.

U.S. Department of Labor. Dictionary of occupational titles. Washington, DC: Government Printing Office, 1990.

U.S. Department of Labor, Occupational Safety & Health Administration. Guidelines on workplace safety and health program man-agement: Issuance of voluntary guidelines. Federal Register, *54:* 3904–3918, 1989.

U.S. Office of Management and Budget. Standard industrial classification manual. Springfield, VA: National Technical Information Service, 1987.

Verma, D & Verrall, B. Principles of industrial hygiene. AAOHN Update Series, *2*(26): 2–11, 1985.

Williams, P & Burson, J. Industrial toxicology. New York: Van Nostrand Co., 1985.

APPENDIX
9–1

Worksite Assessment Guide

DATE _____

NAME OF INDUSTRY/WORKSITE _____

ADDRESS: _____

TELEPHONE: (   ) _____ Hours of Operation _____

Days of Operation _____

SIC Code _____

Parent Company _____

Name/Location of Corporate Offices _____

PERSON COMPLETING GUIDE _____

Describe the historical development of the company (including parent company and subsidiaries). _____

_____

_____

THE WORK

Identify the major products of the industry:

_____

_____

_____

Describe each stage of the operational processes, raw materials used and byproducts produced.
Is there an inventory of chemicals used in the processes? How is this managed? How are materials stored?

_____

_____

_____

_____

Is the work considered stimulating? (Describe) _____

_____

_____

THE WORK *Continued*

Do workers take pride in the final product? _____

_____

In general, what are the different types of jobs? _____

_____

_____

THE WORK ENVIRONMENT

Describe the general conditions of the work environment including physical (temperature, lighting, noise, ventilation), and psychosocial (stress) characteristics, eating & hygiene facilities, and housekeeping.

_____

_____

_____

_____

_____

_____

Describe the mechanism for disposal of waste products. Are there problems with pollution? _____

_____

_____

Are safety signs posted and apparent where needed? _____

Is there a company union? If yes, please describe the relationship.

_____

_____

Please describe the physical arrangements of the health unit (equipment, space, and location within the organization).

_____

_____

_____

_____

WORKER POPULATION

Total Number Employees _____

    Percent men _____

    Percent women _____

    Age range _____

    Average age _____

    Percent non-production _____
      employees

    Percent production _____
      employees

Additional comments about the characteristics of the workforce:

_____

_____

_____

Do workers rotate shifts? _____

    Shift Work: Percent Employees first shift _____

             Percent Employees second shift _____

             Percent Employees third shift _____

HUMAN RESOURCES/MANAGEMENT

	Number Full-time	Number Part-time (Hours per week)	Job Descriptions Available($\sqrt{}$)
OHN			
Nurse Practitioner			
LPN			
Physician			
Industrial hygienist			
Safety Specialist			
Clerical Support			
Other			
(Specify) _____			

Describe the corporate/company philosophy and commitment to the occupational/safety program.

_____

_____

_____

Are there written policies and procedures regarding operation of the health unit? If yes, describe how these were developed (i.e. decision-making process).

_____

_____

_____

_____

Describe narratively the management style and line and staff functions that operate with respect to the occupational health and safety program. Provide a diagram of the organizational structure (attach).

_____

_____

_____

_____

_____

Please indicate if an employee/manager health and safety committee exists and describe the committee composition, functions, frequency of meetings and outcomes.

_____

_____

_____

_____

_____

Describe the focus, frequency and outcomes of industrial hygiene and safety inspections.

_____

_____

_____

_____

HUMAN RESOURCES/MANAGEMENT *Continued*

Describe the record system in the health unit (including logs, records, reports). What is the policy regarding confidentiality of health records and is this observed?

_____
_____
_____
_____
_____

HEALTH/DISABILITY INSURANCE

What type of employee health insurance does the company have (e.g. third party, self-insured)? _____
What are average annual company expenditures for health insurance claims? _____
$ _____
        Percentage hospital claims   _____
        Percentage ambulatory care claims   _____
What are the major categories of expenditures for these claims (indicate specific illnesses, injury, etc.)?
_____

What are the average annual company expenditures for worker's compensation claims? $ _____

What are the major categories of expenditure for worker's compensation claims (specify illness, injury)?
_____
_____

OCCUPATIONAL HEALTH & SAFETY PROGRAMS

Give an overall description of the occupational health and safety program and health promotion activities. What are the major objectives for the health program? Describe monitoring/surveillance activities, disability and disaster preparedness programs.

_____
_____
_____
_____
_____
_____

Health/Safety Programs/Services

Please indicate which of the following services are provided: (check)

_____ breast cancer screening
_____ cervical cancer screening
_____ chest x-ray
_____ cholesterol screening
_____ colon cancer screening
_____ diabetes management
_____ diabetes screening
_____ disability management
_____ emergency care and follow-up
_____ employee assistance program
_____ exercise/fitness program
_____ first aid/CPR for employees
_____ general health counseling
_____ general health education
_____ glaucoma screening
_____ hazardous materials management (Haz Com)
_____ healthy back program
_____ health risk appraisals
_____ hearing protection program
_____ hepatitis screening

_____ home visiting
_____ hypertension management
_____ hypertension screening
_____ immunizations
_____ monitoring/surveillance of employees
_____ periodic exams by nurse
_____ periodic exams by physician
_____ physical therapy
_____ prenatal instruction
_____ preplacement exams by nurse
_____ preplacement exams by physician
_____ pulmonary function tests
_____ reproductive health
_____ respiratory protection program
_____ retirement planning
_____ return to work
_____ smoking cessation program
_____ stress management program
_____ treatment of non-occupational illness/injury
_____ treatment of occupational illness/injury

_____ tuberculin testing

_____ urine drug screening

     _____ preplacement

     _____ for cause

     _____ random

_____ vision protection program

_____ weight reduction program

_____ other (specify) _____

_____

_____ other (specify) _____

When are group health education/promotion programs conducted?

     _____ Percent on company time

     _____ Percent on employee time

     _____ Not offered

Comments: _____

_____

_____

Please indicate what, if any, mandated programs are in place and to what extent they are observed and enforced.

_____

_____

_____

_____

_____

Do workers use personal protective equipment? (Describe)

_____

_____

What other control measures are in place? (Describe)

_____

_____

Are OSHA regulations adhered to? (Describe) _____

_____

_____

Is there a fire safety program; how often are fire drills and inspections conducted?

_____

_____

Estimate the number of visits made to the health unit by employees.

     _____ Number of weekly visits

     _____ Percent of visits for preventive screening

     _____ Percent of visits for illness injury

     _____ Percent of visits handled by nurse staff

     _____ Percent of visits handled by physician

What are the most common illnesses reported?

_____

_____

What are the most common injuries reported?

_____

_____

HEALTH HAZARD SURVEY

Describe potential/actual health hazards to which workers are exposed, the extent of the exposure and the mechanism for hazards, abatement, and jobs that are high risk. Identify the nursing role in handling these hazards and your recommendations for improvement, if any. Use back of this page or additional sheets if needed.

10

WORKERS AS CLIENTS: HEALTH ASSESSMENT AND SURVEILLANCE

Central to occupational health nursing professional practice is the management, surveillance, and promotion of worker health. The development and conduct of worker health assessment, monitoring, and surveillance programs may be a joint effort among several health care disciplines; however, in most occupational health settings the occupational health nurse assumes major responsibility for the implementation and management of these programs. Depending on the skills, experience, and knowledge level of the occupational health nurse and/ or specific conditions being evaluated, some functions, such as physical assessment/examination, may be performed by or shared collaboratively with other health care professionals. Written guidelines should be available to detail the processes and procedures necessary to carry out programs specific to each occupational health setting.

A health assessment, monitoring, and surveillance program for workers is multidimensional, the purposes of which are to provide for the:

- assessment of the compatibility of the worker with the demands of the job without risk to the worker or coworkers;
- proper placement of prospective workers in jobs that will match their capabilities;
- collection and recording of baseline health status data for future comparative purposes, particularly in the event of disability, illness, or injury;
- documentation of preexisting or concurrent illnesses and injuries to be included in the worker health status data profile;
- promotion of continued safe and healthful employment for employees within the context of the work and working environments;
- detection of infectious or communicable diseases and referral for appropriate medical management;
- detection of nonoccupationally related conditions, acute and chronic, for appropriate management, referral, and/or monitoring;
- evaluation of any evidence of impaired health as a result of harmful ex-

posures and working conditions, and recommendations for corrective actions/work placement;

* maintenance of compliance with government-mandated regulations; and
* maintenance, improvement, or rehabilitation of employee health.

Several benefits have been associated with the assessment and monitoring of worker health. These include the early recognition of work-related illness and injury and prevention of recurrence, decreased absenteeism as a result of hiring workers who can safely perform the job, and the identification of health status and lifestyle risk factors. The risk factors may be reduced through early medical referral and health counseling techniques (Kemerer & Raniere, 1990; Levy & Wegman, 1988; Matte et al., 1990).

benefits

Depending on the work environment, exposures and related health hazards, government-mandated surveillance activities, and company philosophy related to health, several types of health management programs may be performed at the worksite. The most common types include worker placement assessments, preventive/periodic health monitoring, and health surveillance. Various definitions for these types of assessments have been provided (Table 10–1) (Brown, 1981; Burkeen & Cooper, 1985; Felton, 1990; Freeman, 1983; Guidotti et al., 1989; McCunney, 1988). Special health assessments such as fitness for duty or retirement assessments may also be conducted.

■ WORKER PLACEMENT ASSESSMENT

Worker placement assessments are conducted in order to ensure that employees are able to perform a job without hazard to themselves or coworkers. There are various reasons for performing worker placement assessments; however, the most common reasons include preplacement, return to work, and job transfer assignment.

Preplacement Assessment

The preplacement assessment is conducted once an offer of employment is made and is designed to recommend placement of prospective workers into their positions of hire in accordance with their physical and emotional capacities, and

■ TABLE 10–1   Common Workplace Assessments

Preplacement assessment   conducted in order to match the employee's capabilities with the demands of the job and to evaluate existing health conditions with respect to potential aggravation by job duties, and provide baseline data for future comparisons.

Return-to-work assessment   conducted to evaluate any change in the employee's health status that might require a change in the worker's duties and to assure proper placement to prevent further illness and injury.

Job transfer assessment   conducted to match the employee's capabilities with proposed new job, when there has been a change in the employee's health status or in the work conditions that place the employee at health risk.

Periodic health monitoring   conducted, at intervals, to detect any previously unrecognized health problems or undiagnosed health effects and determine if work-related health effects have occurred.

Health surveillance   conducted to target specific high-risk groups for specific adverse health effects tied to a particular occupational exposure.

the physical, psychosocial and environmental demands of the job (Felton, 1990). The assessment is also conducted to ensure that the worker examined does not have any health-related condition that may be aggravated by the job duties or that may affect the health and safety of coworkers. The critical determinants in the decision-making processes are the individual's health, a thorough understanding of the job duties to be performed, and the work environment (McCunney, 1988). Preplacement assessments also provide baseline data against which future evaluative data can be measured, and they may also be part of certain legally mandated Occupational Safety and Health Administration (OSHA) standards' requirements (e.g., asbestos, benzene, lead).

In order to complete an accurate health and occupational history and physical examination, it is imperative that the employer furnish the occupational health professional with current information about the worker's job, such as a job, task, and safety analysis. This will help to focus data collection relative to specific target body systems that may be impacted by job demands. The analysis provides a definition of the work, how it is to be performed, the duration and frequency of the tasks, any specific activities to be conducted, such as repetitive movements and lifting or operation of equipment, the potential for exposure to hazardous agents, and recommendations for abatement (Fig. 10–1).

The preplacement assessment actually incorporates subjective and objective data to arrive at a nursing diagnosis and plan of care to facilitate worker placement and health (Bates, 1988; Jarvis, 1993). Subjective data include information obtained from a comprehensive personal and family health history, a detailed occupational health history, and general review of systems, and the occupational health nurse should be thoroughly familiar with these components. Various formats for obtaining pertinent historical and health status information are available and can be modified or tailored to guide the data collection process and meet the needs of employees completing the forms in terms of understanding and terminology. A thorough family and personal history can help the health care provider to determine if a health condition exists that makes the employee incompatible with the job (i.e., a job requiring heavy lifting and back injury). It also provides an opportunity to do health teaching and counseling (Burkeen & Cooper, 1985). An example of a comprehensive health history is shown in Table 10–2.

It is vital that the occupational health nurse/examiner know the prospective employee's job title, a description of the job, duties, tasks, and related demands, potential work-related hazards, and any physical and/or emotional capacities required (Felton, 1990). The occupational health history (Table 10–3) is designed to determine previous work experiences and to assist the occupational health care provider in discovering preexisting conditions that may be exacerbated by the workplace (Coyle & Rosenstock, 1983; Ginetti & Greig, 1981; Goldman & Peters, 1981; LaDou, 1990; Stein & Franks, 1985). For example, the same job title may mean entirely different job responsibilities in two different companies and the occupational history can add to the description of the actual work performed with associated hazards. In addition, external to the workplace exposures (e.g., home use pesticides) can also be noted. Questions relevant to occupational health history taking are listed in Appendix 10–1.

As part of the history taking, a complete review of systems should be performed in order to further explicate data needed for a complete assessment. If previous health records need to be obtained, they should be requested with the

Text continued on page 217

INSTRUCTIONS FOR COMPLETING JOB SAFETY ANALYSIS FORM

Job Safety Analysis (JSA) is an important accident prevention tool that works by finding hazards and eliminating or minimizing them *before* the job is performed, *and before* they have a chance to become accidents. Use your JSA for job clarification and hazard awareness, as a guide in new employee training, for periodic contacts and for retraining of senior employees, as a refresher on jobs which run infrequently, as an accident investigation tool, and for informing employees of specific job hazards and protective measures.

Set priorities for doing JSAs: jobs that have a history of many accidents, jobs that have produced disabling injuries, jobs with high potential for disabling injury or death, and new jobs with no accident history.

Here's how to do each of the three parts of a Job Safety Analysis:

SEQUENCE OF BASIC JOB STEPS

Break the job down into steps. Each of the steps of a job should accomplish some major task. The task will consist of a set of movements. Look at the first set of movements used to perform a task, and then determine the next logical set of movements. For example, the job might be to move a box from a conveyor in the receiving area to a shelf in the storage area. How does that break down into job steps? Picking up the box from the conveyor and putting it on a handtruck is one logical set of movements, so it is one job step. Everything related to that one logical set of movements is part of that job step.

The next logical set of movements might be pushing the loaded handtruck to the storeroom. Removing the boxes from the truck and placing them on the shelf is another logical set of movements. And finally, returning the handtruck to the receiving area might be the final step in this type of job.

Be sure to list *all* the steps in a job. Some steps might not be done each time—checking the casters on a handtruck, for example. However, that task is a part of the job as a whole, and should be listed and analyzed.

POTENTIAL HAZARDS

Identify the hazards associated with each step. Examine each step to find and identify hazards—actions, conditions and possibilities that could lead to an accident.

It's not enough to look at the obvious hazards. It's also important to look at the entire environment and discover every conceivable hazard that might exist.

Be sure to list health hazards as well, even though the harmful effect may not be immediate. A good example is the harmful effect of inhaling a solvent or chemical dust over a long period of time.

It's important to list *all* hazards. Hazards contribute to accidents, injuries and occupational illnesses.

In order to do part three of a JSA effectively, you must identify potential and existing *hazards*. That's why it's important to distinguish between a hazard, an accident and an injury. Each of these terms has a specific meaning:

HAZARD—A potential danger. Oil on the floor is a *hazard*.

ACCIDENT—An unintended happening that may result in injury, loss or damage. Slipping on the oil is an *accident*.

INJURY—The *result* of an accident. A sprained wrist from the fall would be an injury.

Some people find it easier to identify possible accidents and illnesses and work back from them to the hazards. If you do that, you can list the accident and illness types in parentheses following the hazard. But be sure you focus on the *hazard* for developing recommended actions and safe work procedures.

RECOMMENDED ACTION OR PROCEDURE

Using the first two columns as a guide, decide what actions are necessary to eliminate or minimize the hazards that could lead to an accident, injury, or occupational illness.

Among the actions that can be taken are: 1) engineering the hazard out; 2) providing personal protective equipment; 3) job instruction training; 4) good housekeeping; and 5) good ergonomics (positioning the person in relation to the machine or other elements in the environment in such a way as to eliminate stresses and strains).

List recommended safe operating procedures on the form, and also list required or recommended personal protective equipment for each step of the job.

Be specific. Say exactly what needs to be done to correct the hazard, such as, "lift, using your leg muscles." Avoid general statements like, "be careful."

Give a recommended action or procedure for *every* hazard.

If the hazard is a serious one, it should be corrected immediately. The JSA should then be changed to reflect the new conditions.

■ **Figure 10–1. A** Instructions for completing job safety analysis form. (Reprinted with permission from the National Safety Council. National Safety Council. *Job Safety Analysis: Instructor's Manual.* Itasca, Ill: NSC 1991.)

JOB SAFETY ANALYSIS

JOB TITLE (and number if applicable): Banding Pallets	PAGE 1 OF 2	JSA NO 105	DATE: 1/1/95	☒ NEW ☐ REVISED

INSTRUCTIONS ON REVERSE SIDE

TITLE OF PERSON WHO DOES JOB: Bander	SUPERVISOR: James Smith	ANALYSIS BY: James Smith

COMPANY/ORGANIZATION: Metal Fabricating Corp.	PLANT/LOCATION: Chicago	DEPARTMENT: Packaging	REVIEWED BY: John Martin

REQUIRED AND/OR RECOMMENDED PERSONAL PROTECTIVE EQUIPMENT: Gloves; eye protection; long sleeves; safety shoes

APPROVED BY: Joe Bottom

SEQUENCE OF BASIC JOB STEPS	POTENTIAL HAZARDS	RECOMMENDED ACTION OR PROCEDURE
1. Position portable banding cart and place strapping guard on top of boxes.	1. Cart positioned too close to pallet (strike body & legs against cart or pallet; drop strapping gun on foot).	1. Leave ample space between cart and pallet to feed strapping; have firm grip on strapping gun.
2. Withdraw strapping and bend end back 3".	2. Sharp edges of strapping (cut hands, fingers & arms). Sharp corners on pallet (strike feet against corners).	2. Ware gloves, eye protection, & long sleeves; keep firm grip on strapping; hold end between thumb & forefinger; watch where stepping.
3. Walk around load while holding strapping with one hand.	3. Projecting sharp corners on pallet (strike feet on corners).	3. Assure a clear path between pallet and cart; pull smoothly; avoid jerking strapping.
4. Pull and feed strap under pallet.	4. Splinters on pallet (punctures to hands and fingers). Sharp strap edges (cuts to hands, fingers, and arms).	4. Wear gloves, eye protection, & long sleeves. Point strap in direction of bend; pull strap smoothly to avoid jerks.
5. Walk around load. Stoop down. Bend over, grab strap, pull up to machine, and streighten out strap end.	5. Protruding corners of pallet (splinters, punctures to feet and ankles).	5. Assure a clear path; watch where walking; face direction in which walking.
6. Insert, position and tighten strap in gun.	6. Springy and sharp strapping (strike against with hands and fingers).	6. Keep firm grasp on strap and on gun; make sure clip is positioned properly.

■ **Figure 10–1.B** Job safety analysis.

JOB SAFETY ANALYSIS	JOB TITLE (and number if applicable): banding Pallets		PAGE _2_ OF _2_ JSA NO._105_	DATE: 1/1/95	☒ NEW ☐ REVISED
INSTRUCTIONS ON REVERSE SIDE	TITLE OF PERSON WHO DOES JOB: Bander		SUPERVISOR: James Smith	ANALYSIS BY: James Smith	
COMPANY/ORGANIZATION: Metal Gabricating Corp.	PLANT/LOCATION: Chicago		DEPARTMENT: Packaging	REVIEWED BY: John Marting	
REQUIRED AND/OR RECOMMENDED PERSONAL PROTECTIVE EQUIPMENT:	Gloves, eye protection; long sleeves; safety shoes			APPROVED BY: Joe Bottom	

SEQUENCE OF BASIC JOB STEPS	POTENTIAL HAZARDS	RECOMMENDED ACTION OR PROCEDURE
7. Tighten clip with gun and cut strapping.	7. Loose strap ends not adequately clamped (cut hands, fingers, and arms).	7. Assure presence of clips in gun before operating gun to clamp; hold strap down with free hand.
8. Repeat steps 1-7 if additional bandings are needed.	8. Same	8. Same

■ **Figure 10–1.B** *Continued*

■ **TABLE 10-2**   Comprehensive Health History

Identifying data   date of history, demographic information such as date of birth, sex, race/ethnicity, marital status, education, and occupation.

Major concerns   detailed description of pertinent health problems or concerns. This should include the onset and manifestation of the problem and treatment, if any, received.

Health history   general state of health; all previous childhood and adult illnesses/injuries, immunizations; mental illness; hospitalizations and operations; allergies; current medications; living patterns including diet, sleep, exercise, and use of coffee, alcohol, other drugs, and tobacco.

Family history   age and health status of each immediate family member, and cause of death. Occurrence of relevant health conditions within the family such as arthritis, blood disorders, cardiovascular disease (i.e., stroke), diabetes, headaches, hypertension, kidney dysfunction, mental illness, or tuberculosis.

Psychosocial history   an outline or description of important, relevant information about the employee such as recreation and leisure activities, lifestyle, and social support system.

Occupational history   see Table 10-3.

Review of systems

General	Usual weight or recent change, weakness, fatigue, fever
Skin	Rashes, itching, irritation, injury, color change, changes in hair or nails
Head	Headaches, head injury
Eyes	Pain, redness, itching, excessive tearing, discharge, vision blurred/impaired, cataracts, glaucoma, glasses, last eye examination
Ears	Pain, infection, discharge, tinnitus, vertigo, earaches, hearing loss, hearing aid
Nose/sinuses	Stuffiness, hay fever, epistaxis, sinus trouble
Mouth/throat	Condition of teeth and gums, frequent sore throats, hoarseness
Neck	Pain, swollen nodes, goiter, limited range of motion
Respiratory	Cough, sputum (color, quality), dyspnea, wheezing, asthma, pneumonia, tuberculosis, bronchitis, emphysema, smoking history, allergies
Cardiovascular	Coronary heart disease, hypertension, murmurs, dyspnea, orthopnea, edema, varicosities, thrombophlebitis, past electrocardiogram
Breasts	Pain, nipple discharge, dimpling, lumps, mastectomy
Gastrointestinal	Difficulty swallowing, change in appetite, pain, nausea, vomiting, diarrhea, constipation, change in bowel habits, rectal bleeding, hemorrhoids, jaundice, liver/hepatitis, gallstones
Urinary	Frequency of urination, dysuria, hematuria, nocturia, infections, incontinence
Genitoreproductive	
Male	Discharge from or sores on penis, history of sexually transmitted diseases, tecticular pain/masses, sexual/reproductive difficulties, hernias
Female	Menstrual history/dysfunction, menopausal symptoms, post-menopausal bleeding, discharge, itching, history of sexually transmitted diseases, last Pap smear, obstetrical history, birth control methods, sexual/reproductive difficulties
Musculoskeletal	Back or neck pain, stiffness, injury, or abnormality; stiff, painful (arthritis), locking, dislocated, trick, or weak joints; flat feet; bone fracture, deformity, infection, or disease; amputations; difficulty working in certain body positions; bursitis.
Neurologic	Fainting, blackouts, dizziness, loss of balance or poor coordination, seizures, paralysis, local weakness, numb places or situations
Mental status	Nervousness, depression, mood changes, anxiety, tension
Endocrine	Thyroid trouble, diabetes, heat or cold intolerance, excessive sweating, thirst, hunger, urination
Hematologic	Anemia, bleeding tendencies, past transfusions

■ **TABLE 10-3** Occupational Health History

What is your current job?

Job title _____

How long at this job? _____ years, months

Description of the work:

In your current job, have you had regular exposure to any of the following substances? Please circle them.

Fumes or dusts:	silica	asbestos	talc	fiberglass	cotton dust
	graphite	sawdust	plastics	other: ___	
Metals:	lead	mercury	nickel	cadmium	beryllium
	chromium	arsenic	aluminum	other: ___	
Solvents:	benzene	carbon disulfide	carbon tetrachloride	methyl chloroform	
	naphtha	toluene	trichloroethylene	xylene	other: ___
Chemicals or gases:	ammonia	formaldehyde	hydrogen sulfide	cyanide	
	sulfur dioxide	fluorides	nitrogen oxides	other: ___	
Infectious Agents:	hepatitis B	HIV			
	cytomegalovirus	tubercle bacillus			
		(tuberculosis)			
	other virus/bacteria				
Miscellaneous:	radiation	insecticides	cutting oils or mists		
	auto or truck exhaust	noise	temperature extremes		

Table continued on following page

■ **TABLE 10–3** Occupational Health History *Continued*

Starting with the job before your current job and working back in time, please provide the information requested below. Please list all of the jobs you have held including military occupations.

Job Title	Dates From–To	Description of Work	Exposures (see list above)	Frequency of Exposures (daily, weekly)	Protective Equipment Used (specify)	Any Illnesses or Injuries Experienced (describe)	Any Co-workers Ill or Injured from Similar Exposures (Yes or No)

Do you have any health problems that you feel are associated with your work?

Have you or a family member lived near any other industrial facilities, waste dump sites, etc. where hazardous substances may have been brought home? Yes ____ No ____
If yes, please describe.

Do you have any hobbies? Yes _____ No _____
If yes, please describe.

Smoking History:

employee's written permission. A synthesis of data obtained from the personal and occupational histories, and review of systems can facilitate accurate diagnoses, prevent occupational disease and the aggravation of underlying medical conditions by workplace factors, identify potential workplace hazards, detect new associations between exposure and disease, and establish the basis for compensation of work-related disease (Kemerer & Raniere, 1990; Rosenstock & Cullen, 1986).

As part of the health assessment, objective data are obtained through a physical examination, systematically conducted to examine each organ system, and through appropriate laboratory tests (McCunney, 1988). The examination must be performed by a practitioner skilled in physical assessment and one who has knowledge of the job demands and related exposures in question. The extent of the examination and tests should be determined by the details of the specific job and emphasis should be placed on functional status capacity, particularly if warranted by the job demands. In other words, not every body system needs to be examined unless so indicated by the job requirements and working conditions. For example, workers who drive heavy equipment or large trucks will generally require a fairly detailed physical examination and extensive laboratory and special clinical testing (i.e., audiogram, CBC, blood chemistry, EKG, urinalysis, vision/depth perception), whereas workers who perform office functions may require musculoskeletal, audiometric, visual, and manual dexterity assessments. Workers in jobs where silica or asbestos may be present will require special emphasis on pulmonary functioning including spirometric evaluation and chest x-ray examination (Guidotti et al, 1989). It is important to remember that the preplacement assessment does not constitute a substitute for a complete health assessment by one's personal health care provider, but is directed at defining the applicant's abilities to perform the job and detecting conditions that prevent the employee from performing the work safely.

Laboratory and clinical measurements are often done during the preplacement assessment to establish baseline data that can be used for future comparison, as part of mandated regulations, and to obtain information needed to prevent adverse health end points. As with the physical examination, only laboratory tests necessary for an accurate assessment of the worker's ability to perform her or his job should be performed. This generally includes a complete blood count, urinalysis, and blood chemistry. Other clinical measurements such as spirometric and audiometric testing should be performed as appropriate to the job demands. These measurements require special practitioner knowledge and skills, and certification in these areas may be required. Chest roentgenograms and special blood testing (e.g., lead levels, carboxyhemoglobin levels) may also be part of the assessment package when tied to certain job exposures. With the rise of tuberculosis, tuberculin skin testing should be considered part of the overall preplacement assessment. Whatever the situation, the employee should be informed of the examination findings and referred for necessary follow-up of any abnormal finding.

Appropriate recommendation as to the employee's compatibility with the job requires professional judgment reflecting an evaluation of all parts interacting as a whole (i.e., job demands, health history, and health status). If an employee is judged able to work in a specific job with reasonable modifications made, an attempt should be made to make these accommodations. The occupational health nurse has a key role in suggesting alternative modifications. In addition to substantial knowledge about the job duties and tasks, this requires good communication skills between the supervisor, employee, and occupational health professional.

Refusal to hire based on a health and physical examination should be based on an applicant's inability to perform the job safely. A prospective employee cannot be refused hire if the assessment reveals a chronic disease that may increase health insurance costs or if the employee is disabled but can do the job with reasonable accommodation (Kemerer & Raniere, 1990). The occupational health nurse should make certain that appropriate health information is fully documented and records are stored, maintained, and adequately secured.

Personal health information should be kept confidential and data obtained from the assessment should not be given to the employer as this specific information is not needed for the worker placement decision. A recommendation as to applicant's suitability for the position, with requirements for work modification if appropriate, is all that is needed. In some situations the applicant has a right, within the parameters of state laws, to refuse the physical examination or parts of the examination, and this right must be observed. The occupational health nurse needs to be cognizant of these laws and document appropriately. In all instances the occupational health professional must act ethically and protect the individual's right to confidentiality of medical and health information and reveal only outcome information pertinent to the hiring decision.

Return to Work Job Transfer Assessment

Return to work assessments and examinations are part of the health program of some companies and are performed in order to evaluate a worker after a severe illness or injury, and/or one that has kept the worker absent from work for an extended duration. This assessment is similar to the preplacement assessment with a focus on whether there has been a change in the employee's health status that would potentiate risk to the worker or to coworkers. The employee health problem can be such to require the employee to have limited duty or work restrictions and this should be determined and recommended by the occupational health professional. On occasion, a worker may be unable to return to her or his usual job but may be able to perform less demanding work until fully recovered (Weeks et al., 1991). Depending on the company philosophy and policies, this approach is a useful option in returning the ill/injured employee to work as soon as possible, which may be in the form of light duty or limited duty.

Light duty generally refers to some adaptation of the employee's original job; whereas, limited duty is defined as a job that is appropriate to an injured worker's skills, interests, and capabilities. It is a new job designed for individuals who cannot return to their original work area and is created for either a temporary (specified time period such as a few weeks or months) or permanent placement (Randolph & Dalton, 1989).

Work hardening is used to facilitate or ease workers back into the workplace. It is a progressive, individualized physical conditioning and training program in which the worker simulates work tasks. The intent is to gradually increase all physical and psychological requirements or aspects of the job so that the person will return to the usual job or achieve a level of productivity that is acceptable at the worksite (Matheson et al., 1985; Ogden & Wright, 1985).

To make appropriate recommendations about return to work, the health care provider should know the physical demand characteristics of the job that the worker is expected to perform. This knowledge also will allow the nurse to coordinate temporary alternative work or modified duty assignments for injured workers returning to work. Matching the work abilities and restrictions of the employee to the physical demands of the job is essential in keeping the employee in the position without increased risk of re-injury (Peters, 1990).

Rapid, safe return to work is an important factor in successful rehabilitation. Research has shown that the longer employees are off the job, the less likely it is that they will return at all. Kelsey and White (1980) have reported that the likelihood of return to work after six months of lost work days is only 50%. This drops to 25% after one year, and almost to zero after two years off the job. Return to work in a part-time position or in a modified-duty program can be important in halting the deconditioning and psychological behavior patterns that hamper successful return to work.

When serious occupational injury or inadequate treatment results in chronic or debilitating physical problems and delayed recovery, both physical and psychological barriers must be addressed if the worker is to be returned successfully to previous job demand. Rehabilitative services, referrals, and case management services may be part of the return to work program and can help the employee with a less stressful work return and the employer maintain less lost work time.

Job transfer assessments are conducted when there has been a change in the health status of the employee or when working conditions change, thereby placing the worker at risk of work-related illness or injury. A job transfer assessment is similar to the preplacement assessment in that its purpose is to determine the worker's fit with the proposed new job. Thus, the assessment should be conducted to match the employee with the job while ensuring health protection.

The occupational health nurse will find previously collected baseline data helpful for comparative purposes with respect to job placement parameters and recommendations. In addition, it is important to emphasize the need for adequate recording and documentation of work-related illnesses and injuries that may be used for determination of disability management or worker's compensation claims.

Regardless of the type of worker placement assessment performed, it is important to remember the need for an appropriate match between the worker and the job demands. To complete a worker placement evaluation, one must understand the working conditions and type of work duties performed. Much of this information can be obtained from the job description and job analysis specifications. Talking with employees who occupy the position and with supervisory staff can also help to clarify the details and demands of the job.

■ PREVENTIVE AND PERIODIC HEALTH MONITORING

Periodic health assessments are performed for employees for both preventive health monitoring and health surveillance purposes (to be discussed in the next section) (Miller, 1986; Ordin, 1992). Periodic health assessments are conducted at intervals during the employment period to determine the worker's continued compatibility with the job assignment, and to determine if adverse health effects have occurred that may be attributable to the work or working conditions. Using the occupational health history as a guide, a detailed interval history can be obtained to gather data about significant health events (i.e., pregnancy, illness) that may have occurred since the last evaluation. In addition, changes in lifestyle risk factors such as weight, alcohol or drug consumption, and exercise, and in work conditions such as shiftwork, change in the number of work hours, or increased work stress should be explored. Physical assessment procedures and laboratory tests should be thorough and complement the interval history with respect to new findings and potentially hazardous work exposures identified.

Monitoring focuses on the overall health experience or status of the worker and is aimed at detecting previously unrecognized health problems or undiagnosed health effects (Guidotti, 1989). In 1922, the American Medical Association recommended a routine physical examination accompanied by a battery of laboratory tests be performed annually on all patients as a preventive medical service (American Medical Association, 1947). In recent years, controversy has existed about the relative value of conducting annual physical examinations in healthy or asymptomatic individuals with respect to the efficacy and cost-effectiveness of such evaluations. However, the use of preventive or periodic health evaluations and monitoring related to specific epidemiological characteristics of the population, related risk factors, morbidity, and mortality experiences has been beneficial in the early detection of disease. For example, with the widespread use of Papanicolaou testing to detect cervical dysplasia, cervical cancer mortality has been reduced by more than 70% since 1950 (NCI, 1988; Yu et al., 1982). It is now increasingly clear, however, that while routine visits with the primary care clinician are important, performing the same interventions on all individuals and performing them as frequently as every year are not the most clinically effective approaches to disease prevention. Rather, both the frequency and the content of preventive or periodic health examination need to be tailored to the unique health risks of the individual and should take into consideration the quality of the evidence that specific preventive services are clinically effective. This approach to the periodic visit was endorsed by the American Medical Association in 1983 in a policy statement that withdrew support for a standard annual physical examination.

In 1979, the Canadian Task Force on Periodic Health Examination published its findings after an extensive study of the usefulness or value of annual/periodic health evaluations. Recommendations centered on offering health protection packages tied to targeted conditions and selected demographic characteristics (e.g., age-groupings) (Canadian Task Force, 1979). In 1977, Breslow and Sommers proposed a Lifetime Health Monitoring Program (LHMP), which uses epidemiologic data to delineate schedules and parameters for health monitoring according to a person's age and known risk factors. The LHMP offers a sound approach to periodic health evaluation that is unlikely to miss preventable diseases or conditions identifiable by the screening elements selected (Guidotti et al., 1989). While an example of an LHMP is shown in Table 10–4, occupational health professionals can collaboratively construct a program to match the specifics of their industry population (e.g., age, sex, risk factor profile). Parameters to consider in constructing such a program is shown in Table 10–5.

In 1984, the U.S. Preventive Services Task Force, composed of 20 nonfederal panel members, was commissioned by the Department of Health and Human Services to develop recommendations by age group on the appropriate use of preventive interventions based on evidence of clinical effectiveness (Lawrence & Mickalide, 1987). Extensive work of the U.S. Preventive Services Task Force included: defining the services to be examined and the review process; adopting specific criteria for recommending certain preventive services; conducting extensive literature searches and reviewing quality studies; adopting guidelines for clinical practice; and finally, having recommendations reviewed extensively by more than 300 international experts. Several recommendations came forth (U.S. Preventive Services Task Force, 1989):

1. Personal health practices related to primary prevention, such as smoking cessation, exercise, and improved nutrition, are among the most effective interventions available to reduce the incidence and severity of the leading causes of morbidity and mortality and generally are more effective in improving overall personal health than many routine screening measures.

2. Greater selectivity in screening tests should be considered with respect to age, sex, and other individual risk factors in order to minimize the risk of adverse health effects and reduce unnecessary expenditures due to screening.

3. Counseling and health education activities related to personal health behaviors should be an integral component of health care providers' practice profile. For example, emphasizing the use of seat belts in contrast to obtaining a "routine" complete blood count may receive less attention by the primary care provider but should receive more attention given that motor vehicle accidents are the leading cause of death in persons aged 5–44.

4. Individuals must assume more responsibility for their own health, particularly as related to primary prevention activities. Individuals must be empowered by health care professionals to change certain health behaviors.

5. The illness visit should be used as an opportunity to promote wellness and preventive health practices.

Interventions for the prevention of 60 targeted conditions and the content specific for periodic health evaluations by age grouping were identified. These recommendations are based on the recognition that the leading causes of illness and injury in populations are age-, sex-, and risk factor–specific.

It is essential that the health care professional consider the leading causes of mortality (Table 10–6) and morbidity within each age group, so as to target specific interventions appropriate to these groups and set priorities for preventive health services. The Task Force's recommendations for preventive care or periodic health evaluations in the working population ages 40 to 64 are shown in Table 10–7. Their recommendations for other age groups in the working population, including the adolescent population, which may be employed in full-time, part-time, or summer jobs, are shown in Appendix 10–2. The services recommended are carefully defined to be performed on asymptomatic persons within the context of routine health care. The interventions listed are not exhaustive; rather they reflect preventive services (as examined in the report) as having satisfactory evidence of clinical effectiveness. The reader is encouraged to read the report of the Task Force in its entirety for a more detailed description of the preventive services examined.

■ HEALTH SURVEILLANCE

Various authors have sought to define and differentiate the terms monitoring and health surveillance. However, ambiguity regarding conceptual differences

■ **TABLE 10–4** Lifetime Health Monitoring Program

	Age at Entrance into Program (years)											
	30	31	32	33	34	35	36	37	38	39	40	41
Complete history	X										X	
Alcohol intake history	X					X					X	
Tobacco use history	X					X					X	
Emotional and sexual history	X					X					X	
Physical activity and exercise history	X					X					X	
Nutritional history	X					X					X	
Occupational history	X					X					X	
Complete physical examination	X										X	
Blood pressure	X			X		X		X			X	
Weight and height	X			X		X		X			X	
Vision	X					X					X	
Hearing	X										X	
Oral examination	X			X		X		X			X	
Breast examination	X			X		X		X			X	X
Pelvic examination	X	X		X		X		X			X	X
Rectal examination	X					X					X	X
Stool occult blood	X					X					X	
Complete blood count	X					X					X	
Serum glucose	X					X					X	
Serum lipids (cholesterol and triglycerides)	X					X					X	
Urinalysis chemical (Dipstick)	X					X					X	
Urinalysis microscopic	X										X	
VDRL	X					X					X	
Purified protein derivative (tuberculin)	X										X	
Tonometry	X										X	
Spirometry	X										X	
Electrocardiography	X										X	
Pap smear	X			X		X			X		X	
Proctosigmoidoscopy	X										X	
Mammography								X			X	

From Guidotti, TL: Journal of Occupational Medicine, 25: 31-736, 1983.

still exists. Yodaiken (1986) states that the objective of monitoring is to anticipate any disease before it occurs, avoid any pathological consequence, and abort any irreversible tissue change, while the objective of medical/health surveillance is to ensure that disease is detected so that new cases do not occur. Aitio et al. (1988) state that monitoring is a repetitive, regular activity, and is a preventive activity not to be confused with diagnostic evaluation. The authors also provide

Age at Entrance into Program (years)																		
42	43	44	45	46	47	48	49	50	51	52	53	54	55	56	57	58	59	60
								X					X					X
			X					X					X					X
			X					X					X					X
			X					X					X					X
			X					X					X					X
			X					X					X					X
			X					X					X					X
			X					X					X					X
X	X		X		X	X		X		X		X	X	X		X		X
X	X		X		X	X		X		X		X	X	X		X		X
			X					X					X					X
			X					X					X					X
X			X		X			X		X			X		X			X
X	X	X	X	X	X	X	X	X	X	X	X	X	X	X	X	X	X	X
X	X	X	X	X	X	X	X	X	X	X	X	X	X	X	X	X	X	X
X	X	X	X	X	X	X	X	X	X	X	X	X	X	X	X	X	X	X
X		X	X	X		X		X	X	X	X	X	X	X	X	X	X	X
			X					X					X					X
			X					X					X					X
			X					X					X					X
			X					X					X					X
								X			X		X			X		
			X					X					X					X
								X					X					X
								X										X
								X					X					X
	X		X		X		X		X			X			X			X
								X				X				X		
X			X		X			X	X	X	X	X	X	X	X	X	X	X

a definition of monitoring that was developed at a conference sponsored by the European Economic Community (EEC), NIOSH, and the Occupational Safety and Health Administration (OSHA). Monitoring was defined as "a systematic or repetitive health-related activity designed to lead, if necessary, to corrective action." This working group defined health surveillance as "the periodic medicophysiologic examination of exposed workers with the objective of protecting health and preventing disease." Guidotti et al. (1989) defines monitoring as a

■ **TABLE 10–5** Conditions/Parameters to Consider When Modifying a Lifetime Health Monitoring Program in Healthy Adults*

Procedure	Factor	Modification
Complete history	Family history of cancer in several members; possible genetic risk	Increase frequency of history and physical examination to annually if appropriate
History of alcohol intake	Family history of alcoholism, pattern of heavy use	Increase frequency of history of alcohol intake; refer for education or counseling
History of tobacco use	Heavy smoker	Increase frequency of history of smoking; use spirometry as opportunity to counsel patient on cessation
Sexual history	Multiple partners; homosexual lifestyle	Evaluate frequency of Papanicolaou smear, VDRL, rectal examinations
Occupational history	Exposure on job to hazardous substances, continuing or antecedent	Increase frequency of occupational history, considering appropriate surveillance strategy
Complete physical	Family history suggestive of elevated risk	Modify frequency of screening elements accordingly.
Blood pressure	Race—black; family history of essential hypertension	Increase frequency to annually and every visit in between
Breast examination	Family history of breast cancer; female	Increase frequency to annually before age 40; reinforce need for self-examination
Pelvic examination	Family history of malignancy	Increase frequency to annually before age 40; see Papanicolaou smear
Rectal examination	Family history of malignancy	Consider increase in frequency
Stool occult blood	Family history of malignancy	Increase frequency to annually before age 50
Serum glucose	Family history of juvenile-onset diabetes	Increase frequency to annually
Serum lipids	Family history of cardiovascular disease	Consider increasing frequency; emphasize cardiovascular examination
VDRL	Homosexual or heterosexual lifestyle with multiple partners	Consider increasing frequency
Papanicolaou smear†	Multiple sexual partners; proclivity to noncompliance	Consider increasing frequency to annually
Proctosigmoidoscopy	Family history of malignancy	Increase frequency
Mammography	Family history of breast cancer, female	Consider increasing frequency before age 50; emphasize need for breast self-examination
HIV antibody	Men who have sex with other men, intravenous drug users, partners of those in high-risk groups	

*These recommendations apply only to asymptomatic individuals. Positive findings, known preexisting conditions, and unusual exposure opportunities alter the subject risk profile and impose additional requirements for surveillance or monitoring.
†The American Medical Association recommends periodic Pap smears for women starting at age 18 or at time of first sexual intercourse.
From Guidotti, TL. Journal of Occupational Medicine, 25: 731-736, 1983.

■ **TABLE 10–6** Leading Causes of Death by Age Groups

Age Group	Causes of Death
Birth to 18 mo	Conditions originating in perinatal period
	Congenital anomalies
	Heart disease
	Injuries (nonmotor vehicle)
	Pneumonia/influenza
2-6 yr	Injuries (nonmotor vehicle)
	Motor vehicle crashes
	Congenital anomalies
	Homicide
	Heart disease
7-12 yr	Motor vehicle crashes
	Injuries (nonmotor vehicle)
	Congenital anomalies
	Leukemia
	Homicide
	Heart disease
13-18 yr	Motor vehicle crashes
	Homicide
	Suicide
	Injuries (nonmotor vehicle)
	Heart disease
19-39 yr	Motor vehicle crashes
	Homicide
	Suicide
	Injuries (nonmotor vehicle)
	Heart disease
40-64 yr	Heart disease
	Lung cancer
	Cerebrovascular disease
	Breast cancer
	Colorectal cancer
	Obstructive lung disease
≥65 yr	Heart disease
	Cerebrovascular disease
	Obstructive lung disease
	Pneumonia/influenza
	Lung cancer
	Colorectal cancer

strategy for observing the overall health experience of the individual or group without regard to any particular outcome; whereas surveillance is defined as the strategy used to determine the experience of a group of workers when the risk of a particular disease (outcome) is known to be increased in a particular industry. Surveillance programs are targeted to specific high-risk groups defined by workplace assignment and exposure history.

Surveillance as defined by the Centers for Disease Control and Prevention (CDC) and the Council of State and Territorial Epidemiologists (CSTE) is an

■ **TABLE 10–7**   Guide to Clinical Preventive Services

Ages 40–64 Schedule: Every 1–3 Years*	**Leading Causes of Death:** Heart disease Lung cancer Cerebrovascular disease Breast cancer Colorectal cancer Obstructive lung disease

SCREENING	COUNSELING	IMMUNIZATIONS
History Dietary intake Physical activity Tobacco/alcohol/drug use Sexual practices **Physical Exam** Height and weight Blood pressure Clinical breast exam[1] *HIGH-RISK GROUPS* Complete skin exam (HR1) Complete oral cavity exam (HR2) Palpation for thyroid nodules (HR3) Auscultation for carotid bruits (HR4) **Laboratory/Diagnostic Procedures** Nonfasting total blood cholesterol Papanicolaou smear[2] Mammogram[3] *HIGH-RISK GROUPS* Fasting plasma glucose (HR5) VDRL/RPR (HR6) Urinalysis for bacteriuria (HR7) Chlamydial testing (HR8) Gonorrhea culture (HR9) Counseling and testing for HIV (HR10) Tuberculin skin test (PPD) (HR11) Hearing (HR12) Electrocardiogram (HR13) Fecal occult blood/sigmoidoscopy (HR14) Fecal occult blood/colonoscopy (HR15) Bone mineral content (HR16)	**Diet and Exercise** Fat (especially saturated fat), cholesterol, complex carbohydrates, fiber, sodium, calcium[4] Caloric balance Selection of exercise program **Substance Use** Tobacco cessation Alcohol and other drugs: Limiting alcohol consumption Driving/other dangerous activities while under the influence Treatment for abuse *HIGH-RISK GROUPS* Sharing/using unsterilized needles and syringes (HR19) **Sexual Practices** Sexually transmitted diseases; partner selection, condoms, anal intercourse Unintended pregnancy and contraceptive options **Injury Prevention** Safety belts Safety helmets Smoke detector Smoking near bedding or upholstery *HIGH-RISK GROUPS* Back-conditioning exercises (HR20) Prevention of childhood injuries (HR21) Falls in the elderly (HR22) **Dental Health** Regular tooth brushing, flossing, and dental visits **Other Primary Preventive Measures** *HIGH-RISK GROUPS* Skin protection from ultraviolet light (HR23) Discussion of aspirin therapy (HR24) Discussion of estrogen replacement therapy (HR25)	Tetanus-diphtheria (Td) booster[5] *HIGH-RISK GROUPS* Hepatitis B vaccine (HR26) Pneumococcal vaccine (HR27) Influenza vaccine (HR28)[6] --- **This list of preventive services is not exhaustive.** It reflects only those topics reviewed by the U.S. Preventive Services Task Force. Clinicians may wish to add other preventive services on a routine basis, and after considering the patient's medical history and other individual circumstances. Examples of target conditions not specifically examined by the Task Force include: Chronic obstructive pulmonary disease Hepatobiliary disease Bladder cancer Endometrial disease Travel-related illness Prescription drug abuse Occupational illness and injuries --- **Remain Alert For:** Depressive symptoms Suicide risk factors (HR17) Abnormal bereavement Signs of physical abuse or neglect Malignant skin lesions Peripheral arterial disease (HR18) Tooth decay, gingivitis, loose teeth

*The recommended schedule applies only to the periodic visit itself. The frequency of the individual preventive services listed in this table is left to clinical discretion, except as indicated in other footnotes.

1. Annually for women.   2. Every 1–3 years for women.   3. Every 1–2 years for women beginning at age 50 (age 35 for those at increased risk).   4. For women.   5. Every 10 years.   6. Annually.

■ **TABLE 10–7**   Guide to Clinical Preventive Services *Continued*

Ages 40–64	High-Risk Categories

HR1   Persons with a family or personal history of skin cancer, increased occupational or recreational exposure to sunlight, or clinical evidence of precursor lesions (e.g., dysplastic nevi, certain congenital nevi).

HR2   Persons with exposure to tobacco or excessive amounts of alcohol, or those with suspicious symptoms or lesions detected through self-examination.

HR3   Persons with a history of upper-body irradiation.

HR4   Persons with risk factors for cerebrovascular or cardiovascular disease (e.g., hypertension, smoking, CAD, atrial fibrillation, diabetes) or those with neurologic symptoms (e.g., transient ischemic attacks) or a history of cerebrovascular disease.

HR5   The markedly obese, persons with a family history of diabetes, or women with a history of gestational diabetes.

HR6   Prostitutes, persons who engage in sex with multiple partners in areas in which syphilis is prevalent, or contacts of persons with active syphilis.

HR7   Persons with diabetes.

HR8   Persons who attend clinics for sexually transmitted diseases, attend other high-risk health care facilities (e.g., adolescent and family planning clinics), or have other risk factors for chlamydial infection (e.g., multiple sexual partners or a sexual partner with multiple sexual contacts).

HR9   Prostitutes, persons with multiple sexual partners or a sexual partner with multiple contacts, sexual contacts of persons with culture-proven gonorrhea, or persons with a history of repeated episodes of gonorrhea.

HR10   Persons seeking treatment for sexually transmitted diseases; homosexual and bisexual men; past or present intravenous (IV) drug users; persons with a history of prostitution or multiple sexual partners; women whose past or present sexual partners were HIV-infected, bisexual, or IV drug users; persons with long-term residence or birth in an area with high prevalence of HIV infection; or persons with a history of transfusion between 1978 and 1985.

HR11   Household members of persons with tuberculosis or others at risk for close contact with the disease (e.g., staff of tuberculosis clinics, shelters for the homeless, nursing homes, substance abuse treatment facilities, dialysis units, correctional institutions); recent immigrants or refugees from countries in which tuberculosis is common (e.g., Asia, Africa, Central and South America, Pacific Islands); migrant workers; residents of nursing homes, correctional institutions, or homeless shelters; or persons with certain underlying medical disorders (e.g., HIV infection).

HR12   Persons exposed regularly to excessive noise.

HR13   Men with two or more cardiac risk factors (high blood cholesterol, hypertension, cigarette smoking, diabetes mellitus, family history of CAD); men who would endanger public safety were they to experience sudden cardiac events (e.g., commercial airline pilots); or sedentary or high-risk males planning to begin a vigorous exercise program.

HR14   Persons aged 50 and older who have first-degree relatives with colorectal cancer; a personal history of endometrial, ovarian, or breast cancer; or a previous diagnosis of inflammatory bowel disease, adenomatous polyps, or colorectal cancer.

HR15   Persons with a family history of familial polyposis coli or cancer family syndrome.

HR16   Perimenopausal women at increased risk for osteoporosis (e.g., Caucasian race, bilateral oopherectomy before menopause, slender build) and for whom estrogen replacement therapy would otherwise not be recommended.

HR17   Recent divorce, separation, unemployment, depression, alcohol or other drug abuse, serious medical illnesses, living alone, or recent bereavement.

HR18   Persons over age 50, smokers, or persons with diabetes mellitus.

HR19   Intravenous drug users.

HR20   Persons at increased risk for low back injury because of past history, body configuration, or type of activities.

HR21   Persons with children in the home or automobile.

HR22   Persons with older adults in the home.

HR23   Persons with increased exposure to sunlight.

HR24   Men who have risk factors for myocardial infarction (e.g., high blood cholesterol, smoking, diabetes mellitus, family history of early-onset CAD) and who lack a history of gastrointestinal or other bleeding problems, and other risk factors for bleeding or cerebral hemorrhage.

HR25   Perimenopausal women at increased risk for osteoporosis (e.g., Caucasian, low bone mineral content, bilateral oopherectomy before menopause or early menopause, slender build) and who are without known contraindications (e.g., history of undiagnosed vaginal bleeding, active liver disease, thromboembolic disorders, hormone-dependent cancer).

HR26   Homosexually active men, intravenous drug users, recipients of some blood products, or persons in health-related jobs with frequent exposure to blood or blood products.

HR27   Persons with medical conditions that increase the risk of pneumococcal infection (e.g., chronic cardiac or pulmonary disease, sickle cell disease, nephrotic syndrome, Hodgkin's disease, asplenia, diabetes mellitus, alcoholism, cirrhosis, multiple myeloma, renal disease or conditions associated with immunosuppression).

HR28   Residents of chronic care facilities and persons suffering from chronic cardiopulmonary disorders, metabolic diseases (including diabetes mellitus), hemoglobinopathies, immunosuppression, or renal dysfunction.

From U.S. Preventive Services Task Force (commissioned by the U.S. Department of Health and Human Services). Baltimore: Williams & Wilkins, 1989.

ongoing systematic collection, analysis, and interpretation of health data essential to the planning, implementation, and evaluation of public health practice and dissemination of information. The final link in the surveillance chain is the application of these data to prevention and control. Rempel's (1990) definition of (medical) surveillance in the workplace follows closely that of the CDC and CSTE but expands the definition specific to the worksite. Thus, surveillance is defined as a systematic collection and evaluation of employee health data to identify specific instances of illness or health trends suggesting an adverse effect of workplace exposures, coupled with actions to reduce hazardous workplace exposures.

A synthesis of these definitions makes it explicit that monitoring and surveillance are tied to prevention. In occupational health settings, monitoring and surveillance are complementary activities sometimes with overlapping characteristics. Monitoring is aimed at averting potential disease before it occurs, such as with biological monitoring where the ultimate purpose is to detect exposures before a disease process is initiated (Bernard & Lauwerys, 1986; Miller, 1986).

Health surveillance programs in occupational health are conducted when workers are potentially exposed to health hazards. At-risk employees are scheduled for evaluations at regular intervals, usually annually. The nature and scope of occupational health surveillance activities and the timing interval of the evaluation are determined by specific standards set forth by the legislative authority (i.e., OSHA) or in criteria documents developed by the National Institute for Occupational Safety and Health (NIOSH). The health history and physical examination are similar to that of the periodic health assessment with emphasis on the specific exposure being evaluated.

Surveillance activities are directed at "watching over" individuals and groups of workers at high risk for specific adverse health outcomes related to a particular occupational exposure. Surveillance is often referred to as the biological monitoring of health effects and usually involves a number of activities, including biological monitoring, health questionnaires and examinations, and laboratory and other clinical measurements (e.g., chest x-ray examination, pulmonary function tests) involving similarly exposed workers, depending on the job exposure or demands. All data are analyzed and interpreted to determine a causal link between workplace exposure and adverse health outcomes. Thus, surveillance is designed for early detection of health impairments in order to reverse presumptive damage and to prevent other individuals (who may be exposed but have yet to evidence clinical signs and symptoms) from developing disease through appropriate control strategies. The basic concept is that early detection before the development of symptoms will lead to a more favorable health outcome (Cohen, 1984; Garry, 1984; Hennekens, 1987; Schilling, 1986; Travers, 1989; Walter, 1993).

Historically and traditionally these programs have been termed "medical" surveillance, implying that surveillance activities require a "medical" intervention, (medical referring to the practice of medicine or treatment of disease). Surveillance activities may encompass taking an occupational health history, evaluating employee health data through health assessments, or performing screening tests (e.g., blood pressure, PFT) all of which are in the realm of occupational health nursing practice. In addition, surveillance activities are often directed, managed, and implemented by occupational health nurses. The term health surveillance rather than medical surveillance is more accurate and reflective of the nature of the activity. Management of the health surveillance program should be under the direction of a health professional, who is qualified by education, experience, and training to evaluate workers and workplace exposures, detect adverse health outcomes, and design strategies to eliminate or reduce risks (Sutherland et al., 1986; Travers, 1989).

Surveillance Activities

Surveillance programs are targeted to specific high-risk groups defined by job assignment, known exposure history, and environmental monitoring. Health surveillance involves the evaluation of employee health data to identify specific instances of illness or health endpoints suggesting an adverse effect from workplace exposure and employment of interventions to reduce hazardous exposures (Guidotti, 1989; Rempel, 1990). It must be emphasized that the most effective means of protecting workers from adverse workplace exposures include, in order of preference, those which (1) "prevent or contain hazardous workplace emissions at their source" (such as product substitution), (2) "remove the emissions from the pathway between the source and the worker" (such as local exhaust ventilation), and (3) "control the exposure of the worker with barriers between the worker and the hazardous work environment" (such as the use of respirators) (Matte et al., 1990). Health surveillance programs should only be considered as an adjunct to worker health hazard protection, never a substitute.

When developing a health surveillance program, several areas should be considered, including the population at risk, workplace/health hazard assessment, determination of health effects, selection of appropriate surveillance measures, including the availability and reliability of tests, testing procedures and frequency, and interpretation of surveillance data examining trends and patterns that might relate any adverse health-end point to an exposure. These procedures can help to detect aberrant control strategies or particular occupations related to the health effect (Table 10–8).

An effective health surveillance program demands a thorough assessment of workplace hazards by occupation, processes, and work areas in order to identify employees potentially at risk. All categories of hazards should be assessed (Table 10–9). In addition to the worksite walk-through discussed in Chapter 9, environmental monitoring, although limited, can yield exposure levels that can then be measured against existing standards. Ambient monitoring for workplace chemicals assesses the health risk by monitoring the external exposure to the chemical such as its concentration in air, food, and water. The risk is estimated by reference to environmental exposure limits (e.g., threshold limit values or time-weighted averages) (Bernard and Lauwerys, 1986).

The purposes of environmental monitoring are to determine the level of exposure of workers to harmful agents; to assess the need for control measures; and to ensure the efficiency of control measures in use (WHO, 1986). This type of monitoring is aimed at early exposure detection so that controls can be instituted to protect the worker before human harm occurs.

Environmental monitoring such as air sampling for airborne contaminants is usually done by an industrial hygienist. Included in the assessment are all routes of exposure (inhalation, skin absorption, ingestion); mixed exposures that may have synergistic or antagonistic effects; detailed knowledge of job demands, such as the rate of physical exertion, which may increase the uptake of chemical

■ **TABLE 10–8** Health/Medical Surveillance Procedures for Selected Chemical Agents

Agent	Route of Entry	Primary Health Effects	Target Organs	Health Surveillance
Ammonia	Absorption Ingestion Inhalation	Irritation of eyes, skin, respiratory tract	Respiratory system, eyes	Complete history and PE; FVC-FEV; initial CXR
Aniline	Absorption Ingestion Inhalation	Headache, weakness, irritability, SOB, dizziness, anemia, hematopoietic problems	Blood, CVS, liver, kidneys	Complete history and PE; CBC
Benzene	Absorption Ingestion Inhalation	Irritation of eyes, nose, respiratory system, dermatitis, bone marrow depression, CNS depression	CNS; skin; hematopoietic, skeletal, respiratory systems	Complete history and PE; urine phenol; CBC; reticulocyte count
Cadmium Dust	Ingestion Inhalation	Pulmonary edema, dyspnea, cough, muscle aches, emphysema, nephrosis, GI symptoms	Kidney; respiratory, hematopoietic systems; prostate	Complete history and PE; urinalysis with albumin; liver function tests; FVC-FEV; initial CXR
Carbon Disulfide	Ingestion Inhalation	Parkinsonism, psychosis, suicide, peripheral neuropathies, heart disease, dermatitis, nephrotic syndrome, possible reproductive dysfunction	CNS, PNS, CVS, eyes, kidneys, liver, skin	Complete history and PE; ophthalmologic examination; urinalysis; liver function tests; ECG
Carbon Monoxide	Absorption Inhalation	Headache, weakness, double vision, dizziness, tachypnea, cyanosis, syncope	CVS, CNS, blood, lungs	Complete history and PE; carboxy-hemoglobin levels
Chromium	Absorption Ingestion Inhalation	Lung cancer, dermatitis, skin ulcers, nasal septum perforation	Pulmonary, skin	Complete history and PE; CXR; FVC-FEV

Substance	Route	Signs and Symptoms	Target Organs/Systems	Medical Surveillance
Formaldehyde	Inhalation	Skin, eye, respiratory tract irritation, asthma	Skin, eye, pulmonary system	Complete history and PE
Lead	Ingestion Inhalation	Anemia, nephropathy, abdominal pain, palsy, encephalopathy, behavioral manifestations	Kidney; CNS; GI, hematopoietic, reproductive systems	Complete history and PE; CBC, blood lead levels; erythrocyte/zinc, protoporphyrin; urine ALA
Magnesium Oxide	Absorption Inhalation	Irritation of eyes and nose, metal fume fever, cough, chest pain, flulike fever	Respiratory system, eyes	Complete history and PE; CXR; CBC
Nickel	Inhalation	Dermatitis sensitization, allergic asthma, lung/paranasal sinus cancer	Nasal cavities, lung, skin	Complete history and PE; CBC; eosinophil count; LFT; urine nickel
Parathion	Absorption Ingestion Inhalation	Meiosis, chest tightness, wheezing, GI symptoms, sweating, muscle fasiculations, seizures, ataxia, coma	Respiratory, hematopoietic systems; CNS, CVS, eyes, skin	Complete history and PE; RBC cholinesterase
Phosgene	Ingestion Inhalation	Eye, respiratory irritation, vomiting, foamy sputum, dyspnea, cyanosis, skin burns	Respiratory system, skin, eyes	Complete history and PE; CXR; PFT
Styrene	Ingestion Inhalation	Eye and nose irritation, drowsiness, weaknesses, unsteady gait	CNS, respiratory system, eyes, skin	Complete history and PE; blood styrene; urine mandelic acid
Toluene	Absorption Inhalation	Acute and chronic CNS depression, dermatitis	CNS, liver, kidneys, skin	Complete history and PE; urine hippuric acid

Abbreviations: ALA, aminolevulinic acid; CBC, complete blood count; CNS, central nervous system; CVS, cardiovascular system; CXR, chest x-ray examination; ECG, electrocardiogram; FVC-FEV, forced vital capacity–forced expiratory volume; GI, gastrointestinal; LFT, liver function tests; PE, physical examination; PFT, pulmonary function tests; PNS, peripheral nervous system; RBC, red blood cell; SOB, shortness of breath.
Data from USDOL, OSHA, 1981; CDC, NIOSH, 1990; WHO, 1986; LaDou, 1990.

■ **TABLE 10–9**   Categories of Potential or Actual Occupational Hazards

Biological/infectious hazards   infectious/biological agents, such as bacteria, viruses, fungi, or parasites, that may be transmitted via contact with infected patients or contaminated body secretions/fluids.

Chemical hazards   various forms of chemicals that are potentially toxic or irritating to the body system, including medications, solutions, and gases.

Environmental/mechanical hazards   factors encountered in the work environment that cause or potentiate accidents, injuries, strain, or discomfort (e.g., poor equipment or lifting devices; slippery floors; deficient workstations)

Physical hazards   agents within the work environment, such as radiation, electricity, extreme temperatures, and noise, that can cause tissue trauma.

Psychosocial hazards   factors and situations encountered or associated with one's job or work environment that create or potentiate stress, emotional strain, and/or interpersonal problems.

substances in the body and thus decrease the safety margin of applicable standards; and compliance with control measures (see Chapter 6).

Control of exposure is accomplished most effectively through the application of industrial hygiene principles. It may take the form of ventilation or of elimination, substitution, or isolation of the offending agent. In addition to these controls, administrative practices may be implemented, which include job rotation and task rescheduling. Personal protective equipment (PPE) is another form of a control strategy, but it must be used in conjunction with health and education programs geared to workers and supervisors. Moreover, attention must be focused on selecting PPE specific to the work hazards that does not compromise the users' ability to work. For example, respirators must be fit to the workers so that adequate protection can be afforded; gloves must prevent penetration of harmful substances; and protective clothing must be appropriately selected to afford protection from exposure (AAOHN, 1987). Control measures are discussed in more detail in Chapters 6 and 9.

In conjunction with workplace hazard assessment, a determination of the types of adverse health effects or end-organ toxicities that might be expected in exposed workers should be made. Examples are shown in Table 10–8. (See also Table 6–3.) In addition, health complaints from exposed workers should be evaluated within the context of workplace exposures. For example, headache, dizziness, drowsiness, and nausea and vomiting, symptoms consistent with toxic exposure to carbon monoxide, should trigger the need for health surveillance testing of all exposed workers regardless of the absence of obvious complaints.

Workers should be encouraged to report signs or symptoms of illness that gradually develop or occur intermittently, so that early detection of adverse effects can occur and the problem can be ameliorated. Workers must feel free to respond to questions without fear of retribution. Through regular health surveillance activities, job modification can also be recommended to enable a worker to remain in the job. However, if health deterioration is evident, removal may be necessary. Surveillance activities provide the occupational health nurse with the opportunity to reinforce with the employee the importance of symptom recognition and reporting, and the need for safe work practices.

As part of the health surveillance program, physical examinations may be required as appropriate to detect adverse health effects. Examinations should be performed by individuals competent to perform such appraisals. When an employee is placed in a health surveillance program, a baseline examination may suggest that an employee may be at increased risk of adverse health effects due to a potential exposure (e.g., asthmatic reaction from chemical exposure). This needs to be discussed in depth with the employee so that informed decisions regarding appropriate job placement can be made.

Periodic health surveillance examinations should be carried out at regular intervals based on the expected timing of health effects in relation to the exposure. The scope and periodicity of the examination should be relative to the type and degree of risk involved; thus, a total, complete examination may not be warranted, especially if overt signs and symptoms of illness are absent. The examination should emphasize the body system most likely to be affected by the hazardous agents in the work environment. For example, for workers exposed to lead, such as foundry workers or those working in battery manufacturing operations, special emphasis should be placed on the gastrointestinal, hematopoietic, nervous, and renal systems during the examination. Workers exposed to manganese in iron and steel industries and those involved in the production of dry cell batteries and welding rods should have special attention paid to nervous and respiratory systems. Examples of health and medical surveillance activities for selected exposures are shown in Table 10–8.

Although the latency period, that is, the period between exposure to a toxic agent and manifestation of adverse health effects, is a major consideration in scheduling the frequency of examinations, it often is unknown. Screening before sufficient time has elapsed to allow for the health effect to become apparent by the designated test is inefficient and ineffective. However, examinations should be given at short enough intervals in order to detect health problems early on. It should be noted that because of individual biovariation and susceptibility and variations in exposures over time, early detection of health effects may not be ensured. Thus, periodic health surveillance examinations should be scheduled to maximize the chances of detecting a toxic effect. However, if signs or symptoms of exposure toxicity occur prior to the scheduled periodic examination, an intermittent examination should be performed immediately.

To be of use in health surveillance, a screening test must be able to detect an exposure-related abnormality as early as possible, so that early diagnosis can be made and treatment or intervention instituted, as appropriate. Matte et al. (1990) state that for a health effect to be "screenable," a test must be available that can detect the toxic health effect before it would normally cause a worker to present for medical attention (i.e., during the "preclinical" phase), and at a time when intervention (reduction of exposure and/or medical treatment) is more beneficial than for advanced disease. Generally, the preclinical phase of an effect must be of sufficient duration (at least weeks or months) to be detected by a screening test given feasible intervals. Screening is of little help in preventing acute, severe health effects, such as cyanide poisoning, since the preclinical phase is too brief to be detected. Some acute but intermittent health effects, such as solvent intoxication, may be amenable to screening by questionnaire, since the workers may recall symptomatic episodes during screening examinations weeks or months after they occur. This information may be useful, since such episodes may precede the development of chronic central nervous system toxicity (Matte et al., 1990).

In order for a test to be appropriate for screening it must have sufficiently high sensitivity and specificity in order to correctly identify individuals with adverse health effects of exposure. Sensitivity is defined as the probability of the test to correctly identify persons with the problem or disease being investigated (true positives), and specificity is defined as the probability of the test to correctly identify persons without the problem or disease being investigated (true negatives). Given a certain amount of test imprecision and human biologic variation, screening tests should reliably reproduce consistent results upon repeat testing. Underlying principles of health/medical screening are important to consider when instituting any screening program. Halperin et al. (1986) provide an interesting discussion on proposed screening principles applicable to the workplace. A summary of these principles is presented in Table 10–10.

Biological Monitoring of Exposure

Health surveillance programs often utilize biological monitoring as an assessment of exposure through measurement of agents or their metabolites in biological specimens (Rosenberg & Rempel, 1990). Biological monitoring evaluates the health risk by monitoring the internal dose of the chemical, that is, the amount of chemical absorbed by the body (Bernard & Lauwerys, 1986). The rationale is that the estimate of the amount of a chemical which has actually entered the body (internal dose) is likely to yield a better prediction of potential toxic effects than ambient air measurement. The intent of biological monitoring

■ **TABLE 10–10**   Health and Medical Screening Principles Applicable to the Workplace

- Condition should be of importance (i.e., severe or prevalent).
- Accepted treatment exists for recognized disease and/or data will be useful in preventive efforts.
- Facilities for diagnosis and treatment are available; care should be provided for participating workers who demonstrate abnormal screening results.
- Conditions suitable for screening must have recognizable latent, asymptomatic stage or early symptomatic stage.
- Screening test must be simple and cost effective.
- Personnel must be adequately trained to conduct and interpret tests for occupational disease.
- Screening tests should be targeted to the specific risks consistent with the exposure or occupation.
- Timing of the screening test should be determined by the natural history of the disease process.
- Sensitivity, specificity, and predictive value should be considered when choosing a test.
- Test interpretation should be compared to established normal values in the target community—the workforce.
- Proper referral and follow-up with the primary care provider should be arranged.
- Population acceptibility should be considered in terms of personal convenience, risk, and perceived value.
- Test should be analyzed to assess the adequacy of engineering controls and biological monitoring.
- Data should be used to protect other workers similarly exposed.

intent

is to detect potentially toxic exposures before their effects become manifest as adverse health endpoints. As shown in Figure 10–2, biological monitoring is aimed at effects prevention, whereas health surveillance is aimed at effects detection. However, if a quantitative relationship is established between internal dose and adverse effects (i.e., dose-effect or dose-response relationships), biological monitoring allows for a direct health risk assessment and thus for effective prevention of adverse effects (Bernard & Lauwerys, 1986).

Biological monitoring integrates the exposure of all routes, sources, use of personal protective devices, differences in physical activity, working habits, personal hygiene, and nonoccupational exposure, which is not accounted for in environmental monitoring. This is usually done through the evaluation of blood, urine, or exhaled air. For example, carbon monoxide exposure may be detected by measuring carboxyhemoglobin blood concentration, whereas trichloroethylene may be measured as metabolites in the urine by spectrophotometry. Pulmonary function testing is often used to detect the degree of functional lung impairment from dust exposure. The measurement of zinc protoporphyrin from lead exposure and blood cholinesterase from organophosphate pesticide exposure are other examples of blood biological monitoring. Urine, however, is the most common medium used for biological monitoring because it is noninvasive, usually easy to collect, and is more suitable for measurement of most exposures, particularly those with short half-lives. It is important to know the normal standardized values obtained on healthy individuals in order to comparatively evaluate the significance of the values observed in exposed workers. Here again, individual baseline data are important to obtain as this provides a basis for comparison of

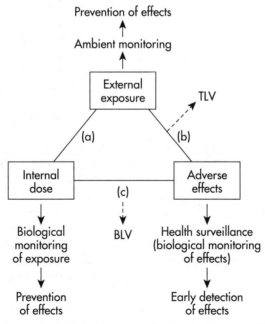

■ **Figure 10–2**   Schemata for monitoring in occupational or environmental health protection. (From Bernard, A & Lauwerys, R. Journal of Occupational Medicine, *28*(8): 558-562, 1986.

data throughout the worker's work life. Examples of substances measured through biological monitoring are shown in Table 10–11.

Samples should be collected at specific times relative to the substance under investigation, such as at the end of the workshift (Droz, 1989). Variation in test results due to multiple factors including diet, medications, alcohol, cigarette smoking, timing of specimen collection, and specimen contamination must be considered limitations when interpreting results. Interpretation of measurement results are usually done by comparing the observed result against an established parameter such as the Biological Exposure Indices (BEI), established by the American Conference of Governmental Industrial Hygienists. The BEI is defined as an "index" chemical that appears in a biological fluid or in exhaled air following an exposure to a workplace chemical (Lowry, 1986). The BEI is a warning of exposure rather than an indicator of a health effect; thus, it can serve as a preventive monitor prior to disease onset. BEIs are intended to correlate with ambient threshold monitoring limit values. Because biological monitoring is in its developmental stages, very few indices are available. Evaluations may then be made from indirect estimates such as dose-response relationships or ambient levels and toxic effects.

Surveillance Data Interpretation and Notification

Interpretation of test results is determined by comparing the observed value (from the exposed worker) against an appropriate reference measure determined statistically from a reference population of healthy, unexposed individuals. (When demographic characteristics impact the test results, e.g., spirometric testing, reference values from the appropriate demographic group should be used when available.) A reference value is usually what is considered within a normal range and whatever falls outside that range may be indicative of a toxic effect.

Baseline examinations are very important as they serve as a comparative reference point for future examination data. Accurate information about the reliability and precision of the test is essential in order to account for any variation in change from baseline results. For example, a 3% decline in FEV over a one-year period may be considered normal variation. However, if this degree of annual decline persisted over several years, pulmonary impairment would be indicated.

Once the health surveillance examination and testing have been completed, all results should be reviewed and any deviations exceeding the accepted threshold should be evaluated by the occupational health nurse and physician. Consultation from other health professionals, such as the industrial hygienist, may be in order, when clinical data are evaluated in reference to an exposure or in concert with sampling data. If an abnormal test result is observed, test errors might be a potential explanation and test confirmation should be considered. Once confirmed, a definitive medical diagnosis should be made by the physician, and further evaluation, testing, or referral to a medical specialist may be in order.

Employees should be notified in writing of test results by the appropriate health care practitioner, according to company policy. Information provided to the employee should include the actual test results, the potential significance of abnormal test results, the risk, if any, from continued exposure to the work environment, recommended changes in work practices and personal habits, any

■ **TABLE 10–11**   Biologic Monitoring for Selected Chemicals

Chemical Determinant	Media (units)
INORGANICS: METALS	
Arsenic	Urine (μg/L)
Cadmium	Urine (μg/g Cr*)
	Blood (μg/L)
Chromium	Urine (μg/g Cr)
Lead	Blood (μg/dl)
	Urine (μg/g Cr)
Zn protoporphyrin (ZPP)	Blood (μg/dl)
Mercury (inorganic)	Urine (μg/L)
Nickel	Urine (μg/L)
	Plasma (μg/dl)
Selenium	Plasma (μg/dl)
	Urine (μg/g Cr)
Vanadium	Urine (μg/g Cr)
INORGANICS: OTHER	
Carbon disulfide (TTCA [2 thiothiazoline 4-carboxylic acid])	Urine (mg/g Cr)
Carbon monoxide Hbco	Blood (%)
Cyanide	
Thiocyanate	Urine (mg/24 h)
Fluorides	Urine (mg/L)
ORGANICS: ALIPHATICS AND ALICYCLICS	
Acetone	Urine (mg/g Cr)
	Blood (mg/dl)
	Alveolar air (mg/m^3)
Ethylene glycol	
Oxalic acid	Urine (mg/g Cr)
Methanol	Urine (mg/L)
Formic acid	Urine (mg/g Cr)
Methyl ethyl ketone	Urine (mg/L)
Propylene glycol monoethyl ether (PGME)	End-exhaled air (ppm)
ORGANICS: AROMATIC	
Benzene	Blood (μg/dl)
Benzene total phenol	Urine (mg/L)
Ethyl benzene	
Mandelic acid	Urine (g/g Cr)
Phenol	Urine (mg/g Cr)
Styrene	
Mandelic acid	Urine (g/g Cr)
Styrene	Mid-exhaled air (ppm)
	Blood (mg/L)
Toluene	
Hippuric acid	Urine (g/g Cr)
	Urine (mg/min)
Toluene	Blood (mg/L)
	End-exhaled air (ppm)
Xylene	
Total methylhippuric acid	Urine (g/g Cr)
	Urine (mg/min)
Xylene	Blood (mg/L)

*Cr, creatinine.

Table continued on following page

■ **TABLE 10–11** Biologic Monitoring for Selected Chemicals *Continued*

Chemical Determinant	Media (units)
ORGANICS: HALOGENATED	
Methyl bromide	
Bromide	Blood (mg/dl)
Methylene chloride	
Hbco	Blood (%)
	End-exhaled air (ppm)
Methylene chloride	Blood (mg/dl)
Perchloroethylene	End-exhaled air (ppm)
	Blood (mg/dl)
Polychlorinated biphenyl	
Total chlorobiphenyl	Blood (μg/L)
Trichloroethylene	
Free trichloroethanol	Blood (mg/L)
ORGANICS: NITROGEN-CONTAINING	
Aniline	
p-Aminophenol	Urine (mg/L)
Methemoglobin	Blood (%)
Dinitrobenzene	
Methemoglobin	Blood (%)
Nitrobenzene	
p-Nitrophenol and *p*-aminophenol	Urine (mg/g Cr)
Methemoglobin	Blood (%)
ORGANICS: PESTICIDES	
Organophosphates	
RBC cholinesterase	Blood (% depression)
Parathion	
RBC cholinesterase	Blood (% depression)
p-Nitrophenol	Urine (mg/L)
Carbamates	
RBC cholinesterase	Blood (% depression)
Carbaryl	
RBC cholinesterase	Blood (% depression)
1-Naphthol	Urine (mg/g Cr)
Chlordane	Blood (g/L)
Dieldrin	Blood (g/L)
Hexachlorobenzene	Blood (mg/L)

medical follow-up or treatment indicated, legal implications of the notification (e.g., workers' compensation), and the need for ongoing testing and surveillance (Matte et al., 1990).

Once an adverse health indicator or effect has been established from a work-place exposure, it is imperative that the work environment be reassessed for hazardous exposure (e.g., environmental sampling, observation), and appropriate modifications and control measures be instituted to reduce or eliminate the exposure. Removal of the employee may need to be considered if sufficient workplace changes cannot be made and the affected employee is left unprotected. This removal may be only temporary until exposures are controlled. In addition, careful monitoring and surveillance of unaffected employees should be a priority. Employers must be appropriately notified; however, only information relevant to the exposure and modifications needed should be given, not confidential health and medical data.

? ? vague

Once workplace modifications are made and the affected employee is returned to the job, continuing surveillance is necessary to ensure adequate protection. It is essential that accurate records be kept, including sampling measurements, examination and testing results, data interpretation, employee and employer notification, workplace reassessment and recommended modifications, and actions regarding those recommendations.

In addition to individual monitoring and surveillance, periodic health surveillance data are usually collected on groups of potentially exposed workers. Depending on the test measure used to detect biological or health effects, data collected before exposure can be compared with postexposure data. This can provide valuable information in determining if any changes have occurred over time that are statistically significant. In addition, individual test results can be compared to group data to observe significant departures from group results. Nonsignificant data, however, should not be discounted, particularly in the face of clinically apparent symptoms. It is important in data interpretation that the emphasis be placed on evaluating the relationship between exposure, test results, and biophysiological effects, not just on whether the test results are normal or abnormal (Tyler, 1992).

While some periodic health surveillance programs are mandated by the Occupational Safety and Health Administration, workers' participation in workplace health surveillance programs is voluntary and will be enhanced by providing employees with information about the purposes of the programs, how the test results will be used, and issues pertaining to confidentiality of health data. Workers must decide for themselves if they choose to participate; however, voluntary nonparticipation should be documented.

Recordkeeping

Maintenance of health records is essential to an effective health surveillance program. This includes individual records on the type of surveillance activities performed, results, and follow-up provided. These records should be kept for the specified period of time according to OSHA regulations in order to compare future test results or to further investigate exposure situations. In addition, group records should be maintained related to exposure data, including the number of employees monitored; types of potential exposures observed; environmental, biological, and other health/medical screening and diagnostic measures performed; written protocols and procedures for surveillance activities implemented; data interpretation; and recommendations and actions taken for exposure abatement.

Confidentiality

Information obtained from health surveillance activities should be treated confidentially and should not be released without the written consent of the employee, except as required by law. Employers should be given information related to surveillance activities when it requires workplace modifications or removal of an affected employee from an exposure situation to protect the worker's health and safety. Confidentiality must be safeguarded and details of the worker's medical or health condition should not be disclosed.

■ CONCLUSION

Occupational health nurses have a major role in the assessment, monitoring, and surveillance of worker health and safety, as has been described in this chapter. Occupational health nurses are performing many of the health assessment and monitoring activities of workers, and making judgments and decisions regarding their health status. Nurses must be knowledgeable about the work-related demands, potential associated hazards, signs and symptoms of acute and chronic exposure, and the need for appropriate and prompt follow-up care to be provided if a health problem develops. The development of a nursing diagnosis and plan of care to facilitate worker placement, as well as to promote and protect health and safety, is essential.

The occupational health nurse needs to be thoroughly involved in the development and management of any health surveillance program. Collaborative efforts, utilizing a team approach, are critical to the initiation and maintenance of a successful program, which includes but is not limited to the following:

- acquisition of resources for an effective health surveillance program;
- development of policies and procedures for management and administration of the program;
- coordination of the health surveillance program including identification of high-risk workers and work areas;
- identification of work areas needing monitoring;
- development, implementation, and evaluation of health surveillance protocols related to specific exposures;
- documentation, interpretation, and communication of health surveillance data and health hazard risks to workers, and appropriate maintenance of confidentiality;
- identification and institution of appropriate control measures;
- education and counseling of workers and management regarding effective strategies for health promotion and protection;
- research and investigation of work-related health problems and recommendations for alteration or modification of risk situations; and
- maintenance of knowledge about work-related hazards and strategies for risk reduction.

Provision of a safe and healthful work environment is the responsibility of the employer, and measures should be implemented to achieve this goal. Workplace health assessment, monitoring, and surveillance programs are designed to aid in identifying hazardous exposures and in recommending risk reduction strategies; however, they should never be considered a substitute for active workplace hazard prevention.

REFERENCES

Aitio, A, Jarvisalo, J, Ruhimaki, V, & Hernberg, S. Biologic monitoring. In: C. Zenz: Occupational medicine. Chicago: Year Book Publishers, 1988.

American Association of Occupational Health Nurses. A comprehensive guide for establishing an occupational health service. Atlanta: Author, 1987.

American Medical Association. Medical evaluations of healthy persons. Council on Scientific Affairs. Journal of the American Medical Association, *249*: 1626–1633, 1983.

American Medical Association. Periodic health examination: A manual for physicians. Chicago: Author, 1947.

Bates, B. A guide to physical examination. Philadelphia: J.B. Lippincott, 1988.

Bernard, A & Lauwerys, R. Present status and trends in biological monitoring of exposure to industrial chemicals. Journal of Occupational Medicine, 28(8): 558–562, 1986.

Breslow, L & Somers, AR. The lifetime health monitoring program: A practical approach to preventive medicine. New England Journal of Medicine, 292: 601–608, 1977.

Brown, ML. Occupational health nursing. New York: Springer, 1981.

Burkeen, O & Cooper, G. Preplacement health assessment: The occupational health nurse's role. AAOHN Update Series, 1(15): 1-8. Princeton, NJ: Continuing Professional Education Center, 1985.

Canadian Task Force on the Periodic Health Examination. The periodic health examination. Canadian Medical Association Journal, 121: 1194–1254, 1979.

Cohen, R. Medical surveillance—which tests? Occupational Health Nursing, 32(5): 244–247, 1984.

Coyle, MJ & Rosenstock, L. The occupational health history in a family practice setting. American Family Practice, 28(5): 229–231, 1983.

Droz, PO. Biological monitoring: Sources of variability in human response to chemical exposure. Applied Industrial Hygiene, 4:(1): 20–24, 1989.

Felton, JS. Occupational medical management. Boston: Little, Brown & Company, 1990.

Freeman, C. Importance of preemployment physicals. Occupational Health Nursing, 31(5): 35–37, 1983.

Garry, M. The nurse's role in medical surveillance. Occupational Health Nursing, 32(5): 248–250, 1984.

Ginetti, J & Greig, A. The occupational health history. Nurse Practitioner, December: 12–13, 1981.

Goldman, R & Peters, J. The occupational and environmental health history. Journal of the American Medical Association, 246(24): 2831–2836, 1981.

Guidotti, T, Cowell, J, & Jamieson, G. Occupational health services: A practical approach. Chicago: American Medical Association, 1989.

Halperin, W, Ratcliff, J, Frazier, T, Wilson, L, Becker, S, & Schulle, P. Medical screening in the workplace: Proposed principles. Journal of Occupational Medicine, 28(8): 547–552, 1986.

Hennekens, CH. Epidemiology in medicine. Boston: Little, Brown & Company, 1987.

Jarvis, C. Physical examination and health assessment. Philadelphia: W.B. Saunders, 1993.

Kelsey, JJ & White, AA. Epidemiology and impact of low back pain. Spine, 5: 133–134, 1980.

Kemerer, S & Raniere, T. Cost effective job placement physical examinations. AAOHN Journal, 38(5): 236–242, 1990.

LaDou, J. Occupational medicine. Norwalk, CT: Appleton & Lange, 1990.

Lawrence, RS & Mickalide, AD. Preventive services in clinical practice. Designing the periodic health examination. Journal of the American Medical Association, 257: 2205–2207, 1987.

Levy, B & Wegman, D. Occupational health: Recognizing and preventing work-related disease. Boston: Little, Brown & Company, 1988.

Lowry, L. Biological exposure index as a complement to the TLV. Journal of Occupational Medicine, 28(8): 578–582, 1986.

McCunney, R. Handbook of occupational medicine. Boston: Little, Brown & Company, 1988.

Matheson, LN, Ogden, LD, Violette, K, & Schultz, K. Work hardening. American Journal of Occupational Therapy, 39(5): 314–321, 1985.

Matte, T, Fine, L, Meinhardt, T, & Baker, E. Guidelines for medical screening in the workplace. Occupational Medicine: State of the Art Reviews, 5(3): 439–456, 1990.

Millar, J. Screening and monitoring: Tools for prevention. Journal of Occupational Medicine, 28(8): 544–546, 1986.

Miller, A. Synthesis of papers on biological monitoring, case studies in screening, and social and economic issues. Journal of Occupational Medicine, 28(8): 782–788, 1986.

National Cancer Institute. 1987 cancer statistics review. Washington, DC: Department of Health & Human Services (Publication # DHHS (NIH) 882789), 1988.

Ogden, LD & Wright, M. Work related programs in occupational therapy: A renaissance. Occupational Therapy in Health Care, 2(1): 109–126, 1985.

Ordin, D. Surveillance, monitoring and screening in occupational health. In: Maxcy-Rosenau-Last: Public health & preventive medicine. Norwalk, CT: Appleton-Lange, 1992.

Peters, P. Successful return to work following a musculoskeletal injury. AAOHN Journal, 38(6): 264–270, 1990.

Randolph, S & Dalton, P. Limited duty work: An innovative approach to early return to work. AAOHN Journal, *37*(11): 446–453, 1989.

Rempel, D. Medical surveillance in the workplace. Occupational Medicine: State of the Art Reviews, *5*(3): 435-438, 1990.

Rosenberg, J & Rempel, D. Biologic monitoring. Occupational Medicine: State of the Art Reviews, *5*(3): 491–498, 1990.

Rosenstock, L & Cullen, M. Clinical occupational medicine. Philadelphia: W.B. Saunders Company, 1986.

Schilling, R. The role of medical examinations in protecting worker health. Journal of Occupational Medicine, *28*(8): 553–557, 1986.

Stein, C & Franks, P. Patient and physician perspectives of work-related illness in family practice. Journal of Family Practice, *20*(6): 561–565, 1985.

Sutherland, J, Clegg, S, & DeCoursey, K. Health hazards in the workplace. AAOHN Journal, *34*(11): 547–553, 1986.

Travers, P. OSHA notice of proposed rulemaking on medical surveillance programs. OEM Report, *3*(5): 34–36, 1989.

Tyler, C & Last, J. Epidemiology. In: Maxcy-Rosenau-Last: Public health and preventive medicine. Norwalk, CT: Appleton & Lange, 1992.

U.S. Preventive Services Task Force. Guide to clinical preventive services. Baltimore: Williams & Wilkins, 1989.

Walter, E. The role of the primary care physician in occupational medicine. In: Zenz, C: Occupational medicine. Chicago: Year Book Publishers, 1993.

Weeks, J, Levy, D, & Wagner, G. Preventing occupational disease and injury. Washington, DC: American Public Health Association, 1991.

World Health Organization. Early detection of occupational diseases. Geneva: WHO, 1986.

Yodaiken, R. Surveillance, monitoring, and regulatory concerns. Journal of Occupational Medicine, *28*(8): 569–571, 1986.

Yu, S, Miller, AB, & Sherman, GJ. Optimizing the age, number of tests, and test interval for cervical screening in Canada. Journal of Epidemiology and Community Health, *36:* 1-10, 1982.

APPENDIX

10–1

Examples of Questions Pertinent to an Occupational Health History

YOUR COMPANY

Is there an occupational health program?
Does the company give physical examinations?
What is the industrial hygiene policy?
Is there a safety program?
Are you informed of the results of examinations or of workroom air samplings?

YOUR JOB

What exactly were you doing when you became ill?
Were you working your regular shift?
What material do you work with?
If it is liquid, does it give off vapor ("fumes") that can be breathed?
Does it ever spill on your skin?
Does it ever soak your clothing?
Has there ever been a spill at your work station?

If you used protective devices, are these maintained by the company?
Has the equipment ever broken down?
Do you exchange your respirator when it gets dirty or when you smell the chemical through the mask?
Does the company ever hold information meetings to tell you about the material you work with?
Is any chemical being used near you by other employees?
Do you become ill during the week at work and then get better over the weekend?
Do you get sick when you return to work? After a weekend off? After your vacation?
Has any new substance been introduced that you work with?
Has the brand of any material been changed?
Has the equipment ever broken down?

Has anything interrupted the usual work process?

Have you ever changed jobs because of your health?

Has there ever been an OSHA inspection of your workplace?

If so, what was found and what action was taken?

Is there an exhaust ventilation system used at your work station?

Does anyone ever take air samples where you work?

YOUR FELLOW WORKERS

Have any of your fellow workers been ill in the same way you are? When?

Have any complained of being unable to have children or having children born with defects?

YOUR HOBBIES AND HABITS

What do you work with at home? Glue? Pesticides? Your car? Furniture refinishers? Photographic chemicals?

Do you smoke? What, where, and how much?

How old when you started? How old when you quit?

Do you drink? What and how much?

Do you use firearms?

Do you play rock music? How long per day?

Do you drive heavy farm machinery?

Where do you have your work clothes washed?

Do you have any pets at home?

Do you take any medicine?

YOUR FEELINGS ABOUT YOUR JOB

Do you like your job?

Are you still good at your job?

Have you had trouble holding a job?

Do you get frustrated at work?

Do you like (odd) shift work?

Is your job more than you can handle?

How do you feel about your foreman?

Is there much stress in your job?

Do you look forward to retirement?

—— APPENDIX ——

10–2

Guide to Clinical Preventive Services

Ages 13–18 Schedule: See Footnote*		Leading Causes of Death: Motor vehicle crashes Homicide Suicide Injuries (nonmotor vehicle) Heart disease
SCREENING **History** Dietary intake Physical activity Tobacco/alcohol/drug use Sexual practices **Physical Exam** Height and weight Blood pressure *HIGH-RISK GROUPS* Complete skin exam (HR1) Clinical testicular exam (HR2) **Laboratory/Diagnostic Procedures** *HIGH-RISK GROUPS* Rubella antibodies (HR3) VDRL/RPR (HR4) Chlamydial testing (HR5) Gonorrhea culture (HR6) Counseling and testing for HIV (HR7) Tuberculin skin test (PPD) (HR8) Hearing (HR9) Papanicolaou smear (HR10)[1]	**COUNSELING** **Diet and Exercise** Fat (especially saturated fat), choles- terol, sodium, iron,[2] calcium[2] Caloric balance Selection of exercise program **Substance Use** Tobacco: cessation/primary preven- tion Alcohol and other drugs: cessation/ primary prevention Driving/other dangerous activities while under the influence Treatment for abuse *HIGH-RISK GROUPS* Sharing/using unsterilized needles and syringes (HR12) **Sexual Practices** Sexual development and behavior[3] Sexually transmitted diseases: partner selection, condoms Unintended pregnancy and contra- ceptive options **Injury Prevention** Safety belts Safety helmets Violent behavior[4] Firearms[4] Smoke detector **Dental Health** Regular tooth brushing, flossing, den- tal visits **Other Primary Preventive Measures** *HIGH-RISK GROUPS* Discussion of hemoglobin testing (HR13) Skin protection from ultraviolet light (HR14)	**IMMUNIZATIONS & CHEMOPROPHYLAXIS** Tetanus-diphtheria (Td) booster[5] *HIGH-RISK GROUPS* Fluoride supplements (HR15) **This list of preventive ser- vices is not exhaustive.** It reflects only those topics re- viewed by the U.S. Preven- tive Services Task Force. Clinicians may wish to add other preventive services on a routine basis, and after considering the patient's medical history and other in- dividual circumstances. Ex- amples of target conditions not specifically examined by the Task Force include: Developmental disorders Scoliosis Behavioral and learning disorders Parent/family dysfunction **Remain Alert For:** Depressive symptoms Suicide risk factors (HR11) Abnormal bereavement Tooth decay, malalignment, gingivitis Signs of child abuse and neglect.

*One visit is required for immunizations. Because of lack of data and differing patient risk profiles, the scheduling of additional visits and the frequency of the individual preventive services listed in this table are left to clinical discretion (except as indicated in other footnotes).

1. Every 1–3 years.   2. For females.   3. Often best performed early in adolescence and with the involvement of parents.   4. Especially for males.   5. Once between ages 14 and 16.

Ages 13–18   High-Risk Categories

HR1 Persons with increased recreational or occupational exposure to sunlight, a family or personal history of skin cancer, or clinical evidence of precursor lesions (e.g., dysplastic nevi, certain congenital nevi).

HR2 Males with a history of cryptorchidism, orchiopexy, or testicular atrophy.

HR3 Females of childbearing age lacking evidence of immunity.

HR4 Persons who engage in sex with multiple partners in areas in which syphilis is prevalent, prostitutes, or contacts of persons with active syphilis.

HR5 Persons who attend clinics for sexually transmitted diseases; attend other high-risk health care facilities (e.g., adolescent and family planning clinics); or have other risk factors for chlamydial infection (e.g., multiple sexual partners or a sexual partner with multiple sexual contacts).

HR6 Persons with multiple sexual partners or a sexual partner with multiple contacts, sexual contacts of persons with culture-proven gonorrhea, or persons with a history of repeated episodes of gonorrhea.

HR7 Persons seeking treatment for sexually transmitted diseases; homosexual and bisexual men; past or present intravenous (IV) drug users; persons with a history of prostitution or multiple sexual partners; women whose past or present sexual partners were HIV-infected, bisexual, or IV drug users; persons with long-term residence or birth in an area with high prevalence of HIV infection; or persons with a history of transfusion between 1978 and 1985.

HR8 Household members of persons with tuberculosis or others at risk for close contact with the disease; recent immigrants or refugees from countries in which tuberculosis is common (e.g., Asia, Africa, Central and South America, Pacific Islands); migrant workers; residents of correctional institutions or homeless shelters; or persons with certain underlying medical disorders.

HR9 Persons exposed regularly to excessive noise in recreational or other settings.

HR10 Females who are sexually active or (if the sexual history is thought to be unreliable) aged 18 or older.

HR11 Recent divorce, separation, unemployment, depression, alcohol or other drug abuse, serious medical illnesses, living alone, or recent bereavement.

HR12 Intravenous drug users.

HR13 Persons of Caribbean, Latin American, Asian, Mediterranean, or African descent.

HR14 Persons with increased exposure to sunlight.

HR15 Persons living in areas with inadequate water fluoridation (less than 0.7 parts per million).

Ages 19–39
Schedule: Every 1–3 Years*

Leading Causes of Death:
Motor vehicle crashes
Homicide
Suicide
Injuries (nonmotor vehicle)
Heart disease

SCREENING

History
Dietary intake
Physical activity
Tobacco/alcohol/drug use
Sexual practices

Physical Exam
Height and weight
Blood pressure
HIGH-RISK GROUPS
  Complete oral cavity
    exam (HR1)
  Palpation for thyroid nod-
    ules (HR2)
  Clinical breast exam
    (HR3)
  Clinical testicular exam
    (HR4)
  Complete skin exam
    (HR5)

**Laboratory/Diagnostic
Procedures**
Nonfasting total blood cho-
  lesterol
Papanicolaou smear[1]
HIGH-RISK GROUPS
  Fasting plasma glucose
    (HR6)
  Rubella antibodies (HR7)
  VDRL/RPR (HR8)
  Urinalysis for bacteriuria
    (HR9)
  Chlamydial testing (HR10)
  Gonorrhea culture (HR11)
  Counseling and testing for
    HIV (HR12)
  Hearing (HR13)
  Tuberculin skin test (PPD)
    (HR14)
  Electrocardiogram (HR15)
  Mammogram (HR3)
  Colonoscopy (HR16)

COUNSELING

Diet and Exercise
Fat (especially saturated fat), choles-
  terol, complex carbohydrates, fiber,
  sodium, iron[2], calcium[2]
Caloric balance
Selection of exercise program

Substance Use
Tobacco: cessation/primary preven-
  tion
Alcohol and other drugs:
  Limiting alcohol consumption
  Driving/other dangerous activities
    while under the influence
  Treatment for abuse
HIGH-RISK GROUPS
  Sharing/using unsterilized needles
    and syringes (HR18)

Sexual Practices
Sexually transmitted diseases: partner
  selection, condoms, anal intercourse
Unintended pregnancy and contraceptive options

Injury Prevention
Safety belts
Safety helmets
Violent behavior[3]
Firearms[3]
Smoke detector
Smoking near bedding or upholstery
HIGH-RISK GROUPS
  Back-conditioning exercises (HR19)
  Prevention of childhood injuries
    (HR20)
  Falls in the elderly (HR21)

Dental Health
Regular tooth brushing, flossing, dental visits

**Other Primary
Preventive Measures**
HIGH-RISK GROUPS
  Discussion of hemoglobin testing
    (HR22)
  Skin protection from ultraviolet light
    (HR23)

IMMUNIZATIONS

Tetanus-diphtheria (Td)
  booster[4]
HIGH-RISK GROUPS
Hepatitis B vaccine
  (HR24)
Pneumococcal vaccine
  (HR25)
Influenza vaccine[5] (HR26)
Measles-mumps-rubella
  vaccine (HR27)

**This list of preventive ser-
vices is not exhaustive.**
It reflects only those topics
reviewed by the U.S. Pre-
ventive Services Task
Force. Clinicians may wish
to add other preventive services on a routine basis,
and after considering the
patient's medical history and
other individual circum-
stances. Examples of target
conditions not specifically
examined by the Task Force
include:
  Chronic obstructive pul-
    monary disease
  Hepatobiliary disease
  Bladder cancer
  Endometrial disease
  Travel-related illness
  Prescription drug abuse
  Occupational illness and
    injuries

Remain Alert For:
Depressive symptoms
Suicide risk factors (HR17)
Abnormal bereavement
Malignant skin lesions
Tooth decay, gingivitis
Signs of physical abuse

*The recommended schedule applies only to the periodic visit itself. The frequency of the individual
preventive services listed in this table is left to clinical discretion, except as indicated in other
footnotes.

1. Every 1–3 years. 2. For women. 3. Especially for young males. 4. Every 10
years. 5. Annually.

Ages 19–39   High-Risk Categories

HR1 Persons with exposure to tobacco or excessive amounts of alcohol, or those with suspicious symptoms or lesions detected through self-examination.

HR2 Persons with a history of upper-body irradiation.

HR3 Women aged 35 and older with a family history of premenopausally diagnosed breast cancer in a first-degree relative.

HR4 Men with a history of cryptorchidism, orchiopexy, or testicular atrophy.

HR5 Persons with family or personal history of skin cancer, increased occupational or recreational exposure to sunlight, or clinical evidence of precursor lesions (e.g., dysplastic nevi, certain congenital nevi).

HR6 The markedly obese, persons with a family history of diabetes, or women with a history of gestational diabetes.

HR7 Women lacking evidence of immunity.

HR8 Prostitutes, persons who engage in sex with multiple partners in areas in which syphilis is prevalent, or contacts of persons with active syphilis.

HR9 Persons with diabetes.

HR10 Persons who attend clinics for sexually transmitted diseases; attend other high-risk health care facilities (e.g., adolescent and family planning clinics); or have other risk factors for chlamydial infection (e.g., multiple sexual partners or a sexual partner with multiple sexual contacts, age less than 20).

HR11 Prostitutes, persons with multiple sexual partners or a sexual partner with multiple contacts, sexual contacts of persons with culture-proven gonorrhea, or persons with a history of repeated episodes of gonorrhea.

HR12 Persons seeking treatment for sexually transmitted diseases; homosexual and bisexual men; past or present intravenous (IV) drug users; persons with a history of prostitution or multiple sexual partners; women whose past or present sexual partners were HIV-infected, bisexual, or IV drug users; persons with long-term residence or birth in an area with high prevalence of HIV infection; or persons with a history of transfusion between 1978 and 1985.

HR13 Persons exposed regularly to excessive noise.

HR14 Household members of persons with tuberculosis or others at risk for close contact with the disease (e.g., staff of tuberculosis clinics, shelters for the homeless, nursing homes, substance abuse treatment facilities, dialysis units, correctional institutions); recent immigrants or refugees from countries in which tuberculosis is common; migrant workers; residents of nursing homes, correctional institutions, or homeless shelters; or persons with certain underlying medical disorders (e.g., HIV infection).

HR15 Men who would endanger public safety were they to experience sudden cardiac events (e.g., commercial airline pilots).

HR16 Persons with a family history of familial polyposis coli or cancer family syndrome.

HR17 Recent divorce, separation, unemployment, depression, alcohol or other drug abuse, serious medical illnesses, living alone, or recent bereavement.

HR18 Intravenous drug users.

HR19 Persons at increased risk for low back injury because of past history, body configuration, or type of activities.

HR20 Persons with children in the home or automobile.

HR21 Persons with older adults in the home.

HR22 Young adults of Caribbean, Latin American, Asian, Mediterranean, or African descent.

HR23 Persons with increased exposure to sunlight.

HR24 Homosexually active men, intravenous drug users, recipients of some blood products, or persons in health-related jobs with frequent exposure to blood or blood products.

HR25 Persons with medical conditions that increase the risk of pneumococcal infection (e.g., chronic cardiac or pulmonary disease, sickle cell disease, nephrotic syndrome, Hodgkin's disease, asplenia, diabetes mellitus, alcoholism, cirrhosis, multiple myeloma, renal disease, or conditions associated with immunosuppression).

HR26 Residents of chronic care facilities or persons suffering from chronic cardiopulmonary disorders, metabolic diseases (including diabetes mellitus), hemoglobinopathies, immunosuppression, or renal dysfunction.

HR27 Persons born after 1956 who lack evidence of immunity to measles (receipt of live vaccine on or after first birthday, laboratory evidence of immunity, or a history of physician-diagnosed measles).

Ages 65 and Over
Schedule: Every Year*

Leading Causes of Death:
Heart disease
Cerebrovascular disease
Obstructive lung disease
Pneumonia/influenza
Lung cancer
Colorectal cancer

SCREENING

History
Prior symptoms of transient
  ischemic attack
Dietary intake
Physical activity
Tobacco/alcohol/drug use
Functional status at home

Physical Exam
Height and weight
Blood pressure
Visual acuity
Hearing and hearing aids
Clinical breast exam[1]
HIGH-RISK GROUPS
  Auscultation for carotid
    bruits (HR1)
  Complete skin exam
    (HR2)
  Complete oral cavity
    exam (HR3)
  Palpation of thyroid nod-
    ules (HR4)

**Laboratory/Diagnostic
Procedures**
Nonfasting total blood cho-
  lesterol
Dipstick urinalysis
Mammogram[2]
Thyroid function tests[3]
HIGH-RISK GROUPS
  Fasting plasma glucose
    (HR5)
  Tuberculin skin test (PPD)
    (HR6)
  Electrocardiogram (HR7)
  Papanicolaou smear[4]
    (HR8)
  Fecal occult blood/Sig-
    moidoscopy (HR9)
  Fecal occult blood/Colon-
    oscopy (HR10)

COUNSELING

Diet and Exercise
Fat (especially saturated fat), choles-
  terol, complex carbohydrates, fiber,
  sodium, calcium[3]
Caloric balance
Selection of exercise program

Substance Use
Tobacco cessation
Alcohol and other drugs:
  Limiting alcohol consumption
  Driving/other dangerous activities
    while under the influence
  Treatment for abuse

Injury Prevention
Prevention of falls
Safety belts
Smoke detector
Smoking near bedding or upholstery
Hot water heater temperature
Safety helmets
HIGH-RISK GROUPS
  Prevention of childhood injuries
    (HR12)

Dental Health
Regular dental visits, tooth brushing,
  flossing

**Other Primary
Preventive Measures**
Glaucoma testing by eye specialist
HIGH-RISK GROUPS
  Discussion of estrogen replacement
    therapy (HR13)
  Discussion of aspirin therapy
    (HR14)
  Skin protection form ultraviolet light
    (HR15)

IMMUNIZATIONS

Tetanus-diphtheria (Td)
  booster[5]
Influenza vaccine[1]
Pneumococcal vaccine
HIGH-RISK GROUPS
  Hepatitis B vaccine
    (HR16)

**This list of preventive ser-
vices is not exhaustive.**
It reflects only those topics
reviewed by the U.S. Pre-
ventive Services Task
Force. Clinicians may wish
to add other preventive services on a routine basis,
and after considering the
patient's medical history and
other individual circum-
stances. Examples of target
conditions not specifically
examined by the Task Force
include:
  Chronic obstructive pul-
    monary disease
  Hepatobiliary disease
  Bladder cancer
  Endometrial disease
  Travel-related illness
  Prescription drug abuse
  Occupational illness and
    injuries

Remain Alert For:
Depression symptoms
Suicide risk factors (HR11)
Abnormal bereavement
Changes in cognitive func-
  tion
Medications that increase
  risk of falls
Signs of physical abuse or
  neglect
Malignant skin lesions
Peripheral arterial disease
Tooth decay, gingivitis,
  loose teeth

*The recommended schedule applies only to the periodic visit itself. The frequency of the individual
preventive services listed in this table is left to clinical discretion, except as indicated in other
footnotes.

1. Annually.   2. Every 1–2 years for women until age 75, unless pathology detected.   3. For
women.   4. Every 1–3 years.   5. Every 10 years.

Ages 65 and Over

High-Risk Categories

HR1 Persons with risk factors for cerebrovascular or cardiovascular disease (e.g., hypertension, smoking, CAD, atrial fibrillation, diabetes) or those with neurologic symptoms (e.g., transient ischemic attacks) or a history of cerebrovascular disease.

HR2 Persons with a family or personal history of skin cancer, or clinical evidence of precursor lesions (e.g., dysplastic nevi, certain congenital nevi), or those with increased occupational or recreational exposure to sunlight.

HR3 Persons with exposure to tobacco or excessive amounts of alcohol, or those with suspicious symptoms or lesions detected through self-examination.

HR4 Persons with a history of upper-body irradiation.

HR5 The markedly obese, persons with a family history of diabetes, or women with a history of gestational diabetes.

HR6 Household members of persons with tuberculosis or others at risk for close contact with the disease (e.g., staff of tuberculosis clinics, shelters for the homeless, nursing homes, substance abuse treatment facilities, dialysis units, correctional institutions); recent immigrants or refugees from countries in which tuberculosis is common (e.g., Asia, Africa, Central and South America, Pacific Islands); migrant workers; residents of nursing homes, correctional institutions, or homeless shelters; or persons with certain underlying medical disorders (e.g., HIV infection).

HR7 Men with two or more cardiac risk factors (high blood cholesterol, hypertension, cigarette smoking, diabetes mellitus, family history of CAD); men who would endanger public safety were they to experience sudden cardiac events (e.g., commercial airline pilots); or sedentary or high-risk males planning to begin a vigorous exercise program.

HR8 Women who have not had previous documented screening in which smears have been consistently negative.

HR9 Persons who have first-degree relatives with colorectal cancer; a personal history of endometrial, ovarian, or breast cancer; or a previous diagnosis of inflammatory bowel disease, adenomatous polyps, or colorectal cancer.

HR10 Persons with a family history of familial polyposis coli or cancer family syndrome.

HR11 Recent divorce, separation, unemployment, depression, alcohol or other drug abuse, serious medical illnesses, living alone, or recent bereavement.

HR12 Persons with children in the home or automobile.

HR13 Women at increased risk for osteoporosis (e.g., Caucasian, low bone mineral content, bilateral oopherectomy before menopause or early menopause, slender build) and who are without known contraindications (e.g., history of undiagnosed vaginal bleeding, active liver disease, thromboembolic disorders, hormone-dependent cancer).

HR14 Men who have risk factors for myocardial infarction (e.g., high blood cholesterol, smoking, diabetes mellitus, family history of early-onset CAD) and who lack a history of gastrointestinal or other bleeding problems, or other risk factors for bleeding or cerebral hemorrhage.

HR15 Persons with increased exposure to sunlight.

HR16 Homosexually active men, intravenous drug users, recipients of some blood products, or persons in health-related jobs with frequent exposure to blood or blood products.

Pregnant Women[1]

FIRST PRENATAL VISIT

SCREENING

History
Genetic and obstetric history
Dietary intake
Tobacco/alcohol/drug use
Risk factors for intrauterine
  growth retardation and
  low birthweight
Prior genital herpetic lesions

**Laboratory/Diagnostic
Procedures**
Blood pressure
Hemoglobin and hematocrit
ABO/Rh typing
Rh(D) and other antibody
  screen
VDRL/RPR
Hepatitis B surface antigen
  (HBsAg)
Urinalysis for bacteriuria
Gonorrhea culture
HIGH-RISK GROUPS
  Hemoglobin electrophore-
    sis (HR1)
  Rubella antibodies (HR2)
  Chlamydial testing (HR3)
  Counseling and testing for
    HIV (HR4)

COUNSELING

Nutrition
Tobacco use
Alcohol and other drug use
Safety belts
HIGH-RISK GROUPS
  Discuss amniocentesis (HR5)
  Discuss risks of HIV infection (HR4)

Remain Alert For:
Signs of physical abuse

This list of preventive services is not exhaustive.
It reflects only those topics
reviewed by the U.S. Pre-
ventive Services Task
Force. Clinicians may wish
to add other preventive services on a routine basis,
and after considering the
patient's medical history and
other individual circum-
stances. Examples of target
conditions not specifically
examined by the Task Force
include:
  Counseling on warning
    signs and symptoms
  Physical findings of ab-
    dominal and cervical
    examination
  Tay-Sachs disease
  Childbirth education
  Teratogenic and fetotoxic
    exposures

FOLLOW-UP VISITS

Schedule: See Footnote*

SCREENING

Blood pressure
Urinalysis for bacteriuria

**Screening Tests at Specific
Gestational Ages**

14–16 Weeks:
  Maternal serum alpha-fetoprotein
    (MSAFP)[2]
  Ultrasound cephalometry (HR8)

24–28 Weeks:
  50 g oral glucose tolerance test
  Rh(D) antibody (HR9)
  Gonorrhea culture (HR10)
  VDRL/RPR (HR11)
  Hepatitis B surface antigen
    (HBsAg) (HR12)
  Counseling and testing for HIV
    (HR13)

36 Weeks:
  Ultrasound exam (HR14)

COUNSELING

Nutrition
Safety belts
Discuss meaning of upcom-
  ing tests
HIGH-RISK GROUPS
  Tobacco use (HR6)
  Alcohol and other drug
    use (HR7)

Remain Alert For:
Signs of physical abuse

1. See also Tables 4–6 for
other preventive services for
women.
2. Women with access to
counseling and follow-up services, skilled high-resolution
ultrasound and amniocentesis
capabilities, and reliable,
standardized laboratories.

*Because of lack of data and differing patient risk profiles, the scheduling of visits and the frequency
of the individual preventive services listed in this table are left to clinical discretion, except for
those indicated at specific gestational ages.

Pregnant Women   High-Risk Categories

HR1 Black women.

HR2 Women lacking evidence of immunity (proof of vaccination after the first birthday or laboratory evidence of immunity.)

HR3 Women who attend clinics for sexually transmitted diseases, attend other high-risk health care facilities (e.g., adolescent and family planning clinics), or have other risk factors for chlamydial infection (e.g., multiple sexual partners or a sexual partner with multiple sexual contacts).

HR4 Women seeking treatment for sexually transmitted diseases; past or present intravenous (IV) drug users; women with a history of prostitution or multiple sexual partners; women whose past or present sexual partners were HIV-infected, bisexual, or IV drug users; women with long-term residence or birth in an area with high prevalence of HIV infection in women; or women with a history of transfusion between 1978 and 1985.

HR5 Women aged 35 and older.

HR6 Women who continue to smoke during pregnancy.

HR7 Women with excessive alcohol consumption during pregnancy.

HR8 Women with uncertain menstrual histories or risk factors for intrauterine growth retardation (e.g., hypertension, renal disease, short maternal stature, low prepregnancy weight, failure to gain weight during pregnancy, smoking, alcohol and other drug abuse, and history of a previous fetal death or growth-retarded baby).

HR9 Unsensitized Rh-negative women.

HR10 Women with multiple sexual partners or a sexual partner with multiple contacts, or sexual contacts of persons with culture-proven gonorrhea.

HR11 Women who engage in sex with multiple partners in areas in which syphilis is prevalent, or contacts of persons with active syphilis.

HR12 Women who engage in high-risk behavior (e.g., intravenous drug use) or in whom exposure to hepatitis B during pregnancy is suspected.

HR13 Women at high risk (see HR4) who have a nonreactive HIV test at the first prenatal visit.

HR14 Women with risk factors for intrauterine growth retardation (see HR8).

From U.S. Preventive Services Task Force (commissioned by the U.S. Department of Health and Human Services). Baltimore: Williams & Wilkins, 1989.

11

CLINICAL PRACTICE IN
OCCUPATIONAL HEALTH NURSING

In most occupational health settings, the occupational health nurse is the sole provider of health care to worker populations, and thus is responsible for the clinical management of many occupational and nonoccupational health-related problems. Although much of the occupational health nurse's practice focuses on health promotion, maintenance, and protection, the occupational health nurse has a major role in the provision of primary health care, management of emergencies, implementation of urgent/critical health interventions occurring as a result of work-related incidents, and counseling related to occupational and nonoccupational health problems. The nurse's interventions focus on the individual's response to altered functioning and require critical thinking about the types of nursing activities that are both appropriate and effective. This chapter will focus on the development of clinical nursing guidelines for occupational health nursing practice, with several examples presented, and on counseling and employee assistance programming in the occupational health setting.

■ OCCUPATIONAL HEALTH NURSING GUIDELINES FOR PRACTICE

As nursing has expanded its scope of practice, new tools are being developed and utilized to help delineate parameters of care and management. Guidelines for clinical nursing practice for certain health-related entities specify nursing actions within the legal limits of defined practice, and are particularly helpful in occupational settings where the occupational health nurse largely practices autonomously. For many health care problems seen in the occupational health unit, independent nursing strategies, which stem from nursing diagnoses, are appropriate. The nurse is not dependent on the physician's medical diagnosis, but rather looks to the individual's response as a directive for nursing interventions. However, because of the interdependent nature of nursing and medicine, some nursing activities are medical interventions prescribed by the physician and delegated to the nurse (Glasgow, 1990). Standing orders from the physician should be used appropriately and within the scope of legal limits.

The quality and consistency of nursing care will be improved by standardizing care. Diagnostic labels help the nurse to develop a concept of the particular health problem within the context of the health state of the individual, and to make assessments to identify the problem, including problem characteristics (signs and symptoms) manifested by the individual. These standardized approaches of nursing interventions provide for a definitive goal-directed outcome rather than a hit-or-miss approach (Glasgow, 1990). Although the individualization of each (person's) plan of care is pivotal to effective nursing care, certain problems are common to many people. This commonality provides an opportunity to develop creative but consistent strategies that can be applied to meet the clinical needs of a given "patient" population (Akers, 1991). It should be noted, however, that care of individuals is a dynamic process and challenges may appear without warning.

In the delivery of effective health care at the worksite, the ability to exercise sound clinical judgment is contingent upon the diagnostic reasoning strategies of the occupational health nurse clinician. Gathering and organizing employee health data in a systematic manner are essential to the delivery of safe and competent care (Tanner et al., 1987). This process is demonstrated by skilled actions or interventions designed to achieve a favorable outcome and involves:

1. setting a specific goal to effect the change or outcome;
2. choosing the appropriate intervention to meet the goal;
3. considering situational factors prior to implementing the interventions;
4. implementing the interventions with skill based on knowledge (Gant, 1986); and
5. knowing the parameters for medical intervention and referral.

Clinical nursing care guidelines and/or protocols enable the nurse to help clients maintain health, as well as treat those with chronic or acute self-limiting illnesses/injuries, both occupational and nonoccupational (Williams, 1984).

In the development of clinical nursing guidelines or protocols, it is important to emphasize that the legal requirements as specified by individual state nurse practice acts must be maintained. In addition, nurses must be cognizant of other legal parameters that may impact on nursing practice, such as the state pharmacy and medical practice acts. The nurse must be fully aware of all limitations of nursing practice in the state within which she or he practices. Benefits of clinical nursing guidelines are outlined in Table 11–1 (Rogers et al., 1992).

Guidelines and protocols are helpful in the decision-making process as they provide a series of clear, step-by-step recommendations to help delineate the problem and intervene appropriately. However, they are not intended to take the place of critical thinking and active nursing judgment; rather, they serve as a reference of essential elements for management of a specific problem. For example, if an employee presents with a headache, there should always be room for healthy suspicion regarding chemical exposure, especially if a cluster effect is apparent and/or if there is a temporal relationship between workplace exposure and symptom onset. Thus, clinical assessment needs to be complete and appropriately documented.

Based on an assessment of the health problems and conditions in the workforce, clinical nursing practice guidelines or protocols can be developed that are reflective of the health needs of that particular population. This can easily be done through a review of employee health records and logs. The occupational health nurse, in collaboration with other health care professionals such as the

■ **TABLE 11–1**   Benefits of Clinical Nursing Guidelines

* Define the parameters of nursing care and treatment
* Guide the systematic collection of data
* Help to focus the nurse's thinking about a health problem or need and ensure that required treatment is not omitted
* Enable the nurse to practice independently and facilitate interdependent functioning as appropriate
* Improve the quality of care through use of a consistent standardized approach
* Enhance the collaborative communication between health care team members

physician and/or physical therapist, can then develop or obtain guidelines or protocols specific to the needs of the workforce and in the format she or he finds most useful. For each clinical entity for which guidelines are developed, a literature review should be conducted to obtain information on the most current and appropriate assessment techniques, management modalities, and follow-up approaches. Consultation with medical and other nursing professionals, such as the state occupational health nurse consultant, should be utilized when needed.

Nursing clinical guidelines or protocols may be developed by diagnostic category or presenting problem, and generally follow a specific format such as an algorithm or the SOAP format, which is patterned to identify *s*ubjective and *o*bjective data and arrive at an *a*ssessment and *p*lan of action. A narrative or some other standard format, which best meets the needs of the practitioner, may also be utilized. The algorithm format specifies a logic or decision-tree approach wherein decision points direct further investigation and action. Examples of these two types of formats are demonstrated in Table 11–2 and Figure 11–1. Once developed, the guidelines or protocols should be reviewed by clinical experts for accuracy, modification, or refinement. Guidelines/protocols should be dated and maintained in the occupational health unit and other satellite settings where they are used, and should be reviewed annually for currency and updated as appropriate.

Another type of guideline format has been developed by Rogers et al. (1992). The intent of these guidelines is to provide a format that defines and characterizes the clinical problem, gives direction as to a policy perspective, identifies assessment needs and specific interventions, delineates conditions requiring medical referral, and specifies follow-up actions. A survey of approximately 500 practicing occupational health nurses identified nearly 65 specific clinical entities related to common occupational health problems and needs for which clinical nursing guidelines were developed (Rogers et al., 1992). Twelve examples are given in Appendix 11–1. For a more complete inventory, see Rogers et al. (1992).

Regardless of the problem, timely and targeted interventions are needed to effect a positive outcome. Although clinical nursing or protocol guides cannot guarantee a positive outcome, they can provide a consistent care approach appropriate to the clinical problem. Clinical nursing guidelines provide the nurse with a foundation for decision making that is critical to prevent, detect, and minimize complications and contribute to better clinical management (Akers, 1991). In addition, these guides can be effective teaching aids, provide the occupational health nurse with cues to enhance clinical assessment and man-

■ **TABLE 11–2** Sample Protocol: Narrative SOAP Format

Acute Sinusitis

Definition:	A condition in which the mucous membrane lining of the paranasal sinuses is inflamed causing obstruction of normal sinus drainage and subsequent bacterial infection.
Etiology:	Commonly occurs following an upper respiratory infection; common causative agents are group A Strep, Hemophilus Influenza, *Staph. aureus,* and Pneumococcus. Bacterial sinusitis commonly occurs as a complication of viral nasopharyngitis.
Demographics:	Most often affects persons who currently or recently have had an upper respiratory tract infection with marked inflammation of the paranasal sinuses. Less frequently may afflict persons who have recently sustained local injuries to the area within or surrounding the paranasal sinuses.
S:	Present History: Client may complain of nasal congestion, sneezing, headache, and sore throat—symptoms of common cold. May also complain of pain and tenderness over affected sinuses, such as forehead and/or maxillary area. If sphenoidal sinuses are involved, the client may complain of pain at base of skull. Involvement of ethmoidal sinus commonly evokes complaint of pain in temples and around the eyes. Headache/pain may be worse in the early morning or at night and may vary with change in position. Complaints of purulent nasal discharge, postnasal drip, and sore throat may be elicited. The client may report fever, feeling of tiredness, and a night cough.
O:	Vital signs: *Temp:* Mild fever (101°F or 38.2°C). *Pulse, Resp and B/P:* May be slightly elevated for clients according to age, intensity of pain, and level of anxiety. HEENT: *Viral:* Findings congruent with those of common cold. *Bacterial:* May note edema and redness of nasal mucous membrane and yellow mucopurulent nasal discharge beneath the superior or middle turbinates. (If occlusion of the passage from the sinus to the nasal cavity occurs, discharge may be absent). Tenderness over involved sinus may be elicited on palpation and percussion; transillumination decreased over the involved sinus. *Lab:* None indicated in the absence of mucopurulent nasal discharge. (Culture if present.)
A: Diagnosis:	
Nursing:	Alteration in comfort due to bacterial infection of the paranasal sinus(es).
Medical:	Acute Sinusitis.
P: Diagnostic:	Consult with physician regarding client management (if bacterial sinusitis present, X-ray will show cloudiness of involved sinus) or if unsure of diagnosis. *Refer* any clients who are acutely or severely ill, those with chronic or recurrent bacterial sinusitis, or those with any signs of orbit or CNS involvement (any protrusion of the eyeball or neurological changes).
Therapeutic:	1. Tylenol and Aspirin may be prescribed as needed for fever and pain. 2. Decongestants such as Chlortrimeton or Sudafed may be prescribed to reduce congestion and promote sinus drainage. 3. For bacterial sinusitis Ampicillin 500 mgm p.o. every 6 hours for 10 days; if *allergic to Penicillin,* use Tetracycline 250 mgm p.o. every 6 hours for 10 days (prescribed).

Table continued on following page

■ TABLE 11–2   Sample Protocol: Narrative SOAP Format *Continued*

	Note: Tetracycline is contraindicated in pregnant women and young children. 4. Increase oral fluid intake and use humidifier to promote liquifying of sinus drainage. 5. *Follow-up:* Call or return to clinic in 3 days if no improvement or condition worsens; if bacterial, return for HEENT exam 1 week following completion of antibiotics.
Education:	1. Explain the underlying etiology, the rationale for treatment, and the importance of taking entire course of medications particularly if on antibiotics. 2. Alert client to signs/symptoms of complications (increasing fever, chills, epistaxis, or change in level of consciousness). If any of these occur, client should return to clinic or nearest emergency room immediately. 3. Encourage the client to rest as much as possible. 4. Provide the client with information regarding treatment regimen and potential side effects of drugs; include written instructions. 5. Inform client of side effects of: 　a. *Aspirin:* G.I. distress, nausea, vomiting, and increased bleeding tendency. 　b. *Tylenol:* G.I. distress, nausea, and vomiting. 　c. *Decongestants:* Mild nervousness, restlessness, and dry mouth. *Note:* Decongestants should be used with caution if high blood pressure, diabetes, heart disease, or thyroid disease are present. 　d. *Antibiotics:* Discuss how and when to take medication. (Take 1 hour before or 2 hours after meals). 　*Ampicillin:* Skin rash, nausea, vomiting, and diarrhea, sneezing or wheezing should be reported immediately. 6. If Tetracycline is recommended: 　a. Instruct regarding side effects of drug: nausea, vomiting, diarrhea, and skin rash. 　b. Advise that drug may cause photosensitivity (increased sensitivity to sun). 　c. Advise that milk and milk products (cheese, yogurt, ice cream, etc.) and antacids should not be taken at the time the drug is ingested.

From Thompson, CE, Jones, JM, Cox, AR, & Levy, EY. Adult health management: Guidelines for nurse practitioners. Reston, VA, Reston Publishing Company, 1984.

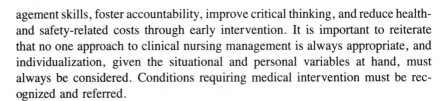

agement skills, foster accountability, improve critical thinking, and reduce health- and safety-related costs through early intervention. It is important to reiterate that no one approach to clinical nursing management is always appropriate, and individualization, given the situational and personal variables at hand, must always be considered. Conditions requiring medical intervention must be recognized and referred.

■ COUNSELING AND EMPLOYEE ASSISTANCE

Employee counseling is offered as an integral component of the occupational health service. In providing health care to workers, the occupational health nurse will find that she or he is involved not only in counseling employees with respect to prevention and management of work-related illnesses and injuries, but also about interpersonal or situational problems that are nonoccupational in origin. The nurse may be involved in counseling about any number of issues, such as nutrition, exercise, substance abuse, marriage and divorce, birth and death, or other health-related events, including breast cancer, HIV/AIDS, or parenting, that may affect not only the employee but also family members or significant others. For example, Fernsler (1989) presents recommendations for counseling

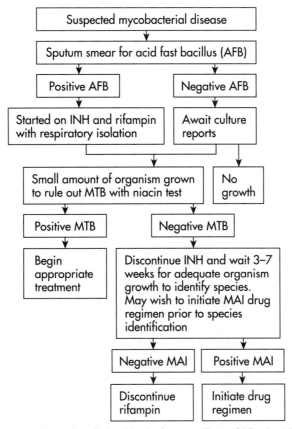

■ **Figure 11–1** Example of algorithmic format. (From O'Grady, M., & Frasier, J. Nurse Practitioner, *17*(7): 41–42, 1992.)

employees regarding breast cancer risks, which includes knowledge of risk factors; methods for early detection of breast cancer including breast self-examination, mammography, physical examination, and biopsy; dietary, exercise, and weight control recommendations; issues related to childbearing or menopause; and fear related to diagnostic procedures or self-identification of a lump.

Nelson and Hellman (1989) state that the occupational health nurse has a role in providing the counseling and voluntary testing of persons whose behavior puts them at high risk for HIV infection, who are planning marriage, who are of childbearing age, or who have unusual illnesses that persist. The purposes of the counseling are to increase the employee's understanding of HIV infection and AIDS, assess the employee's risk of HIV acquisition and transmission, and affect the worker's behavior to reduce the risk of acquiring and transmitting HIV infection.

Another example would include an employee who appears in the occupational health unit with symptoms of depression (i.e., fatigue, decreased energy, loss of appetite, sleep dysfunction). In discussing the situation with the employee, the nurse determines the probable reason is a grief reaction due to loss of a family member. The nurse can proceed to offer support to the employee, and also asks the employee if she or he desires therapy intervention. The nurse can probably assume this is a normal grief reaction but should continue to monitor the employee and offer support. If the depression worsens, a referral for intervention, such as to an employee assistance program or the employee's private physician would be in order. It is also important to determine if any physiologic or organic causes are the basis for any behavioral problems.

These are but a few examples of counseling situations in which the occupational health nurse may be involved. Some of these problems may interfere with the worker's ability to perform the job and the employee will probably benefit from some form of intervention such as listening, supporting, or referral, if indicated. The nurse's role is to help the employee find a solution to an immediate presenting problem and/or refer the employee for appropriate assistance. The role the nurse plays should not be confused with that of a therapist, unless the nurse is specifically trained and credentialed in this area. Thus, the nurse must be skilled to recognize problems, intervene, and refer as required. The nurse will need to have specific knowledge and skills, as identified by Csiernik (1990) (Table 11–3) in order to effectively provide assistance to the employee. When counseling employees, the occupational health nurse should arrange for space or facilities that provide for adequate privacy. The nurse needs to be supportive and demonstrate a sensitive, nonjudgmental, and caring attitude, as well as communicate respect for the employee.

It is important to recognize behavioral signs and symptoms that may be indicative of a "troubled" employee. Csiernik (1990) and Felton (1990) identify behavioral indicators suggestive of emotional distress or impairment, which are summarized in Table 11-4. If signs of behavioral changes or stress appear, which may be observed by the occupational health nurse directly or are reported by the employee's supervisor or a coworker, the occupational health nurse can initiate contact with the employee to determine if she or he needs or desires

■ **TABLE 11–3** Checklist of Knowledge and Skills for Occupational Health Nurses Involved in Employee Assistance Counseling

KNOWLEDGE OF
1. Various problems associated with abuse of substances.
2. Other health and personal problems.
3. Personal attitudes, skills, and limitations.
4. Counseling and crisis intervention.
5. Intervention strategies to help employees.
6. Referral approaches.
7. Follow-up approaches.
8. Community agencies and resources.

SKILL IN
1. Building a helping relationship (initiating, intervening, contracting, building rapport).
2. Interpersonal communication (active listening, verbal and nonverbal skills, attending, paraphrasing, and feedback).
3. Assessment and referral.
4. Case management.
5. Adult education (teaching and consulting).

From Csiernik, RP. AAOHN Journal, *38*(8): 381-384, 1990.

■ **TABLE 11-4**   Some Behavioral Indicators Suggestive of Emotional Distress

- Increased or chronic absenteeism and more frequent absence on Mondays, Fridays, and day after payday.
- Sleeping at work or increased general fatigue.
- Increased number of injuries or accidents at work.
- Increased errors/decreased concentration ability and task completion.
- Decreased interpersonal and/or communication relationships with co-workers, peers, managers.
- Lack of recognition of contributions made by others.
- Increased criticism of others.
- Change in mood and/or appearance.
- Physical symptoms of stress disorder (e.g., weight loss, gastritis) and other complaints or signs (e.g., headache, pharyngitis, petechiae).
- Substance abuse problems and excessive use of prescribed medications.

---

assistance. While employees may not share feelings and thoughts with fellow workers or their supervisors, they frequently will discuss their problems with the occupational health nurse or physician, assuming a trusting and confidential relationship has been established.

It is also important for the nurse to identify employees at risk for psychiatric emergencies, such as suicidal, homicidal, or psychotic behavior, and to have pre-identified community resources and referral options available if emergency hospitalization or care is required (Hughes, 1991). In these instances, the employee may be too incapacitated to handle the situation and the occupational health nurse must be prepared to initiate appropriate action.

Mistretta and Inlow (1991) point out that for any counseling services, whether performed in-house or through referral to an Employee Assistance Program, the employee must feel that the program is a safe environment where problems are dealt with in a professional manner, and that she or he is protected against job loss, criminal sanctions, or embarrassment. Accurate documentation is extremely important and all data collected must remain confidential. When providing aggregate information to management, care should be taken to delete demographic descriptions that could identify a client/employee.

Stress

Stress in the work environment is pervasive and insidious, and may be characterized by physical, psychological, and behavioral manifestations (Table 11-5). The National Center for Health Statistics (1985) reported that more than half of the 40,000 workers they questioned indicated that they felt either "a lot of stress" or "moderate stress" related to their jobs. As depicted in Figure 11-2, several factors in the work environment influence the stress state and generally fall into six broad areas.

Personal factors are related to individual characteristics or conditions that affect personal motivation, such as health status, personality, performance ability, coping and communication skills, value systems, and conflict between demands of the job and home life. More widely recognized than ever before as sources of stress are the multiple roles women find themselves in, such as mother, worker, and student.

■ **TABLE 11–5**   Stress-related Symptoms and Disorders

Physical	Psychological	Behavioral
Fatigue	Irritability	Smoking
Headaches	Anger	Overeating
Musculoskeletal disorders	Depression	Substance abuse
Hypertension	Apathy	Insomnia
Heart disease	Anxiety	Hostility
Gastrointestinal problems	Worry	Burnout
Infection	Withdrawal	Absenteeism

Situational factors are related to events or conditions of the job, such as quality of social support systems, work load, and conflicts with managers, peers, or colleagues. Social support systems at work influence psychological well-being, job satisfaction, health status, and work absenteeism. Conflict issues must be handled quickly and fairly without favoritism for one group or individual over another (Cronin-Stubbs & Rooks, 1985).

Organizational factors are related to policy and operational controls such as lack of shared decision making when job demands exceed worker control, role ambiguity, poor communication, ineffective organizational and managerial leadership, inadequate resources, job depersonalization, and lack of opportunity provided for professional growth. Workers may be faced with too many demands and vigilant tasks without enough help or adequate, state-of-the-art equipment and supplies. The politics of the institution in terms of corporate culture and level of productivity expected may also result in varying degrees of stress.

Technological factors are related to new or advanced systems for delivery of services, such as handling sophisticated equipment, interacting with computers and communication networks, and complex advances in high technology fields (e.g., engineering, medicine). For example, in a study conducted by Grout (1980), literature on air traffic controllers was reviewed and an analogy was drawn between this type of work and the nursing profession. Both professions were seen as demanding, performing critical and managing complex tasks crucial to the lives of others.

Environmental factors are concerned with the quality of the work setting. This category includes the physical design of the work station, overload of stimuli

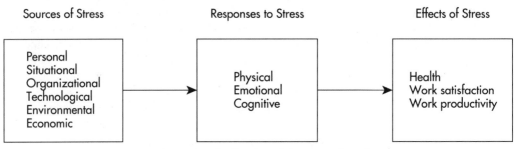

■ **Figure 11–2**   Psychosocial stress and work.

such as lights, noise, and odors, and the general tension level in the environment.

The physiological, psychological, and sociological issues related to shift work and worker health have been the focus of increased attention during the last several years. Studies of shift workers have shown that shift work, especially night and rotating shift work, has a negative impact on the worker's general well-being and performance because of the constant disruption of the individual's circadian rhythms. Loss of sleep, alterations in eating habits, headaches, stomach problems, and disturbances in elimination and relaxation patterns have been reported. Other physiological and psychological complaints include "feeling tired and worn out," feeling like a "nervous wreck," "being quickly angered," and experiencing anxiety and depression (Jung, 1986). Rotating shifts and working night shifts also affect the worker's interactions with family and friends.

Economic factors can cause considerable stress particularly when the worker's economic security is in jeopardy, such as with company downsizing or reduction in pay or benefit. In addition, when one spends more than what she or he earns in order to maintain a certain standard of living, financial crises can ensue.

These various sources of stress can result in one or more clinical manifestations, including physical, emotional, or cognitive disruption, and can cause health dysfunction or a decrease in work satisfaction and performance or both. It may be anticipated that even larger numbers of persons in the future will be at risk for stress responses and stress outcomes, such as chronic fatigue, loss of interest, and alcoholism or drug abuse, which also interfere with their work productivity. Strategies to deal with stress in the workplace and the offering of employee assistance programs to aid in counseling must be encouraged.

Employees may present to the occupational health unit with stress-related symptoms. The occupational health nurse can assist the employee through individual counseling about the specific stress-producing situation, and managing stress through enhanced coping skills, relaxation skills, and lifestyle modification such as physical fitness skills. In addition, the occupational health nurse will want to work with management to create a more satisfying organizational climate through supervisory training programs and more functional policies and structures, such as the establishment of flexible work schedules, encouraging participative management, providing social support and feedback, team building, improved career development, redesign of work tasks and demands, and shared rewards (Elkin & Rosch, 1990).

■ CONCLUSION

In the occupational setting, assessment and management of clinical problems and counseling of employees regarding work-related and nonoccupational health and related concerns is a key component within the scope of occupational health nursing practice. Employees will present to the occupational health unit with various complaints of a physical, emotional, or psychological nature, and the occupational health nurse needs to be skilled in making asessments and judgments regarding necessary care and appropriate referral. The development and use of clinical nursing guidelines will help to provide a systematic approach to nursing care; however, individual judgments are always required. The nurse must always practice within the legal limits of her or his state nurse practice act and utilize appropriate and current resources to provide safe and effective care.

References

Akers, P. An algorithmic approach to clinical decision making. Oncology Nursing Forum, *18:* 1159–1163, 1991.

Cronin-Stubbs, D & Rooks, C. Stress, social support, and burnout of critical care nurses: The results of research. Heart & Lung, *14:* 31–39, 1985.

Csiernik, RP. An EAP intervention protocol for occupational health nurses. AAOHN Journal, *38*(8): 381–384, 1990.

Elkin, AJ & Rosch, PJ. Promoting mental health at the workplace. Occupational Medicine: State of the Art Review, *5*(4): 739–754, 1990.

Felton, J. Occupational medical management. Boston: Little, Brown & Company, pp. 245–270, 1990.

Fernsler, JI. Employee counseling with respect to lifestyle, life events, and breast cancer risks. AAOHN Journal, *37*(5): 158–166, 1989.

Gant, DA. Evaluating caring competencies in nursing practice. Topics in Clinical Nursing, *8:* 77–82, 1986.

Glasgow, G. Quality of care in occupational health through nursing diagnosis. AAOHN Journal, *38:* 105–109, 1990.

Grout, JW. Stress and the nurse: Selected bibliography. Journal of Nursing Education, *19:* 58–63, 1980.

Hughes, KH. Psychiatric emergencies in the workplace. AAOHN Journal, *39*(6): 265–269, 1991.

Jung, F. Shiftwork: Its effect on health performance and well-being. AAOHN Journal, *34:* 160–164, 1986.

Mistretta, EF & Inlow, LB: Confidentiality and the employee assistance program professional. AAOHN Journal, *39*(2): 84–86, 1991.

National Center for Health Statistics. Health promotion and disease prevention. Hyattsville, MD: Author, 1985.

Nelson, LM & Hellman, SL. Counseling employees at risk for HIV. AAOHN Journal, *37*(10): 404–411, 1989.

O'Grady, M, & Frasier, J. Recognizing and managing mycobacterial diseases in clients with AIDS. Nurse Practitioner, *17*(7): 41–42, 1992.

Rogers, B, Mastroianni, K, & Randolph, S. Occupational health nursing guidelines for primary clinical conditions. Boston: OEM Press, 1992.

Tanner, CA, Padrick, KP, & Westfall, VE: Diagnostic reasoning strategies of nurses and nursing student. Nursing Research, *36:* 358–363, 1987.

Williams, G. Protocols for nursing practice. AAOHN Update Series, *1*(2): 1–8, 1984.

───────────── APPENDIX ─────────────

11–1

Examples of Clinical Nursing Guidelines for Common Occupational Health Problems*

---

*Copyright 1990 by Bonnie Rogers.
For additional guidelines, see Rogers, B, Mastroianni, K, & Randolph, S. Occupational health nursing guidelines for primary clinical conditions. Boston: OEM Press, 1992.

ABRASIONS/LACERATIONS

DEFINITION An **abrasion** is a scraping trauma resulting in a break in the skin and removal of epidermis. A **laceration** is a slice or tear in the skin or mucosa. Trauma usually occurs from contact with sharp objects, machinery, or from falls or other injuries.

CHARACTERISTICS Lacerations may have sharp or jagged edges. Tissue, nerves or blood vessels may be involved. Bleeding is usually slight. Any break in the skin involves the risk of infection and contamination with the tetanus organism.

POLICY Employees should be evaluated in the occupational health unit to determine degree and severity of the injury. In caring for abrasions/lacerations the occupational health nurse should ALWAYS assess the worker's immunization status against tetanus.

Clinical Assessments/Interventions

- Assess the extent and location of the injury.
- Control bleeding by applying firm pressure; may need to elevate extremity and utilize pressure points.
- Cleanse area with mild antiseptic solution and water, and rinse.
- Approximate edges of laceration with steri-strips if indicated.
- Apply antibiotic ointment per standing order.
- Apply nonadherent dry sterile dressing (e.g., Telfa, Jellnet); minor abrasions may be left undressed.
- Assess immunization status for tetanus and proceed as outlined in tetanus protocol. If required, immunizations should be received within 24 hours.
- Counsel employee regarding care of the wound on and off the job (e.g., hygiene, avoid repeat injury).
- Advise employee to keep the dressing clean and dry to prevent infection and to change dressing daily (allows for observation of wound).
- Instruct employee on signs and symptoms of infection (e.g., redness at site, warmth at site, tenderness, swelling, pain, etc.)

Referral for Medical Action

Wound involves:
- > 2 cm in length or is deep
- gaping or jagged edges
- embedded material
- cut producing a flap
- serious cut to fingers, hands, toes, feet or is over joints
- human/animal bites
- facial lacerations
- functional disturbance
- uncontrolled bleeding
- gross contamination.

Follow-up Actions

- Evaluate wound for infection/healing.
- If wound is infected, refer employee for medical evaluation.
- Evaluate worksite for potential hazards.

ANAPHYLACTIC SHOCK

DEFINITION An antigen-antibody reaction that occurs when a foreign protein substance enters the body of a sensitized person. The reaction may cause a histamine release with subsequent arteriole/capillary dilation, capillary permeability, intravascular fluid leak, and hypovolemia resulting in inadequate profusion of the cells.

CHARACTERISTICS Respiratory difficulty, bronchospasm, wheezing, warm skin, blotching red skin areas, urticaria, rapid weak pulse, facial swelling, cardiovascular collapse. The reaction is considered life-threatening. Common sensitizing agents include antibiotics or other medications, insect bites, seafood or blood transfusions.

POLICY Immediate treatment should be administered in the occupational health unit and/or on site by the occupational health nurse or appropriately licensed person. The employee should then be immediately referred for medical treatment.

Clinical Assessments/Interventions

INSTITUTE EMERGENCY ACTION
- Maintain an open airway.
- Administer epinepherine 0.3 to 0.5 ml of 1:1000 solution subcutaneously or intramuscularly per standing order.
- Administer oxygen as indicated.
- Start intravenous solution of normal saline or Lactated Ringers per standing order.
- Monitor employee's vital signs.

Referral for Medical Action

- Immediate medical evaluation and treatment required (i.e., transfer to hospital).

Follow-up Actions

- Counsel employee regarding prevention of recurrence.
- Note sensitivity reaction in prominent place on employee's health record.

BURNS - CHEMICAL

DEFINITION

Injury to the tissues as a result of exposure to chemical agents such as strong acids or alkalies which are corrosive. The severity of the burn is determined by the amount of body surface area (BSA) involved and the depth of the burn. First degree burns involve the epithelial layer (erythema); second degree burns include a partial thickness of the dermal skin layer (erythema with blister); third degree burns involve full thickness of the dermal skin layer (white or leathery with no blisters and/or charred appearance), and may extend to muscle and bone (sometimes considered fourth degree burns).

CHARACTERISTICS

First degree burns are usually superficial and initially result in reddening of the skin and pain. Second degree burns (partial thickness) are accompanied by severe pain, erythema, latent blister formation and cell fluid loss. In third degree burns the area may be black, white or leathery in appearance. Excessive fluid loss may cause shock.

POLICY

An employee who experiences a chemical burn should have the burn site immediately irrigated with copious amounts of water or normal saline solution, except when powdered chemicals are present which may be activated by water. Check Material Safety Data Sheets (MSDS). Powdered chemicals should be carefully brushed from the skin. Special caution should be taken to avoid contaminating the eye. Employee should then be evaluated in the occupational health unit. Guidelines should be developed for specific chemicals used at the worksite.

Clinical Assessments/Interventions

- Assess degree and severity of injury.
- Brush dry powder chemicals from the skin before flushing with copious amounts of water; be particularly careful with the eye.
- Gently flush the burned area with cool water or saline for a minimum of 30 minutes; advise employee to shower, if needed.
- Remove contaminated clothing from employee.
- Estimate total extent of burn injury (*See Rule of Nines*).
- Remove constricting jewelry from employee.
- Obtain accurate history of burn event (e.g., sudden flash, scald).
- Review MSDS; cleanse area with mild soap and water—exceptions to this may be dependent on chemical involved.
- Apply topical and other medications if warranted per standing order.
- Apply dressing.
- Assess tetanus immunization status and proceed per tetanus protocol.
- Transport to hospital as indicated.

Referral for Medical Action

- Burns involving face, eyes, feet or perineum.
- Electrical and/or inhalation burns.
- Burns with associated major trauma.
- Second degree burns >10% of BSA or any third degree burn.
- Elderly employees or those with chronic disease.
- Hydroflouric acid burns.

Follow-up Actions

- Change dressing as needed.
- Conduct worksite assessment for hazard control.
- Review MSDS for chemical exposures and safe handling practices.

RULE OF NINES

The Body is Divided Into Multiples of Nine.

Head and Neck =	9%
Each upper extremity = 9% i.e., 9 X 2 =	18%
Each lower extremity = 18% i.e., 18 x 2 =	36%
Each anterior and posterior trunk surfaces = 18% i.e., 18 x 2 =	36%
Perineum and genitalia =	1%
	100%

9%

9%

18% Front

18% Back

9%

9%

1%

18%

18%

CONTUSION

DEFINITION   Injury to soft tissue in which the skin is not broken (a bruise); caused by blunt force, blow, kick or fall.

CHARACTERISTICS   Hemorrhage into injured parts (ecchymosis), pain, swelling, and discoloration are usually present.

POLICY   Employee should be evaluated in the occupational health unit.

Clinical Assessments/Interventions

- Assess injury.
- Elevate affected part.
- Apply cold compresses to area for 10 minutes, remove for 5 minutes, then reapply 3 to 4 times to reduce edema formation.
- Apply elastic or elastic adhesive pressure bandage to reduce swelling and edema.
- Assess neurovascular status distal to injury:
  — look for digital cyanosis
  — assess for peripheral nerve damage.
- Apply warm moist heat, as needed, to affected area after swelling is reduced, usually after 48 hours.

Referral for Medical Action

- Soreness or disability persists.

Follow-up Actions

Advise employee to:
  — continue cold compresses or ice packs periodically during first 24 hours or until swelling is reduced
  — keep affected part at rest and elevated
  — apply heat after swelling has stopped
  — report if soreness or disability persists.

CONVULSION/SEIZURE

DEFINITION   Paroxysms of involuntary muscular contractions and relaxations. They may be caused by epilepsy, meningitis, acute infectious disease, heat cramps, brain lesions, eclampsia, hypoglycemia (related to diabetes), and poisoning from camphor, cyanides, strychnine or other chemical agents.

CHARACTERISTICS   Intermittent contractions and relaxations of muscles, periodic lapses of consciousness, incontinence.

POLICY   Employee should be evaluated in the occupational health unit and referred for medical care.

Clinical Assessments/Interventions

- Assess employee's status.
- Keep employee from injuring self during seizure.
- Keep employee in lying position.
- Maintain open airway after seizure; turn employee prone or in semiprone position; turn head to side.
- Monitor employee's vital signs.
- Record the following:
  — time of onset
  — duration of seizure
  — origin of convulsion (i.e., started in certain area of body or became generalized from the start)
  — type of contractions
  — incontinence
  — injury to head or other areas
  — abnormal odor to breath.
- Arrange for medical care.

Referral for Medical Action

- Any occurrence of seizure activity.

Follow-up Actions

- Collaborate with private physician regarding follow-up treatment plan.
- Educate employee about importance of taking medication as directed.
- Counsel employee about communicating to supervisor and co-workers about procedure if seizure occurs.
- Review appropriate placement of worker to ensure safety.

CUMULATIVE TRAUMA DISORDER (CTD)

DEFINITION   Work-related conditions that generally affect the upper extremities of the musculoskeletal system; physical symptoms which result from trauma or work strain from repeated or continuous application of ergonomic work stress, which for short periods of time or a single application would usually not be harmful.

CTDs may be caused by fatigue from lack of sufficient rest; job requiring level of physical exertion that exceeds person's capacity; repetitive gripping, twisting, reaching, moving; chronic repetition in a forceful and awkward manner without rest or sufficient recovery time.   Other factors are mechanical stress, posture and vibration, and low temperatures.

CHARACTERISTICS   Manifestations include pain, tenderness, swelling, numbness, tingling, burning, or "pins and needles" feeling, and itchy skin surface on affected extremity.

POLICY   Employee should be evaluated in the occupational health unit and referred for medical care.

Clinical Assessments/Interventions

- Assess employee's status.
- Take history of complaint, type of work performed, frequency of symptoms and hobbies.
- Implement medical management protocol for cumulative trauma disorders.
- Administer medications per standing order.
- Apply hot soaks for 10-15 minutes, 4 times daily as needed.
- Bandage or splint injury per standing order.
- Refer employee to physician if symptoms continue after 3 days.

Referral for Medical Action

- Continued pain or limited movement.
- Several workers in same area with similar complaint.

Follow-up Actions

- Educate employee about signs/symptoms and causes of CTD; return to occupational health unit if symptoms reoccur.
- Review with employee exercises which may help.
- Instruct employee about proper techniques for individual job.
- Conduct workplace assessment (i.e., ergonomic assessment) with other members of occupational health team.
- Counsel employee about return to work, limited duty or job rotation.

DERMATITIS

DEFINITION

Inflammation of the skin which may be caused by irritants or sensitizing agents.

Primary Chemical Irritants

Includes acids; alkalis; solvents; such as turpentine, gasoline, kerosene, cutting oils, greases, and lubricants, all of which may cause dermatosis in any individual and after only one or a few contacts. The result is an irritant contact dermatitis.

Sensitizing Agents

Includes various dyes, fabrics, rubber, insecticides, cosmetics, oils, resins, plants, woods, and sunlight, which may cause dermatosis in a few susceptible individuals, following repeated contacts over a period of time. The result is an allergic contact dermatitis.

CHARACTERISTICS

Clinical manifestations include itching, redness, and various skin lesions; dryness, cracking and scaling; burning sensation over affected area.

POLICY

Employee should be evaluated in the occupational health unit.

Clinical Assessments/Interventions

- Assess injury or inflammation.
- Remove employee from source of exposure.
- Obtain accurate history of exposure, location of occurrence and treatment, if any has been given; previous skin problems; hobbies and secondary (other) employment; new clothing, detergents, etc.
- Document any family history of asthma or hay fever.
- Treat mild cases of dermatitis as indicated:
  — cleansing procedure - wash with superfatted soap and water
  — topical medication per standing order
  — cool, wet compresses
  — prevention of exposure to additional irritants.

Referral for Medical Action

- Acute, severe case; persistent or recurrent cases; or complications such as infection.

Follow-up Actions

- Educate employee about:
  — self-care of dermatitis
  — avoidance of exposure to irritants
  — importance and proper method of good personal hygiene
  — use of personal protection (e.g., may need specific gloves for certain agents).
- Collaborate with occupational health team to develop strategies to reduce exposure to irritants or sensitizing agents, including choice of PPE.
- Counsel employee on return to work regarding exposure to irritants/sensitization.
- Review MSDS for chemical exposures and safe handling practices.

PRIMARY LESIONS OF THE SKIN

LESION	DEFINITION
MACULE	flat, circumscribed discoloration of the skin or mucous membrane up to 1 cm.
PAPULE	solid, elevated lesion of the skin or mucous membrane up to 1 cm.
NODULE	solid, elevated lesion of the skin or mucous membrane up to 1 cm. in diameter but extending into the underlying tissues.
TUMOR	solid, elevated lesion of the skin or mucous membrane greater than 1 cm. but extending into underlying tissues.
VESICLE	elevated superficial, fluid-filled lesion of the skin or mucous membrane less than 1 cm. in diameter.
BULLA	fluid-filled superficial or elevated lesion of the skin or mucous membrane larger than 1 cm.
PATCH	flat circumscribed discoloration of the skin or mucous membrane larger than 1 cm.
PLAQUE	solid, elevated lesion of the skin or mucous membrane greater than 1 cm. Example: papules that coalesce form a plaque.
PUSTULE	pus containing lesion of varying size.
WHEAL	"hive," elevated, solid lesion of the skin or mucous membrane that changes in shape and size due to cutaneous edema; a transient lesion.
TELANGIETASIA	permanently dilated capillary that would otherwise be normally invisible.

EYE INJURY - BURN

CHEMICAL BURN TO THE EYE

DEFINITION   Chemical burns to the eye in the form of tissue injury. May be a result of acid, alkali, irritant, or detergent, or material entering the eye causing damage.

While acid burns are usually instantaneous, alkaline burns are always progressive and require diligent treatment. Irritants and detergents do not produce burns, but can damage the eyes by inflammation or drawing water from the tissues. Chemicals may be in the form of vapor, dust particles, or liquid.

CHARACTERISTICS   Clinical manifestations include pain, sensation of burning, blurring, photophobia, tearing, decreased visual acuity, exudates, erythema, and edema of surrounding tissues.

POLICY   Employee should be evaluated in the occupational health unit; arrange for immediate medical care.

Clinical Assessments/Interventions

- Assess injury to eye and surrounding areas.
- Arrange for immediate irrigations of eye with copious amounts of water at the scene (eye wash if available).
- Have employee brought to the occupational health unit. Determine what happened and what the substance was.
- Check eye for contact lenses and remove.
- Administer eye anesthetic per standing order.
- Inspect eye thoroughly; remove any remaining particulate matter by irrigation with water or wet cotton-tipped applicator.
- Determine employee's visual acuity, if able.
- Continue eye irrigation with copious amounts of cool water for at least 15 minutes, making sure that all parts of the eye have been irrigated.
- Arrange for immediate medical care.

Referral for Medical Action

- Any burn to eye.

Follow-up Actions

- Inspect eye thoroughly.
- Educate employee about proper safety procedures and personal protective equipment.
- Instruct employee about eye protection.
- Review signs/symptoms of eye injury with employee.
- Treat employee as specified by medical order.
- Counsel employee about return to work or limited duty as indicated.
- Determine employee's visual acuity.
- Review MSDS for chemical exposure and safe handling practices.

FRACTURE

DEFINITION   Break or crack in a bone caused by motor vehicle accidents, injury related to a fall, or as a result of direct or indirect violence.

Closed: No open wound on the surface of the body; usually simple fracture; neighboring muscles and other tissues may remain largely undamaged.

Open: Associated directly with open wounds; compound fracture; damage to surrounding soft tissues.

CHARACTERISTICS   Deformity, swelling, discoloration, pain or tenderness to the touch, and loss of range of motion in extremity is evident.

POLICY   Provide initial stabilization of employee injury and arrange for immediate medical care.

Clinical Assessments/Interventions

- Assess extent and degree of injury.
- Immobilize the injury; do not move the employee unless there is danger of fire, carbon monoxide poisoning, explosion, or other life-threatening conditions.
- Control any bleeding and prevent contamination of wound; if fragment of bone is protruding, cover the entire wound with large sterile bandage, compress or pads.
- Treat employee for shock.
- Give nothing to eat or drink.
- Apply cold or ice packs to the area.
- If splinting, avoid interference with circulation and be sure that the splint is long enough to immobilize the joints proximal and distal to affected part.
- Elevate the limb slightly to reduce hemorrhage and swelling.
- Arrange for immediate medical care or transfer to hospital.

Referral for Medical Action

- Fracture suspected.

Follow-up Actions

- Counsel employee on return to work, limited duty, or job transfer as indicated.

HYPERCHOLESTEROLEMIA

DEFINITION   Elevated blood cholesterol which increases the risk of atherosclerosis and coronary heart disease. Cholesterol is transported in the blood by lipoproteins. Low density lipoproteins (LDL) deposit cholesterol outside the liver while high density lipoproteins (HDL) transport cholesterol to the liver where the waxlike susbstance is metabolized and eliminated. Increased levels of LDL and low levels of HDL are causally related to an increased risk of coronary heart disease (CHD).

CHARACTERISTICS   Most individuals with hypercholesterolemia are asymptomatic. *See Classification*

POLICY   All employees evaluated for cholesterol or presenting to the occupational health unit with prior cholesterol results should also be evaluated for other risk factors and recommended for follow-up actions.

Clinical Assessments/Interventions

• Maintain calibrated equipment and sound quality assurance practices when doing cholesterol tests.
• Evaluate employee for cardiac risk factors during cholesterol screening, or when presenting with cholesterol results from a prior test.
• For employees who have a desirable blood cholesterol, discuss diet and give educational materials.
• Advise employees with a desirable cholesterol to repeat the serum cholesterol evaluation within 5 years.
• For employees whose values exceed 200 mg/dL, obtain a repeat total cholesterol within 1-8 weeks. If the two values are within a 30 mg/dL range, average the values or obtain a third value in another 1-8 weeks and average all three values; discuss dietary changes designed to lower serum cholesterol and advise annual follow-up.
• For employees with high blood cholesterol or borderline high cholesterol levels plus CHD or 2 risk factors, advise immediate lipoprotein analysis.

Referral for Medical Action

• Unable to reevaluate employee in the occupational health unit.
• Definite CHD or 2 additional risk factors (schedule for lipoprotein analysis).

Follow-up Actions

• For employees with hypercholesterolemia:
— Define cholesterol and dietary cholesterol, and provide information on how to limit cholesterol intake
— Provide information based on the current dietary guidelines, including the role of protein, carbohydrates, fiber, alcohol intake, exercise, and maintenance of desirable weight
— Emphasize importance of continued follow-up treatment
— Describe and differentiate between types of fat, emphasizing foods to avoid and foods to consume
— Discuss a nutritionally adequate diet consisting of a variety of foods.
• See *General Follow-up Information*

HYPERCHOLESTEROLEMIA

CLASSIFICATION

Total

< 200 mg/dL	Desireable Level
200 to 239 mg/dL	Borderline high cholesterol
≥ 240 mg/dL	High blood cholesterol

LDL

< 130 mg/dL	Desireable Level
130 to 159 mg/dL	Borderline high LDL cholesterol
≥ 160 mg/dL	High Risk blood cholesterol

RISK FACTORS

1. Definite CHD: Prior Myocardial infarction (MI) or angina

   OR

2. Two other CHD risk factors:

   • Male gender

   • Family history (MI before age 55 for parent or sibling)

   • Cigarette smoking (> 10 cigarettes/day)

   • Hypertension

   • Low HDL (< 35 mg/dL)

   • Diabetes

   • History of definitve cerebrovascular or occlusive peripheral vascular disease

GENERAL FOLLOW-UP INFORMATION

Total cholesterol: < 200mg/dL	Dietary information and repeat cholesterol within 5 years.
200 - 239 mg/dL: Without CHD or 2 other CHD risk factors	Dietary information and repeat cholesterol annually.
With Definite CHD or 2other CHD risk factors or ≥ 240 mg/dL	Lipoprotein analysis: further action based on LDL-cholesterol level.

DIETARY THERAPY

Nutrient	Step-One Diet	Step-Two Diet
Total Fat	< 30% of total calories	< 20% of total clories
Saturated	< 10% of total calories	< 7% of total calories
Polyunsaturated	≤ 10% of total calories	≤ 10% of total calories
Monounsaturated	10% - 15% of total calories	10% to 15% of total calories
Carbohydrates	50% to 60% of total calories	50% to 60% of total calories
Protein	10% to 20% of total calories	10% to 20% of total calories
Cholesterol	< 300 mg/day	< 200mg/day
Total Calories	To achieve and maintain desireable weight.	

HYPERTENSION

DEFINITION   Sustained, elevated pressure exerted on arterial walls. The etiology is usually unknown (essential or idiopathic) but a small percentage of individuals have a secondary cause originating from the kidneys, adrenal glands, neurogenic causes, coartation of the aorta and toxemia.

CHARACTERISTICS   Onset of hypertension is usually insidious. In severe hypertension or blood pressure sensitive employees, symptoms can include headache, epistaxis, tinnitus, syncopy, fatigue, shortness of breath, failing vision and chest pain.

POLICY   Control of hypertension begins with detection and is maintained through continued surveillance. Blood pressure should be measured at each client visit as appropriate. Hypertension requires medical attention. Maintain current American Heart Association recommendations, including calibration of equipment. Follow-up care is crucial when providing blood pressure screening for employees. Medical treatment should be documented for confirmed hypertensive employees before returning to work.

Clinical Assessments/Interventions

- Assess and monitor employee's blood pressure.
- Confirm high blood pressure by obtaining blood pressure readings on three different visits during the same week with average levels of diastolic pressure of 90mm Hg or greater, or systolic pressure of 140mm Hg or greater.
- Seat employee with arms bare, supported and positioned at heart level.
- Instruct employee not to smoke or ingest caffeine within 30 minutes prior to measurement.
- Measure blood pressure after 5 minutes of quiet rest. Check both arms.
- Use appropriate cuff size (child, adult, large adult) with the rubber bladder encircling at least two-thirds of the arm.
- Average two or more blood pressure readings during same visit. If the first two readings differ by 5mm Hg, additional readings should be obtained; record the averaged measurements.
- Inform employee of blood pressure reading and advise of the need for periodic remeasurement.
- Obtain health history to include medication useage.

Referral for Medical Action

- Confirmed blood pressure of 140/90 or greater.
- Severe blood pressure.
  See Classification and Follow-up Criteria for Blood Pressure in Adults 18 Years or Older

continued

Follow-up Actions

- Collaborate with private physician regarding treatment plan.
- Discuss disease etiology, course and treatment with the employee.
- Emphasize importance of medical treatment/follow-up.
- Discuss the importance of low fat, low salt diet and weight reduction with employee.
- Instruct employee in prescribed medication sechedule and possible side effects.
- Advise employee to initiate an aerobic exercise program gradually, after appropriate clinical evaluation and physician consult.
- Advise employee in other healthy lifestyle changes (i.e., tobacco avoidance, restriction of alcohol and relaxation techniques).
- Consult with family/significant others as necessary with employee permission.
- Maintain flow chart of employee blood pressure recordings.

CLASSIFICATION AND FOLLOW-UP CRITERIA FOR BLOOD PRESSURE IN ADULTS 18 YEARS OR OLDER

Classification of Blood Pressure in Adults Age 18 Years or Older

Range, mm Hg	Category
Diastolic	
<85	Normal blood pressure
85-89	High normal blood pressure
90-104	Mild hypertension
105-114	Moderate hypertension
≥115	Severe hypertension
Systolic, when diastolic blood pressure is < 90	
<140	Normal blood pressure
140-159	Borderline isolated systolic hypertension
≥160	Isolated systolic hypertension

Follow-up Criteria for Initial Blood Pressure Measurements Age 18 Years or Older

Range, mm Hg	Recommend Follow-up
Diastolic	
<85	Recheck within 2 years
85-89	Recheck within 1 year
90-104	Confirm within 2 months
105-114	Refer promptly to source of care
>115	Refer immediately to source of care
Systolic, when diastolic blood pressure is < 90	
<140	Recheck within 2 years
140-199	Confirm within 2 months
≥200	Refer promptly to source of c are wihin 2 weeks

(Adopted from 1988 Report of the Joint National Committee)

INSECT STINGS

DEFINITION   An antigen-antibody reaction, usually occurring from the sting of a bee, wasp, yellow jacket, or hornet, that can result in anything from a local reaction to anaphylactic shock. The greater the incidence of stings, the greater the possibility of severe reaction.

CHARACTERISTICS   Usually a localized reaction of redness, itching and swelling.

POLICY   Employee should be evaluated in the occupational health unit for severity of reaction and possible anaphylaxis. Stings around the mouth or throat or multiple stings may cause airway constriction and unconsciousness. These types of stings are potentially life threatening and should be treated as an emergency situation.

Clinical Assessments/Interventions

- Assess employee's vital signs.
- Assess employee for mild reaction (stinging, burning, swelling, itching) or severe reaction (extremity edema, urticaria, pruitis, brochospasm, hypotension); if anaphylaxis is imminent institute shock protocol.
- Remove the stinger gently from the site under magnification.
- Cleanse the sting site with soap and water.
- Apply preparation of aluminum salt (e.g., Burrow's Solution or an antiperspirant) which may relieve pain/swelling by inactivating venom.
- Apply ice or cold packs to the site to limit swelling.
- Apply antiseptic cream per standing order to the site.
- Elevate employee's limb.
- Administer oral antihistamine or steroid to the employee per standing order.
- Advise employee regarding signs and symptoms of systemic allergic reaction including:
    — airway tightness
    — weakness
    — generalized itching
    — red skin blotches
    — numbness and tingling
    — anxiety
    — gastrointestinal distress.
- Caution employee to avoid areas where bees are usually present, and advise against wearing bright clothing and perfumes particularly outdoors.

Referral for Medical Action

- Severe reaction.
- Previous history indicative of allergic sensitivity or evidence of general allergic response seems apparent.
- Stings around mouth or throat or multiple stings.

Follow-up Actions

- Reevaluate employee in 24 hours if needed.
- Reinforce teaching and prevention strategies with employee.
- Note sensitivity in prominent place on employee's health record.
- Advice employee to wear Medic Alert if known to be hypersensitive and/or carry insect sting kit, and to wear shoes, long sleeves and pants when walking/working outdoors.

12

HEALTH PROMOTION AND HEALTH PROTECTION

The roots of health promotion are grounded in the epidemiological revolution of the 19th century, in which the reduction of morbidity and mortality was brought about through social and environmental reforms in hygiene, housing, sanitation, and improvement of working conditions (Burnham, 1984). This movement extended into the 20th century, which has witnessed an even greater emphasis on health promotion and disease prevention through legislative acts such as the Health Maintenance Organization Act of 1973 and the National Health Planning and Resource Development Act of 1974. Both acts stress the importance of preventive health and health education efforts in improving the health of our society. In addition, more emphasis has been placed on self-care and self-responsibility for health, and the need for behavioral change to control chronic and communicable diseases.

While preventive interventions have resulted in overall health improvements in society, preventable illness and injury continue to plague society with respect not only to our health and quality of living but also to health-related costs. It is estimated that for every health care dollar spent, 97% is spent on illness treatment, and only 3% is spent on health promotion and prevention activities (Pender, 1987). This point is exemplified by examining the cost of U.S. health care, which has risen dramatically in the past few decades. Health care services represented 5% of the Gross National Product (GNP) in 1960 compared to an estimated 12% in 1990 (USDHHS, 1991) and a predicted 18% in the year 2000 without cost controls. Preventable health-related conditions such as cardiovascular disease, cancer, and injuries have resulted in an annual health care cost of more than $300 billion (Rice et al., 1989; Hodgson & Rice, 1992).

In addition, in 1991 American employers paid approximately $355 billion in health care costs, with a rate of increase of 21% annually. If health care costs continue to climb at this rate, it is estimated that the annual health care bill to business will double in less than five years (Taming, 1992), and health care costs will be nearly one fifth of the GNP by the year 2000. Table 12–1 depicts various preventable conditions with related per patient capita costs (USDHHS, 1991).

■ **TABLE 12–1** Preventable Health Conditions and Economic Impact

Condition	Overall Magnitude	Avoidable Intervention[1]	Cost per Patient[2]
Heart disease	7 million with coronary artery disease 500,000 deaths/yr 284,000 bypass procedures/yr	Coronary bypass surgery	$ 30,000
Cancer	1 million new cases/yr 510,000 deaths/yr	Lung cancer treatment Cervical cancer treatment	$ 29,000 $ 28,000
Stroke	600,000 strokes/yr 150,000 deaths/yr	Hemiplegia treatment and rehabilitation	$ 22,000
Injuries	2.3 million hospitalizations/yr 142,500 deaths/yr 177,000 persons with spinal cord injuries in the United States	Quadriplegia treatment and rehabilitation Hip fracture treatment and rehabilitation Severe head injury treatment and rehabilitation	$570,000 (lifetime) $ 40,000 $310,000
HIV infection	1–1.5 million infected 118,000 AIDS cases (as of Jan 1990)	AIDS treatment	$ 75,000 (lifetime)
Alcoholism	18.5 million abuse alcohol 105,000 alcohol-related deaths/yr	Liver transplant	$250,000
Drug abuse	Regular users: 1–3 million: cocaine 900,000: IV drugs 500,000: heroin Drug-exposed babies: 375,000	Treatment of drug-affected baby	$ 63,000 (5 years)
Low birth weight baby	260,000 LBWB born/yr 23,000 deaths/yr	Neonatal intensive care for LBWB	$ 10,000
Inadequate immunization	Lacking basic immunization series: 20–30%, aged 2 and younger 3%, aged 6 and older	Congenital rubella syndrome treatment	$354,000 (lifetime)

[1]Examples (other interventions may apply).
[2]Representative first-year costs, except as noted. Not indicated are nonmedical costs, such as lost productivity to society.
From USDHHS. Healthy People 2000: Washington, DC: DHHS publication No. 91-50212, 94–110, 1991.

On a national level, efforts to address preventable causes of disease, disability, and premature mortality are addressed in *Healthy People 2000*. This effort emphasizes health promotion, protection, and disease prevention as a more humane and economical route to good health than the more costly, painful, and life-disruptive procedures necessitated by after-the-fact treatment and curative measures (Sullivan, 1991). Many Americans have bought into the health promotion philosophy as demonstrated by efforts to become better informed about health problems and to change lifestyle behaviors to improve their health and quality of life. However, a recent article by the (former) Secretary of Health and Human Services, Dr. Louis Sullivan, reports data, summarized below, which reflect a considerable need for much more improvement in the health and well-being of society (Sullivan, 1991):

- Of the 10 leading causes of death in America, half are related to improper diet and lack of exercise.
- Nearly 400,000 deaths each year are related to smoking. In 1989, direct and associated health care costs for smoking-related illnesses were $23 billion and $52 billion respectively.
- More than 18 million Americans abuse alcohol and more than 100,000 deaths each year are alcohol-related. Nearly half of the motor vehicle deaths and drowning deaths are alcohol-related. Alcohol-related health problems cost about $70 billion annually.
- Between 1 and 3 million individuals are regular users of cocaine and half a million are heroin users. In 1989, approximately half of all arrested men and women tested positive for drugs.
- Between 1 and 1.5 million U.S. citizens have been infected with the HIV virus, 242,000 have been diagnosed with AIDS, and the number of deaths exceeds 162,000.
- Injuries result in 2.3 million hospitalizations per year with more than 140,000 deaths annually.
- In 1988, the infant mortality rate for black male and female infants was 2.5 and 2.7 times the rate for white male and female infants, respectively. Since 1985, the black infant mortality rate, which had begun to decline, began to rise. The black female infant mortality rate has increased 1.9% annually whereas for white female infants the rate declined by 4.2% annually.
- Violence in America is increasing. During the first six months of 1990, reported violent crimes increased by 10% compared to the same period in 1989. In 1989, 19,000 Americans were murdered. Overall life expectancy rates have begun to decline.

The *Healthy People 2000: National Health Promotion and Disease Prevention Objectives* presents a blueprint or plan for action to combat the leading preventable diseases and health-related problems. Priority areas identified are all-encompassing and are segmented into health promotion, health protection, preventive services and surveillance and data systems. In addition, objectives within these areas have been categorized and are presented separately as age-related and special population objectives (Table 12–2). Efforts to achieve these priorities will require a commitment on the part of society and its members to promote and adopt healthy lifestyles and behaviors conducive to optimal health, and by business and government to develop strategies, opportunities, and resources required to support the behavioral and environmental changes needed. The health objectives specific for occupational safety and health are identified in Chapter 1; however, the reader should refer to the reference source for a detailed description.

Previous to the advent of health promotion activities and program initiatives, the employer's responsibility for employee health care was viewed primarily as providing for hospitalization benefits for its employees, monitoring work-related illnesses and injuries, and providing treatment for injuries at the worksite (McGovern, 1991). In a recent survey, as reported in the *National Survey of Worksite Health Promotion Activities* (1987), 66% of U.S. worksites with 50 or more employees offered some type of disease prevention or health promotion activity. However, Golaszewski (1992) points out that while this number sounds

■ **TABLE 12–2** National Health Promotion and Disease
Prevention Objectives

Health promotion
 1. Physical activity and fitness
 2. Nutrition
 3. Tobacco
 4. Alcohol and other drugs
 5. Family planning
 6. Mental health and mental disorders
 7. Violent and abusive behavior
 8. Educational and community-based programs

Health protection
 9. Unintentional injuries
10. Occupational safety and health
11. Environmental health
12. Food and drug safety
13. Oral health

Preventive services
14. Maternal and infant health
15. Heart disease and stroke
16. Cancer
17. Diabetes and chronic disabling conditions
18. HIV infection
19. Sexually transmitted diseases
20. Immunization and infectious diseases
21. Clinical preventive services

Surveillance and data systems
22. Surveillance and data systems

Age-related objectives
• Children
• Adolescents and young adults
• Adults
• Older adults

Special population objectives
• People with low income
• Blacks
• Hispanics
• Asians and Pacific islanders
• American Indians and Native Americans
• People with disabilities

---

impressive, the findings could be overstated as the survey design did not allow
for the differentiation of type activity, which could have referred to a poster
display, pamphlet distribution, or a full-fledged program initiative. Thus, while
it is encouraging to note a presumed increase in employer-sponsored health
promotion-related activities, the importance of a comprehensive approach to
worker health must be emphasized and facilitated. This can best be accomplished
through developing a concept of health at the worksite and operationalizing this

concept through program planning, implementation, and evaluation. This includes not only a corporate and company-wide commitment to health but a combination of educational, organizational, economical or other environmental supports, rather than only appeals for changes in specific behaviors (Fielding, 1988; Jacobson et al., 1990; Green & Kreuter, 1991).

The occupational health nurse is uniquely positioned to facilitate a worksite health concept and to perform the skills required for the establishment of worksite health promotion programs (Popp, 1989; Spellbring, 1991). The nurse will find it beneficial to be familiar with health promotion definitions and models which propose a conceptual framework for understanding variables related to health behavior, health promotion and health protection. This can provide a foundation for developing programs for health enhancement and disease prevention.

■ DEFINITIONS AND MODELS

Definitions for the concepts of health promotion and disease prevention or health protection have been provided by experts in the field. Several definitions of health promotion are contrasted in Table 12–3. In addition, models to identify conceptual linkages to support measures for health promotion and health protection program planning as well as strategies for risk reduction have also been delineated. Several definitions and models will be briefly presented; however, the reader is referred to the reference source for an in-depth description and discussion.

■ LEVELS OF PREVENTION

More than 25 years ago, Leavell and Clark (1965) first described the concept of levels of prevention within the medical context of preventing or halting disease, previously described in Chapter 3. Shamansky and Clausen (1980) further explicated the concept to provide for a nursing application. While Leavell and Clark (1965) describe health promotion activities within the context of primary prevention, Pender (1987) distinguishes health promotion from prevention and argues that underlying conceptual differences for each exist. Pender notes that health promotion is neither disease nor health-problem specific whereas prevention is, and further that health promotion is "approach" behavior while primary prevention is "avoidance" behavior. Health promotion seeks to expand positive potential for health, while prevention is considered synonymous with health protection behaviors that seek to thwart the occurrence of pathogenic insults to health. Both health promotion and illness prevention/health protection are considered complementary processes aimed at enhancing or altering person-environment interactions.

Pender defines health promotion as "activities directed toward increasing the level of well-being and actualizing the health potential of individuals, families, communities, and society." Health promotion behaviors are described as continuing activities that must be an integral part of one's life-style and include examples, such as engaging in physical exercise or nutrition eating practices directed at maximizing optimal health. For example, some individuals may exercise and/or reduce their cholesterol and fat intake because they are at risk for cardiovascular disease (avoidance behavior), whereas others engage in the same type of activities primarily from a proactive health-promoting motivation.

Prevention is best described as health-protecting behavior because primary

■ **TABLE 12–3** Definitions of Health Promotion

- Pender (1987): Health promotion is neither disease nor health-problem specific. Health promotion is activities directed toward increasing the level of well-being and actualizing the health potential of individuals, families, communities, and society.
- Goodstadt et al. (1986): Health promotion is the maintenance and enhancement of existing levels of health, through the implementation of effective programs, services, and policies.
- Green and Kreuter (1991): Health promotion is the combination of educational and environmental supports for actions and conditions of living conducive to health that influence the determinants of health. The purpose of health promotion is to enable people to gain greater control over the determinants of their own health.
- O'Donnell (1989): Health promotion is the science and art of helping people change their lifestyle to move toward a state of optimal health. Optimal health is defined as a balance of physical, emotional, social, spiritual, and intellectual health. Life-style change can be facilitated through a combination of efforts to enhance awareness, change behavior, and create environments that support good health practices.
- WHO (1988): Health promotion is the process of enabling individuals and communities to increase control over the determinants of health and thereby improve their health. Such a process requires the direct involvement of individuals and communities in the achievement of change, combined with political action directed toward the creation of an environment conducive to health.

emphasis is placed on guarding or defending an individual or group against specific illness or injury (Shamansky & Clausen, 1980; Tripp & Stachowiak, 1992). Primary prevention activities are aimed at eliminating or reducing the risk of disease through specific protective actions. Effective primary prevention measures include providing worksite immunizations to control infectious disease onset, counseling and education directed at weight control and proper nutrition to avoid, for example, cardiovascular or diabetic disease onset, and education and training regarding the appropriate use of personal protective equipment for health hazard reduction.

Secondary prevention is directed at early case-finding and diagnosis of individuals with disease, in order to institute prompt interventions to halt the progression of the disease and limit disability. For employees and employee groups, secondary prevention activities involve screening examinations (e.g., preplacement, periodic) and medical and health surveillance in order to identify illness or injury and institute measures to eliminate the problem. For example, through reviewing Material Safety Data Sheets, the occupational health nurse may become aware of the potential for health effects related to specific chemical exposures. This would support the design and implementation of health surveillance programs/measures for early detection of harmful effects.

Screening for hypertension or cancer (e.g., mammography) represents examples of other types of traditional early detection screening activities that may be performed at the worksite. The provision of health care and prompt treatment to ill and injured employees, whether for occupational or nonoccupational health problems, in order to interrupt the disease process and limit further deterioration, are also considered secondary prevention activities. Screening programs and early referral or treatment provide educational opportunities for employees and a measure of cost containment for the employer through reduction in progressive morbidity and premature mortality.

Tertiary prevention comes into play when a health problem or disability is fixed, stabilized, or irreversible. Tertiary prevention activities are directed at rehabilitating and restoring individuals to an optimal level of health and functioning within the constraints of their health problem or disability (Shamansky & Clausen, 1980; Wachs, 1991). The occupational health nurse can assist the ill or injured worker to return to limited or full-duty work as soon as feasible, so they may continue to function as a productive member of the workforce. The occupational health nurse should be involved in the counseling and rehabilitative processes/programs, such as with an employee following a stroke, in order to help minimize any residual disability and to work with community agencies to optimize resources available to the worker and her or his family. In addition, the occupational health nurse can work with management to develop, where necessary, policy initiatives with respect to job modifications or restructuring in order to accommodate an employee with a residual disability.

Chronic disease monitoring, including education and counseling about and reinforcement of the medical regime, enables workers to exercise more control over their disease and remain on the job (Ray, 1985). The occupational health nurse can work to assure continuity of health care and provide the employee with information regarding signs and symptoms of exacerbation of a health problem. Cardiac rehabilitation programs and employee substance abuse programs that emphasize life-style changes and occupational and environmental modifications are excellent examples of tertiary prevention programs. Several examples of health promoting and protecting/prevention activities are shown in Table 12–4.

O'Donnell (1989) defines health promotion as follows:

> Health promotion is the science and art of helping people change their life-style to move toward a state of optimal health, that is, a balance of physical, emotional, social, spiritual, and intellectual health. Life-style change can be facilitated through a combination of efforts to enhance awareness, change behavior, and create environments that support good health practices.

■ **TABLE 12–4**   Examples of Health Promotion–Health Protection Activities

Primary Prevention		Secondary Prevention	Tertiary Prevention
Health Promotion ↔	**Risk Reduction/Prevention**	**Secondary Prevention**	**Tertiary Prevention**
Nutrition enhance-ment	Immunization	Preplacement, periodic examination	Disability/case management
Exercise/fitness	Stress management	Health surveillance	Early return to work
Reproductive health	Smoking cessation	Screening programs	Chronic illness monitoring
Health motivation enhancement	Risk factor appraisal (e.g., weight, smoking, sun exposure)	Monitoring health/illness trend data	Substance abuse rehabilitation
	Seat belt use	Nutrition education to control illness (e.g., diabetes, hypertension)	
	Worksite walk-throughs		
	Personal protective equipment use		

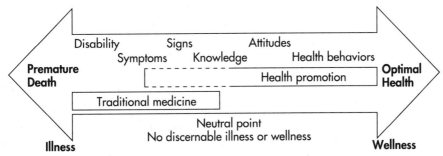

■ **Figure 12–1**   Health continuum model. (From O'Donnell, MP. American Journal of Health Promotion, *1:* 4-5, 1986a.)

O'Donnell (1986a) presents a health continuum model (Fig. 12–1), adapted from the work of John Travis, M.D., which at the extreme left end represents a state of severe illness or premature death; the midpoint represents a neutral point of no discernible illness; and the right end depicts a state of optimal wellness. O'Donnell points out (1) that traditional medicine has focused on the far left side of the continuum, treating patients with chronic disabilities and disease and moving them toward the continuum's midpoint of a healthy state or a state where the disease process can be managed and controlled, and (2) that health promotion has traditionally focused on the right side of the continuum to support strategies/behaviors aimed at optimum health. These strategies are focused on changing, modifying, or enhancing health-related behaviors and lifestyle practices of individuals who are presumed healthy, but may be at risk of health-damaging consequences. He further emphasizes that health promotion activities should also be directed at individuals who may be in a process of rehabilitation in order to promote life-style changes to facilitate recovery and enhance health. In this definition, health promotion and health protection are not explicitly differentiated.

As part of a task force for the Addiction Research Foundation of Ontario, Canada, Goodstadt et al. (1987) propose a conceptualization of health promotion as a planning and operations framework. The conceptual definition was reviewed by 100 individuals in various disciplines who were employees of the Foundation and 40 health promotion experts who were not affiliated with the Foundation. Comments from this group were reviewed and integrated, as appropiate, by the authors.

In defining health promotion, Goodstadt and colleagues acknowledge conceptual problems related to the narrowness of the traditional biomedical model of health and disease prevention. Also, they express concern that health promotion not be viewed so broadly as to encompass anything that might enhance any aspect of health, thereby lacking sufficient definitional specificity. In addition, they point out problems in differentiating terms, whereas health is sometimes used synonymously with wellness and at other times it is defined with respect to absence of disease.

In order to arrive at a definition of health promotion, Goodstadt et al. adopt a holistic perspective of health that involves four domains including:

- *Physical health:* the absence of disease and disability; functioning adequately from the perspective of physical and physiological abilities; the biological integrity of the individual.
- *Psychological health:* sometimes referred to as mental health; may include emotional health; may make explicit reference to intellectual capabilities; the subjective sense of well-being.
- *Social health:* the ability to interact effectively with other people and the social environment; satisfying interpersonal relationships; role fulfillment.
- *Spiritual health:* this dimension engenders the greatest degree of disagreement. In addition to spiritual health, it has been labelled "personal health;" it has been associated with the concept of self-actualization; it sometimes relects a concern for issues related to one's value system; alternatively, it may be concerned with a belief in a transcending unifying force (whether its basis is in nature, in scientific law, or in a godlike source).

Based on an examination of the interrelatedness of these domains and comments received from the interdisciplinary group of reviewers and experts, Goodstadt and colleagues offer the following definition: *health promotion is the maintenance and enhancement of existing levels of health, through the implementation of effective programs, services, and policies.*

Further, they discuss health promotion related to health maintenance and health enhancement within the context of what they describe as a health promotion network and health recovery network (Fig. 12–2). The health promotion network is concerned with programs, policies, and services directed at maintaining or increasing levels of health among those who are not ill, while the health recovery network is primarily concerned with the ill. Thus, the definition of health promotion is extended to span the traditional prevention and treatment networks.

The health promotion network is concerned with strategies aimed at risk avoidance and risk reduction. Risk avoidance strategies such as immunizations are primarily directed at low-risk populations to effect the prevention of disease (primary prevention). Risk reduction strategies such as smoking cessation programs are aimed at persons already at risk, in an effort to reduce or eliminate the risk.

The health recovery network is concerned with strategies directed at the ill,

- **Figure 12–2**   Health promotion–health recovery network. (From Goodstadt MS, Simpson RI, & Loranger, PO. American Journal of Health Promotion, *1:* 58-63, 1987.)

designed to stabilize their condition and to introduce interventions to move individuals toward some level of optimal wellness within the constraints of their disease or disability (secondary and tertiary prevention). For example, increased exercise for individuals with cardiovascular disease may be viewed as part of a restorative health program and as a health enhancement initiative. However, many would argue that integration of health promotion within the context of health restoration serves to further confuse and blur the conceptual differences between health promotion, health protection, and health restoration. This in turn may result in health objectives and strategies that may be ineffective if they are targeted inappropriately. For example, developing objectives and a fitness program for persons returning to work after myocardial infarction or other cardiac problems will be quite different than objectives and program strategies for individuals engaging in fitness activities because they enjoy exercise and simply want to stay fit. Thus, strategies specifically targeted and effective for one group may be minimally effective for another group with different motives.

Goodstadt and colleagues acknowledge and support the need to define the boundaries of health promotion strategies for the ill without jeopardizing the value of the concept for health promotion. This will require much more research in determining both conceptual and practical differences with respect to program planning and health motivation as related to effective interventions.

Green and Kreuter (1991) offer a definition of health promotion as "the combination of educational and environmental supports for actions and conditions of living conducive to health. The actions or behaviors in question may be those of individuals, groups, or communities, policymakers, employers, teachers, or others whose actions control or influence the determinants of health. The purpose of health promotion is to enable people to gain greater control over the determinants of their own health." Further, the authors discuss the life-style construct and place caution on the use of the term. They describe life-style as a complex of related practices and behavioral patterns, in a person or group, that is maintained with some consistency over time and when considered within the context of health-related behaviors and practices, can be viewed as having either health-promoting or health-damaging consequences. In addition to self-responsibility for health, life-style changes require a multifaceted approach including attention to cultural, socio-economic, and environmental influences, and regulatory, policy, and organizational initiatives (Allen & Allen, 1986). While Green and Krueter (1991) point out that changing life-style behaviors requires a long-term commitment involving complex health promotion strategies, they advocate that actions and practices which affect even one determinant of health, such as smoking cessation or getting an immunization, should be emphasized within the context of health promotion program planning.

Green and Krueter offer a comprehensive multi-phase model termed PRECEDE-PROCEED (Fig. 12–3), designed through the use of specific data benchmarks and analyses, to help the health-promotion planner and/or occupational health nurse develop programs with targeted objectives, interventions, and evaluation processes. The PRECEDE framework considers the multiple factors that shape health status (e.g., health, life-style, environment), and focus on those targets for intervention through development of specific objectives and criteria for evaluation. The PROCEED framework continues with the development of additional steps for policy formulation and the initiation of implementation and evaluation

PRECEDE

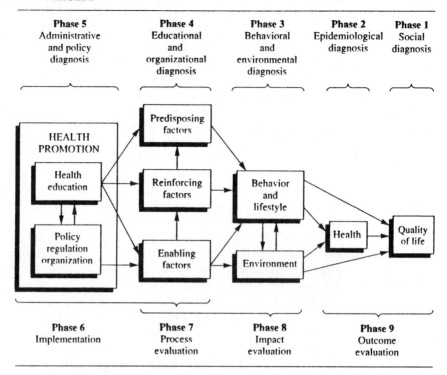

■ **Figure 12–3**   Precede–Proceed: a health promotion planning and evaluation model. (From Green, L & Kreuter, M. Health promotion planning: An educational & environmental approach. Mountain View, CA: Mayfield Publishing Co., 1991.)

processes. The model is briefly described here; however, the reader is referred to the reference for an in-depth discussion of the model and its application.

The model begins with *Phase I,* which is a social diagnosis of the quality of life or health concerns of the target population within the context of the community or organizational environments in which people live and work. The perceptions of health and related problems of the target group are critical to analyze if there is any hope of having a successful program; otherwise, programs developed apart from the group to be involved may not succeed. For example, when Lichter and colleagues (1986) examined consumers' and health professionals' perceptions regarding the importance of health topics needing attention, discrepancies were found, as shown in Table 12–5. Within the context of social diagnosis in the occupational setting, the occupational health nurse should consider an assessment of concerns regarding occupational health problems and related issues of productivity, morale, and safety (i.e., absenteeism, medical claims, injuries, substance abuse) from both the workers' and management's perception.

Phase 2 involves an analysis of epidemiologic data, such as morbidity, mortality, and disability patterns and trends, and other relevant health information, such as population risk factors, in order to target and prioritize specific health

■ **TABLE 12–5** Contrasting Perceptions of Consumers and Health Care Professionals Regarding Health Concerns

Topic	Consumers		Professionals	
	Very Concerned (%)	Rank	Very Concerned (%)	Rank
Health care insurance	49	1	59	7
CPR	46	2	62	6
First aid	46	3	39	15
Use of medication	45	4	73	2
Accident prevention	43	5	52	10
Auto safety	43	6	63	5
Diet and nutrition	41	7	53	9
Immunization	40	8	64	4
Poison control	40	9	56	8
Stress management	37	10	45	11
Physical fitness	37	11	42	13
Weight control	33	12	41	14
Smoking	30	13	83	1
Birth control	29	14	44	12
Prenatal care	25	15	70	3

From Lichter, M. Health Care Management Review, *11:* 75–87, 1986.

problems needing intervention. In addition, an epidemiologic assessment should consider which behavioral and environmental factors might contribute to the health problems. Programmatic goals and objectives in terms of mortality/morbidity reduction can then be developed. At the work setting, a determination of the incidence and prevalence of work-related diseases and health problems, such as high blood pressure, stress, or reproductive disorders, which may be aggravated by working conditions and/or family problems, will be beneficial in helping the occupational health nurse target interventions to reduce risk. Further, morbidity and premature mortality may be ultimately reduced through screening programs for early detection.

Phase 3 involves a systematic analysis of the behavioral and environmental links related to the health problems targeted in *Phase 2*. For example, controllable risk factors such as smoking, elevated cholesterol, obesity, and lack of exercise are related to cardiovascular diseases. An inventory of specific behavioral and environmental risks can be developed, which will then lead to the development of objectives to promote behavioral/environmental changes. In the work setting, behavioral actions might include use of personal protective equipment, compliance with safety programs, and participation in voluntary health programs. Environmental influences relate to industrial monitoring and control of safety and hygiene conditions, and issues related to concern for working conditions such as work schedules and security.

Phase 4 involves the educational and organizational diagnosis. Behavioral and environmental factors that are linked to health concerns become the target of the health promotion program. These include predisposing, reinforcing, and enabling factors. Predisposing factors include one's knowledge, attitudes, beliefs, values, and perceptions that facilitate or hinder motivation to change. Reinforcing factors are rewards and/or positive feedback used to encourage or discourage continuation of the behavior. These include social support, peer influences, or a feeling of well-being (or pain) from exercise. Enabling factors are those skills or resources that facilitate or hinder the performance of the desired behavioral and environmental changes, such as the ability to physically participate in a fitness program.

The occupational health professional will find it helpful to examine factors that influence one's willingness, desire, or ability to participate in an educational intervention. For example, participation in a worksite skin cancer screening program could be influenced by predisposing factors such as knowledge and awareness of the risks associated with sun exposure, personal experience, such as with a relative with skin cancer, and/or the perceived value of early detection. Reinforcing factors that influence motivation to continue to participate in the program might include management's support, attitude and role modeling performance related to program participation, timely feedback about results of screening, and assured maintenance of confidentiality of the findings. Enabling factors include influences such as program accessibility and convenience. For example, offering the screening program on company time at the worksite can greatly influence participation. In addition, the ease or lack of discomfort related to the method of examination, such as skin observation in this example, the company-borne cost of the screening, and perhaps an incentive for participation such as giving sunblock lotion, would be considered enabling factors.

Phase 5 is an analysis of organizational and administrative capabilities and resources needed for the development and implementation of a program. Issues related to personnel, space, equipment, money, and policy initiatives to support worker health and safety, such as release or flex time, are important to determine. In addition, the nurse will want to identify barriers, such as lack of commitment or a negative attitude, in order to develop strategies to deal with these hindrances. For example, if a goal is to establish a smoke-free work environment, a determination needs to be made regarding resources available to conduct or offer smoking cessation programs as well as the viability of establishing policy directives to support the change.

The implementation component, *Phase 6*, will employ a combination of methods and strategies including staffing and marketing techniques appropriate to the intervention. The implementation phase may follow these steps:

1. Introduction of the overall program to management
2. Announcement of the program to the employees
3. Recruitment and organization of a worker-management committee
4. In-house communication planning
5. Employee interest and risk-factor surveys
6. Formation of subcommittees for each risk factor
7. Exploration of community risk-factor reduction programs
8. Committee review and program selection
9. Development of a program proposal
10. Discussion of the proposal with management
11. Promotion of programs and recuitment of employees
12. Scheduling of programs
13. Program implementation, modification, and maintenance.

The final *Phases 7–9* include the evaluation components that will be dependent upon the objectives established during the initial phases of program development. Evaluation should target the effectiveness of educational and organizational resources available, program satisfaction, and behavioral and environmental changes made. For example, in a worksite skin cancer screening program, performance variables to measure knowledge/skill development and utilization might include doing a self-skin assessment, avoiding sun exposure and using sunscreens. In addition, the evaluation of health-related outcomes such as increased productivity, improved performance, enhanced well-being, reduced morbidity and premature mortality, and improved quality of life will be important indicators to measure. The occupational health nurse may find this model helpful in the overall assessment, diagnosis, implementation, and evaluation of health promotion and protection programs. It can provide a comprehensive framework to guide practice options and evaluate findings in order to improve programming efforts.

■ THE HEALTH BELIEF MODEL

The Health Belief Model is one of the most widely used models to explain why people do or do not take preventive health actions (Nemcek, 1990). The model was first developed in the early 1950s by Hochbaum (1958), Kegeles (1965), and Rosenstock (1966) to determine causes for nonparticipation in preventive measures, such as Pap smears and tuberculosis screening. Becker et al. (1974, 1977) later modified the model (Fig. 12–4) to include the influence of health motivation. The model is comprised of three primary components, including individual perceptions, modifying factors, and factors affecting the likelihood of initiating or engaging in an action. These are briefly described. Individual perceptions include:

- Perceived susceptibility: an individual's estimated probability of encountering a specific health problem.
- Perceived seriousness: the degree of concern one experiences created by the thought of disease or problems associated with a given health condition.
- Perceived threat: the combined impact of perceived susceptibility and perceived seriousness.

Modifying factors include a variety of demographic, sociopsychological and structural factors that predispose one to take preventive action, and cues to action are factors that purport to trigger preventive health actions, depending on one's level of readiness to engage in such activities. Examples of modifying factors are included in Figure 12–4.

The likelihood of action component of the model is driven by the positive difference between perceived benefits and perceived barriers (Becker et al., 1977). Perceived benefits are beliefs about the effectiveness of recommended preventive health actions such as the ability of a screening test to detect a health problem and discomfort. Perceived barriers are possible blocks or hindrances to engaging in preventive behaviors and include such factors as cost, inconvenience, and discomfort.

Several studies have been conducted that both support and negate the various constructs of the Health Belief Model. Rundall (1979) surveyed 500 senior citizens regarding taking the swine flu inoculation. While perceived susceptibility, benefits, and barriers were significantly correlated with obtaining the

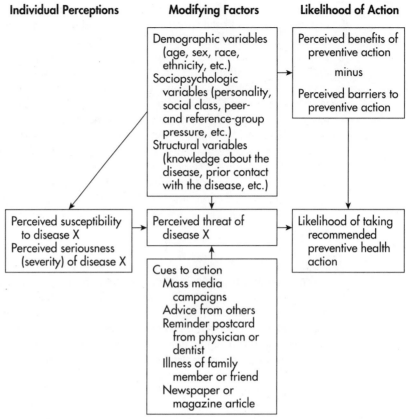

Individual Perceptions	Modifying Factors	Likelihood of Action

Figure 12–4 Health belief model. (From Becker, MH, Drachman, RH, & Kirscht, JP. American Journal of Public Health, *14*(3):205-216, 1974.

vaccination, perceived seriousness was not. However, vaccination studies conducted by Cummings et al. (1979) and Larson et al. (1979) found all four constructs to be significantly correlated.

Weinberger et al. (1981) examined smoking behaviors of 120 adult outpatients and found that ex-smokers, as compared to two groups of smokers, were significantly more likely to perceive themselves susceptible to health problems and viewed smoking as a serious health problem. Becker et al. (1974) examined compliance with recommended medical regime and appointment-keeping practices of mothers with respect to child health practices, and found positive significant relationships with perceived susceptibility, seriousness, benefits, barriers, and health motivation constructs.

Several investigators have examined breast self-examination practices (BSE) using the Health Belief Model. The model proposes that women who practice BSE regularly will exhibit positive beliefs with respect to perceived susceptibility, seriousness, benefits and health motivation. Perceived barriers are predicted to be minimal or absent. Champion (1985) studied 301 women regarding BSE practices and found that perceived barriers to preventive actions were the most important variable in explaining BSE behavior followed by health motivation. The variables of perceived susceptibility, seriousness, and benefits were not significant. Massey (1986) found that perceived susceptibility and demographic variables of younger age and higher education correlated positively with the frequency of BSE practice in a sample of 225 women.

Studies such as these suggest that certain demographic characteristics and beliefs regarding health and illness influence one's use of preventive health measures (O'Dell et al., 1991). The occupational health nurse can use this model to identify factors in the worker population that can facilitate or hinder compliance with health and safety programs. Programs and strategies can then be developed to meet specific workforce needs in order to increase participation in health promotion/protection activities.

The Health Belief Model offers some insight into utilization of preventive health; however, concern has been expressed that the model lacks specificity in defining relationships between variables and lacks consistency in operationalizing and measuring variables across studies (Wallston & Wallston, 1984). Thus, further research is needed to test and refine the constructs to increase the validity of the model, in order to fully operationalize health promotion programming efforts at the worksite. The occupational health nurse can help in this process through collecting and analyzing data when using the model for preventive health programming.

Pender (1987) states that the Health Belief Model is a model for health protecting (preventive) behaviors and is directed at decreasing the probability of experiencing illness by active protection of the body against pathological stressors or detection of illness in the asymptomatic stage. Pender suggests the Health Promotion Model as a complementary counterpart that is directed at increasing the level of well-being and self-actualization of an individual or group. Health promoting behaviors are viewed as proactive rather than reactive.

The Health Promotion Model (Fig. 12–5) is structurally similar to the Health Belief Model and is composed of three major components: cognitive-perceptual factors, modifying factors, and likelihood of action factors. Cognitive-perceptual factors include seven constructs that exert a direct influence on engaging in health promoting actions. These factors are:

- Importance of health: the impact of valuing health as related to the performance of health-promoting behaviors.
- Perceived control: the degree to which an individual believes she or he has personal/internal control over self-health behavior.
- Perceived self-efficacy: the ability of the individual to implement behavioral skills to enhance health.
- Definition of health: the achievement of optimal or higher levels of health.
- Perceived health status: the extent to which individuals consider themselves in good (or poor) health.
- Perceived benefits of health promoting behaviors: the frequency of or continued participation in health promoting behaviors.
- Perceived barriers to health promoting behaviors: the influence of barriers (i.e., inconvenience, discomfort) in reducing engagement in health promoting behaviors.

Modifying factors include several constructs that influence health promoting behaviors indirectly through their impact on cognitive-perceptual mechanisms. These include:

Cognitive-Perceptual
Factors

Modifying Factors

Participation in
Health-Promoting Behavior

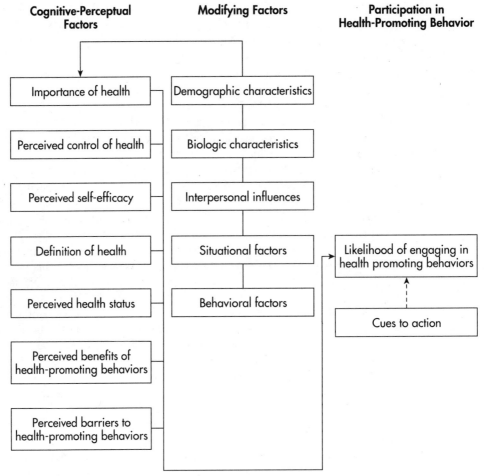

■ **Figure 12–5**   Pender's health promotion model. (From Pender, N. Health promotion in nursing practice [2nd ed]. Norwalk, CN: Appleton & Lange, 1987.)

- Demographic factors: characteristics such as age, sex, race, ethnicity, and education.
- Biological characteristics: physiological factors related to engaging in health promoting activities (e.g., weight, blood pressure).
- Interpersonal influences: expectations and/or supports of significant others and health care professionals, and family patterns of health care.
- Situational factors: environmental or situational conditions or options that enhance or hinder health promoting alternatives (e.g., availability of vending machines with low or non-nutrient foods).
- Behavioral factors: previous experience with or knowledge and skills about health promotion activities.

According to the model, participation in health promoting behavior is concerned with the likelihood of implementing health promoting actions. This may involve internal cues, such as personal growth from repeatedly utilizing health promoting behaviors, and external cues, including interaction with family or

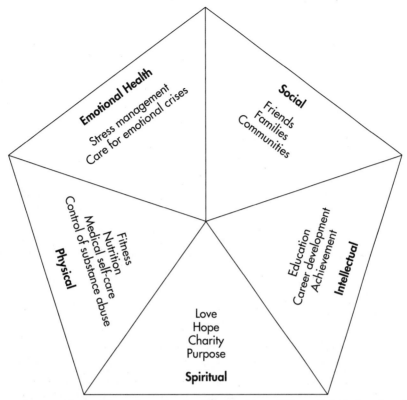

Emotional Health
Stress management
Care for emotional crises

Social
Friends
Families
Communities

Fitness
Nutrition
Medical self-care
Control of substance abuse
Physical

Education
Career development
Achievement
Intellectual

Love
Hope
Charity
Purpose
Spiritual

■ **Figure 12–6**   Dimensions of optimal health. (From O'Donnell, MP. American Journal of Health Promotion, *1:* 6-9, 1986b.)

others regarding health promotion activities or the effects of mass media on behavioral actions (e.g., advertisements).

The occupational health nurse can use this model to evaluate facilitators and barriers that either enhance or negate preventive health activities. Programs can then be designed to effectively reduce the barriers to participation (e.g., cost, time) and increase strategies that support health improvement.

While this model serves as an explanation to determine factors that influence one's engagement in health promoting activities, empirical testing of the model is needed and is in progress. The extent to which the Health Promotion Model can explain or predict specific health promoting behaviors remains to be determined (Pender, 1987).

■ HEALTH PROMOTION PROGRAM PLANNING

Worksite health promotion programs are designed to enhance employee well-being and movement toward a state of optimal health as well as to reduce health risks. As demonstrated in Figure 12–6, optimal health represents a balance between physical, emotional, social, spiritual, and intellectual health (O'Donnell, 1986b). Pruitt (1987) and Scofield (1990) also points out that health promotion encompasses various activities such as physical fitness, weight and stress management, and smoking cessation in order to improve the quality of life.

O'Donnell (1986b) indicates that health promotion (and protection) programs

■ **TABLE 12–6** Examples of Activities by Health Promotion Program Levels

Level I Awareness	Level II Behavioral Change	Level III Environmental Support
Posters	Health building programs	Physical environment
Pamphlets/brochures	Smoking cessation	Healthy food offerings
Fact sheets	Stress management	No cigarette vending
Newsletters	Nutrition/exercise fitness	Safety hazard control
Health screening	Support groups	Organizational culture
		Role models
		Health/wellness commitment
		Employee partnership in decision-making
		Policies that support health
		Flex-time
		Employee assistance
		Employee health leadership
		Program planning
		Program sponsorship
		Program teaching

should be targeted at three levels, including awareness, life-style behavioral change, and supportive environments. Awareness programs are targeted at individuals and groups to increase their understanding of health and related risk factors. Awareness programs are most appropriate for those who need to increase their knowledge and reflect on attitudes and/or beliefs in order to effect a behavior change.

Life-style change programs are directed at assisting individuals in making behavioral changes such as starting and sustaining exercise, eating nutritious foods, and enhancing communication and coping skills. Life-style change programs are most successful if they engage a multi-step process (i.e., introducing one or two programs/activities at a time), include a combination of educational and behavioral modification experiences, and take place over time.

Supportive environments include families, friends, organizational/work cultures, coworkers, communities, and regulations that help to shape these environments (e.g., availability of jogging trails or on-site exercise classes). Fostering a supportive environment or changing an environment to encourage a concept of health will go a long way in improving ultimate health behavior and outcomes. Table 12–6 presents examples of awareness, life-style, and environmental approaches that can be used at the worksite. Occupational health nurses are well-positioned to design programs that will help meet these aims and promote healthy behaviors and wellness (Selleck et al., 1989).

To assist the occupational health nurse to develop a comprehensive approach to health promotion programming efforts, Figure 12–7 presents a health promotion program model that can be used as a guide or framework for health promotion program development. The framework comprises four phases: assessment, planning, implementation, and evaluation.

The health promotion program *assessment* phase includes a determination of the following components: corporate commitment and support, needs assessment,

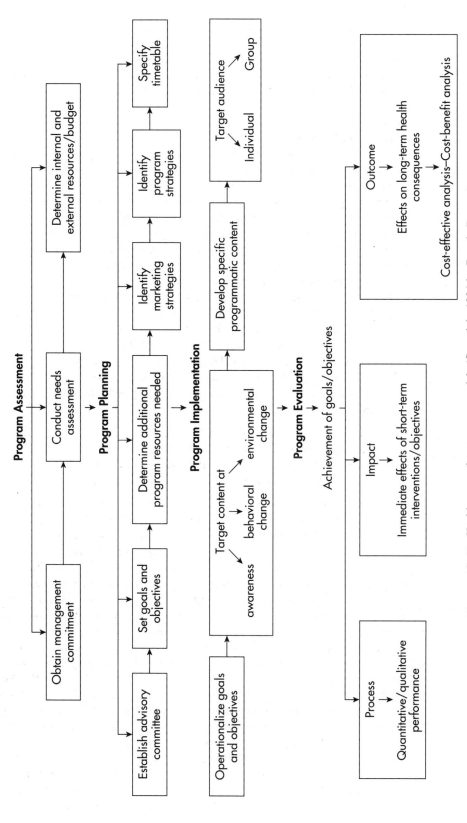

■ **Figure 12–7** Health promotion program model. (Copyright 1994 by Bonnie Rogers.)

299

and internal and external programs/services availability. Determining and obtaining commitment and support from top and middle management is essential to the success of any health promotion program. It is important for the occupational health nurse to assess management's attitude regarding concern for employee health and safety, the company's corporate image, the cost-effectiveness of health programming, and personal attitudes about health promotion and protection activities. In addition, the nurses will want to determine what the organization is willing to contribute in terms of financial and physical support (space, equipment), personnel support, and employee off-duty time. A management survey such as shown in Appendix 12–1 can be useful in making this determination.

The occupational health nurse may find it necessary to persuade management about the benefits of health promotion and wellness programs. This will often entail providing a review of the health indices of the employee population and related health care costs for specific employee illnesses and injuries that may be obtained from the insurance carrier. For example, comparing health care costs of smokers and nonsmokers and related productivity and absenteeism, giving examples of successful programs from other companies, and being prepared to discuss different types of programs (educational, screening, behavior change) and cost options will lend support to the health promotion initiative.

The second component of the assessment phase involves performing an employee needs assessment, which will help to identify employee goals and interests and plan a more effective health promotion program. A health interest survey that can be distributed to all employees or to a targeted group has several advantages, including:

- fostering employee ownership of the program;
- providing some health education awareness;
- reducing resistance to future program participation; and
- evaluating program impact.

Numerous health interest surveys are available from various resources, and several examples from the Wellness Councils of America (1990) are included in Appendix 12–2. The occupational health nurse can also design a simple health interest survey specific to the company style and employee profile. Whatever format is used, the survey form should be limited in length, be graphically attractive, ask relevant questions that are sensitive in tone and give useful information regarding health risks and needs, include a variety of topics from which the employee can choose, allow space for employees to write comments, and indicate a date and to whom the survey form should be returned.

A cover letter should accompany the survey, explaining the concept of health promotion and wellness and pointing out potential benefits. Emphasis should be placed on anonymity to ensure employee confidentiality of responses (McNeil, 1988). A letter of support from the company manager or CEO that accompanies the survey may also help to increase survey participation. After completing the needs assessment, employees should be provided with feedback about the survey results, which will be linked to program implementation.

Another tool to consider using when conducting the needs assessment is a health risk appraisal (HRA) (Terry, 1987). General HRA forms cover many topics such as smoking, substance abuse, eating/nutrition habits, exercise and fitness, stress, safety, and other preventive health activities (e.g., mammography, BSE). HRAs may also be more specific and address each of these areas as singular topics or may be population-focused such as with women's health. By focusing on health behaviors, HRAs can enhance employee's awareness of health risks and thus encourage thinking directed at making life-style changes. For employers, if HRAs disclose major health risks in the employee aggregate, the information can be very useful in program planning.

HRAs are usually self-administered either in paper and pencil format or via computer software packages. Scoring can be done on-site by the occupational health nurse or the completed questionnaires (or computer discs) can be returned to the vendor or HRA source, who in turn completes the scoring and returns both individual and group results. Consideration of the best time for administering the HRA and informing employees about the process for education about the appraisal will help to enhance participation. Many HRA forms come with an instruction manual that serves as a guide in presenting the questionnaire to participants and interpreting the responses. Individual counseling regarding risk factors should be provided as appropriate.

While aggregate data can be shared with management for program planning purposes, strict confidentiality of individual employee responses should be maintained so that only the employee and health professional have data access. Demographic information about employees (age, sex, race, type of job, etc.), past history of claims and payments for health insurance, workers' compensation, and disability, if accessible, can provide additional data about actual and potential health problems within the workplace (Selleck et al., 1989).

The Centers for Disease Control and Prevention, in conjunction with the Carter Center at Emory University, developed an HRA form (Appendix 12–3) that is now available through Computer Outfitters, Tuscon Arizona. In addition, "Healthfinder," published by the Office of Disease Prevention and Health Prevention, Public Health Service, of the U.S. Department of Health and Human Services, presents a review of current information and sources related to HRAs (Appendix 12–4).

Determining availability and capabilities of existing internal and external programs and services is the third component of the assessment phase. The occupational health nurse will want to meet with other department managers such as food service and environment and safety in order to complete an inventory of programs and services currently offered to employees. This will also help make determinations about the need for new programs or modification or expansion of existing programs, and may enhance opportunities for health promotion program support and collaboration.

Making a determination about a supportive environment is part of the internal assessment. For example, is lighting adequate in work areas? Are ergonomics addressed? Do desk chairs cause back problems? Other examples of signs of support for a healthy environment include nonsmoking areas; vending machines stocked with healthful foods; nonalcoholic alternatives at company functions; rooms set aside for exercise classes; availability of shower facilities or bicycle racks; and appropriate security. It is also important to assess the types of space available for holding seminars, conferences, and/or exercise classes, the types of equipment available for specific program implementation (e.g., fitness equipment, scales, hematological instruments), and methods for communication of information (e.g., audiovisual, bulletin boards). Other areas such as a seat belt policy for company vehicles, an absenteeism policy that offers incentives for job attendance (as well as days off for illness), and flexible hours to attend to health and wellness needs can all add up to an environment that shows the company's commitment to good health.

Community resources can provide an enormous array of programs for employees, thus providing a more cost effective and efficient approach to health promotion programming. The occupational health nurse can conduct an assessment of external nonprofit organizations such as the American Heart Association, American Lung Association, American Cancer Society and American Red Cross, to determine the types of educational materials or packaged programs available for cosponsoring with the company. Churches, temples, and community centers often have low-cost recreational facilities available free or for rent. Universities may have students in academic training programs such as nursing, nutrition, or exercise physiology who may be interested in participating in a health promotion program/service as part of a curricular learning requirement. In addition, communication and collaboration with other occupational health nurses and local nursing societies, and exploration of other available resources such as professional journals, newsletters, library references, and the telephone directory may provide valuable information. Thousands of resources are available to the occupational health nurse to assist in the planning and implementation of health promotion and protection programs (Soha & Vickery, 1988), several of which are identified by Chen and Cabot (1988). In addition, a listing of selected resources can be found in Appendix 12–5.

The health promotion *planning* phase includes forming an advisory committee, setting goals and measurable objectives, determining additional program implementation resources, identifying marketing strategies and programmatic strategies/activities, and setting a timeline for completion of activities. Each of these areas will be discussed.

A successful health promotion program requires a high level of employee and employer participation. Thus, forming a health promotion planning and advisory committee can help foster employee rather than management ownership of the program and encourage an environment supportive of health behavior change (Selleck et al., 1989). Committee members should include the occupational health nurse and other appropriate health care professionals (i.e., the physician or industrial hygienist), respected employee leaders, representatives from management who can provide company support, line superivsors, individuals responsible for other program areas (i.e., compensation/benefits, employee assistance, dietary), and union representatives if appropriate. The worksite health promotion manager, who often is an occupational health nurse, should be responsible for coordinating and providing leadership and direction for programmatic activities.

The advisory committee is usually involved with reviewing all pertinent aggregate data relative to health promotion activities, obtaining information about successful health promotion programs in other companies, and reviewing historical information about the successes and failures of previously tried program activities. Specific determinations can then be made about the types and extent of program activities to be developed. In addition, committee members can serve as a sounding board for ideas prior to their implementation, help to market the program to employees, and provide feedback on program operation (Pfeiffer, 1986).

Goals and objectives set the framework for measuring program successes. Setting program goals and objectives are based on priorities identified through employee needs assessment and other available data; however, the prudent planner will pay particular attention to employee interests that scored high on the surveys and supplement it with information from HRAs and other data sources. Goals are broad statements that provide the overall direction for the intended activity while objectives are measurable statements of the intended outcome derived from the goals. For example, the goal might be to increase employees' understanding of HIV/AIDS. Objectives might be stated as programmatic (a statement of activity to be carried out by the program) and/or behavioral (a statement of desired change; e.g., knowledge, behavior, biomedical parameter of the learner) such as:

1. Provide information on HIV transmission and prevention (programmatic).
2. By the end of the teaching session, the employee will be able to state the routes of transmission of HIV (behavioral).

When setting goals and objectives it is important to consider expected outcomes, as one approach will promote health awareness while another will be more conducive to supporting behavior change as previously described.

Determining resources and developing the budget entails reviewing, from the assessment phase, what currently exists within the company in terms of human resources, space, equipment, supplies, etc., and what is available from external community resources. Based on this review, determinations about additional resources needed for new or expanded programs within the context of the goals, objectives, and feasible budget allocations can be made.

When developing the budget, several points should be considered, such as whether a singular or more comprehensive program will be offered; what external resources will be utilized with associated costs anticipated (e.g., consultants, HRAs, educational materials, instructors); the number of employees expected to participate in the program(s); and how costs will be paid, that is, will the company pay all costs (e.g., screening programs) or will cost for some programs be shared (e.g., smoking cessation). When planning for health promotion programs the following costs should be considered: utilization of company personnel such as graphic artists from other departments; additional professional staff such as consultants, instructors, technicians, and support staff; equipment and supplies; audiovisual aides and educational materials such as pamphlets, slides, and video-tapes; refreshments; incentives, marketing materials, and printing; off-site space and travel; and program evaluation. Indirect costs related to employee off-duty time may also need to be factored particularly when determining program cost-effectiveness. Every effort should be made to develop a realistic budget that allows for implementation of the programmatic objectives.

Marketing the health promotion program is critical to program success. Marketing strategies are designed to attract individuals into the program and provide sufficient benefits, incentives, or challenges to maintain commitment to participation. Some strategies for in-house marketing might include the following:

- inviting employees to a healthy breakfast to introduce the program;
- distributing a letter from the CEO promoting the wellness concept and related programs to employees;
- using posters and fliers to advertise the programs;
- publishing a calendar of events to give employees an advance preview;
- capturing photos of the programs and displaying them on a poster in the lunchroom, break room, or employee entrance for viewing; and
- disseminating information about the program and any results in the company newsletter.

In addition, promoting a positive company image is also important to the health promotion effort and this can be done through use of media public service announcements. Marketing activities should be scheduled several weeks in advance of the health promotion program, building from week to week, thus providing a continued stimulus for sustained interest in the program (Kizer, 1987; O'Donnell & Ainsworth, 1984).

Incentives, which are offered to stimulate employee motivation for program participation, may be considered as part of the overall marketing design. Incentives are viewed as something the employee values in exchange for a prescribed action or behavior, which may range from program attendance to a sustained life-style change, such as quitting smoking (Wellness Councils of America, 1990). Incentives may be offered for program participation, program completion, and behavioral change. Examples of such include:

For program participation:

- door prizes for those attending wellness events
- discount fees for early registration
- "bring a buddy" bonus
- free or subsidized lunches
- health snacks
- beverages for brown baggers

For program completion:

- bonuses for perfect attendance
- prize drawings for near perfect attendance
- formal certificates for attendance
- T-shirts, sportswear, other material goods for high attenders

For behavioral changes:

- write-up in newsletter of employee who makes a major health habit change
- fee rebate for sustained weight loss or completing a course
- day off after one year of successful, sustained, behavior change

The advisory committee should make a determination about what incentives will work best for the employee population.

Setting a timetable for health promotion program development will help to foster a logical flow of activities. For most organizations, the best strategy for program implementation is timely or organized planning through which programs can be gradually phased in. This often begins with one or two programs and later develops into a more comprehensive approach to health and wellness. In

■ **TABLE 12–7**   Timeline for Organizing Health and Wellness Programs / Activities

FOLLOWING ARE SOME GENERAL RULES OF THUMB CONCERNING WHEN TO SCHEDULE WELLNESS PROGRAMS:

- Good times to launch wellness programs are in the fall (September), at the new year (January), and any time in the spring (March, April, and May).
- Workshop series should be planned for the same day and time each month.
- Aerobics should be planned for lunch time if showers are available, and at the end of the workday if showers are not available. Eliminate summer scheduling of indoor aerobics because people usually like to be outside in the summer.
- Schedule multiple offerings of the same type of activity. For example, schedule several sessions of a stress management workshop with an evening session offered for spouses and second-shift workers.
- Plan a health and fitness testing activity to take place right before you offer programs such as smoking cessation and weight management so that people have a logical follow-up to the testing process.
- Start out with "lunch and learn" sessions on employees' time. Then later offer activities that are scheduled on work time.
- Publish an article in the employee newsletter on the personal side of a wellness topic and then follow up with a workshop or program.
- Don't plan too much at one time. Spread the program offerings out over the year so that every couple of weeks some event or wellness issue comes to the attention of employees.
- Tag along with national campaigns such as the Great American Smokeout in November of each year or National Employee Health and Fitness Day (held annually in May). Brochures, posters, table tents, fact sheets, and press releases are usually free for the asking. Your Wellness Council can keep you supplied with materials and ideas.
- Start your program and build it slowly. That way you can assure that the quality will be good. Employees will recognize that the wellness program will be around for the long haul.

From Wellness Councils of America. Healthy, Wealthy, Well and Wise. Omaha, Neb: Author, 1990.

addition, organizing programs or activities around national campaigns such as the Great American Smokeout or National Safety Week may add impetus to employee participation. An example of a timeline for program planning development is shown in Table 12–7.

The *implementation* phase of the health promotion program is the actual action phase of the overall program. The implementation phase flows from the planning phase and should run smoothly, assuming planning has been adequate and realistic. Program implementation will be based on the goals and objectives set forth in the plan and will be targeted at awareness and education, behavioral change, and developing supportive environments. A comprehensive approach to worksite health promotion and health protection should fit with the company's commitment and philosophy toward health and wellness and may include a variety of programs focusing on such areas as exercise, nutrition, weight loss, smoking cessation, stress management, coping enhancement, and risk factor screening (Campbell, 1991; Wachs & Parker-Conrad, 1990). Numerous and specific types of programs, such as back care or prenatal education, can be offered that will be dependent upon an analysis of workforce needs (Bigbee & Jonsa, 1991). The occupational health nurse may develop health promotion / protection programs for groups of employees based on aggregate interests or identified needs, as well as provide individual counseling about selected risk factors or health problems. The nurse will want to assess awareness, knowledge, and behavior of the employee(s) so that appropriate counseling and education interventions can be implemented. In addition, the program content and delivery will also vary dependent on the objectives, budget, and whether the program is developed in-house or provided by an external contractor.

Several factors will influence participation in health promotion programs, including age, gender, ethnicity, perception, and social and family support. For example, studies show that women are more likely to engage in preventive health programs, and that family and other forms of social support help to strengthen efforts in the modification of life-style health habits (Rose, 1989; Sandroff et al., 1990). In addition, health promotion activities at the worksite help to create an atmosphere that supports and rewards health-promoting behaviors. The occupational health nurse will want to consider these factors when planning programs.

After reviewing available resources, the occupational health nurse can then decide to offer an in-house or external source program. The latter is often a packaged program, of which there are several to choose. If the nurse decides to develop an in-house program, several considerations need to be explored. As an example, one option for a nutrition program will be discussed.

The decision to implement a nutrition program should take into account previous factors discussed, such as employee interests and needs, available resources, and management's commitment to the program. Adequate nutrition is essential to healthy living and also is implicated in the prevention and control of many types of diseases such as cardiovascular disorders, cancer, diabetes, obesity, and hypercholesterolemia. Convenience type foods constitute a significant portion of the American diet and many of these types of food are high in fat, salt, and refined carbohydrates, and low in fiber. It is important to establish baseline information about what employee's concerns and knowledge are about nutrition and eating practices.

Hunt and Murphy (1986) outline one example of a worksite nutrition program that consists of three levels: employee awareness, employee knowledge, and behavior change. In addition, the need for environmental changes should be emphasized. Nutrition awareness is the first step in working with employees to further their understanding about the nature of different food groups and their relationship to healthy and unhealthy states, and promoting healthy food choices. What is taught or discussed will be dependent on the employee's needs. However, general topics for discussion might include the basics of good nutrition, the consequences of poor nutrition, and the role of exercise as a contributing practice. Other awareness activities might include distributing literature or pamphlets on a certain topic such as cholesterol; posting information on bulletin boards; or publishing information in the company newsletter.

Increasing employee knowledge, which is a higher level activity, is the next step designed to help employees begin to make behavioral change, and expands on information generated through awareness activities. The occupational health nurse may consider asking a registered dietician to help plan and/or participate in the program activities or teaching. This level of program implementation might include:

1. planning and implementing a Nutrition Awareness Month;
2. developing an extended nutrition educational/seminar series over a period of six to ten weeks (Table 12–8), which would involve increased employee participation such as sharing of experiences;

■ TABLE 12–8 Suggested Topics for a Ten-Week
Nutrition-Management Program

Week 1:   Orientation and assessment
- Program goals, methods, and content
- Individual assessment and goal setting
- Nutrition and exercise—weekly participation

Week 2:   Basics of good nutrition
- The role of nutrition in prevention
- Nutrient and caloric density
- Important nutrients
- Food-drug interactions
- Establishing a healthy eating pattern–nutrient balance
- Review food diary–calorie regulation

Week 3:   Factors influencing eating behavior
- Biological factors
- Psychological factors
- Sociocultural factors
- Environmental factors
- Sharing experiences

Week 4:   Review of exercise and nutrition and self-monitoring techniques
- Exercise theory and recommendations
- Exploring variety in exercise
- Exercise activity record
- Food diary relationship

Week 5:   Meal planning
- Shopping strategies
- Menu planning
- Low-fat cooking techniques (microwave, stir-fry)

Week 6:   Behaviors and attitudes about nutrition management
- Behavior-modification and stress-management techniques
- Review of nutrition weight-management myths
- Effects of personal relationships

Week 7:   Body image
- Effect of genetics on body size and shape
- Making peace with your body

Week 8:   Special eating situations
- Eating in restaurants
- Holiday (party/celebration) situations
- Traveling

Week 9:   Relapse prevention
- Coping with problem times
- Support systems

Week 10: Maintaining motivation
- Motivational techniques—highlights of nutrition/exercise
- Review of personal goals
- Overview of weight-maintenance theory

3. inviting family members to participate in nutrition activities;
4. involving employees in newsletter publications such as contributing healthy recipes or providing healthy cooking tips; and
5. obtaining physiological measurements of height/weight for comparative purposes.

Behavioral changes require more intense participation by employees, the occupational health nurse, and others responsible for the program (Best & Cameron, 1986). Nutrition education must remain an integral part of the program, and employees must develop an understanding of the adverse physical and psychological effects of fad and quick weight loss diets. Families should be included in any nutritional education/behavior modification efforts as they significantly influence dietary practices. Examples of activities designed to promote behavioral changes include:

1. self-monitoring of eating practices and habits (e.g., food/behavior diaries);
2. using self, family, or significant other reward reinforcement strategies;
3. contracting for nutrition/eating practice changes;
4. participating in group sessions; and
5. engaging in regular physical activity.

Having a supportive environment is of paramount importance in the program's success. This will usually require enhanced commitment on the part of management in further resource allocation and supporting environmental changes. Examples of environmental strategies include:

1. providing company-sponsored cooking classes for employees and family members;
2. providing nutritious foods in the cafeteria with caloric, sodium, and cholesterol content displayed;
3. providing nutritious foods in vending machines; and
4. providing space/equipment for exercise or developing a walking/jogging trail.

Potential obstacles may interfere with changing eating behaviors, including reaching a plateau, premature cessation of new behaviors, temptation to reward weight loss with food treats, or interpersonal difficulties with significant others because of physical changes (Pender, 1987). The employee should be counseled regarding these potential pitfalls in order to identify and institute preventive strategies to maintain and facilitate goal achievement.

As with any program, evaluation is an important component in order to provide feedback to management and the workers (Lukes, 1992). Examples of evaluation components include participation rates, program satisfaction data, behavioral changes made (e.g., dietary, weight loss), and results of any knowledge testing. Once program data are reviewed, changes for improvement can be instituted.

The final phase of the health promotion program is program evaluation. Evaluation, which actually begins in the planning phase, denotes the extent to which the program has met preestablished goals and objectives and desired program outcomes. O'Donnell and Ainsworth (1984) identify major benefits of worksite health promotion programs to both employees and employers (Table 12–9), which should be considered when developing an evaluation plan. Worksite health promotion programs have been criticized for focusing efforts almost entirely on

■ **TABLE 12–9** Major Benefits to Employers from Health
Promotion Programs

Improved productivity
Reduced absenteeism
Improved morale
Conserved operating costs
Improved ability to perform
Development of higher quality staff

Reduced benefit costs
Reduced health insurance costs
Lowered life insurance costs
Reduced workers' compensation claims
Provision of welfare benefits

Reduced human resources and development costs
Decreased recruiting costs
Decreased costs for educating and training new employees

Improved image of the organization
General visibility
Concerned and responsible employers

Data from O'Donnell, MP & Ainsworth, T. Health promotion in the workplace. New York: John Wiley & Sons, 1984.

changing individual behavior and risk factors (Conrad, 1987). While individuals have responsibility for certain health-related behaviors such as smoking and diet, there are strong social pressures, particularly in some work groups, that condone or encourage smoking, or the cafeteria or vending machines may not offer sufficient healthful food choices (Katz & Showstack, 1990). In addition, social networks, family, community, and institutional policies often influence individual behavior, yet these factors are often neglected both in developing objectives and in the evaluation component.

Green and Kreuter (1991) define three levels of evaluation: process, impact, and outcome. Process evaluation focuses on materials, quantitative adequacy and qualitative performance of staff, and programmatic activities including quantity and quality of programs or services. Evaluative evidence might include the completion of evaluation forms by employees to determine satisfaction with the degree and quality of programs and instructors, and the quality of teaching materials, facilities or any other program components. Other measures frequently examined are the number of program attendees, the number of brochures distributed, and the number of referrals made for further monitoring as a result of the program.

Impact evaluation is concerned with the immediate effects of the program intervention on meeting short-term or intermediate objectives, such as an increase in employee awareness or knowledge, attitudinal changes about health or related risk factors such as smoking, or a behavioral change such as seat belt useage or smoking reduction. This might be measured through a comparison of pre- and post-test measures of knowledge or attitudes, indications of change in the targeted behavior such as self-report of smoking reduction (number of cigarettes smoked) or smoking cessation, or physiological or biochemical changes such as reduction in blood pressure, weight, or cholesterol levels. In addition, the impact of family or social support systems as related to attitudinal or behavioral change could be examined.

Outcome evaluation determines the effects of the program on long-term health consequences including sustained behavioral or life-style changes, and improvements in quality of health, life, and supportive environments. These typically include measures of absenteeism, productivity, morbidity, sustained risk factor reduction for disease prevention, and mortality. Some of these indicators might be measured in a one to three year span; however, long-term outcome measures are more difficult to determine as the time-lag for health effects may be too long when considering employee attrition.

In addition to program evaluation strategies, determinations about cost-analyses may be required. The primary reason for performing evaluations of health promotion programs is to be able to draw inferences about the effectiveness of the program, generally measured by the degree to which specific program activities are associated with desired outcomes. Health promotion programs in a business setting must also be evaluated as to whether the outcomes produced are worth the cost of implementation. For example, do enough employees quit smoking to justify the cost of the intervention (Katz & Showstack, 1990)?

Walsh & Egdahl (1989) reported that the top reasons cited by executive level corporate managers for the establishment of health promotion programs included cost containment (the primary reason cited), increased productivity and morale, promotion of employee health, and enhancement of the corporate image. However, little empirical evidence exists regarding the cost-effectiveness of health promotion programs largely because most companies fail to conduct economic evaluations (Katzman & Smith, 1989), or because valid evaluation methods are not used. Several reasons have been cited with respect to the difficulty in determining the true cost analyses of health promotion programs, including lack of a consistent definition of worksite health promotion; varying degrees of employee participation in both in-house and off-site programs; wide differences in corporate resources and goals; poor definition of outcome measures; significant variation in target populations, program activities, and program continuation follow-up; absence of comparative baseline measures; and failure to deal with self-selection of program participants (Katz & Showstack, 1990; Warner et al., 1988). While these problems need addressing, several programs have demonstrated cost-effective results, such as an evaluation of the Johnson and Johnson Live for Life Program, which showed a decrease in the annual outpatient costs, hospital days, and admission rates for employees who participated in the healthy lifestyles program over a five-year period (Bly et al., 1986). The program's objectives are to "help contain illness costs attributable to unhealthy behavior and life-styles that are amenable to modifications in the work setting, while at the same time promoting improvements in quality of life, work performance, and attitudes of employees" (Holzbach et al., 1990).

Two types of costs analyses used today include cost-effectiveness and cost-benefit analyses (Barry & DeFriese, 1990). The purpose of cost-effective analysis is to determine which activities or interventions, given alternative approaches, will achieve the program objective and yield the most value or greatest impact for the least cost (Eddy et al., 1989). Cost-effectiveness measures the resources consumed in monetary terms as related to planned outcomes, usually in terms of participant successes (Girdano, 1986). For example, Erfurt et al. (1990, 1991) examined the cost-effectiveness of a work-site wellness program for reducing cardiovascular disease risks of employees at four manufacturing sites. Worksites were randomly assigned by intervention strategy. Site 1, the control site, included advice only, where blood pressure screening was done followed by only one health education class post-screening, to provide advice and information; Site 2 offered media-focused health education, which included the use of promotional materials, at least two health education classes, and health foci. Site 3 included individualized support, encouragement, and assistance with problem solving with emphasis on one-on-one and follow-up counseling, in addition to activities offered at Site 2; and Site 4 involved organizational strategies including peer support groups, organized competition, and buddy systems, in addition to activities offered at Sites 2 and 3. For engaging employees into treatment/program participation, Sites 3 and 4 were nine to 10 times more cost-effective than Site 2; for reducing risks/preventing relapse, Sites 3 and 4 were five to six times more cost-effective than Site 2. At Sites 3 and 4, the total direct cost per percent of risks reduced/relapse prevented was less than $1 (67¢ and 74¢, respectively) per employee per year.

Cost-benefit analysis is a technique whereby both costs and benefits or outcomes of a program are represented in monetary terms, thus permitting a comparison between unlike elements and yielding a benefit-to-cost ratio (Eley, 1989). For example, one can determine the benefit of a smoking cessation program in terms of reduction in per capita and aggregate health care costs. The cost of implementing a smoking cessation program for X number of employees can be compared to costs assigned to insurance, absenteeism, and productivity of smoking employees. For example, Kristein (1982) reported a potential company savings of $349 per year per smoker in health care costs when a smoking cessation program intervention was provided.

■ ADULT LEARNING

In preparing to offer a health promotion or protection program, the occupational health nurse must be cognizant of the characteristics of the audience and the best methods to present the material. In order to be effective in teaching and communicating health promotion and protection strategies in the work environment, one must be familiar with principles of adult education. Knowles (1984) extensively describes the differences between adult and child patterns of learning and emphasizes the importance of teaching adults based on a framework of andragogy (teaching of adults) rather than pedagogy (teaching of children). Knowles suggests that adults, because of their greater independence and more extensive backgrounds, bring more to the learning experience, and that the instructor should serve as a facilitator and enhancer of the teaching-learning process (Table 12–10).

Knowles' principles of adult education focus on four areas: independent learning, usefulness of past experiences, readiness to learn, and problem-oriented learning. They are summarized as follows:

Independent Learning. Padberg and Padberg (1990) emphasize that it is important for the health care professional to respect the independence of the learners and include them as active self-directed participants rather than passive

■ **TABLE 12–10**   Role of the Teacher/Facilitator

Conditions of Learning	Principles of Teaching
The learners feel a need to learn.	1. Exposes students to new possibilities of self-fulfillment. 2. Helps each student clarify her or his own aspirations for improved behavior. 3. Helps each student diagnose the gap between her or his aspiration and present level of performance. 4. Helps the students identify the life problems they experience because of the gaps in their personal equipment.
The learning environment is characterized by physical comfort, mutual trust, respect, and helpfulness, freedom of expression, and acceptance of differences.	5. Provides physical conditions that are comfortable (as to seating, smoking, temperature, ventilation, lighting, decoration) and conducive to interaction (preferably, no person sitting behind another person). 6. Accepts each student as a person of worth and respects her or his feelings and ideas. 7. Seeks to build relationships of mutual trust and helpfulness among the students by encouraging cooperative activities and refraining from inducing competitiveness and judgmentalness. 8. Exposes own feelings and contributes resources as a co-learner in the spirit of mutual inquiry.
The learners perceive the goals of a learning experience to be their goals.	9. Involves the students in a mutual process of formulating learning objectives in which the needs of the students, of the institution, of the teacher, of the subject matter, and of the society are taken into account.
The learners accept a share of the responsibility for planning and operating a learning experience, and therefore have a feeling of commitment toward it.	10. Shares thinking about options available in the designing of learning experiences, the selection of materials and methods, and involves the students in deciding among these options jointly.
The learners participate actively in the learning process.	11. Helps the students to organize themselves (project groups, learning-teaching teams, independent study, etc.) to share responsibility in the process of mutual inquiry.
The learning process is related to and makes use of the experience of the learners.	12. Helps the students exploit their own experiences as resources for learning through the use of such techniques as discussion, role playing, case method, and so forth. 13. Gears the presentation of own resources to the levels of experience of her or his particular students. 14. Helps the students to apply new learning to their experience, and thus to make the learnings more meaningful and integrated.
The learners have a sense of progress toward their goals.	15. Involves the students in developing mutually acceptable criteria and methods for measuring progress toward the learning objectives. 16. Helps the students develop and apply procedures for self-evaluation according to these criteria.

From Knowles, M. The adult learner; A neglected species. Houston: Gulf Publishing, 1984.

recipients. This can be done by finding out what they already know about a topic, what they need to know to do the job better and safer, or what more they would like to learn about the topic.

Previous Experience.   Puetz (1988) points out that adults have a wealth of life experiences on which to base new learning. For example, an employee may have a relative who has had a heart attack and may be able to share related information about the rehabilitation process. This also presents an opportunity to assess employee baseline knowledge and to focus on areas of special concern.

Readiness to Learn.   At certain times in life or related to critical incidents or situations, adults present with a readiness to learn or a teachable moment. For example, a woman who becomes pregnant may be more interested in learning about workplace hazards or the effects of related life-style hazards such as smoking, and an employee recently diagnosed with high blood pressure may be more interested in learning about dietary control strategies.

Preventive information on topics such as AIDS or diabetes may not have a direct impact unless the employee knows someone affected. In addition, other changes or concerns in the individual's life such as family or career issues may take precedence over the learning event. The occupational health nurse will need to be astute to this and use this barrier as an opportunity for other teaching or counseling.

Problem-Oriented Learning.   Knowles (1984) suggests that adults' learning is usually in response to a problem. For example, employees who have had difficulty in quitting smoking will probably consider it a heatlh problem and thus be more amenable to a smoking cessation clinic or educational program. Adult education will be most effective when it responds as directly as possible to an individual's concerns (Padberg & Padberg, 1990).

The occupational health nurse can use Knowles' framework as a guide to structure the teaching/learning process and facilitate the motivation to learn. Puetz (1988) suggests that the occupational health nurse concentrate motivational efforts on enhancing the beginning learning situation, stimulating sustained interest, and providing for skill/knowledge reinforcement. Motivational strategies directed at these aims may include:

- providing visual marketing strategies such as photos and posters to stimulate interest;
- structuring simulated activities such as a mock disaster drill or actually learning to take blood pressures;
- being enthusiastic (by the teachers) about the topic;
- using a variety of teaching methods (e.g., films, videos, discussions);
- inviting participants to share experiences;
- providing skill laboratory exercises;
- testing for skill/knowledge acquisition to provide for learning feedback; and
- recognizing employee participation and program completion through newsletters, bulletin board photos, and so forth.

Knowles (1984) encourages mutual respect in the teaching/learning process. Applied to the occupational health setting, employees are seen as independent learners and both the nurse and the employees learn from each other. Previous experiences are considered valuable and useful resources for teaching opportunities, and employee learning should be structured to be responsive to problems or concerns. The occupational health nurse can use this framework to assist employees to achieve learning goals rather than manipulating the learning experience. Using this approach, both the employees and the occupational health nurse will benefit.

■ CONCLUSION

In summary, concepts and principles of health promotion and health protection are fundamental to occupational health nursing practice. In applying these concepts, the nurse will spend a good deal of her or his time in planning, developing, implementing, and evaluating strategies that will enhance worker health and productivity and reduce work-related and life-style risks. The models and approaches discussed in this chapter can offer a guide to developing health promotion and health protection programs that are worker-driven, cost-effective, and health-enhancing. The aim is to achieve the goal of a healthy workforce within the framework of quality living and work.

References

Allen, J & Allen, RF. From short-term compliance to long-term freedom: Culture-based health promotion by health professionals. American Journal of Health Promotion, *1*(2): 39–47, 1986.

Barry, PZ & DeFriese, GH. Cost-benefit and cost-effectiveness analysis for health promotion programs. American Journal of Health Promotion, *4*(6): 448–452, 1990.

Becker, MH, Maiman, LA, Kirscht, JP, Haefner, DP, & Drachman, RH. The health belief model and prediction of dietary compliance: A field experiment. Journal of Health and Social Behavior, *18:* 348–366, 1977.

Becker, MH, Drachman, RH, & Kirscht, JP. A new approach to explaining sick-role behavior in low-income populations. American Journal of Public Health, *64*(3): 205–216, 1974.

Best, JA & Cameron, RC. Health behavior and health promotion. American Journal of Health Promotion, *1:* 48–57, 1986.

Bigbee, JL & Jonsa, N. Strategies for promoting health protection. Nursing Clinics of North America, *26*(4): 895–913, 1991.

Bly, JL, Jones, RC, & Richardson, JE. Impact of worksite health promotion on health care costs and utilization. Journal of the American Medical Association, *256:* 3235–3240, 1986.

Burnham, JC. Change in the popularization of health in the United States. Bulletin of the History of Medicine, *58:* 183–197, 1984.

Campbell, K. Worksite health promotion: Prevention for the future. AAOHN Update Series, *4(19): 1–8, 1991.*

Champion, VC. Use of the health belief model in determining frequency of breast self examination. Research in Nursing and Health, *8*(4): 373–379, 1985.

Chen, MS & Cabot, EL. Organizational resources for worksite health promotion. AAOHN Journal, *36*(6): 282–284, 1988.

Conrad, P. Wellness in the work place: Potentials and pitfalls of work-site health promotion. Milbank Quarterly, *65:* 255–275, 1987.

Cummings, KM, Jette, AM, Brock, BM, & Haefner, D. Psychosocial determinants of immunization behavior in a swine influenza campaign. Medical Care, *17*(6): 639–649, 1979.

Eddy, JM, Gold, RS, & Zimmerli, WH. Evaluation of worksite health enhancement programs. Health Values, *13:* 3–9, 1989.

Eley, JW. Analyzing costs and benefits of mammography screening in the workplace. AAOHN Journal, *37*(5):171–177, 1989.

Erfurt, JC, Foote, A, Heinrich, MA, & Gregg, W. Improving participation in worksite wellness programs: Comparing health education classes, a menu approach, and follow-up counseling. American Journal of Health Promotion, *4*(4): 270–278, 1990.

Erfurt, JC, Foote, A, & Heinrich, MA. The cost-effectiveness of work-site wellness programs for hypertension control, weight loss, and smoking cessation. Journal of Occupational Medicine, *33*(9): 962–970, 1991.

Fielding, JE. The proof of the health promotion pudding is . . .. Journal of Occupational Medicine, *30*(2): 113–115, 1988.

Girdano, D. Occupational health promotion. New York: Macmillan Publishing Company, 1986.

Golaszewski, T. What is a program: Thoughts

on definitions in worksite health promotion. Journal of Occupational Medicine, *34:* 162–163, 1992.

Goodstadt, MS, Simpson, RI, & Loranger, PO. Health promotion: A conceptual integration. American Journal of Health Promotion, *1:* 58–63, 1987.

Green, L & Kreuter, M. Health promotion planning: An educational & environmental approach. Mountain View, CA: Mayfield Publishing Company, 1991.

Hochbaum, GM. Public participation in medical screening programs: A socio-psychological study. Public Health Service Publication (No. 572). Washington, DC: U.S. Government Printing Office, 1958.

Hodgson, TA & Rice, DP. Economic impact of cancer in the United States. In Cancer epidemiology and prevention, D. Schottenfeld, Ed. 1992.

Holzbach, RI, Piserchia, PV, McFadden, DW, Hartwell, TD, Herrmann, A, & Fielding, JE. Effect of a comprehensive health promotion program on employee attitudes. Journal of Occupational Medicine, *32:* 973–978, 1990.

Hunt, PE & Murphy, KE. Nutrition counseling in the workplace. AAOHN Update Series, 2(13): 1–8, 1986.

Jacobson, MI, Yenney, SL, & Bisgard, JC. An organizational perspective on worksite health. Occupational Medicine: State of the Art Reviews, 5(4): 653–664, 1990.

Katz, PP & Showstack, JA. Is it worth it? Evaluating the economic impact of worksite health promotion. Occupational Medicine: State of the Art Reviews, 5(4): 837–850, 1990.

Katzman, MS & Smith, KJ. Occupational health-promotion programs: Evaluation efforts and measured cost savings. Health Values, *13*(2): 3–10, 1989.

Kegeles, SS, Kirscht, JP, & Haefner, DP. Surveys of beliefs about cancer detection and taking Papanicolaou tests. Public Health Reports, *80*(9): 815–823, 1965.

Kizer, WM. The healthy workplace: A blueprint for corporate action. New York: John Wiley & Sons, 1987.

Knowles, M. The adult learner: A neglected species. Houston: Gulf Publishing, 1984.

Kristein, MM. The economics of health promotion at the worksite. Health Education Quarterly, *9:* 27–35 (suppl), 1982.

Larson, EB, Olsen, E, Cole, W, & Shortell, S. The relationship of health beliefs and a postcard reminder to influenza vaccination. Journal of Family Practice, *89:* 1207–1211, 1979.

Leavell, H & Clark, E. Preventive medicine for the doctor in his community. New York: McGraw-Hill, 1965.

Lichter, M. Oakwood Hospital community health promotion program. Health Care Management Review, *11:* 75–87, 1986.

Lukes, EN. Program evaluation: Demonstrating cost savings. AAOHN Update Series, 4(12): 1–8, 1992.

Massey, V. Perceived susceptibility to breast cancer and practice of breast self examination. Nursing Research, *35*(3): 183–185, 1986.

McGovern, PM. Managing health care costs: The first step. AAOHN Update Series, 4(1): 1–12, 1991.

McNeil Consumer Products Company. Worksite wellness. Fort Washington, PA: Author, 1988.

National Survey of Worksite Health Promotion Activities. Office of Disease Prevention and Health Promotion, U.S. Department of Health and Human Services, 1987.

Nemcek, MA. Health beliefs and preventive behavior. AAOHN Journal, *38*(3): 127–138, 1990.

O'Dell, C, Mangin, RJ, Leavitt, LE, Levine, TC, Maloney, S, Schwartz, F, & Winton, R. Teaching employees breast self-examination. AAOHN Journal, *39*(8): 385–391, 1991.

O'Donnell, MP & Ainsworth, T. Health promotion in the workplace. New York: Wiley & Sons, 1984.

O'Donnell, MP. Definition of health promotion. American Journal of Health Promotion, *1:* 4–5, 1986a.

O'Donnell, MP. Definition of health promotion: Part II: Levels of programs. American Journal of Health Promotion, *1:* 6–9, 1986b.

O'Donnell, MP. Definition of health promotion: Part III: Expanding the definition. American Journal of Health Promotion, *3*(3): 5, 1989.

Padberg, RM & Padberg, LF. Strengthening the effectiveness of patient education: Applying principles of adult education. Oncology Nursing Forum, *17*(1): 65–69, 1990.

Pender, N. Health promotion in nursing practice (2nd ed). Norwalk, CN: Appleton & Lange, 1987.

Pfeiffer, GJ. Management aspects of fitness program development. American Journal of Health Promotion, *1*(2): 10–18, 1986.

Popp, RA. An overview of occupational health promotion. AAOHN Journal, *37*(4): 113–119, 1989.

Pruitt, RH. Economics of health promotion. Nursing Economics, *5*(3): 118–120, 1987.

Puetz, BE. Theories of adult education and their application to occupational health nursing. AAOHN Update Series, *3*(19): 1–8, 1988.

Ray, L. Community health nursing at the worksite. In Community Health Nursing, S.

Archer & R. Fleshman, Eds. Monterey, CA: Walsworth Health Sciences, 394–403, 1985.

Rice, DP, MacKenzie, EJ, Jones, AS, Kaufman, SR, deLissovoy, GV, Max, W, McLoughlin, E, Miller, TR, Robertson, LS, Salkever, DS, & Smith, GS. Cost of injury in the United States: A Report to Congress, 1989. San Francisco, CA: Institute for Health and Aging, University of California and Injury Prevention Center, Johns Hopkins University, 1989.

Rose, MA. Health promotion and risk prevention: Application for cancer survivors. Oncology Nursing Forum, 16(3): 335–340, 1989.

Rosenstock, IM. Why people use health services. Milbank Memorial Fund Quarterly, 44: 94–127, 1966.

Rundall, TG & Wheeler, JR. Factors associated with utilization of the swine flu vaccination program among senior citizens. Medical Care, 17: 191–200, 1979.

Sandroff, OJ, Bradford, S, & Guligan, VF. Meeting the health promotion challenges through a mode of shared responsibility. Occupational Medicine: State of the Art Reviews, 5(4): 677–690, 1990

Scofield, M. Worksite health promotion. Occupational Medicine: State of the Art Reviews, 5(4): xiii–xiv, 1990.

Selleck, CS, Sirles, AT, & Newman, KD. Health promotion at the workplace. AAOHN Journal, 37(10): 412–422, 1989.

Shamansky, SL & Clausen, CL. Levels of prevention: Examination of the concept. Nursing Outlook, 28: 104–108, 1980.

Soha, C & Vickery, CE. Guide for assessing wellness programs. AAOHN Journal, 36(10): 417–418, 1988.

Spellbring, AM. Nursing's role in health promotion. Nursing Clinics of North America, 26(4): 805–814, 1991.

Sullivan, LW. Partners in prevention: A mobilization plan for implementing Healthy People 2000. American Journal of Health Promotion, 5(4): 291–297, 1991.

Taming the health cost monster. Workplace Health, 1 (October): 5, 1992.

Terry PE. The role of health risk appraisal in the workplace: Assessment versus behavior change. American Journal of Health Promotion, 1: 18–21, 1987.

Tripp, SL & Stachowiak, B. Health maintenance, health promotion: Is there a difference. Public Health Nursing, 9(3): 155–161, 1992.

USDHHS. Healthy People 2000: National Health Promotion & Disease Prevention Objectives (DHHS Pub No 91-50212, 94–110). Washington, DC: U.S. Government Printing Office, 1991.

Wachs, JE & Parker-Conrad, JE. Occupational health nursing in 1990 and the coming decade. Applied Occupational and Environmental Hygiene, 5(4): 200–203, 1990.

Wachs, JE. Levels of prevention: A framework for cost-effective occupational health programs. AAOHN Update Series, 4(7): 1–8, 1991.

Wallston, BS & Wallston, KA. Social psychological models of health behavior: An examination and integration. In Handbook of psychology and health, Vol IV, Social psychological aspects of psychology, A. Baum, S. Taylor & JE Singer, Eds. Hillsdale, NJ: Erlbaum Associates, 1984.

Walsh, DC & Egdahl, RH. Corporate perspectives on worksite wellness programs: A report on the seventh Pew Fellows Conference. Journal of Occupational Medicine, 31: 551–556, 1989.

Warner, KE, Wickizer, TM, Wolfe, RA, et al. Economic implications of workplace health promotion programs: Review of the literature. Journal of Occupational Medicine, 30: 106–112, 1988.

Wellness Councils of America. Healthy, Wealthy, Well and Wise. Omaha, NE: Author, 1990.

Weinberger, M, Greene, J, Mamlin, J, & Jerin, M. Health beliefs and smoking behavior. American Journal of Public Health, 71: 1253–1255, 1981.

12–1

MANAGEMENT SURVEY

We are currently undertaking a study to determine the amount of interest and the kinds of feelings and assumptions that employees have about the development of a worksite health promotion program. Please answer the questions honestly. The survey is completely confidential. You do not need to give us your name.

AGREE OR DISAGREE?	Agree	Disagree
It is cheaper to prevent disease than to treat it after the fact.	☐	☐

People need accurate health information and education about their

	Agree	Disagree
1. health risks	☐	☐
2. behaviors that create risks	☐	☐
3. health care costs	☐	☐
4. health choices	☐	☐
5. how to change their behaviors	☐	☐

	Agree	Disagree
People will choose to change their behavior if they are informed, motivated, and supported.	☐	☐
Healthy people do their best and are more productive on and off the job.	☐	☐
The people I associate with have an influence on my choices.	☐	☐
My work environment has an impact on my health, my behaviors, and my choices.	☐	☐

Because of the influence of the company's work environment, I have changed or I have seen coworkers change the following:

1. Started and maintain a regular exercise program?	T	F
2. Stopped or cut back on my smoking?	T	F
3. Developed skills to manage the stress in my life?	T	F
4. Adopted new eating habits to maintain healthy body weight?	T	F
5. Adopted new eating habits to lower cholesterol?	T	F
6. Avoid the overuse of caffeine, sugar, salt?	T	F
7. Avoid the overuse or misuse of alcohol and/or drugs?	T	F
8. Have regular medical and dental check-ups?	T	F
9. Maintain healthy blood pressure?	T	F
10. Understand the importance of and need for good mental and emotional health as well as physical health?	T	F

What is your reaction to the prospect of a worksite health promotion program in our company?

☐ Excited
☐ Moderately interested
☐ Neutral
☐ Slightly disinterested
☐ Opposed

If a worksite health promotion program is implemented here, would you:

personally participate in any programs or activities?	Y	N
encourage the employees you supervise to participate?	Y	N

12–2

Health Interest Surveys

■ **TABLE A** Employee Health Promotion Survey

From the following list of Programs and Activities, circle the number that shows your level of interest for each, "1" being the lowest level and "5" the highest.

Priority

I. PROGRAMS:

Least				*Highest*	
					A. Understanding Personal Health
1	2	3	4	5	1. Nutrition
1	2	3	4	5	2. Healthy Life-style
1	2	3	4	5	3. Physical Fitness Education
1	2	3	4	5	4. Alcohol and Other Drug Control
1	2	3	4	5	5. Healthy Back
1	2	3	4	5	6. Men's Health Issues
1	2	3	4	5	7. Women's Health Issues
1	2	3	4	5	8. Stress Management
1	2	3	4	5	9. Blood Pressure Management

Least				*Highest*	
					B. Reducing Risks
1	2	3	4	5	1. Safety-Accident Prevention:
1	2	3	4	5	a. Home
1	2	3	4	5	b. Gun
1	2	3	4	5	c. Water
1	2	3	4	5	d. Automobile
1	2	3	4	5	e. Motorcycle
1	2	3	4	5	f. Other
1	2	3	4	5	2. Cancer Risk Reduction
1	2	3	4	5	3. Dental Disease Prevention
1	2	3	4	5	4. Heart Attack Risk Reduction

Least				*Highest*	
					C. Developing Healthy Relations with Others
1	2	3	4	5	1. Caring for and Understanding Aging Parents
1	2	3	4	5	2. Parenting Issues: Caring for and Understanding Children
1	2	3	4	5	3. Dealing with Difficult People
1	2	3	4	5	4. Positive Mental Attitude

Priority

II. ACTIVITIES:

Least				*Highest*	
					A. Promoting Health Through Actions
1	2	3	4	5	1. Physical Fitness Activities (Circle the type(s) of physical fitness activities you would like to take part in.)
1	2	3	4	5	a. Aerobics–Exercises that bring the heart rate up to a certain level for a period of time.
1	2	3	4	5	b. Calisthenics–Exercises that increase strength, balance, coordination, and joint movement.

1	2	3	4	5	c. Flexibility and Stretching–Exercises that increase blood supply to the muscles. Improves range of motion.
1	2	3	4	5	d. Walking/Jogging
1	2	3	4	5	e. Other
1	2	3	4	5	2. Smoking Cessation
1	2	3	4	5	3. Weight Management
1	2	3	4	5	4. Arthritis (Help for self and family)
1	2	3	4	5	5. Blood Pressure Control (Managing high blood pressure)

Least			*Highest*		**B. Screening for Specific Health Concerns**
1	2	3	4	5	1. Glaucoma
1	2	3	4	5	2. Cholesterol
1	2	3	4	5	3. Blood Pressure
1	2	3	4	5	4. Cancer
1	2	3	4	5	5. Back Problems

Least			*Highest*		**C. Developing Skills to Help Others**
1	2	3	4	5	1. CPR (Cardiopulmonary Resuscitation)
1	2	3	4	5	2. First Aid

Would you attend one or more of the above programs if they were offered at a convenient time?

☐ YES ☐ NO

III. ADDITIONAL CONSIDERATIONS

Would you prefer a health promotion program at the worksite or some other place? (If other, please write down the location you would prefer.)

☐ Worksite ☐ Other, where?

_____

_____

Would your spouse and/or family take part in a health promotion program? ☐ Yes ☐ No

Would you be willing to share in the cost for some programs? ☐ Yes ☐ No

Would you take part in a weekend program? ☐ Yes ☐ No
Would you take part in a lunch hour program? ☐ Yes ☐ No

What hours do you work? _____ a.m./p.m. to _____ a.m./p.m.

What hours are best for you to take part in a health promotion program?
_____ a.m./p.m. to _____ a.m./p.m.

In the space below, let us know about any other health care or health promotion ideas or concerns that you may have.

_____

_____

_____

_____

_____

_____

_____

Return Survey to: _____ By _____

Thank You!

■ **TABLE B**   Health Interest Survey

Please circle the answer or answers that best fit the question.

1. Are you presently involved in some regular form of physical fitness? YES   NO
   If yes, how often?

   a. three or more times per week
   b. once a week
   c. once a month

   In what type of physical activity are you currently involved?

   a. running/walking   d. tennis/racquetball
   b. weight/strength training   e. team sports
   c. aerobics/jazzercize   f. other _____

   Would you use an on-site jogging/aerobic walking trail? YES   NO

   Would you use exercise stations strategically placed along the trail? YES   NO

2. Which of the following would encourage your regular participation in physical fitness activities?

   a. par course   e. weight/strength training
   b. bicycling   f. tennis/racquetball
   c. swimming   g. team sports
   d. indoor ski equipment   h. other _____

3. Do you consider your diet a healthy one? YES   NO

   Would you like to have information on:

   a. appropriate caloric intake
   b. dietary salt, sugar, and fiber
   c. healthy intake of cholesterol
   d. special diets such as diabetic, sports diets, bland ulcer diet
   e. vitamin and mineral supplements

   Are you overweight? YES   NO

4. Are you subject to daily stress? YES   NO
   If yes, would you consider it?

   a. high
   b. medium
   c. minimal

   What is the likely source of your stress?

   a. marital/other relationship
   b. financial
   c. work-related
   d. parenting
   e. other

■ **TABLE B** Health Interest Survey *Continued*

5. Do you smoke cigarettes? YES   NO
   If yes, how many packs per day?

   a. less than one
   b. one to two
   c. three or more

   How long have you smoked?

   a. less than 1 year
   b. 2–5 years
   c. 6–10 years
   d. 1–20 years
   e. greater than 20 years

   Are you interested in quitting? YES   NO
6. Do you need information or assistance in coping with alcohol/drug abuse problems?
   YES   NO

7. Would information on the prevention of certain diseases such as cancer, heart disease, stroke, diabetes, and arthritis be helpful? YES   NO

   Circle any activities you feel are important:

   a. availability of pamphlets and audiovisual materials
   b. learning of self-examination techniques such as those for breast and testicular cancers
   c. presentation of worksite educational sessions
   d. worksite screening for blood sugar, cholesterol, and blood pressure

8. Would you complete a generalized HEALTH RISK APPRAISAL to advise you of your own health risk factors? YES   NO

9. Consider the following health promotion programs that could be offered at the workplace. Please rank them #1 through #7 in the order that you feel they should be offered.

Program	Rank (1–7)
a. High blood pressure workshop	_____
b. Stress management seminar	_____
c. Weight management program	_____
d. Smoking cessation program	_____
e. Fitness testing	_____
f. Nutrition program to encourage a healthy diet	_____
g. Neck and back pain prevention	_____

10. Other health-related information can also be important. For each item below, please indicate your level of interest by marking a "0" if no interest, a "1" if interested, and a "2" if extremely interested.

    Sexually transmissable diseases (AIDS, herpes, etc.) _____
    Prenatal care _____   Birth control _____
    Parenting _____   Day care centers _____

                                                                              Continued.

■ **TABLE B**   Health Interest Survey *Continued*

Choosing the right doctor _____   "How to talk with your doctor" _____
Dental health _____   Cardiovascular fitness _____
Skin cancer _____   Food additives _____

Please complete the following information:

Age: _____   Sex: F _____   M _____
Educational level: _____
Position (circle):   Clerical   Technical   Professional
Marital Status (circle):   Married   Single   Divorced   Separated
Number of children _____   Ages:

Thank you for your participation.

Comments/Suggestions: _____
_____
_____
_____
_____
_____
_____
_____
_____
_____

■ **TABLE C1**   Employee Health Promotion Survey

This information is for future program design purposes only. Please do not sign your name.

1. Please specify your work location:

2. If the following health promotion programs were offered by [Company Name] please indicate in
   which programs, if any, you would participate? Please circle the programs of most interest to you and
   rank them in order of preference 1 through 10 with #1 of most importance to you, #2 is second, and
   #10 is of least importance.

   _____ Physical fitness
   _____ Weight management
   _____ Nutrition
   _____ Smoking cessation
   _____ Stress management
   _____ Blood pressure control
   _____ Coping/interpersonal skills
   _____ Home and auto safety
   _____ Cardiac resuscitation and first aid
   _____ Medical self-care and wiser use of medical services
   _____ Other (specify) _____

■ **TABLE C1**   Employee Health Promotion Survey *Continued*

3. Would you participate in the health promotion programs of interest you specified if they were offered after working hours?

_____ Yes   _____ No

4. Which health practices are important to you for staying healthy? Check all that apply.

_____ Physical fitness
_____ Proper nutrition
_____ ideal body weight
_____ Not smoking
_____ Stress management
_____ Having a good relationship with family
_____ Having a good relationship with coworkers
_____ Controlling blood pressure
_____ Safety on the job
_____ Using seat belts and child safety restraint devices
_____ Moderate use of alcohol

5. How often do you use seat belts?

_____ Every time
_____ Usually
_____ Half of the time
_____ Occasionally
_____ Never

6. If [Company Name] offered preventive health examinations periodically (e.g., every three years) would you participate?

Yes _____   _____ No

7. Do you think that people in good health are happier with their daily lives?

_____ Agree   _____ Disagree   _____ Neutral

8. Do you think people in good health are more productive?

_____ Agree   _____ Disagree   _____ Neutral

9. Do you think that you could improve your health by changing some habits or health practices?

_____ Agree   _____ Disagree   _____ Neutral

10. Would you consider the offering of screening and health promotion programs by [Company Name] a significant employment benefit?

_____ Agree   _____ Disagree   _____ Neutral

11. Do you favor providing smoking and nonsmoking areas in the workplace?

_____ Yes   _____ No

Continued.

■ **TABLE C1**   Employee Health Promotion Survey *Continued*

12. Do you favor a no smoking policy when smokers and nonsmokers must meet in closed rooms?

    _____ Yes   _____ No

13. Do you favor a total no smoking policy at the workplace?

    _____ Yes   _____ No

14. Do you smoke now?

    _____ Yes   _____ No

15. Do you feel your job is stressful?

    _____ Always   _____ Much of the time   _____ Occasionally   _____ Rarely

16. Do you feel your life away from the job is stressful?

    _____ Always   _____ Much of the time   _____ Occasionally   _____ Rarely

17. Do you participate in an exercise program now?

    _____ Yes   _____ No

19. In what fitness activities do you participate?

    _____ Jogging Trail
    _____ Swimming
    _____ Racketball
    _____ Aerobics
    _____ Nautilus Equipment
    _____ Other _____ (specify)

20. Your age is _____ . (optional)

21. Are you: (circle one)

    Salary Exempt
    Salary Nonexempt
    Hourly

Please make any additional comments you may have _____
_____
_____
_____
_____
_____

■ TABLE C2 For Good Health Practices

Listed below are a number of health practices that could be supported at [Company Name]. Please circle the number that best indicates the level of support you perceive exists for these practices at your worksite.

If a Coworker Were to	Most Other Employees Would				
	Approve and Encourage It	Approve but Do Nothing to Encourage It	Consider It Not Important	Disagree but Do Nothing to Discourage It	Disagree and Discourage It
1. engage in a regular, planned program of physical exercise	1	2	3	4	5
2. stop smoking	1	2	3	4	5
3. understand the significance of stress and engage in stress management techniques	1	2	3	4	5
4. achieve her or his correct weight and maintain it on a sustained basis	1	2	3	4	5
5. understand and follow sound nutritional practices, including eating a nutritional breakfast every day	1	2	3	4	5
6. avoid the overuse of caffeine, saccharin, sugar, salt and cholesterol-producing foods	1	2	3	4	5
7. avoid the overuse and misuse of alcohol	1	2	3	4	5
8. avoid the overuse and misuse of drugs	1	2	3	4	5
9. have regular health and dental examinations or health screenings and follow-up on the recommendations given	1	2	3	4	5
10. maintain their proper blood pressure	1	2	3	4	5
11. follow sound safety practices at home, at work, and on the highway	1	2	3	4	5
12. understand the importance of good mental health and deal effectively with mental and emotional problems	1	2	3	4	5

■ **TABLE D**

HEALTH RISK INTEREST SURVEY

Please indicate which of the following areas you have a need or interest by placing a check in the appropriate column which indicates the type of program that would best meet your needs or interests. This survey will help us determine the kinds of programs that will be offered.

If a health promotion program were made available to you, which of the following would you be most likely to attend?

PLEASE CHECK ONE

	YES	YES AT A SMALL COST	NO
1. Cardiovascular fitness/exercise			
2. Personal stress management			
3. Organizational stress management			
4. Smoking cessation			
5. Weight control & nutrition education			
6. High blood pressure management			
7. Medical self-care approaches			
8. Alcohol/drug use			
9. Mental/emotional problems (depression, nervousness)			
10. Parenting skills			
11. Marital problems			
12. Assertiveness training			
13. Educational/career planning			
14. Spiritual or philosophical values			
15. Interpersonal communication skills			
16. Home budgeting/financial planning			
17. Automobile safety			
18. Time management			

■ **TABLE D**   Health Risk Interest Survey *Continued*

PLEASE CHECK ONE

	AFTER WORK	LUNCH	EVENINGS
19. When would you most likely attend a class or activity?			

	ONE TIME	6-8 WEEKS	EITHER
20. Would you be most likely to attend:			

	YES		NO
21. Would you be interested in programs that could include family members?			

	YES		NO
22. Could changes be made in your work behaviors? (example: choice of fruit and/or fruit juices as well as soft drinks and coffee) If yes, please describe: _____			

_____
_____

	YES	NO
23. Would you be willing to assist in the planning and delivery of programs? If yes, give topics:_____		

_____
_____

	YES	NO
24. Any suggestions for additional health promotion programs? If yes, suggestions:_____		

_____
_____

Thanks for your interest

Name _____

Department _____

Telephone _____

From Wellness Councils of America, Omaha, NE, 1993.

■ **TABLE E**

EMPLOYEE WELLNESS SURVEY

We are considering the development of an employee wellness program and would like to learn more about your interests in wellness and health-related activities. Your responses will be used in planning the program and deciding what types of activities should be included.

Please take a few minutes to complete this survey. Since we want to keep individual survey information confidential, please do not put your name on it.

1. Sex: ____Male   ____Female

2. Age Group: ____Under 21   ____21-30   ____31-40   ____41-50
                   ____51-60   ____Over 60

3. Check any of the following that apply regarding your current health habits:

Yes   No

Exercise
____   ____ I exercise vigorously for at least 20 minutes three times a week.
____   ____ I exercise once in a while.
____   ____ I rarely exercise.

Eating
____   ____ I usually eat three nutritious meals daily.
____   ____ I often eat on the run, dropping meals.
____   ____ I avoid eating too much fat.
____   ____ I make an effort to eat enough high fiber foods.
____   ____ I like a lot of salt on my food.
____   ____ I eat breakfast every day.

Weight
____   ____ I am about the right weight.
____   ____ I would like to lose weight.
____   ____ I am more than 20 pounds over my ideal weight.

Sleep
____   ____ I usually get a good night's sleep.
____   ____ I average at least two nights of inadequate sleep per week.
____   ____ I often have trouble getting enough sleep.

Smoking/Alcohol/Drugs
____   ____ I regularly smoke cigarettes.
____   ____ I have at least three drinks daily containing alcohol.
____   ____ I sometimes drive after drinking alcohol.
____   ____ I avoid drinking too many caffeinated drinks.
____   ____ I regularly use tranquilizers and similar drugs.

Other
____   ____ I regularly practice some type of stress management.
____   ____ I have had lower back pain in the last six months.
____   ____ I usually consult a medical self-care book when I am sick.

■ **TABLE E**   Employee Wellness Survey *Continued*

---

4. List any health concerns you have about yourself or your family:

_____

5. Would you like the organization to conduct a wellness program?

       ____Yes   ____No   ____Don't know

6. In which of the following activities would you consider participating?

Yes	Maybe		Yes	Maybe	
____	____	Aerobic exercise	____	____	Other exercise
____	____	Weight management	____	____	Health fair
____	____	Smoking cessation	____	____	Blood test for
____	____	Confidential health			cholesterol
		screening	____	____	Cancer screening
____	____	Coping with stress	____	____	CPR training
____	____	Alcohol/drug abuse	____	____	Regular wellness
		education			presentations
____	____	Safety/accident	____	____	Retirement
		prevention			planning
____	____	Parenting	____	____	Back pain
____	____	Walking program	____	____	Medical self-care
____	____	Other, please specify_____			

7. When would you be most likely to participate? (Please check all that apply.)

____Monday	____Spring	____A.M., before work
____Tuesday	____Summer	____Lunchtime
____Wednesday	____Fall	____P.M., after work
____Thursday	____Winter	____Evening
____Friday		____Other, specify_____

8. Where would you be most likely to participate? (Check as many as apply.)
    ____Worksite   ____School
    ____YMCA/YWCA   ____Private health club

9. Would you be willing to share the cost of participating in these programs?
    ____Yes   ____No

10. Any additional comments?_____

Thank you for your help in completing this survey!

From Wellness Councils of America, Omaha, NE, 1993.

■ **TABLE F**   Needs and Interest Survey

The purpose of this survey is to obtain employee input for our health promotion program. It includes needs, interests, and other information to be used in deciding what programs to offer and when to offer them. There are no right or wrong answers. Please use an "X" to respond to questions. Your completion of the survey is completely voluntary. The surveys are completely anonymous; there is no identifying number on the form.

A. TOBACCO USE

1. Do you chew or dip tobacco now?

☐ Yes   ☐ No, but former user   ☐ No, never used

2. Do you smoke a pipe or cigars?

☐ Yes   ☐ No, but former user   ☐ No, never used

3. How would you classify your current use of cigarettes?

☐ Current cigarette smoker (____cigarettes per day)

☐ Never smoked/smoked less than 100 cigarettes in my lifetime

☐ Ex-smoker, years quit____ or ____ months if less than one year

B. NUTRITION AND PHYSICAL ACTIVITY

Please rate how often you do each of the following

	Never	Seldom	Sometimes	Often	Very Often
4. Eat fresh fruits, vegetables, whole grain bread.	☐	☐	☐	☐	☐
5. Eat food high in cholesterol or fat, such as fatty meat, cheese, fried foods, or eggs?	☐	☐	☐	☐	☐
6. Eat foods at home that are already prepared (like TV dinners, pizzas, frozen main courses, canned soup).	☐	☐	☐	☐	☐
7. Eat food at a fast food outlet such as Kentucky Fried Chicken, McDonald's, or canteen trucks.	☐	☐	☐	☐	☐

8. Please check below the category that best describes your physical activity level for the previous year.

☐ No physical activity.

☐ Moderate to vigorous exercise 1 time/week for at least 20 minutes.

■ **TABLE F**   Needs and Interest Survey *Continued*

☐ Moderate to vigorous exercise 1-2 times/week for at least 20 minutes each time.

☐ Moderate to vigorous exercise 3 times/week for at least 20 minutes each time.

☐ Moderate to vigorous exercise 5 times/week for at least 30 minutes each time.

C. HEALTH SCREENINGS

Please indicate whether you have had the following screenings or examinations in the past year.

	Yes	No	Not sure
9. Cholesterol check	☐	☐	☐
10. Blood sugar check	☐	☐	☐
11. Rectal exam	☐	☐	☐
12. Stool check	☐	☐	☐

Exams for women only (men skip to 16)

	Yes	No	Not sure
13. Breast physical exam by doctor	☐	☐	☐
14. Mammogram (x-ray of breasts)	☐	☐	☐
15. Pap smear during pelvic exam	☐	☐	☐

Exams for men only (women skip to 17)

	Yes	No	Not sure
16. Prostate exam	☐	☐	☐

D. PROGRAM INTERESTS

Please indicate how likely you would be to participate in each of the following programs if they were offered at work during the next year.

	Extremely Likely	Somewhat Likely	Somewhat Unlikely	Extremely Unlikely
17. Nutrition and cancer	☐	☐	☐	☐
18. Cancer awareness for women	☐	☐	☐	☐
19. Cancer awareness for men	☐	☐	☐	☐
20. Smoking cessation	☐	☐	☐	☐

■ **TABLE F**　Needs and Interest Survey *Continued*

	Extremely Likely	Somewhat Likely	Somewhat Unlikely	Extremely Unlikely
21. Walking program	☐	☐	☐	☐
22. Weight loss and nutrition program	☐	☐	☐	☐
23. Managing chronic health conditions (e.g., diabetes, hypertension)	☐	☐	☐	☐
24. Blood pressure screening	☐	☐	☐	☐
25. Cholesterol screening	☐	☐	☐	☐

Please indicate how likely you would be to participate in a health promotion program during the following times.

	Extremely Likely	Somewhat Likely	Somewhat Unlikely	Extremely Unlikely
26. Before work	☐	☐	☐	☐
27. During lunch	☐	☐	☐	☐
28. After work	☐	☐	☐	☐

E. DEMOGRAPHIC INFORMATION

29. What was your age on your last birthday?　____years

30. What is your sex?　☐ male　☐ female

31. Your job category:

☐ Management/professional

☐ Clerical

☐ Technical

☐ Service/Labor

THANK YOU FOR COMPLETING THIS SURVEY

From Wellness Councils of America, Omaha, NE, 1993.

--- APPENDIX ---

12–3

No. _____

Healthier People
Health Risk Appraisal

Detach this coupon and put it in a safe place.
You will need it to claim your appraisal results.

✂ —

Healthier People
Health Risk Appraisal
The Carter Center of Emory University

No. _____

_____

Health risk appraisal is an educational tool. It shows you choices you can make to keep good health and avoid the most common causes of death for a person your age and sex. This health risk appraisal is not a substitute for a check-up or physical exam that you get from a doctor or nurse. It only gives you some ideas for lowering your risk of getting sick or injured in the future. It is NOT designed for people who already have HEART DISEASE, CANCER, KIDNEY DISEASE, OR MOST OTHER SERIOUS CONDITIONS. If you have any of these problems and you want a health risk appraisal anyway, ask your doctor or nurse to read the report with you.

DIRECTIONS: Your answers will be treated as confidential. Please keep the coupon with your participant number on it. You will need it to claim your computer report. To get the most accurate results answer as many questions as you can and as best you can. If you do not know the answer leave it blank. Questions with a ★ (star symbol) are important to your health, but are not used by the computer to calculate your risks. However, your answers may be helpful in planning your health and fitness program.

Please put your answers in the empty boxes.   (Examples: ☒ or ☐125☐)

1. SEX	1 ☐ Male 2 ☐ Female
2. AGE	☐☐ Years
3. HEIGHT	(Without shoes) (No fractions) ☐☐ Feet ☐☐ Inches
4. WEIGHT	(Without shoes) (No fractions) ☐☐ Pounds
5. Body frame size	1 ☐ Small 2 ☐ Medium 3 ☐ Large
6. Have you ever been told that you have diabetes (or sugar diabetes)?	1 ☐ Yes 2 ☐ No
7. Are you now taking medicine for high blood pressure?	1 ☐ Yes 2 ☐ No
8. What is your blood pressure now?	☐☐ / ☐☐ Systolic (High number)/Diastolic (Low number)
9. If you *do not* know the numbers, check the box that describes your blood pressure.	1 ☐ High 2 ☐ Normal or Low 3 ☐ Don't Know
10. What is your TOTAL cholesterol level (based on a blood test)?	☐☐ mg/dl
11. What is your HDL cholesterol (based on a blood test)?	☐☐ mg/dl
12. How many cigars do you usually smoke per day?	☐☐ cigars per day
13. How many pipes of tobacco do you usually smoke per day?	☐☐ pipes per day
14. How many times per day do you usually use smokeless tobacco? (Chewing tobacco, snuff, pouches, etc.)	☐☐ times per day

Continued.

Health risk appraisal is an educational tool. It shows you choices you can make to keep good health and avoid the most common causes of death for a person your age and sex. This health risk appraisal is not a substitute for a check-up or physical exam that you get from a doctor or nurse. It only gives you some ideas for lowering your risk of getting sick or injured in the future. It is NOT designed for people who already have HEART DISEASE, CANCER, KIDNEY DISEASE, OR MOST OTHER SERIOUS CONDITIONS. If you have any of these problems and you want a health risk appraisal anyway, ask your doctor or nurse to read the report with you.

Your report may be picked up at _____ on _____ .

✂ ---

15. **CIGARETTE SMOKING** How would you describe your cigarette smoking habits?	1 ☐ Never smoked 2 ☐ Used to Smoke 3 ☐ Still Smoke	☛ Go to 18 ☛ Go to 17 ☛ Go to 16
16. **STILL SMOKE** How many cigarettes a day do you smoke? ☛ GO TO QUESTION 18	[ ] cigarettes per day	☛ Go to 18
17. **USED TO SMOKE** a. How many years has it been since you smoked cigarettes fairly regularly? b. What was the average number of cigarettes per day that you smoked in the 2 years before you quit?	[ ] years [ ] cigarettes per day	

18. In the next 12 months how many thousands of miles will you probably travel by each of the following? (NOTE: U.S. average = 10,000 miles) a. Car, truck, or van: b. Motorcycle:	[ ] ,000 miles [ ] ,000 miles

19. On a typical day how do you USUALLY travel? (Check one only)	1 ☐ Walk 2 ☐ Bicycle 3 ☐ Motorcycle 4 ☐ Sub-compact or compact car 5 ☐ Mid-size or full-size car 6 ☐ Truck or van 7 ☐ Bus, subway, or train 8 ☐ Mostly stay home

20. What percent of the time do you usually buckle your safety belt when driving or riding?	[ ] %

21. On the average, how close to the speed limit do you usually drive?	1 ☐ Within 5 mph of limit 2 ☐ 6-10 mph over limit 3 ☐ 11-15 mph over limit 4 ☐ More than 15 mph over limit

22. How many times in the last month did your drive or ride when the driver had perhaps too much alcohol to drink?	[ ] times last month

23. How many drinks of alcoholic beverage do your have in a typical week? ☛ **(MEN GO TO QUESTION 33)**	(Write number of each type of drink) [ ] Bottles or cans of beer [ ] Glasses of wine [ ] Wine coolers [ ] Mixed drinks or shots of liquor

WOMEN 24. At what age did you have your first menstrual period?	[ ] years old

25. How old were you when your first child was born?	[ ] years old (If no children write 0)

26. How long has it been since your last breast x-ray (mammogram)?

1 ☐ Less than 1 year ago
2 ☐ 1 year ago
3 ☐ 2 years ago
4 ☐ 3 or more years ago
5 ☐ Never

27. How many women in your natural family (mother and sisters only) have had breast cancer?

☐ women

28. Have you had a hysterectomy operation?

1 ☐ Yes
2 ☐ No
3 ☐ Not sure

29. How long has it been since you had a pap smear?

1 ☐ Less than 1 year ago
2 ☐ 1 year ago
3 ☐ 2 years ago
4 ☐ 3 or more years ago
5 ☐ Never

★ 30. How often do you examine your breasts for lumps?

1 ☐ Monthly
2 ☐ Once every few months
3 ☐ Rarely or never

★ 31. About how long has it been since you had your breasts examined by a physican or nurse?

1 ☐ Less than 1 year ago
2 ☐ 1 year ago
3 ☐ 2 years ago
4 ☐ 3 or more years ago
5 ☐ Never

★ 32. About how long has it been since you had a rectal exam?

☛ (WOMEN GO TO QUESTION 34)

1 ☐ Less than 1 year ago
2 ☐ 1 year ago
3 ☐ 2 years ago
4 ☐ 3 or more years ago
5 ☐ Never

MEN
★ 33. About how long has it been since you had a rectal or prostate exam?

1 ☐ Less than 1 year ago
2 ☐ 1 year ago
3 ☐ 2 years ago
4 ☐ 3 or more years ago
5 ☐ Never

★ 34. How many times in the last year did you witness or become involved in a violent fight or attack where there was a good chance of a serious injury to someone?

1 ☐ 4 or more times
2 ☐ 2 or 3 times
3 ☐ 1 time or never
4 ☐ Not sure

★ 35. Considering your age, how would you describe your overall physical health?

1 ☐ Excellent
2 ☐ Good
3 ☐ Fair
4 ☐ Poor

★ 36. In an average week, how many times do you engage in physical activity (exercise or work which lasts at least 20 minutes without stopping and which is hard enough to make you breathe heavier and your heart beat faster)?

1 ☐ Less than 1 time per week
2 ☐ 1 or 2 times per week
3 ☐ At least 3 times per week

★ 37. If you ride a motorcycle or all-terrain vehicle (ATV) what percent of the time do you wear a helmet?

1 ☐ 75% to 100%
2 ☐ 25% to 74%
3 ☐ Less than 25%
4 ☐ Does not apply to me

Continued.

| ★38. Do you eat some food every day that is high in fiber, such as whole grain bread, cereal, fresh fruits or vegetables? | 1 ☐ Yes   2 ☐ No |

| ★39. Do you eat foods every day that are high in cholesterol or fat such as fatty meat, cheese, fried foods, or eggs? | 1 ☐ Yes   2 ☐ No |

| ★40. In general, how satisfied are you with your life? | 1 ☐ Mostly satisfied
2 ☐ Partly satisfied
3 ☐ Not satisfied |

| ★41. Have you suffered a personal loss or misfortune in the past year that had a serious impact on your life? (For example, a job loss, disability, separation, jail term, or the death of someone close to you.) | 1 ☐ Yes, 1 serious loss or misfortune
2 ☐ Yes, 2 or more
3 ☐ No |

| ★42a. Race | 1 ☐ Aleutian, Alaska native, Eskimo or American Indian
2 ☐ Asian
3 ☐ Black
4 ☐ Pacific Islander
5 ☐ White
6 ☐ Other
7 ☐ Don't know |

| ★42b. Are you of Hispanic origin such as Mexican-American, Puerto Rican, or Cuban? | 1 ☐ Yes   2 ☐ No |

| ★43. What is the highest grade you completed in school? | 1 ☐ Grade school or less
2 ☐ Some high school
3 ☐ High school graduate
4 ☐ Some college
5 ☐ College graduate
6 ☐ Post graduate or professional degree |

★I.

A ☐
B ☐
C ☐
D ☐
E ☐
F ☐
G ☐
H ☐
I ☐
J ☐
K ☐
L ☐

★II.

A ☐
B ☐
C ☐
D ☐
E ☐
F ☐
G ☐
H ☐
I ☐
J ☐
K ☐
L ☐

| Last Name | First Name | M.I. |

| Address | City | State | Zip |

Courtesy Computer Outfitters, Tucson, Arizona.

12–4

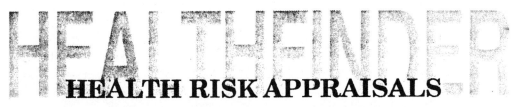

HEALTH RISK APPRAISALS

Health Risk Appraisals (HRA's) are instruments that analyze a person's health history and current lifestyle to determine his or her risk for preventable death or chronic illness. They are gaining popularity in community, school, and workplace health promotion programs as tools to help people recognize the importance of a healthy lifestyle, and they are also being used by physicians in clinical settings. A typical HRA asks questions about habits such as smoking, diet, and exercise, as well as some physiological data, such as weight, cholesterol levels, and blood pressure. The HRA analyzes the individual's responses and compares them to a database of epidemiological and mortality statistics. This analysis shows the individual's risk of death or disease through the "current health age," and gives an "achievable health age" that the person can attain through appropriate changes in health behavior.

HRA's can help motivate people to take responsibility for their own health and to change health-damaging behavior, bringing the added benefit of reduced medical costs and fewer hospitalizations. But there are concerns. HRA's could be used by employers to discriminate against workers, and confidentiality of employee health records is a major issue. Furthermore, HRA's themselves are not completely accurate because occurrence of disease can be only partially explained by exposure to risk factors and because the databases lack adequate information on different age and ethnic groups.

Indeed, the results of some HRA's may not be comparable because they are based on different databases. For example, a person could enter the same personal information for two HRA's and yet receive two very different current health ages and achievable ages. The self-reported information may be inaccurate as well. Another concern is the effectiveness of these health promotion tools. Do they really motivate people to change their habits or is it inappropriate to consider them as vehicles of behavior change?

One aim of current research is to increase accuracy, both by updating the statistical database and by improving the methods used to compute risk. Researchers are also working to develop appraisals for specific populations, such as senior citizens, adolescents, and minority groups. Experts continue to study the risk appraisal process to deal with these issues, but most agree that HRA's must be used in conjunction with counseling or health promotion programs to maximize their effectiveness.

This *Healthfinder* divides HRA's into three categories:

▼ Computer-scored, which are mailed to a central facility where computers score the questionnaires all at one time. This procedure is known as batch processing.

▼ Microcomputer-based, which can be analyzed on a personal computer. Some of these popular HRA's may be scored through either batch processing or the interactive mode, in which the individual answers questions on the computer and the results are displayed on the screen.

▼ Self-scored, which are usually brief and can be scored by the individual.

Most vendors offer volume discounts and package pricing on evaluations and software. Information and materials should be requested directly from the vendors, whose addresses appear on pages 5 and 6.

COMPPUTER-SCORED HRA'S

COSTPREDICT and HEALTHPREDICT
CompuHealth Associates

Developed for organizations, these HRA's calculate costs and savings related to 51 health-related conditions and 44 risk factors.
Questionnaire: Approximately 200 items collect data on habits, stress, medical history, and women's health.
Profile: Reports give predicted costs and savings related to risks, absenteeism, and hospitalization. Individuals receive reports on major health conditions with contributing risk factors. (By Ralph T. Overman, Ph.D.) $6-$8 per evaluation for one PREDICT; an additional $2-$3.50 if both are used; group profiles available.

GENERAL WELL-BEING QUESTIONNAIRE
CompuHealth Associates

This instrument assesses fitness and quality of life as well as future health. It emphasizes research findings rather than mortality statistics.
Questionnaire: Clients are asked to respond to 143 questions and statements covering health attitudes and lifestyle.
Profile: The report provides numerical scores and graphs for a comprehensive set of 30 indicators of general well-being and health. (By Robert Wheeler, Ph.D.) $3 per evaluation; group profiles available.

HEALTH AND LIFESTYLE QUESTIONNAIRE
Health Enhancement Systems

This is another HRA that emphasizes current quality of life over long-term risks.
Questionnaire: The 54 questions collect data on health habits, psychological and job attitudes, and social relationships.
Profile: The resulting 2-page profile does not report statistics but assigns scores ranging from "excellent" to "immediate attention" and discusses the individual's risks. $4-$7.50 per evaluation; $10 with laboratory data; group profiles included.

HEALTH HAZARD APPRAISAL
Prospective Medicine Center

This appraisal is the statistically updated version of the original HRA developed at Methodist Hospital by Drs. Jack Hall and Lewis Robbins.
Questionnaire: The approximately 80 questions cover medical history, family history, lifestyle, stress, and women's health.
Profile: Computer analysis provides a 4-5 page report that is a combination of narrative, bar graph, and tabulated data, including summaries of health age, projected health cost, and stress. $10-$15 per evaluation; group profiles available.

HEALTHLINE
Health Logics

Questionnaire: Forty-four questions gather data on medical history and lifestyle, women's health, stress, and psychological and social factors, exercise, and nutrition.
Profile: A 4-page report uses graphs to display the leading probable causes of death and descriptions of alterable risk factors. A 15-page report displays bar graphs on specific risks such as frustrations, satisfactions, and stresses. $7.50 per 4-page report, $12.50 per 15-page report; group profiles and software available.

HEALTHLOGIC
HMC Software Inc.

Questionnaire: The 17-page booklet includes questions on health history, men's and women's health, stress, and motor vehicle safety.
Profile: A 20-page report focuses on the impact of lifestyle changes on health, fitness, and risk of chronic disease. $15 per evaluation; group reports and software available.

HEALTHPATH
Control Data Corp.

HealthPath is a comprehensive health risk assessment tool designed to serve the cost-containment objectives of a corporation.
Questionnaire: The HRA's 72 questions cover 13 risk/lifestyle areas. Physical measurements and laboratory data are optional.
Profile: The 14-page report scores participants in 11 health habit areas and compares the current scores to that of the baseline profile and the most recent report. $12 per evaluation; group reports available.

HEALTHPLAN and HEALTHPLAN PLUS
General Health, Inc.

Questionnaire: A total of 111 items collect data on personal and family medical history, behavior habits, socioeconomic status, and women's health.
Profile: This 12-page booklet provides brief narrative and graphic information on eight important health areas, current risk as compared to average and achievable risk, and specific recommendations for behavior change. A summary of the individual's five leading health problems in order of importance is also included. Healthplan Plus features a longer and more detailed profile. $16 per evaluation, $26 per Plus evaluation; group profiles and software available.

HEALTH RISK APPRAISAL
University of Michigan

This HRA covers a flexible range of behaviors.
Questionnaire: The basic form includes 50 items covering health habits and medical status. A wider-ranging Lifestyle Development Questionnaire is available.
Profile: The standard 4-page report tabulates risks for five leading causes of death, gives appraisal and achievable ages, recommends ways to reduce risks, and gives a 20-year future projection. A deluxe version includes extensive background information on risk factors. $3-$8 per evaluation; group profiles available.

HEALTH RISK APPRAISAL QUESTIONNAIRE
St. Louis County Health Department

This HRA is based on the Methodist Hospital instrument (see Health Hazard Appraisal, previously cited).
Questionnaire: The 39 questions cover personal and family medical history, health habits, and women's health.
Profile: The 2-page report, a combination of narrative and tabular data, explains the client's risk factors for the 12 leading causes of death as percentages by which he or she deviates from the average; appraisal and achievable ages are also given as are behavioral changes that could reduce risks. $5 per evaluation.

HEALTH RISK ASSESSMENT
University of California

Questionnaire: Personal and family medical history are substantial parts of this 85-question instrument, but it also includes sections on alcohol, smoking, and driving. A special section for women is included.
Profile: The computer analysis gives appraisal and achievable ages, recommends ways to reduce risks, and compares the client's risk factors with those of others of the same age, sex, and race. $5 per evaluation; group profiles available.

HEALTH RISK ASSESSMENT QUESTIONNAIRE
Wisconsin Center for Health Risk Research

Questionnaire: Topics covered in this 96-question HRA on premature mortality risk factors include medical history, physical examination, family history, women's health, and personal health habits.
Profile: A 3-page report is standard; a 5-page report is available at the client's request, describing risks in tabular form. The standard report gives information on health age, achievable age, and top 10 mortality causes and risk factors sorted into four categories, i.e., ideal, average, risky, and not-modifiable. Interactive and batch versions for IBM-PC are expected by 1989. $6.75 per evaluation; group profiles included.

HEALTH RISK QUESTIONNAIRE
Health Enhancement Systems

This program is modifiable for volume users.
Questionnaire: The 39 questions ask about lifestyle, medical history, and some physical and laboratory measurements.
Profile: The report is a combination of narrative and tabulated data, discussing risk factors for 15 major diseases with an emphasis on cancer. A "General Well-Being Questionnaire" to measure stress is also included. $6 per evaluation; group profile included; software available.

HEALTH STATUS PROFILE
Health Evaluation Programs, Inc.

Volume users may modify this instrument also.
Questionnaire: The 21-page questionnaire collects information on current symptoms, medications used, and medical history, and probes nutrition, stress, and exercise habits in detail.
Profile: The individual feedback averages 10 pages, gives appraisal and achievable ages, and discusses individual findings in detail. It also provides suggested readings for each section. $15 per evaluation.

HEALTH WRAP
Lifestyle and Health Promotion
Questionnaire: This HRA contains 93 questions.
Profile: Both a standard risk profile and a "wellness index" are provided. The 3-4 page printout uses a narrative format. This instrument is also distributed by Random House in conjunction with its college textbook series, *Life and Health*. A free, 24-hour computer database and bulletin board is available; the modem line is (504)588-5743. (By Michael Pejsach, Ed.D.) $3.75-$6 per evaluation; group profiles, educational materials, and consultation are available.

INNERVIEW PERSONAL HEALTH ASSESSMENT
Medical Datamation, Inc.

Questionnaire: InnerView Health Assessment is an information gathering system utilizing machine readable questionnaires to gather input on individual lifestyles and health histories.
Profile: Output reports are based on data from the InnerView Health Assessment questionnaire, and are available in a wide variety of formats. Reports for individuals and caregivers provide a comprehensive assessment of health status and recommendations for improved well-being. $8-$12 per evaluation; group profiles available.

LIFE
Wellsource
This HRA is available in batch-processing and interactive formats.
Questionnaire: Included in the 16-page questionnaire are sections on personal and family medical histories, habits and lifestyle, attitudes about health, and physical measurements. Diet, exercise, and other health habits are explored in detail.
Profile: The printout lists 20 major risk indicators (mostly physical measurements), the client's values for these, and the recommended values. It also lists the 20 leading causes of death for the client's age and sex, making recommendations to reduce risks where appropriate. A nutrition profile, a stress profile, and appraisal and achievable ages are included. $12 per evaluation; group profiles and software available.

LIFESCORE PLUS
Center for Corporate Health Promotion

Questionnaire: This 62-question program provides employees with detailed feedback on their health risks. It is based on biomedical measurements (e.g., cholesterol levels and blood pressure), lifestyle habits, and health history.
Profile: Employees receive a computerized report projecting their lifespan and identifying risks. A booklet suggests guidelines to reduce or eliminate these health risks. $5-$9 per evaluation; group profiles are also available.

LIFESTYLE ASSESSMENT QUESTIONNAIRE (LAQ)
National Wellness Institute
Information on resources is an unusual feature of this HRA.
Questionnaire: The 270 questions are divided into two sections. The "Wellness Inventory" section assesses the individual in six dimensions of wellness. The "Personal Growth" section asks the client to select topics on which to receive more information.
Profile: The printout suggests specific resources on topics selected and compares the level of wellness to the average of others who have taken the LAQ. The top 10 risk factors are listed, as well as ways to reduce them. $10 per evaluation; group profiles and software available.

LIFESTYLE DIRECTIONS
Lifestyle Directions, Inc.
Questionnaire: The 30 questions cover diet, exercise, and health.
Profile: The short report presents graphic information on risk for five major diseases. The long report adds recommendations on stress management, diet, and exercise. $15 per short report, $25 per long report.

THE LIFESTYLE MANAGEMENT SYSTEM-
Lifestyle Management Reports, Inc.

This company has seven HRA's which vary in size and complexity.
Questionnaire: The different versions range in size from 75 to 242 questions.
Profile: The personal report, 7 to 45 pages, provides health and lifestyle information with positive feedback comparing the individual's health status to optimal status. The group report, provided for 50 or more individuals, may be used as a management tool in establishing cost-effective health promotion/wellness programs and to measure their effectiveness from year to year. $4.95-$24.95 per individual assessment (health screening costs not included).

PERSONAL STRESS PROFILE
General Health, Inc.
Questionnaire: The 167 questions collect data on personal and family medical history, lifestyle behaviors, socioeconomic status, and stress factors.
Profile: A 12-page booklet aimed at employees in a workplace environment contains explanations on stress and specific recommendations for behavior change. $16 per evaluation.

PULSE
International Health Awareness Center

Questionnaire: The PULSE questionnaire includes 87 questions on nutrition, exercise, stress, personal and family medical history, lifestyle, and habits.
Profile: The 8-page narrative report describes personal health status and compares the individual's mortality risks with those of others in the same demographic group. It includes appraisal and achievable ages and ways to reduce risks in addition to the individual's top five health risks. $8.50-$15 per evaluation; group profiles available.

RHRC HEALTH RISK APPRAISAL
Regional Health Resource Center

In addition to assessing individual risks, this HRA estimates the impact of workplace wellness programs.
Questionnaire: The 39 questions cover lifestyle, medical history, frequency of medical screening, optional laboratory data, and women's health. An additional "General Well-Being Questionnaire" measures stress.
Profile: The 5-page report, a combination of narrative and tabular data, includes 10-year mortality estimates for the 12 leading causes of death, estimated annual hospital days, and advice on reducing risks. A group profile includes the estimated reduction in work force mortality and hospitalization achievable through wellness programs. $4-$6 per evaluation; group profiles available.

WELL AWARE HEALTH RISK APPRAISAL
Well Aware About Health

The emphasis of this HRA, developed under a 5-year Kellogg Foundation research grant, is on quality of life and current risks.
Questionnaire: The questionnaire gathers information on health habits and lifestyle, health knowledge, stress, and women's health.
Profile: The 16-page report includes mortality predictions but stresses practical measures to improve health. Topics include diet, motor vehicle safety, alcohol use, stress index, and sociability index, as well as the results of physical and laboratory measurements. $15 per evaluation; group profiles and supplementary courseware available.

MICROCOMPUTER-BASED HRA'S

A-HRA
Health Enhancement Systems

This is an interactive or batch processing program for the Macintosh.
Questionnaire: 46 questions cover the standard lifestyle and health history areas.
Profile: printout includes narrative, graphics, and group report. License fee will vary.

AVIVA
Center for Research in Medical Education and Health Care Jefferson Medical College

This interactive HRA is designed to assess hospitalization risks, but concerns only those risks which an individual can modify.
Questionnaire: A short (5-10 minutes) or a long (15-20 minutes) version can be chosen. The program screens users to ensure that the interview is appropriate; for example, it is inappropriate for pregnant women. Questions cover alcohol consumption, driving habits, weight, blood pressure, cholesterol levels, depression, and smoking. The user can ask why certain information is requested and receive explanations.
Profile: The online profile gives an overall risk score adjusted for age and sex, the contribution of each risk factor to the score, and suggestions for modifying risks. For IBM-PC; $75. The program listing has been printed in the journal *Medical Care* (July 1987).

COSTPREDICT and HEALTHPREDICT
CompuHealth Associates

See entry under "Computer-scored HRA's." May be used with the Automated Physician's Management System. For IBM-PC; $450.

GENERAL WELL-BEING QUESTIONNAIRE
CompuHealth Associates

See entry under "Computer-scored HRA's." For Apple II and IBM-PC; $150.

HEALTH AGE AND LONGEVITY
Wellsource

Questionnaire: Ten items collect information on seven health habits in this program which can be run in either interactive or batch processing mode.
Profile: The report computes a health age in contrast to

chronological age. It also gives achievable age and suggests ways to reduce risks. For IBM-PC; $250. Corporate/Statistical Summary Option; $75.

HEALTH APPRAISAL
University of Michigan

See entry under "Computer-scored HRA's." For IBM PC; $295. Customization available.

HEALTH AWARENESS GAMES
Queue Inc.

This is a set of five microcomputer programs that draw on statistics about lifestyle and health as they relate to life expectancy.
Questionnaire: The five programs are Coronary Risk, Why Do You Smoke?, Exercise and Weight, Life Expectancy, and Lifestyle.
Profile: Separate profiles and recommendations for change are displayed with each program. The distributor states that it is appropriate for audiences from junior high school through college and is suitable for home use as well. (By Lynda Ellis, Ph.D.) For Apple II+, IIE, and IIC; TRS-80, Model III and 4; IBM-PC and PC Jr.; teaching guide included; $99.

HEARTCHEC and HEARTCHEC PLUS
Wellsource

Questionnaire: This is a 79-question profile on heart health and includes the following subjects: eating habits, smoking, exercise, stress, and other lifestyle factors.
Profile: The test also includes subjects on blood pressure and pulse, blood tests for total cholesterol and blood sugar. The HeartChec Plus version also tests for HDL cholesterol and triglycerides. For IBM-PC. HeartChec, $245; HeartChec Plus, $295; corporate report, $125 Exam packet, $5.

HEALTH RISK APPRAISAL
University of Minnesota Media Distribution

Questionnaire: This interactive HRA is based on the old CDC HRA and asks up to 40 questions on lifestyle and physiological indicators.
Profile: It displays the user's risks for 10 leading causes of death and provides a 1-page summary printout. (By John Raines, M.D., and Lynda Ellis, Ph.D.) For Apple II, II+, IIe, and IBM-PC; $97.

HEALTH RISK QUESTIONNAIRE
Health Enhancement Systems

See entry under "Computer-scored HRA's." For IBM-PC; $750.

HEALTHSTYLE
Wellsource

Based on *HealthStyle: A Self Test*, a self-scoring questionnaire, this program is designed for individual and interactive users. The scores are printed out, rather than being displayed on the screen.
Questionnaire: The 24 items cover the health habits listed under *HealthStyle: A Self Test* in the next section.
Profile: The printout displays the scores in bar graphs, with values ranging from unhealthful to healthful. The individual's and the group's scores are compared to those of the general population. An explanation sheet interprets the scores and gives advice on reducing risks. For IBM-PC; $190; corporate report, $75.

LIFESCAN
National Wellness Institute

LifeScan is available in interactive or batch-processing format.
Questionnaire: The 40 questions cover physical activity, drug usage, driving habits, cholesterol level, medical history, and women's health issues.
Profile: Each individual receives a printout listing his or her top 10 risk factors and suggested methods to reduce these risks. A special feature of this HRA is a listing of the individual's positive lifestyle behaviors. For IBM-PC; $695.

LIFESCORE M
Center for Corporate Health Promotion

This interactive program is based on Lifescore-C, a self-scoring questionnaire described in the next section.
Questionnaire: In addition to habits and lifestyle, the questions cover environmental factors, utilization of health care, and family medical history.
Profile: Scores are interpreted in items of general health and life expectancy. For IBM-PC; $250.

LIFE STRESS ANALYSIS
MedMicro

This interactive program correlates stressful events of the past year with the probability of illness in the next year.
Questionnaire: There are 15 questions about stressful events of the past year.
Profile: The program gives a Life Stress score and the probability of illness in the next year. For IBM-PC; $29.

MacWRAP
Lifestyle and Health Promotion

See HEALTH WRAP entry under "Computer-scored HRA's." For Macintosh Plus, SE, or II; $295 until November 15, 1988, $325 thereafter.

MICRO-HRA
Planetree Medical Systems

This program employs the Carter Center HRA. It may be used interactively or in a batch-processing mode.
Questionnaire: The 62 questions cover nutrition, stress, family history, lab tests, and women's health.
Profile: Five reports are possible, including a detailed epidemiological report and group summaries. (By Arden Ashton, M.D.) For IBM-PC; $485.

PERSONAL HEALTH APPRAISAL
MedMicro

There are two versions: The personal version is interactive, and the professional version can be used in either an interactive or batch-processing mode and can store and update profiles.
Questionnaire: The 84 items cover medical history and occupational health information as well as lifestyle. An additional 20 questions concern women's health.
Profile: In the interactive mode, feedback is given throughout the interaction, and the user's life expectancy is calculated at the end. The professional version also allows for an 8-page, explanatory printout, on which an organization's logo may be imprinted. This HRA includes an analysis of the user's "Cancer Early Warning Signs" (American Cancer Society) and preventive health practices. For IBM-PC; $59.50 (personal version), $259.50 (professional version). A $100 utility will transfer all user data directly to Lotus 1-2-3.

RHRC HEALTH RISK APPRAISAL

See entry under "Computer-scored HRA's." Group reports can be generated. For IBM-PC; $795.

SPHERE
University of British Columbia

This interactive or batch-processed program is available in English and French versions based on Canadian statistics, and in an English version based on U.S. statistics.
Questionnaire: The 25 items cover medical and lifestyle characteristics.
Profile: Graphic displays as well as narratives explain each user's risks and appraisal and achievable ages. For IBM-PC; $100 (interactive or batch).

TESTWELL
National Wellness Institute

Questionnaire: The 100-question program measures strength in each of six dimensions of wellness: social, occupational, spiritual, physical, intellectual, and emotional.
Profile: A printout lists each category along with the percentile score. For IBM-PC; $195; also available as a self-scoring questionnaire, $.75.

WELLNESS INVENTORY - INTERACTIVE
Wellness Associates

Adapted from the self-scoring questionnaire of the same name, this interactive program emphasizes stress, personal relationships, and social attitudes. It is based on Wellness Associates' Wellness Workbook, not statistical data. Statistical norms are being developed.
Questionnaire: The 120 items assess the user's lifestyle in 12 areas of personal energy expenditure, such as "Eating," "Feeling," and "Transcending."
Profile: The resulting report shows the balance or lack of balance in the 12 areas, prints an individualized list of priorities for personal growth, and cites references for further reading. (By John W. Travis, M.D., M.P.H.) For IBM-PC; Macintosh Plus, SE, and II (requires Hypercard software); $45.

SELF-SCORED QUESTIONAIRES

HEALTHSTYLE: A SELF-TEST
ODPHP National Health Information Center

This 2-page, 24-question form, published by the U.S. Public Health Service, includes an introductory section explaining how personal habits influence one's health and a concluding section that gives specific suggestions for reducing risks. Areas covered in this HRA are nutrition, alcohol and drug use, smoking, fitness, stress, and safety. Each section is scored on a scale of 1 to 10, and the scores are explained in general terms with ideas for improvement. A single copy or reproducible master is available free of charge.

HOPE HEALTH APPRAISAL
International Health Awareness Center

A complete health kit designed to help an individual manage his health risk and improve his lifestyle. Includes 12 self-scoring tests and some informational brochures. $3.95.

HOW DO YOU RATE AS A HEALTH RISK?
Channing L. Bete Co., Inc.

This HRA booklet includes 40 questions on the following topics: smoking, alcohol and other drugs, nutrition, weight control, exercise, stress, and safety. The booklet also offers suggestions on ways to improve an individual's present condition. Minimum order of 25 copies. $19.75.

LIFESCORE-C
Center for Corporate Health Promotion

Designed for employee health programs, this questionnaire comes with an attached carbon copy. Each employee keeps a self-scored copy, while the carbons are batch-processed to yield a group profile. Questions cover lifestyle, environmental factors, family medical history, and utilization of health care. Scores are given for general health and life expectancy. See also "Lifescore M" under "Micro-computer-Based HRA's." (Adapted from *Lifeplan for Your Health* by Donald M. Vickery). $1.55-$3 per evaluation; group profiles included.

WELLNESS INDEX/ WELLNESS INVENTORY
Wellness Associates

Both the Index with 380 questions and the Inventory with 120 questions assess wellness in 12 areas of personal energy expenditure, emphasizing stress factors, personal relationships, and social attitudes. Scores are entered on a "Wellness Index Wheel" to demonstrate graphically the balance or lack of balance among the 12 areas. Followup is provided in the *Wellness Workbook* by J.W. Travis and R. Ryan, Ten Speed Press, 1988, $11.95. (By John W. Travis, M.D., M.P.H). $1.50-$2.90.

VENDOR LIST

Center for Corporate Health Promotion
1850 Centennial Park Drive
Suite 520
Reston, VA 22091
(703)391-1900

Center for Research in Medical Education and Health Care
Jefferson Medical College
Philadelphia, PA 19107
(215)928-8907
Attn: Dr. Farrokh Alemi

Channing L. Bete Co., Inc.
200 State Road
South Deerfield, MA 01373
(800)628-7733; (413)665-7611 in MA

CompuHealth Associates
13795 Rider Trail
Earth City, MO 63045
(314)291-5958

Control Data Corp.
StayWell/EAR Division
901 East 78th Street
Minneapolis, MN 55420
(612)853-3772
Attn: G.L. Anderson

General Health, Inc.
3299 K Street, NW.
Washington, DC 20007
(800)424-2775
(202)965-4881 in DC area

Health Evaluation Programs, Inc.
808 Busse Highway
Park Ridge, IL 60068
(312)696-1824
Attn: John F. Joyce

Health Enhancement Systems
9 Mercer Street
Princeton, NJ 08540
(800)437-6668
(609)924-7799 in NJ
Attn: John Rassweiler

Health Logics
111 Deerwood Place
San Ramon, CA 94583
(415)831-4881
Attn: Linda Hojnacki

HMC Software Inc.
4200 North MacArthur Boulevard
Irving, TX 75038
(800)255-6809
(214)255-5430 in TX
Attn: John Ellis

International Health Awareness Center
157 South Kalamazoo Mall
Suite 482
Kalamazoo, MI 49007-4895
(616)343-0770
Attn: Shawn M. Connors

Lifestyle and Health Promotion
59 Monterrey Avenue
Kenner, LA 70065
(504)443-4958
Attn: Michael Pejsach

Lifestyle Directions, Inc.
300 Ninth Street
Conway, PA 15027-1696
(412)869-2164
Attn: John Alan Conte

Lifestyle Management Reports, Inc.
368 Congress Street
Boston, MA 02210
(800)531-2348
(617)451-0440 in MA
Attn: James Gillis

Medical Datamation, Inc.
3299 K Street, NW.
Third Floor
Washington, DC 20007
(202)337-7795
Attn: Steve Pederson

MedMicro
6701 Seybold Road
Suite 220A
Madison, WI 53719
(608)274-9599
Attn: Carol Schwartz

I n 1986, the Carter Center of Emory University joined with the Centers for Disease Control (CDC) to update the CDC's HRA instrument, a program that had been adapted from a Canadian product in the 1970's. Twenty major health organizations and a network of State health departments cosponsored the project, which was aimed at updating and expanding the database and at improving accuracy by using multivariate statistical techniques instead of actuarial formulas where possible. The project was completed 2 years later, and the Carter Center assumed full responsibility for user support and program maintenance of this public domain HRA.

The Carter Center HRA has five volumes of documentation which include information on the program's structure and the risk calculations, as well as instructions on how to customize portions of the HRA's analysis and output. User support is provided through periodic updates and through "User Network Focal Points," which are contacts in State health departments or collaborating universities.

Carter Center HRA users must pay a network registration fee of $125 before they receive the HRA package. The Carter Center user network provides training workshops in the ethical and professional use of HRA's. The HRA source code is also available on request to registered users. For further information, contact the Carter Center of Emory University: (404)321-4104.

The CDC operates a computer bulletin board for researchers and administrators interested in HRA's. The modem line is (404)639-2127.

VENDOR LIST   (continued)

National Wellness Institute
University of Wisconsin-
Stevens Point
South Hall
Stevens Point, WI 54481
(715)346-2172
Attn: Patrick Salaski

ODPHP National Health
Information Center
P.O. Box 1133
Washington, DC 20013
(800)336-4797
(301)565-4167 in MD

Planetree Medical Systems
3519 South 1200 East
Salt Lake City, UT 84106
(801)486-7640
Attn: Dr. Arden Ashton

Prospective Medicine Center
Suite 219
3901 North Meridian
Indianapolis, IN 46208
(317)923-3600

Queue Inc.
562 Boston Avenue
Bridgeport, CT 06610
(800)232-2244
(203)335-0908 in CT

Regional Health Resource
Center
Medical Information
Laboratory
1408 West University Avenue
Urbana, IL 61801
(217)367-0076

St. Louis County Health
Department
1001 East First Street
Duluth, MN 55805
(218)727-7547
Attn: Jean Mershon

University of British
Columbia
Health Care and
Epidemiology
5804 Fairview Crescent
Mather Building
Vancouver, BC V6T W5
Canada
(604)228-2258

University of California
Epidemiology and
International Health
1699 HSW
San Francisco, CA 94143
(415)476-1158
Attn: Theresa L. Braun

University of Michigan
Fitness Research Center
401 Washtenaw Avenue
Ann Arbor, MI 48109-2214
(313)763-2462
Attn: Terri Goodman

University of Minnesota
Media Distribution
Box 734, Mayo Building
420 Delaware Street, SE.
Minneapolis, MN 55455
(612)624-7906

Well Aware About Health
P.O. Box 43338
Tucson, AZ 85733
(602)297-2960 or 2819
Attn: Sabina Dunton

Wellsource
15431 Southeast 82nd Drive,
Suite E
P.O. Box 569
Clackamas, OR 97015
(503)656-7446
Attn: Forrest Knudson

Wellness Associates
7899-T St. Helena Road
Santa Rosa, CA 95404
(707)539-0507

Wisconsin Center for Health
Risk Research
University of Wisconsin
Center for Health Sciences
600 Highland Avenue, Room
J5/224
Madison, WI 53792
(608)263-9530
Attn: Dr. Norman Jensen

12–5

National Health Promotion and Education Resources

General resources

National AIDS Information
Clearinghouse (NAIC)
P.O. Box 6003
Rockville, MD 20850
1-800-458-5231

American Dental Association
211 East Chicago Ave.
Chicago, IL 60611
(312) 440-2593

American Diabetes Association
(National Headquarters)
Public Relations
1660 Duke Street
Alexandria, VA 22314
1-800-232-2472

American Red Cross
Public Affairs
National Headquarters
17th and D Streets, N.W.
Washington, DC 20006
(202) 737-8300

National Arthritis and Musculoskeletal and
    Skin Diseases Information Clearinghouse
P.O. Box AMS
Bethesda, MD 20892
(301) 468-3235

National Audiovisual Center
8700 Edgeworth Drive
Capitol Heights, MD 20743-3701
(301) 763-1896

Business Coalitions for Health Action
1615 H Street, N.W.
Washington, DC 20062
(202) 463-4970

Centers for Disease Control & Prevention
Center for Health Promotion & Education
Bldg. 3, Room 121
Atlanta, GA 30333
(404) 329-3923

Centers for Disease Control and Prevention
Educational Resources Branch
Bldg. 1 South, Room SSB 249
Atlanta, GA 30333
(404) 329-3492

Channing L. Bete Co., Inc.
200 State Road
South Deerfield, MA 01373
1-800-628-7733

Office of Consumer Affairs
Consumer Inquiries Section
5600 Fishers Lane
Rockville, MD 20857
(301) 443-3170

Consumer Information Center
General Services Administration
Pueblo, CO 81009
(202) 501-1794

Consumer Product Safety Commission (CPSC)
5401 Westbard Ave., Room 332
Bethesda, MD 20207
1-800-638-2772

Department of Health & Human Services
Office of Disease Prevention & Health Promotion
Health Information Center
P.O. Box 1133
Washington, DC 20013-1133
1-800-336-4797

Environmental Protection Agency (EPA)
Public Information Center, PM
211B, 401 M Street SW
Washington, DC 20460
(202) 382-2080

Family Information Center
National Agricultural Library
Room 304, Department of Agriculture
10301 Baltimore Boulevard
Beltsville, MD 20705
(301) 344-3719

National Health Information Clearinghouse
P.O. Box 1133
Washington, DC 20013-1133
1-800-336-4797

Health Research, Inc.
Health Education Services Division
P.O. Box 7126
Albany, NY 12224
No number listed

Health Systems Resources
601 Valley Street, Suite #201
Seattle, WA 98109
(206) 464-6143

National Heart, Lung and Blood Institute
National Institutes of Health
Bldg. 31, Room 4A21
Bethesda, MD 20892
(301) 496-4236

National Injury Information Clearinghouse
U.S. Consumer Product Safety Commission
5401 Westbard Ave., Room 625
Washington, DC 20207
(301) 492-6424

National Kidney and Urologic Diseases
Information Clearinghouse (NKUDIC)
Box NKUDIC
9000 Rockville Pike
Bethesda, MD 20892
(301) 468-6345

Krames Communications
Dept. 388
312 90th Street
Daly City, CA 94015-1898
1-800-228-8347;
1-800-445-7267 in CA

March of Dimes Birth Defects Foundation
1275 Mamaroneck Ave.
White Plains, NY 10605
(914) 428-7100

Metropolitan Insurance Co.
Health and Safety Education Division
One Madison Ave.
New York, NY 10010
(212) 578-2211

Clearinghouse for Occupational Safety & Health
Information
Technical Information Branch
4676 Columbia Parkway
Cincinnati, OH 45226
(513) 533-8326

Planned Parenthood Federation of America
NFSEM
810 Seventh Ave.
New York, NY 10019
(212) 541-7800

National Clearinghouse for Primary Care
Information
8201 Greensboro Drive, Suite 600
McLean, VA 22102
(703) 821-8955

Public Affairs Pamphlets
381 Park Ave., South
New York, NY 10016-8884
(212) 736-6629

National Safety Council
444 North Michigan Ave.
Chicago, IL 60611
(312) 527-4800

National Sudden Infant Death Syndrome
Clearinghouse
8201 Greensboro Drive, Suite 600
McLean, VA 22102
(703) 821-8955

Superintendent of Documents
U.S. Govt. Printing Office
Washington, DC 20402
(202) 783-3238

National Second Surgical Opinion Program
Health Care Financing Administration
200 Independence Ave., SW
Washington, DC 20201
(202) 245-6183

National Technical Information Service
U.S. Department of Commerce
Springfield, VA 22161
(703) 487-4600

National Wellness Institute
1045 Clark Street, Suite 210
Stevens Point, WI 54481
(715) 342-2969

National Resource Center for Worksite
  Health Promotion
777 North Capitol Street, NE
Suite 800
Washington, DC 20002
(202) 408-9320

Aging resources
Administration on Aging
330 Independence Ave. SW
Washington, DC 20201
(202) 245-0351

American Association of Retired Persons
1909 K Street NW
Washington, DC 20049
(202) 872-4700

National Center for Health Promotion and Aging
National Council on Aging
600 Maryland Ave., SW
West Wing 100
Washington, DC 20024
(202) 479-1200

National Resource Center on Health Promotion
  and Aging
1909 K Street NW
5th Floor
Washington, DC 20049
(202) 728-4476
1-800-729-6686

National Institute on Aging
Building 31, Room 5C35
Bethesda, MD 20205
(301) 496-4000

Cancer/smoking resources
American Cancer Society (National Headquarters)
Public Information Department
90 Park Ave.
New York, NY 10016
(212) 736-3030

American Lung Association (National Headquarters)
1740 Broadway
New York, NY 10019
(212) 315-8700

Cancer Information Service
National Cancer Institute
Building 31, Room 10A-24
9000 Rockville Pike
Bethesda, MD 20892
1-800-4-CANCER;
(808) 524-1234 in Oahu, HI

Office on Smoking and Health
Technical Information Center
Park Building, Room 1-16
5600 Fishers Lane
Rockville, MD 20857
(301) 443-1690

Child health resources
Association for the Care of Children
3615 Wisconsin Ave. NW
Washington, DC 20016
(202) 244-1801

Clearinghouse on Child Abuse and Neglect
P.O. Box 1182
Washington, DC 20013
(703) 821-2086

Health and Human Development
National Institutes of Health
Building 31, Room 2A-32
9000 Rockville Pike
Bethesda, MD 20892
(301) 496-5133

Department of Health and Human Services
Division of Maternal and Child Health
Parklawn Building, Room 6-05
5600 Fishers Lane
Rockville, MD 20857
(301) 443-2170

National Center for Education in
  Maternal and Child Health
38th and R Streets, NW
Washington, DC 20057
(202) 625-8410

Exercise and fitness resources
American College of Sports Medicine
1440 Monroe St.
Madison, WI 53706
(608) 262-3632

American Alliance for Health, Physical Education,
Recreation and Dance
1900 Association Drive
Reston, VA 22091
(703) 476-3488

American Running and Fitness Association
2001 S. Street NW
Suite 540
Washington, DC 20009
(202) 667-4150

Association for Fitness in Business
1312 Washington Blvd.
Stamford, CT 06902
(203) 359-2188

President's Council on Physical
Fitness & Sports
Judiciary Plaza
405 Fifth St. NW
Suite 7103
Washington, DC 20001
(202) 272-3424

Womens Sports Foundation
Eisenhower Park
East Meadow, NY 11554
1-800-227-3988

Heart-related resources
American Heart Association
7320 Greenville Ave.
Dallas, TX 75231
(214) 750-5414

Citizens for the Treatment of High Blood Pressure
Citizens for Public Action on Cholesterol
888 17th St. NW
Suite 904
Washington, DC 20006
(202) 466-4553

National Cholesterol Education Program
National Heart, Lung and Blood Institute
C-200 Bethesda, MD 20892
(301) 496-0554

National High Blood Pressure Information Center
120/80 National Institutes of Health
Bethesda, MD 20892
(301) 496-1809

Mental health resources
American Institute of Stress
124 Park Ave.
Yonkers, NY 10703
(914) 963-1200

Institute of Stress Management
United States International University
School of Human Behavior
10455 Pormerado Road
San Diego, CA 92131
(619) 271-4300

Mental Health Association
1021 Prince Street
Alexandria, VA 22314
(703) 276-8800

National Institute of Mental Health
Public Inquiries Branch
Office of Scientific Information
Praklawn Bldg., Room 15C-05
5600 Fishers Lane
Rockville, MD 20857
(301) 443-3513

Nutrition resources
American Dairy Association
6300 North River Road
Rosemont, IL 60018
(312) 696-1880

Center for Science in the Public Interest
1501 16th St., NW
Washington, DC 20036-1499
(202) 332-9110

Food and Drug Administration
Office of Consumer Affairs
5600 Fishers Lane
HFE-88
Rockville, MD 20857
(301) 443-1544

Food and Nutrition Information Center
National Agricultural Library
Room 304
Beltsville, MD 20705
(301) 344-3719

General Foods Consumer Nutrition Services
North Street
White Plains, NY 10625
1-800-431-1004

Giant Foods Inc.
Consumer Affairs Dept.
P.O. Box 1804
Washington, DC 20013
1-800-638-0268

ILSI International Life Sciences Institute
Nutrition Foundation
1126 16th Street, NW
Suite 111
Washington, DC 20036
(202) 659-0074

Mazola Nutrition/Health Information Services
Box 307
Coventry, CT 06238
No number listed

North Dakota Wheat Comm.
Education Materials
1305 East Central Ave.
Bismark, ND 58505
(701) 224-2498

The Pennsylvania State University
Nutrition Information and Resource Center
Beecher House
University Park, PA 16802
(814) 865-6323

The Pillsbury Company
Box 5876
Minneapolis, Minn 55480
1-800-328-4466

Society for Nutrition Education
1700 Broadway, Suite 300
Oakland, CA 94612
No number listed

United Fresh Fruit & Vegetable Association
727 N Washington Street
Alexandria, VA 22314
(703) 836-3410

Substance abuse resources
Alcoholics Anonymous World Services
P.O. Box 459
Grand Central Station
New York, NY 10163
(212) 683-3900

American Council on Alcoholism
National Executive Offices
8501 LaSalle Rd. Suite 301
Towson, MD 21204
(410) 931-9393

National Clearinghouse for Alcohol and Drug
Information
P.O. Box 2345
Rockville, MD 20852
(301) 468-2600

National Council on Alcoholism
12 West 21st
New York, NY 10010
(212) 206-6770

National Federation of Parents for Drug-Free Youth
8730 Georgia Ave., Suite 200
Silver Spring, MD 20910
No number listed

Women's health resource
ACOG Resource Center
American College of Obstetricians and
Gynecologists
600 Maryland Avenue, SW
Suite 300 East
Washington, DC 20024-2588
(202) 863-2518

American Fertility Society
2140 11th Avenue South
Suite 200
Birmingham, AL 35205-2800
(205) 251-9764

Anorexia Bulimia
Treatment and Education Center
(800) 33-ABTEC;
(301) 332-9800 in MD

Bulimia Anorexia
Self-Help
6125 Clayton Avenue
Suite 215
St. Louis, MO 63139
1-800-227-4785
24-hour Crisis Line:
1-800-762-3334

Center for Women Policy Studies
2000 P Street, NW
Suite 508
Washington, DC 20036
(202) 872-1770

C-Sec Inc.
Cesarean/Support Education and Concern
22 Forest Road
Framingham, MA 01701
(617) 877-8266

Endometriosis Association
P.O. Box 92187
Milwaukee, WI 53202
(415) 962-8972;
1-800-992-ENDO in WI

Family Life Information Exchange
P.O. Box 10716
Rockville, MD 20850
(301) 770-3662

Maternity Center Association
48 East 92nd Street
New York, NY 10128
(212) 369-7300

National Osteoporosis Foundation
1625 Eye Street, NW
Suite 1011
Washington, DC 20006
(202) 223-2226

9 to 5; National Association of Working Women
614 Superior Avenue, NW
Cleveland, OH 44113
(216) 266-9308

PMS Access
P.O. Box 9326
Madison, WI 53715
1-800-222-4767;
(608) 833-4767 in WI

Women's Occupational Health
Resource Center
117 St. Johns Place
Brooklyn, NY 11217
(718) 230-8822

Women's Sports Foundation
342 Madison Avenue
Suite 728
New York, NY 10173
1-800-227-3988;
(212) 972-9170 in AK, HI, and NYC metro area

13

MANAGEMENT CONCEPTS, PRINCIPLES, AND APPLICATIONS

In many occupational health settings, the occupational health nurse functions as a manager or member of the management team. In addition, the occupational health manager must have a good understanding of organizational culture and dynamics as described in Chapter 8, and possess knowledge and skills about concepts related to leadership, quality improvement and cost management, and the importance of change in a dynamic environment. The occupational health nurse manager must be thoroughly familiar with the organization's purpose, goals, and structures that support the organization's mission. This chapter will focus on a discussion of concepts and skills important to effective managerial guidance.

■ DEFINITIONS

There are many definitions of management; however, two common threads that permeate these definitions are organizational goal achievement and people orientation. A discrete, yet targeted and encompassing definition is offered by Hersey and Blanchard (1993), who define management as working with and through individuals and groups to accomplish organizational goals. The terms management and leadership are often used synonymously or interchangeably; however, the concept of leadership is broader and is not bound by organizational structures and boundaries. Thus, it involves the process of influencing the behavior of other persons in their efforts toward goal setting and achievement, whether the goals are personal, organizational, or professional (Yura et al., 1986; Yukl, 1989).

■ MANAGERIAL SKILLS

In a classic article by Katz (1955), three management skill levels are identified as important to the managerial role, including technical, interpersonal, and conceptual skills:

1. Technical skills emphasize the use of knowledge, methods, processes, procedures, techniques, and equipment necessary for the performance of specific tasks and activities.

2. Interpersonal skills utilize knowledge about human behavior and interpersonal processes, including an understanding of motivational and leadership concepts and effective communication techniques.

3. Conceptual skills are concerned with the ability to understand organizational complexities and dynamics, analyze internal/external trends that impact the organization, and develop and conceptualize ideas that provide a visionary direction for the organization as a whole.

Managers need all three skills to fulfill their role requirements, but the relative importance of each skill depends on the situation and the manager's position in the authority hierarchy of the organization.

As illustrated in Figure 13–1, the manager's skill mix is dependent on the role and level at which she or he functions in the organization. As one advances in the management/organizational structure, less technical and more conceptual skills are needed (Yukl, 1989). However, top level executives need to have an understanding of how these skills interrelate. The occupational health nurse may find herself or himself in the role of manager of the occupational health unit, manager of occupational health services, or as a regional or corporate nurse or health director. Managerial skills should be developed to reflect the level and scope of responsibilities attached to the position.

As described by Katz and Kahn (1978), conceptual skills, the major responsibility of top executives, are essential to move the organization forward. This is accomplished through promoting effective strategic planning, policy formulation and program development, recognizing the influence and impact of the external environment, and understanding inter and intra relationships among and within the organizational units. In order to effectively lead the organization, input must be actively sought from all levels in the organization.

The authors describe the role of middle managers as primarily focused on furthering organizational goals and developing plans to implement policies established at higher levels. While this requires some skill in visioning and technical competence, good communication and interpersonal skills are essential to empower workers to assume increased responsibility for accomplishing the work

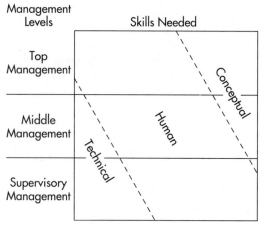

■ **Figure 13–1** Managerial skill mix at various organizational levels. (From Paul Hersey/Kenneth H. Blanchard, MANAGEMENT OF ORGANIZATIONAL BEHAVIOR: Utilizing Human Resources, 6e, © 1993, pp. 8, 195. Reprinted by permission of Prentice-Hall, Englewood Cliffs, New Jersey.)

goals and objectives. Technical skills are particularly important at the supervisory level in order to train, develop, and direct workers regarding specialized activities, and to evaluate their performance. Supervisory level managers are mainly responsible for implementing policy and maintaining the workflow within the organizational structure.

Of course, the type, size, and structure of organizations need to be considered with respect to managerial skill levels. For example, in organizations where decision making is highly decentralized, technical skills are less important for top level executives; whereas in smaller organizations that operate with highly centralized decision-making authority, top level executives may require more intense technical skill abilities. Although middle managers may be placed in the position to deal with human relations problems and situations, interpersonal or human relations skills fall within the domain of all levels of managers. Organizations are social systems that require both individual productivity and teamwork to achieve organizational goals. As the occupational health unit manager, the occupational health nurse must possess the ability to relate to people, communicate clearly, manage conflict, and promote productivity through motivation, which is central to human resource management.

■ DECISION MAKING

In order to function effectively the manager needs to be skilled in making effective decisions (Kerfoot, 1988); thus, the occupational health nurse manager needs to be familiar with the decision-making process. As described by Gillies (1989) and Marriner Tomey (1991) decision making is a dynamic, deliberate, cognitive process consisting of sequential steps that allow for more rational and accurate problem solving and action. One decision ultimately affects other decisions. Steps in the decision-making process, as modified from Gillies (1989) and Marriner-Tomey (1991), are illustrated in Figure 13–2. A discussion of this process within the context of occupational health follows.

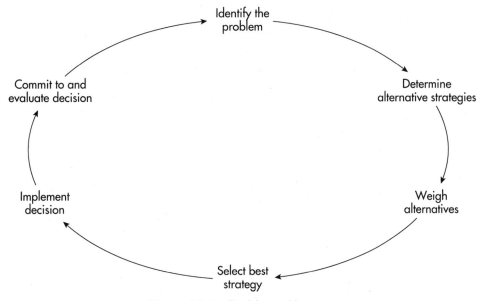

■ **Figure 13–2** Decision-making process.

1. **Identify the problem.** The occupational health nurse manager needs to be perceptive to problem awareness and gather as much data as needed in order to fully identify the problem. For example, if there appears to be a turf issue at work, the real problem may be an inadequate job description or ill-defined task delineation. Once the real problem is identified, effective decision making can begin.

2. **Determine alternative courses of action.** Usually there are a number of ways to solve a problem. The occupational health nurse manager should first determine if a policy exists to handle the situation. If no policy exists, the manager should explore various avenues, such as experience, literature, consultation, and brainstorming with staff members. Creative ideas are likely to emerge from examination of these various sources. The greater the number of alternatives identified, the higher the probability of problem resolution.

3. **Weigh alternatives.** The pros and cons of each alternative should be considered and measured against the current method of handling the problem or situation in order to determine which proposed strategy is potentially the most effective. Resources and constraints such as manpower, human relations, finances, facilities, and equipment must be evaluated to determine potential pitfalls that might be avoided if they can be managed up front.

4. **Select an alternative.** The nurse manager and/or group should select the alternative that will yield the best results within a cost-efficient framework. Multiple factors should be considered in selecting a strategy, including worker acceptance, morale, time, and risk of failure.

5. **Implement decision.** Hopefully, coworkers have been involved in the decision-making process so that implementation of the decision will not create undue antagonism. Often situations that require change will arouse uncomfortableness so the manager will need to communicate with staff regarding the best approaches to decision implementation. Involvement of staff will help to increase ownership and decrease resistance.

6. **Commit to and evaluate decision.** The manager should allow for some time to pass in order for the decision to be integrated. There may be resistance to the decision; however, if the decision was made thoughtfully, management should adhere to the decision commitment. If after time it is recognized that the decision is not workable, alternative strategies may need to be invoked.

There are many tools and techniques to help the occupational health nurse manager in the decision-making process such as brainstorming, nominal group process, decision trees, PERT models (program evaluation and review techniques), Delphi methods, critical path analyses, and simulated computer applications and analyses. The nurse manager may make independent decisions or involve the group responsible for decision implementation. This will be dependent on the manager's knowledge and expertise relative to the area under consideration, degree of commitment from the group, time constraints, and impact and importance of the decision.

■ MANAGERIAL FUNCTIONS

The managerial process engages the five major functions of planning, organizing, staffing/coordinating, leading/directing, and controlling. The planning function is the most important and provides the groundwork for all other functions. Although these functions are described separately, they are interrelated. As an effective manager, the occupational health nurse will need to possess skills in all areas (Marriner-Tomey, 1991).

Planning

Planning is the first managerial function and is critical to the management process. Planning requires conceptual thinking, the results of which set the stage for effective strategic and operational functioning (Goodstein, Nolan, & Pfeifer, 1992; Simyar & Lloyd-Jones, 1988). Planning is a continuous process of assessing and analyzing organizational needs (Chapter 8); establishing the organization's mission, goals, and objectives; determining organizational capabilities and potential courses of action; and evaluating achievement and results of goal attainment. It involves the effective use of human and fiscal resources.

Establishing Goals and Objectives

When planning for occupational health programs and services, it is important for the occupational health nurse manager to identify and/or review the organizational mission, goals, and objectives, and determine where in the structure the occupational health unit fits. The nurse manager should be familiar with the organization's history, structure, value system, and organizational culture, particularly with respect to health care, existing occupational health and safety programs, leadership/management styles, trends in illness/injury, health care costs, professional attitudes, role behaviors, communication lines and patterns, and productivity measures (Gillies, 1989; Hersey & Blanchard, 1993). Although it may seem evident, it is essential for the occupational health nurse manager to clarify the purpose of the occupational health service and/or program. For example, does the occupational health service exist to reduce work-related risk, improve worker health, prevent premature disability and mortality, or for a combination of these reasons or for other reasons?

In congruence with the organization's mission and goals, occupational health unit goals and objectives should be established in order to achieve the unit's purpose. Goals are broad statements central to the whole management process, and the planning process explicitly defines the goals. Objectives are specific aims set to achieve the goals and they should be measurable. Goals and objectives may address, for example, existing programs and services or use of resources or innovations and should be prioritized as to order of importance. Personnel involved in setting goals and objectives should be familiar with the needs of the organizational unit. For example, the board of directors and top level administrators usually set organizational goals and objectives, whereas the corporate nurse or occupational health nurse manager sets the goals and objectives for the occupational health/nursing service in collaboration with other staff members. Goals and objectives should be reviewed periodically to assess progress toward achievement and/or need for modification. Examples of occupational health goals and programmatic objectives are shown in Table 13–1.

Management by Objectives, first introduced by Peter Drucker in the 1950s, is a tool and philosophy used for both planning and control functions and is aimed at improving worker motivation and productivity (Drucker, 1982). It is widely used by American business and in the health care sector. The purpose of Management by Objectives is to aid workers and managers to negotiate

■ **TABLE 13–1**   Examples of Occupational Health Goals and Objectives for 1994

GOAL: IMPROVE THE HEALTH OF PREGNANT WORKING MOTHERS
Objectives:
• Provide prenatal education programs stressing the importance of prenatal care and healthy habits.
• Develop communication mechanisms with personal health care providers for appropriate prenatal care monitoring and facilitation of prenatal care.
• Develop strategies to provide emotional support and counseling.
• Reduce the proportion of pregnant women who smoke (by 80%).
• Increase the percentage of women who improve their nutritional intake (by 50%).

GOAL: TO IMPROVE HEALTHY LIFESTYLE HABITS IN THE WORKFORCE
Objectives:
• Provide two health promotion programs targeted to meet the health needs of the workforce.
• Reduce the proportion of workers who smoke by 50%.
• Increase the proportion of workers who exercise regularly by 40%.

---

mutually acceptable goals and performance objectives that are results-oriented and measurable. It helps to broaden participation in day to day decision making and focuses on work outcomes.

Management by Objectives encourages employee growth, strengthens employee identification with organizational goals, promotes self-direction, and builds self-esteem. In Management by Objectives, the manager does not set goals and objectives for the employee; rather, she or he acts as a mentor, collaborator, or coach for the employee. Goal setting is a deliberate act wherein the employee analyzes strengths and weaknesses, reviews the work plan, and establishes measurable objectives. The process allows for feedback and an option to modify objectives and thus provides a more fair evaluation of employee performance (Beyers, 1984; Moss-Kanter, 1989).

In developing objectives, the employee should review job duties and existing responsibilities, outline proposed or expansion initiatives, discuss with the manager key areas needing accomplishment, and construct performance objectives related to these areas along with a target date for achievement of each objective and an action plan.

Specifically, each objective should be:

• written and should address an observable behavior;
• attainable but sufficiently challenging;
• measurable with a target date for completion; and
• mutually agreed upon by the employee and manager.

To determine the outcome of each objective, evaluation criteria must be established in advance against which measurements can be made.

Policies and Procedures

The development of policies and procedures is aimed at facilitating the work toward achievement of the goals and objectives set forth. The occupational health nurse manager should be involved in setting policies and procedures relative to the occupational health unit. Policies are designed to guide workers in their functions and should be comprehensive in scope, stable, fair, unambiguous, and written. Policies are approved and often developed by top management but may originate at any level in the organization (Marriner-Tomey, 1991). Policies should be consistent with the overall goals of the organization, help to solve recurring problems, establish areas of authority, and be accessible and available usually in a policy manual. They should be identified by source, dated, regularly reviewed, modified, and updated. Elements found in a policy manual will vary depending on the organization and its size.

Procedures define specific actions, help define steps in the activity being undertaken, and are often departmental in nature rather than organizational. Procedures serve to standardize operations, provide a basis for orientation and staff development, help to simplify the work, and increase productivity. Before developing a procedure, the nurse manager should consider if a procedure is really needed, as goals can be achieved in different ways. However, if procedures are deemed to be necessary, staff input, if available, should be obtained in their development. Procedures should be dated and written in a consistent format that considers definition, purpose, materials/equipment, steps in the procedure, and documentation. Procedures should be placed in a manual with a table of contents and should be easily accessible. They should be reviewed and updated periodically for accuracy and provided to all staff. Examples of procedures would include chain of custody procedures for urine drug screening, referral and follow-up procedures for employees needing medical evaluation, and procedures for conducting a walk-through.

Budgets

Budgeting is a financial control system defined as a tool for planning, monitoring, and controlling costs (Douglas, 1988). A budget is a quantitative plan, the primary purpose of which is to ensure the most effective use of scarce resources over a period of time. The budget is tied to the formal organizational plan set forth to meet the goals and objectives established in the planning process. Participation in the budget from individuals at all levels in the organization is more likely to produce a budget that is realistic. The presumption is that individuals who are operationally responsible for meeting a part of the overall budget are allowed to help determine budget allocations and have some control over expenditures and outcomes (Finkler, 1992).

Preparation of the annual budget requires the manager to think and plan ahead, anticipate costs, and monitor and control expenditures. Through monitoring the budget, deviations from the budget line can be detected and corrective actions taken quickly. There are many types of budgets (e.g., operating, program, performance, capital, strategic); however, the operating budget is probably the one most familiar to the occupational health nurse manager. Numerous computer software programs are available for organizing and preparing budget spread sheets.

The operating budget is specified for a period of time and is designed to plan for the daily operation of the cost center, a functional unit within the organization that generates costs, in this case the occupational health unit. The budget projects salary and nonsalary expenditures.

In developing the operating budget, the occupational health nurse manager will need to know historical budget data, unit goals and objectives reflecting projected needs and growth, and quantifiable indicators of resource consumption (e.g., numbers and types of personnel, pieces of equipment, supplies) necessary to accomplish the goals and objectives identified in the program plan.

A review of historical data can help the occupational health nurse understand how resources were previously used (Bozman & Childres, 1991), if allocations and expenditures were cost-effective, if unexpected deviations occurred, and if performance objectives were met (Finkler, 1992). Goals and objectives are closely tied to the budget so that resource allocation is appropriate to conduct the work needed to achieve programmatic/unit goals. Here, the nurse manager will want to plan for such areas as inflationary costs, new or expansion services or programs (e.g., health screening, surveillance activities), new or updated computer systems, advanced health/medical therapeutics and technologies, and the cost impact of regulatory mandates.

Armed with historical data, a unit/program plan, and expense data, the occupational health nurse can prepare an operating budget. The actual preparation of the operational budget translates goals and objectives into numbers. Although terms or categorical labels may vary from organization to organization, typical cost or line item categories to include in the budget are personnel, materials/supplies, equipment, communication, professional/staff development, travel, consultants, and small capital items. Examples of items usually considered within the line item categories are shown in Table 13-2. However, it is important to note that line item categories will vary from organization to organization, and the occupational health nurse manager will need to be skilled in budget preparation specific to the company.

Preparation of the budget should begin several months in advance of the fiscal (or calendar) year of expenditure, at the time the unit/program plan is developed. During the annual planning process, goals and objectives are established, and the budget is then finalized and readied for approval by top management.

As previously mentioned, projected costs to operate the occupational health unit will in part be derived from historical usage levels. The nurse manager should review all line item expenditures from the previous year to determine the cost-effectiveness in meeting goals and objectives. The review should indicate if resources were adequate to operate the occupational health unit. If not, adjustments should be factored in to meet actual needs for the next budget period. Inflationary costs, anticipated bonuses, and costs associated with proposed, expanded, or new mandated programs should be budgeted. This might include projected costs for mammography screening for women employees and/or spouses or family members of male employees, expansion of occupational health services to the night shift, or start-up costs associated with implementation of a new satellite occupational health service. All line item costs must be considered in any projected budget preparation. For example, projected personnel expenditures should include all mixes and the quantity (full-time, part-time, contractual) of personnel needed by shift. An example of an occupational health service cost center budget is shown in Table 13-3.

The next step in the budgeting process is obtaining formal approval from top management. It is important that the occupational health nurse fully justify the budget in terms of growth related to projected goals and objectives, outlining

■ **TABLE 13–2**   Examples of Line Items Included in a Occupational Health Unit Budget

Personnel
Full-time staff
Part-time staff
Fringe benefits for each individual (e.g., life insurance, pension, vacation/sick pay)
Taxes
Contract personnel
Substitute personnel
Overtime pay
Shiftwork differential
Merit/bonus supplements

Materials/supplies
Office supplies (forms, paper, pens, etc.)
Health care supplies
Pharmaceuticals
Health education materials
Xeroxing

Equipment
Desks/chairs
File cabinets
Xerox machine
Laboratory items/instruments
Equipment rental/maintenance/repair

Communication
Telephone
Postage/Overnite mail
FAX
Print materials (e.g., brochures)
Computer

Professional/staff development
Conferences/seminar fees
Professional dues
Journals
Certification

Special programs/projects
Health promotion activities
Research

Travel
Conferences/seminars and related business trips
Site or other satellite visits

Consultant
In-house site services
External fees (preparatory work, reports)
Travel/lodging

■ **TABLE 13–3** Example of Budget Spreadsheet

BS32A

Rev.

(even dollars)

Cost Center   5600   Health Center

Budget System
Budget Worksheet
Fiscal Year 1992/93

Page: 1
Date: 1-09-92
Time: 16:15:53

Acct Code	Description	1990/91 Actual	(1991/92 – 03 Mos.) YTD Actual	YTD Bud	1991/92 Est Actual	1991/92 Budget	1992/93 Budget	1993/04 Forecast
611110	Salaries: Office							
611210	Sick pay: Office							
611310	Overtime: Office							
616450	Fringe charge: Office							
621111	T & E: Lodging							
621222	T & E: Meals							
621333	T & E: Trans/Tips—No air							
621339	T & E: Air travel							
621444	T & E: Entertainment							
621666	T & E: Other							
621810	T & E: RTP/Greenville							
623110	Employee medical services							
623190	Other employee services							
624240	Dues & registration fees							
625100	Temporary help							
631160	USA forms							
631180	Other printed matter							
632110	Office equipment not capital							
632310	Stationary stock supplies							
632320	Office supplies: O/S purchase							
633110	Chemicals							
633410	Scientific apparatus/supp							
639110	Computer operating supplies							
639120	Subscriptions & pamphlets							
639130	Books							
639220	Photographic supplies							
639244	Other audiovisual							
639250	Reprints, photostat & transl.							
639260	Multilith & offset supplies							
639310	Fin gds inv by IT-med							

Code	Description
639315	Fin gds inv by IT-diag
639410	Art supplies
639540	Cleaning supplies
639910	Sundry supplies
644110	Electrical supplies
644310	Hardware supplies
653110	Consulting fees
656210	O/S repairs-bldg/mach/equipment
656510	O/S maint-comp hrdw & sftw
656610	O/S repairs-office mach
656710	O/S repairs-scientific
659110	O/S laundry service
659910	Other outside services
661110	Telephone & telegraph
683150	Comp hardware-purchases
683180	Computer software
683190	CIS hardware charges
683210	O/S computer charges
684210	Sales tax on purchases
685110	Postage
685910	Sundry freight
689910	Sundry expenses
699107	Travel contingency
699117	Other O/S serv contingency
699134	Sundry supplies contingency
699154	Training & meetings contingency
699155	Office supplies contingency
699162	M & R supplies contingency
	Cost center subtotals
662110	Deprec-building & improve
662210	Deprec-machinery & equipment
662310	Deprec-computer hardware
662410	Amortz-comp. software
662510	Amortz-land improvements
	Below the line totals
	Cost center totals

Courtesy Burroughs-Wellcome Co., Research Triangle Park, NC.

359

the rationale for program initiation or expansion, and emphasize the contribution the occupational health service makes in health care cost reduction. This can be carried out by providing data relative to trends in work-related illness and injury, workers' compensation costs, insurance claims, and lost work time and disability management.

Once the budget is operationalized, the occupational health nurse manager is responsible for the ongoing monitoring and controlling of actual expenditures. The occupational health nurse manager should be provided with regular computerized budget statements or spreadsheets that specify each line item actually budgeted, current expenditures, any variance (amount spent over or under budget), and the balance available. This scrutiny should be done at least monthly to be certain that projected and actual expenditures are compatible. If deviations are apparent, the nurse manager can identify problem areas and minor modifications can then be made to adjust expenditures.

Although the budget process is relatively straightforward, unforeseen problems can occur because organizations are always changing. Examples of unanticipated costs might be associated with regulatory changes, staff turnover, budget cuts, or cost overruns. Problems should be analyzed for cause and solutions determined to prevent recurrence.

Business Proposals/Plans

In the current health care and business environment, the occupational health nurse manager is challenged with developing new or expanding existing health programs and services. This is part of the nurse manager's planning function. The formal business plan or proposal is the vehicle often used to acquire resources and gain approval for program implementation (Jarrett, 1989). The plan is a written document that specifies concisely, but in sufficient detail, what the proposed venture or program is and the expectations to be achieved from its implementation. The nurse executive must always keep in mind that she or he will be competing with other departments for scarce funding and should produce evidence of the potential cost-effectiveness of the proposed services, such as how the program will improve employee health and reduce health insurance premiums, workers' compensation claims, or absenteeism. The business plan serves as a guide for efficient project operation and management; an information source; and a document that will facilitate decision making, motivation, and the measurement of performance (Vestal, 1989).

The specific elements, format, and length of a business plan or proposal are not universal and the occupational health nurse should be familiar with the organizational expectations. However, a basic set of components that should be considered for inclusion in any plan or proposal (Table 13–4) is described here.

Title Page. This page should include the title of the proposed project, the author or project leader, organizational unit, date of submission, and anticipated date of project implementation.

Project Summary. This section should provide a clear, brief overview of the entire project. This component is often considered the most critical piece of the plan since many reviewers will read only this initial summary and financial plan (to determine if there is any interest in the proposal project). The essence of the project must be condensed into one or two pages that clearly state the project's

■ **TABLE 13-4**   Typical Elements of a Business Proposal or Plan

* Title page
* Project summary
* Table of contents
* Need and justification
* Alternative approaches
* Project description/purpose
* Operational plan (implementation plan)
* Financial plan
* Marketing plan
* Evaluation plan
* Appendices

purpose and value in relation to the organization's mission and goals, the need or rationale for the project, and the financial implications that provide a brief summary of the initial or start-up costs and expected return on investment.

Table of Contents. The table of contents should provide an easy reference guide to the major components of the document so that the reader can quickly access specific components as desired.

Rationale/Identification of Need. This component of the plan or proposal provides the justification for the project or program and includes evidence to support the need. For example, if a program for cholesterol and/or high blood pressure screening and monitoring is proposed, supporting evidence might include epidemiologic data such as demographic, risk factor, morbidity and mortality indicators compared to known population parameters, health insurance claims data, and absenteeism trends for cardiovascular-related illnesses. In addition, the nurse can review a sample of health charts or actively sample the workforce via questionnaires to determine if relative risk factors exist and then provide these data in aggregate form.

Alternative Options. Alternative approaches to addressing the problem should be discussed. This will provide the reviewer with information that the problem and alternative solutions have been carefully explored. Cost-benefit data for varying alternatives should also be presented. If alternative propositions are of roughly equal cost, the occupational health nurse should state why one alternative is recommended over another. For example, if the proposed project is to offer a fitness and exercise program, alternative strategies might include exercise classes offered on-site that might entail hiring a fitness instructor or creating or renovating space. In addition, factors associated with employee release time versus off-work time should be considered. Another option could be to contract with a fitness center to have employees utilize the center through a limited voucher system. Each alternative should be described along with anticipated benefits and costs estimated.

Project Description. The purpose of this section is to clearly describe the exact purpose of the project. In addition, goals and objectives, expected outcomes, how the project fits with the overall organization's goals, the impact of the project on the company's image, timetables, and flowcharts should be presented succinctly and in a logical order.

Operational Plan. This component of the plan should be tied to the objectives and is intended to describe activities of how the plan will be carried out. The exact content, of course, will reflect how the objectives will be implemented in terms of human and physical facilities/material resource needs. Information regarding organizational management/charts, personnel to be hired along with targeted activities or responsibilities, plans for training, and how the program or project will be organized to produce the desired outcome should be presented. The physical facilities/materials should be described in terms of new or existing space needs, including renovation or remodeling, capital expenditures for equipment or furniture and maintenance, and consumable supplies and materials. If a contractual arrangement is proposed, it should also be thoroughly described with respect to the operational procedure. Resumés for key personnel and proposed job descriptions can be included in the Appendix.

Financial Plan. The budget or financial plan should address all costs associated with the project that are tied to meeting the goals and objectives including operating and capital expenditures. In the operating budget, personnel costs should include compensation and benefits, training, travel, and any other related expenditures such as professional dues or insurance. If consultant services are expected, these will also need to be allocated in the financial plan. Nonpersonnel items can be categorized and include space (e.g., rent, lease), small supplies, communications (i.e., telephone, postage, computer), and promotional and project materials (e.g., brochures, handouts, videos, refreshments, data analysis). A capital budget should be developed for large expenditures such as construction or remodeling of physical facilities and high-cost equipment such as a Reflotron. Often a budget is prepared for the start-up first-year costs plus the second- and third-year estimated budgets (which might include additional or replacement inventory). Standardized organizational budget forms should be utilized.

Marketing Plan. This section should describe how the program or project will be marketed to the target group, including a promotional schedule or calendar, media selection, and advertising plans and materials. Costs for marketing materials need to be included in the financial or budget plan.

Evaluation Plan. This component should spell out in detail how the outcomes of the project will be measured, which should be reflective of the original objectives specified. A plan for evaluating anticipated costs of achieving the objectives should be included. For example, measuring programmatic costs of identifying individuals with high blood pressure and referral for treatment versus the costs of potential cardiovascular morbidity and mortality could be specified. A plan for data analysis and written report should be included. The appendix should include all supporting documents related to the plan such as charts, job descriptions (Appendix 13–1), and resumés.

Writing business plans or proposals is a process the occupational health nurse will increasingly use in planning and providing for health care programs to the workforce. If not already acquired, the occupational health nurse will need to develop skills to formulate a persuasive business plan utilizing the appropriate organizational format. The occupational health nurse can use the business plan as a tool to obtain the resources necessary to achieve the goals and objectives of the occupational health department (Jarrett, 1989).

Organizing

Organizing is the second managerial function, wherein the manager organizes personnel to accomplish the plan. This involves establishing a formal structure that provides for the coordination of resources to accomplish objectives and determining position qualifications and descriptions (Marriner-Tomey, 1991). While planning is the key to effective management, the organizational structure provides the formal framework for getting the job done.

Organizational Concepts

The occupational health nurse manager should be fully familiar with the formal organizational structure that shows the relationship among people and positions, and depicts hierarchical structures which define authority relationships and accountability. This is dramatized by an organizational chart or schematic that shows how the parts of an organization are linked, areas of responsibility, persons to whom one is accountable, and channels of communication. The visual diagram of a chart is often a more effective means of communicating the organization's structure than is a written description. Vertical charts depict the chief executive at the top with formal hierarchical lines of authority, often referred to as the chain of command (McClure, 1984; Tappen, 1989). Within this context, line authority represents a chain of command, and is a direct line from the manager to the worker depicted by a solid line on organizational charts. Line positions are related to the direct achievement of organizational objectives.

In contrast, staff authority supports line-authority relationships, and its functions are advisory or service oriented, such as locating required data and offering counsel on managerial problems. Staff individuals function through influence; they do not have the authority to accept, use, modify, or reject plans.

When communicating with employees, the organizational chart may be used for several purposes, such as outlining administrative authority, defining relationships with other departments and agencies, describing policy and operational levels of the organization, and evaluating strengths and weaknesses of the current structure. It can also be used by the nurse manager to orient new personnel or to present the agency's structural design to others external to the organization (Hein & Nicholson, 1986). In addition, organizational principles help guide the occupational health nurse manager to clarify relationships and maximize organizational efficiency. These principles are outlined in Table 13–5.

In addition to the formal organizational structure, informal networks exist that comprise the personal and social relationships not identified on the organizational chart (e.g., individuals who lunch or take breaks together). These networks or structures help employees to meet personal and social needs and to gain recognition. Informal structures have their own modes of communication and are often referred to as the "grapevine" (Hein & Nicholson, 1986). Management should recognize this structure, its value, and how it operates.

■ **TABLE 13–5** Principles for Organizational Efficiency

1. Clear lines of authority
2. Unity of command with each person having only one boss
3. Authority and responsibility relationships clearly defined in writing (reduces role ambiguity)
4. Clear role definition for each worker
5. Delegation of responsibility to the lowest effective level in the organization along with appropriate authority for decision making and goal achievement

Span of Management

The concept of span of management or span of control is important in determining effective manager/worker relationships and reflects the scope of coordination of employee activities, that is, the number of workers that can be effectively managed (Marriner-Tomey, 1991). The span of control will vary within the organization and is influenced by the pace and type of work as well as the knowledge and skill of the workers. Supervising routine work performance requires less time than supervising innovative work performance because people know what is expected of them. However, it can be expected that as the degree of difficulty increases for performing a task satisfactorily, so will the demand on the manager's time and effort (Yukl, 1989). For example, if a new health promotion program such as mammography screening is to be developed, the occupational health nurse manager will need to spend considerable time in determining how the program should be organized for implementation, including the training of nurses and other health care personnel with respect to the screening procedures. In addition, as the variability or number of different functions increases, the manager must consider more performance factors and interrelationships, which consumes more time. Interdependent functions of workers require more management time than independent functions because of the increased need for managerial coordination within and across departments.

The greater the geographical separation of personnel reporting to the occupational health nurse manager, the more limited will be the span of control. Increased emphasis on nonmanagerial responsibilities will also lessen the time the manager has for managing (Jones, 1968). Supervisors in flat organizational structures have a broader range of management responsibilities than those in tall structures, and lower level managers have a broader range of responsibility than do top level managers. In addition, managers of positions where tasks are shared will most likely have a smaller span of control than first-line managers who coordinate employees who do the same task (Gillies, 1989; Yukl, 1989).

Decentralization Versus Centralization

One characteristic of an organization that influences both productivity and staff morale is the degree of centralization or decentralization of management responsibility. A highly centralized organization is one in which most decisions are made by the chief executive officer. Decisions made at the top of an organization must then be filtered down through intermediaries to reach occupational health personnel. Retention of major decision making by top level administrators decreases the need for critical thinking and problem solving by middle and supervisory level personnel and does not increase growth in decision-making abilities. Eventually, these workers may become passive and unenthusiastic about their jobs. Usually agencies tend to be more centralized during their early formative years.

Decentralization is the degree to which decision making is diffused throughout the organization (Salmond, 1985). In order for this to be effective, top managers must adopt a positive attitude toward decentralization, and they need competent personnel to whom they can delegate authority and responsibility. Decentralization of responsibility leads to improvement in worker morale, as it demonstrates a certain degree of trust and confidence in the decision-making abilities of others. When middle managers are given the responsibility for managerial decision making, they too may decentralize decision making still further, enabling direct caregivers to help formulate organizational plans, policies, and procedures.

The advantages of decentralization seem to outweigh the disadvantages. When people have a voice in governance, they feel empowered, more ownership, and are more willing to contribute. This increased motivation provides a feeling of individuality and freedom that in turn encourages creativity and commits the individual to making the system more successful. Decentralization brings decision making closer to the action. Thus, decisions may be more effective because people who know the situation and have to implement the decision are the ones who make it.

Decentralization develops managers by allowing them to manage and releases top management from the burden of daily administration, freeing them for long-range planning, goal and policy development, and systems integration (Marriner-Tomey, 1991). On the down side, because decentralization requires more managers and larger staffs, it is more costly.

Delegation

Delegation is the process of assigning work from one organizational level to another (i.e., manager to a subordinate) and should be recognized by the occupational health nurse manager as an opportunity to maximize the utilization of the talents of those to whom the task has been delegated. It is the manager's responsibility to assess the results of the delegated activity. Learning to live with differences may be difficult for a manager, especially if the manager once performed the tasks now assigned to another worker and finds that the tasks are not performed in the same way (Poulin, 1984).

Assignment of responsibility, delegation of authority, and creation of accountability are the three concepts most often mentioned in relation to the delegation process with which the occupational health nurse manager must be familiar. Responsibility denotes obligation and refers to what must be done to complete a task.

Authority is the power to make final decisions and give commands. The person to whom responsibility has been assigned needs authority in sufficient scope to direct delegated duties without frequent consultation with her or his manager. The granting of too little authority is a common problem, and should be avoided. Although authority is delegated so that responsibilities can be fulfilled, the nurse manager maintains control over the delegated authority and may recall it at any time.

Accountability refers to an obligation to complete work satisfactorily and to accept the consequences for the outcome. In authority relationships, the occupational health nurse manager is accountable for the performance of the task, the selection of the individual to complete it, and both the individual's and her or his own performance.

Underdelegating is often evident and there are numerous reasons for this (Marriner-Tomey, 1991). The manager may believe she or he can do the job quicker, may resent interruptions to answer questions from those delegated the task, or may not want to take the time to check what has been done. In addition, the occupational health nurse manager may feel that those to whom the task has been delegated will not keep them adequately informed or the manager may be unwilling to take risks for fear of being blamed for others' mistakes.

Position/Job Description

The position or job description is derived from a job analysis and is the key organizational tool that provides a written summary of the principal duties and scope of responsibility for a particular position (Simms et al., 1985). Position descriptions are developed by the occupational health nurse manager with input from the staff as appropriate, and are used to define the job, assist with recruitment and orientation procedures, and provide criteria elements for performance evaluation. The job position is organized according to a standard format that meets the needs of the organization. However, common elements generally include the following: position title, summary purpose statement of the position describing the overall concept and nature of the position, span of responsibility and accountability, list of duties, and qualifications for the position (e.g., knowledge, skills, education, experience). Duties should be arranged in a logical order, with the primary duties listed first and stated clearly, specifically, and concisely. Position descriptions should be accurate, realistic, current, and dated. Examples are shown in Table 13–6 and Appendix 13–1.

Staffing/Coordinating

In order to accomplish the organizational goals set forth in the plan, the manager must staff the unit to coordinate and carry out the work of the organization. Staffing involves the following:

- identifying the type and amount of services and number of staff needed to deliver services;
- recruiting, interviewing and selecting personnel; and
- orienting staff and scheduling the work.

The majority of occupational settings is staffed by one occupational health nurse; therefore, some issues to be discussed with regard to affecting nursing staffing will be more applicable to multinurse units, regional or corporate settings. However, in occupational health settings the nurse manager may also be responsible for managing clerical, support (e.g., laboratory), and professional staff (e.g., physicians and counselors).

Staffing Needs and Recruitment

When planning how to staff the occupational health unit, the type of setting, number and demographics of workers, types of hazards, worker and management orientation toward health care, and budgeting constraints will influence the type and number of personnel needed. For example, an assessment of the organization and workforce by the occupational health nurse manager may reveal the need for health promotion activities related to lifestyle changes, chemical exposure monitoring, ergonomics, and employee assistance. The types of personnel recruited should reflect this need, although the categories of personnel utilized may be part-time, full-time, or contractual.

Recruitment, Interviewing, and Selection

Active recruitment of qualified personnel is essential for the growth of the organization (Marriner-Tomey, 1991). Prior to recruitment, the nurse manager should review the job description for accuracy and revise the document appropriately. Appropriate advertising and marketing should be done including word of mouth and in-house.

■ **TABLE 13–6**   Example of Job Description for Occupational Health Nurse

Job Title:	Senior Occupational Health Consultant
Department:	Occupational Health Services
Classification:	Exempt
Job Summary:	Direct, manage and supervise the occupational health unit and staff. In addition, develop and manage health promotion and safety programs in consultation with other members of the Occupational Health Team and community resources.
Educational Requirements:	Graduate from an accredited school with a Bachelor of Science in Nursing and licensed as a registered nurse in North Carolina. Prefer a master's degree in occupational health nursing, or public health.
Work Experience:	2-3 years nursing experience and an additional 1-2 years experience in occupational health.
Knowledge, Skills, and Abilities Required:	Must be able to assess, plan, develop, implement, and evaluate health promotion programs. Must possess effective management and leadership techniques and advanced communication and interpersonal relationship skills.

The following described job functions are not meant to be all-inclusive but to reflect the general work description for this job.

Position:	Senior Occupational Health Consultant

DESCRIPTION OF WORK

1. Plan, develop, implement, manage, and evaluate occupational health and health promotion programs.
2. Perform needs assessment of the workplace and the employees for the purpose of determining need, interest, and scope of occupational health and health promotion programs.
3. Prepare and deliver written and oral presentations/reports for management regarding occupational health and health monitoring programs.
4. Develop written policies, procedures, goals, objectives, and protocols for the occupational health and health promotion program to be updated annually.
5. Plan, develop, and promote the necessary facilities, equipment, supplies, and records system to operate the employee health service.
6. Orient, supervise, and evaluate nursing and/or support staff in the Occupational Health unit. Assign the staff's work, duties, and schedules and provide in-service education and professional growth opportunities for staff.
7. Prepare an annual budget for an occupational health unit/program.
8. Consult with management and other members of the occupational health team such as industrial hygiene, safety, toxicology, and human resources.
9. Use epidemiological methods to determine the major health and safety needs of a group of workers.
10. Calculate the cost-effectiveness of different types of occupational health services and health safety programs.
11. Conduct and/or supervise on-site health promotion programs including classes, individual counseling sessions, and health screenings.
12. Provide treatment for work- and non-work-related injuries and illnesses.
13. Assist with or conduct accident and injury investigation of workers.
14. Continuously update knowledge of federal, state, and local laws, regulations, and requirements that are applicable to an occupational health and safety program.
15. Develop written proposal for occupational health and health promotion programs, including a budget for the program.
16. Participate in the service delivery, educational programs, and research projects of the Occupational Health Service.
17. Assist with management of the safety committee and programs.
18. Supervise the First Responder and Emergency Teams.
19. Utilize community resources with company support by establishing good work relations, relationships with the universities, and with the community emergency planning committee.

All applicants should submit resumés and references when appropriate. Reference letters should be used cautiously when evaluating the applicant as the authors may be unfamiliar with the applicant's current work performance and are seldom critical. More emphasis should be placed on comments by previous employers, co-workers and colleagues. However, letters from personal references may attest to the applicant's character and integrity, which should be highly valued.

A preemployment interview is a critical function requiring much skill and should be conducted with the most qualified applicants. The purposes of the interview are to obtain and give information and judge the applicant on predetermined criteria specific for that job. The interview should be considered by the occupational health nurse manager as a reciprocal experience, with both parties prepared to ask questions as well as to discuss issues relevant to the position (Wallace & Ventura, 1991). Information from the resumé and references can serve to initiate and facilitate discussion during the interview process.

The interview process should have an introduction, body, and closure. The environment and behavioral aspects related to the interview should be considered. The occupational health nurse manager provides introductory information about the job and any relevant historical data. A pre-planned set of questions based on criteria established from the job description should be developed to facilitate the interview process (Wallace & Ventura 1991). Certainly information about the applicant's knowledge, skills, ability to work with others, congruence of professional goals with that of the organization, willingness to perform the job responsibilities, and other skill areas specific to the position should be addressed. Open-ended questions are probably the most valuable method for information gathering as they allow the applicant to express ideas and encourage self-disclosure. Problem-solving approaches particular to situations can also be explored. The nurse manager should be prepared to answer questions from the applicant about the organizational structure and culture, policies and procedures, working conditions and benefits, and specific questions pertinent to the position under consideration. Interviewing principles shown in Table 13–7 should be observed.

Verbal and nonverbal behavior by the manager during the interview can affect

---

■ **TABLE 13–7** Interviewing Principles

1. Create and maintain a comfortable environment throughout the interview.
2. Conduct the interview according to a preplanned outline.
3. Explore the applicant's background and future plans before describing the available position.
4. Encourage the applicant to talk freely by asking nondirective, open-ended questions.
5. Listen actively and talk sparingly while the applicant describes his background and future plans.
6. Be aware of your own and the applicant's nonverbal communications.
7. When describing the available position, give information about job responsibilities and working environment, and withhold opinion about the applicant's ability to fill the position.
8. Identify both positive and negative aspects of the job in detail.
9. In concluding the interview, clarify subsequent steps in the selection procedure.

From Gillies, DA. Nursing management: A systems approach. Philadelphia: W.B. Saunders, 1989.

the applicant's comfort. Therefore, the nurse manager should demonstrate respect for the applicant's ideas, listen carefully, and maintain eye contact. Behavioral characteristics of the applicant should also be observed as to style of relationships and comfort with the interview process. For example, the applicant might be asked to interview with several people in a group format, conduct a formal presentation, or attend a social reception. This will provide an opportunity to witness both formal and informal interactions. At closure, the interview discussion should be summarized and clarifications made. The applicant should be told what to expect in terms of a decision.

After all applicants have been interviewed, strengths and weaknesses can be evaluated. Education and experience can be easily compared; however, other characteristics such as interpersonal skills, social style, creativity, and integrity may be more difficult to measure. Once this is done a selection should be made quickly.

Coordinating the Work

After an employee has been hired, a planned orientation program should be provided. The employee is acquainted with policies and procedures, work surroundings, and job functions and should have an opportunity to ask questions for clarification. The occupational health nurse manager will then want to plan and coordinate the work schedule, taking into consideration the number of staff needed, programs offered, especially if they are seasonal or special programs, vacation schedules, absenteeism, professional education needs, turnover, rotation, shift schedules, and special needs of the staff. In addition, consideration should be given to the need for substitute and/or additional personnel if workload demands increase for special programs.

The staffing/coordinating function is very important in determining the correct mix and number of workers needed to achieve the organizational goals and carry out the program plans. When determining the number of staff needed in an occupational setting, there is no specific rule. This will vary, depending on the needs and relative health of the workforce and industry. For a work setting with 300 employees or less, AAOHN recommends one full-time equivalent (FTE) of an occupational health nurse. For nonindustrial employers, one occupational health nurse FTE is recommended for 750 employees (AAOHN, 1989).

Leading

In order to accomplish the organizational goals, the occupational health nurse manager must apply leadership skills and facilitate the work of the staff efficiently and effectively (McClure, 1984). In order to facilitate the activities, the nurse manager needs to be aware of management and leadership styles, her or his own leadership style, and how this style influences the relationship with and performance of those being managed. For the most part, the occupational health nurse manager will be managing and working with knowledge workers who usually require a great deal of autonomy in carrying out the responsibilities of the job. Colleagueship and collaboration are essential ingredients in the management experience.

Management Theories

There are various management theories that describe the relationship and impact of management and leadership styles on the motivation and productivity of workers/staff. Contrary to early management theories that emphasized autocratic leadership and rules and regulations, human relations management focuses on encouraging and empowering workers to develop their potential and enhancing worker efforts to meet their needs for recognition and accomplishment (Flarey, 1991; Lorsch & Mathias, 1987; Patz, 1991). The occupational health nurse manager will find that understanding and applying principles related to these theories will help in discovering strategies to stimulate worker motivation and creativity. Several theories will be briefly discussed; however, reference to a good management text is suggested for a fuller description.

Maslow developed the hierarchy-of-needs theory in which he classifies a human needs structure into five categories: physiological/survival, safety and security, belongingness/social, self-esteem, and self-actualization (Maslow, 1954). The essence of the theory is that lower-level needs (i.e., eating, shelter) must be met before moving onto higher-level needs (i.e., recognition, achievement). Although many types of needs or motivators are apparent in the work setting, the occupational health nurse manager needs to recognize that people are different and what satisfies one may not satisfy another. For example, one person may desire social affiliation while another good pay and work hours, and yet another, work performance recognition. Depending on one's circumstances, one's motivators will change; that is, recognition and achievement are likely to be valued by most employees at different points in time. The occupational health nurse manager should be attuned to recognizing staff needs.

Herzberg's theory of job enrichment was based on interview research conducted with 200 engineers and accountants regarding job situations they found satisfying or dissatisfying. The research indicated that workers are most satisfied with job factors associated with what he called motivators, including achievement, recognition, advancement, responsibility, growth potential, and the work itself. Factors that produced dissatisfaction are termed hygiene factors and are associated with supervision, policy, work status, work conditions, interpersonal relationships, and job security. Job dissatisfaction leads to increased absenteeism, turnover, and reduced productivity resulting in excessive recruitment, orientation, and job development, which is costly in time and money (Marriner-Tomey, 1991). Herzberg believed that these more personal and environmentally related hygiene factors do not necessarily motivate but can lower job performance. Although there is some controversy surrounding this theory based on the research methodology, human relations conditions identified as satisfiers and dissatisfiers comparably reflect Maslow's work. A comparison is shown in (Fig. 13–3).

McGregor's Theory X and Theory Y (Table 13–8), which describes one's philosophy of human nature as applied to managerial relationships, shares some of the same concepts as Maslow's hierarchy of needs and Herzberg's motivation theory. The basic assumptions underlying Theory X management is that the manager places strong emphasis on the attainment of organizational goals, and that workers must be fully directed, controlled, coerced, and punished into performing their jobs. This type of manager assumes that workers inherently dislike their jobs, and avoid responsibility and new challenges. Theory X managers will do the thinking and planning for and closely supervise the workers.

Theory Y managers emphasize the goals of the individual within the context of the organization. They believe that workers have self-direction and control skills necessary to meet work performance objectives and enjoy personal achieve-

Maslow's Needs Heirarchy	Herzberg's Factors	
Personal Growth	Motivators	Work Itself Achievement
Esteem		Advancement Recognition
Belongingness	Hygiene Factors	Interpersonal and Supervisory Relationships
Safety		Technical Supervision Working Conditions Company Policy/Administration
Physiological		Salary

■ **Figure 13–3** Comparison of Maslow's and Herzberg's theories related to human needs and rewards.

ment and task accomplishment. The Theory Y manager believes that under good working conditions, people seek responsibility and are creative and innovative. This manager encourages worker participation in goal setting, delegates authority, supports and enhances job expansion, and uses positive motivations such as praise and recognition to encourage goal attainment.

Hersey and Blanchard (1993) extended the earlier (1960s) work of Blake and Mouton in examining task/productivity and relationship behavior with maturity levels of workers (Table 13–9). The researchers assert that the most effective leadership is dependent on the maturity of the workers. Groups with below average maturity function best under leaders with high task-low relationship orientations; whereas, groups with average maturity function best under leaders with high task-high relationship or low task-high relationship. Employees' attitudes toward management are an important factor to consider with respect to their perception of the manager's role. Some employees perceive an authoritarian, highly structured role as desirable, some prefer strong interaction with the manager in decision making and control, while others prefer to work autonomously. Individual differences require that the occupational health nurse manager be adaptive.

■ **TABLE 13–8**   List of Assumptions about Human Nature that Underlie McGregor's Theory X and Theory Y

Theory X	Theory Y
1. Work is inherently distasteful to most people.	1. Work is as natural as play, if the conditions are favorable.
2. Most people are not ambitious, have little desire for responsibility, and prefer to be directed.	2. Self-control is often indispensable in achieving organizational goals.
3. Most people have little capacity for creativity in solving organizational problems.	3. The capacity for creativity in solving organizational problems is widely distributed in the population.
4. Motivation occurs only at the physiological and safety levels.	4. Motivation occurs at the social, esteem, and self-actualization levels, as well as physiological and security levels.
5. Most people must be closely controlled and often coerced to achieve organizational objectives.	5. People can be self-directed and creative at work if properly motivated.

■ **TABLE 13–9**   Leadership Styles Appropriate for Varying Maturity Levels of Workers

Maturity Level	Appropriate Style
M1 *Low Maturity* Unable and unwilling or insecure	S1 *Telling* High task and low relationship behavior
M2 *Low to Moderate Maturity* Unable but willing or confident	S2 *Selling* High task and high relationship behavior
M3 *Moderate to High Maturity* Able but unwilling or insecure	S3 *Participating* High relationship and low task behavior
M4 *High Maturity* Able/competent and willing/confident	S4 *Delegating* Low relationship and low task behavior

From Hersey, P & Blanchard, K. Management of organizational behavior, 6th ed. Englewood Cliffs, NJ: Prentice Hall, 1993.

Traditional management theory is based on McGregor's Theory X, Maslow's primary physiological and safety needs, and Hertzberg's hygiene needs. Contemporary management is based on McGregor's Theory Y, Maslow's secondary needs, and Herzberg's motivators. Employee participation in goal direction and planning and empowerment of workers to assume more decision-making responsibility are considered major factors in management philosophy and have been shown to contribute to worker satisfaction.

This overview of management/leadership theories demonstrates a trend toward increased emphasis on human needs, and commitment through participation within the context of the organization, rather than emphasizing efficiency in the absence of human relations, recognition, and personal goal fulfillment. The occupational health nurse manager is encouraged to explore these theories and styles, analyze her or his management style within the context of the organization and determine the most effective management approach that fits the situation, personal style, and objectives. By studying the management process, management and leadership theories, and motivational enhancers, the occupational health nurse manager can gain an increased understanding of effective strategies in working with others in order to accomplish both organizational and personal goals.

Communication

Effective communication techniques are central to the leading function and must flow freely both vertically and horizontally. Vertical communication follows the chain of command and employee input into decision making is critical to satisfaction. Although communication about accomplishing the work tasks may be directive at times from the manager, more successful communication can be accomplished when the worker and manager mutually agree on task assignment and strategy implementation (Gardner et al., 1991). The employee must feel free to communicate solicited and unsolicited information to the nurse manager. Communication cannot be taken for granted and requires effort.

Lateral or horizontal communication occurs between departments on the same level, between coworkers, and is needed primarily to coordinate activities and clarify roles and responsibilities. This type of communication is crucial when multiple departments or parties collaborate on projects. It is also used when staff/advisory personnel provide technical assistance to supervisors or managers.

Informal communication, often referred to as the "grapevine," exists in all organizations and is a method whereby workers at all levels transmit information to each other. The grapevine transports information much faster; however, information received may be distorted as it passes from person to person. Grapevine information has no formal lines of accountability. Nurse managers should pay attention to informal communication channels in order to recognize sources of information, correct deviations and pass on messages. Examples of facilitators and barriers to communication are listed in Table 13–10.

Depending on the type of communication behavior displayed, the occupational health nurse manager may need to utilize special communication skills and techniques to deal with employees who demonstrate difficult communication behaviors, that is, hostile, complaining, unresponsive, negative, or overly agreeable. It is important not to get into a battle with workers who are hostile or aggressive, but rather to deal with them directly and forthrightly and to state

■ **TABLE 13–10**   Effective Communication: Facilitators and Barriers

Facilitators	Barriers
• Clear ideas/purpose	• Lack of clarity or precision
• Well-organized message	• Faulty reasoning/poorly expressed message
• Familiarity with problem	• Omitting facts or filtering information
• Seeking/understanding other's point of view	• Using jargon
• Avoiding arguments/giving advice	• Selective screening/perception
• Positive verbal/nonverbal expressions	• Distrust of sender
• Nonjudging atmosphere	• Potential for punishment
• Appropriate confidentiality	• Poor listening
• Appropriate repetition	• Poor/unsafe working conditions and environment
• Allowing for feedback	• Resistance to change
• Well-written, courteous memos	• Lack of authority
• Timing	• Timing

your position forcefully but in a friendly manner. If an employee has an outburst, the employee should be given the opportunity to calm down, regain control, and then discuss the problem. For workers who continually complain or shed negative thoughts, it is important for the manager to acknowledge the comments but then move on to explore alternatives and engage these workers in problem solving (Marriner-Tomey, 1991).

It is difficult to read silent or unresponsive individuals; however, it is important to try to get their thoughts or opinions by directly asking open-ended questions such as "What do you think about this?" Employees who are overly agreeable have a strong need to be liked and accepted and may agree to tasks that do not get completed. The occupational health nurse manager should try to determine what specific goals are important to this type of worker and recognize clues in hidden messages, humor, and remarks.

Controlling

The function of controlling is key in evaluating overall programmatic effectiveness. It involves setting performance standards and criteria, evaluating performance results, and recommending and taking corrective actions.

Evaluation of Employees

As mentioned previously, Management by Objectives (MBO) is a tool for both planning and evaluation. Its emphasis is on achievement of objectives rather than personality traits; therefore, it reflects a results-orientation. The performance appraisal is a periodic formal evaluation to determine how well the employee has performed her or his duties during a specified period of time. Based on measurable objectives, professional standards of practice and performance criteria established in advance by the manager and employee, the occupational health nurse manager can objectively complete the performance evaluation or appraisal. Both the employee and manager know the standard of performance expected and can discuss modifications that may need to be made. In addition to reviewing and discussing organizational/unit goals and objectives, the evaluation can help determine the employee's aspirations, recognize accomplishments, determine professional growth needs, and reward exceptional performance (Gillies, 1989).

When evaluating the employee, the manager might consider a checklist that can be used to denote the presence or absence (yes/no) of a desired characteristic or behavior. However, checklists have limited utility as they do not measure the degree (e.g., average, above average, exceptional) of the characteristic being measured and are generally not suitable for measurement of interpersonal relationships.

Rating scales can provide much more data about a desired behavior or characteristic and can be constructed numerically using qualitative terms such as poor to excellent, low to high, or almost never to almost always. The following example demonstrates several characteristics measured on a five-point scale from low to high:

		RATING SCALE		
Low (1)	Below Average (2)	Average (3)	Above Average (4)	High (5)

Characteristic/behavior

Works well with others
Demonstrates initiative
Demonstrates creativity
Demonstrates leadership abilities

Using this type of scale, the occupational health nurse manager is able to evaluate each characteristic independently, a set or group of characteristics, or all characteristics combined. Numerical scores can be tallied and the manager can then compare groups or sets of characteristics to help target strengths and limitations.

Evaluation Conference

Although the occupational health nurse manager's formal evaluation of the employee's performance is usually conducted annually, evaluation should be a continuous process so that the employee has sufficient feedback to maximize performance. Both the manager and employee should be prepared for the performance evaluation conference with adequate time scheduled. Privacy should be afforded and interruptions and distractions avoided. Seating arrangements should be comfortable and reflect equality or collegiality (i.e., sitting side by side or at the corners of a table). Emphasis should be placed on achievement of specific objectives, special or outstanding accomplishments, and observed performance. The employee should be asked to identify areas that she or he perceives need improvement, if any, as this will enhance joint evaluation efforts and reduce the potential for defensiveness. A collaborative discussion about performance improvement, goal setting, and new initiatives or job responsibilities should be encouraged.

If the nurse manager must point out a need for performance improvement, this should be interspersed with favorable performance indicators to avoid setting up a barrier during the evaluation process. If the employee becomes defensive the manager should listen and not engage in a battle.

Problem solving and goal setting evaluation approaches are more facilitative and growth stimulating (Dubnicki & Sloan, 1991; Townsend, 1991). Through problem solving, the employee discusses problems and expresses ideas and opinions for solutions while the nurse manager listens, reflects and summarizes. Goal setting is future oriented and focuses on results. It encourages the employee to determine how to achieve objectives and it also enhances teamwork. Before the evaluation is completed, ways in which the manager can help the employee achieve performance goals should be discussed (e.g., additional or reduced responsibilities, resources, time for special projects or research).

The evaluation should be written addressing achievements, accomplishments, and future goals. If weaknesses or performance deviations are evident, these should be documented with recommendations for improvement stipulated within a defined timeframe. In order for changes to be made, recommendations for improvement should be mutually agreed upon and the employee should understand the consequences of failure to perform. In some structures, performance interventions such as positive reinforcement (e.g., recognition, verbal praise), counseling, or referral to an Employee Assistance Program may be helpful and needed. The evaluation report should be signed and dated by both the occupational health nurse manager and the employee and placed in the performance file to be used as a basis for promotions, pay increases, and other rewards, or for disciplinary or termination action if necessary. A progressive disciplinary action program and grievance procedure should be established and should be uniformly applied to personnel.

■ QUALITY ASSURANCE

Quality assurance in nursing has been of concern since nursing's beginnings when Florence Nightingale called for systematic collection and analysis of data and identification of practice standards (Nightingale, 1860). In contemporary times, the impetus for quality assurance programs came about as a result of recognizing the need to improve the quality of health care and at the same time reduce health care costs (Dienemann, 1992). Quality assurance activities also assist the professional in self-regulation and accountability for nursing practice (Migliozzi, 1985). A quality assurance program involves a measurable means of achieving professional goals with a positive impact on the quality of service provided. Setting standards and comparing actual performance/practice to those standards through defining criteria against which performance can be measured, and initiating change to enhance standards compliance is still recognized as the basic foundation for assuring quality performance (Lieske, 1985; Mailbusch, 1984). Quality assurance programs reflect two major purposes: evaluation and improvement of care or services. The intent of quality assurance expresses a commitment to take action that results in the assurance of quality nursing care (and services) to the public (Lang, 1976), efficiently and effectively, with a minimum expenditure of resources (Decker, 1985). It is not intended to be a mechanism for disciplining caregivers or trying to find fault or determine blame.

The general framework for quality assurance mechanisms is based on the classic work of Donabedian (1966). Three major approaches form the basis for evaluative mechanisms in quality assurance: structure, process, and outcome.

Structural elements relate to the physical setting and organizational modalities designed to facilitate the work (e.g., facilities, personnel); process elements relate to the actual performance of work or process of nursing care/service (e.g., performing walk-throughs, recordkeeping, examinations) and decision-making processes involved; outcome elements relate to the results achieved from the work performed or nursing interventions or service delivered (e.g., reduced work-related injuries, improved working conditions, service satisfaction). Evaluative elements for each of these approaches are listed in Table 13–11. In addition, as an example of the application of components of the Donabedian framework, Rogers et al. (1993) describe the results of a survey regarding employee satisfaction with health services as a quality indicator mechanism for service improvement.

Various methods for quality assurance have been utilized, the most common of which include quality assurance audits, peer review, and quality circles. Establishment of standards of performance and related measurement criteria are necessary in order to conduct an effective audit. Most often practice and performance standards are developed by professional societies, wherein the standard(s) reflects the values and beliefs of the collective profession as to what constitutes competent practice. However, organizations or groups may sometimes develop specific standards tailored to the institutional demands; or may develop specific criteria to meet established standards (AAOHN, 1988).

Practice Standards

Deming (1982) encourages the voluntary establishment of standards, thereby avoiding government regulation and allowance for greater freedom of practice.

■ **TABLE 13–11**   Evaluative Elements in Quality Assurance

Structural elements may include
- Physical setting
- Philosophy of health by management, employees, health care professionals
- Organizational mission and structure
- Unit goals and objectives
- Human and financial resources
- Operational resources

Process elements may include
- Management of the operation
- Decision-making processes
- Collaboration
- Nursing interventions/monitoring
- Services provided
- Records and reports

Outcome elements may include
- Improved health
- Compliance with treatment regimen
- Reduced morbidity and mortality
- Positive changes in knowledge and attitudes about health
- Satisfaction with service delivery

The American Nurses Association (1990) states that it is the function of professional associations to establish the scope of practice and desirable qualifications required for general specialty practice. Further, a profession regulates itself through codes of ethics, standards, accreditation agencies, peer review, and certification processes allowing for appropriate expansion commensurate with public needs, research findings, and demands from the practice environment.

ANA defines standards as authoritative statements by which the nursing profession describes the responsibilities for which its practitioners are accountable. Consequently, standards reflect the values and priorities of the profession. Standards provide direction for professional nursing practice and a framework for the evaluation of practice. Written in measurable terms, standards also define the nursing profession's accountability to the public and the client outcomes for which nurses are responsible. Standards are broad statements that address the full scope of professional nursing practice (ANA, 1991).

The American Nurses Association first developed standards of nursing practice in 1973. Numerous specialty organizations also have independently established standards for practice utilizing different definitions, formats, and so forth, creating confusion as to standards' utility. Working collaboratively with specialty nursing organizations, including the American Association of Occupational Health Nurses, the ANA revised its original standards in 1991, and the revised standards were set forth as *Standards of Clinical Nursing Practice*. These standards are considered generic and applicable to all registered nurses engaged in clinical practice, regardless of clinical specialty, practice setting, or educational preparation, and describe a competent level of professional nursing care and professional performance (ANA, 1991).

ANA *Standards of Clinical Nursing Practice* are categorized as "Standards of Care" and "Standards of Professional Practice" as shown in Table 13–12. Standards of Care describe a competent level of nursing care as demonstrated by the nursing process that provides the foundation for clinical decision making, whereas Standards of Professional Performance describe a competent level of behavior in the professional role (Table 13–12). All nurses are expected to engage in professional role activities appropriate to their education, position, and practice setting (ANA, 1991).

Standards developed for specialty practice or advanced clinical practice are further defined and determined by those nursing specialties building on the ANA standards and based upon specific criteria relevant to the practice specialty. *Standards of Occupational Health Nursing Practice* established by the American Association of Occupational Health Nurses are currently under revision. Thus a description and discussion are not appropriate at this time. However, Table 13–13 outlines the standard components. Upon complete revision, these will be further defined as to structure, process, and outcome criteria. Even with the availability of standards, nurses must exercise professional judgment based on education and experience in determining what is appropriate, pertinent, and realistic care at any one time (Dienemann, 1992). The reader should obtain the newly revised standards from AAOHN when they become available (1994).

Standards should remain stable over time as they reflect the values and beliefs of the profession about the practice. However, criteria should be reviewed and revised to reflect advancements in scientific knowledge and technology, and utilization of research findings into practice.

■ **TABLE 13–12**   ANA Standards of Clinical Nursing Practice

Standards of care
- Assessment
- Diagnosis
- Outcome identification
- Planning
- Implementation
- Evaluation

Standards of professional performance
- Quality of care
- Performance appraisal
- Education
- Collegiality
- Ethics
- Collaboration
- Research
- Resource utilization

From American Nurses Association. Standards of clinical nursing practice. Washington, DC: Author, 1991.

■ **TABLE 13–13**   Standards of Occupational Health Nursing Practice

STANDARDS OF CARE

  I. *Assessment:* The occupational health nurse systematically assesses the health status of the client.
 II. *Diagnosis:* The occupational health nurse analyzes data collected to formulate a nursing diagnosis.
III. *Outcome Identification:* The occupational health nurse identifies expected outcomes specific to client.
 IV. *Planning:* The occupational health nurse develops a plan of care that is comprehensive and formulates interventions for each level of prevention and for therapeutic modalities to achieve expected outcomes.
  V. *Implementation:* The occupational health nurse implements interventions to promote health, prevent illness and injury, and facilitate rehabilitation, guided by the plan of care.
 VI. *Evaluation:* The occupational health nurse systematically and continuously evaluates the client's responses to intervention and progress toward the achievement of expected outcomes.

PROFESSIONAL PRACTICE STANDARDS

  I. *Professional Development/Evaluation:* The occupational health nurse assumes responsibility for professional development and continuing education and evaluates personal professional performance in relation to practice standards.
 II. *Quality Improvement/Quality Assurance:* The occupational health nurse monitors and evaluates the quality and effectiveness of occupational health practice.
III. *Collaboration:* The occupational health nurse collaborates with employees, management, other health care providers, professionals, and community representatives in assessing, planning, implementing, and evaluating care and occupational health services.
 IV. *Research:* The occupational health nurse contributes to the scientific base in occupational health nursing and uses research findings in practice.
  V. *Ethics:* The occupational health nurse uses an ethical framework as a guide for decision making in practice.
 VI. *Resource Management:* The occupational health nurse collaborates with management to provide resources that support an occupational health program that meets the needs of the worker population.

From American Association of Occupational Health Nurses, Atlanta, GA: Author, 1994.

Quality Assurance Models and Instruments

Various quality assurance models, often used in auditing approaches, have been developed to evaluate health care. Two models are described as examples. One classic model developed by Norma Lang in 1974 and adopted by the American Nurses Association identifies seven steps (Fig. 13–4). It describes a circular flow of activities and incorporates structure, process, and outcome standards and criteria within a problem-solving process. The components of this model are generic and can be adapted for use in any quality improvement program (Dienemann, 1992).

The model is described as follows (Lang, 1976):

1. Identify and clarify values of the culture, institution, profession, nursing service, and individual nurse, considering the constant incorporation of new knowledge generated by research.
2. Identify structure, process and outcome standards and criteria (these were described previously) in order to measure aspects of quality care given as compared to the standards set.
3. Secure measurements about the degree to which actual performance conforms to established criteria. This can be done through various methods such as self-assessment, performance evaluation, peer review, observations, and record audits.
4. Make interpretations about the strengths and limitations of the current nursing program or practice in meeting the criteria and standards and begin to pinpoint successful and problem areas. For example, if walk-throughs were not conducted to monitor workplace hazards, information may reveal that the problem lies with management (e.g., insufficient nurses) rather than a limitation in nursing practice (e.g., insufficient knowledge).
5. Identify possible courses of action to correct deviations from meeting the standard, such as administrative changes, continuing education, self-initiated change, environmental change, or research.
6. Choose a course of action that best meets the need for the change, considering the organizational resources.
7. Take action to improve the quality of care. This may require both individual and organizational behavioral change (i.e., increasing self knowledge, providing better resources, developing effective policies/procedures).

Continued monitoring of actions is important to assess progress toward meeting criteria and standards and whether the action taken needs modification.

The Marker Quality Assurance Umbrella Model (Fig. 13–5) (1987) offers another approach to quality assurance. Marker describes this model as reflecting nine interdependent universal activities that constitute professional practice in any practice setting. Although Marker advocates that all nine areas be implemented, all should not be implemented at the same time and priorities for implementation should be established. The nine activities include the following:

1. Standards development for professional practicing directed at structure, process, and outcome. Standards should be validated periodically with mechanisms determined for their implementation.
2. Credentialing means validating competency both legally and professionally, including licensure, performance monitoring, certification, and skill-based testing.

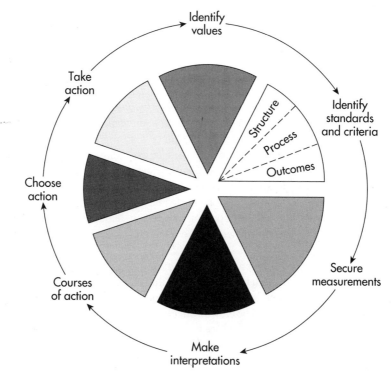

■ **Figure 13–4** ANA Model for Quality Assurance in Nursing. (From American Nurses Association: *A Plan for Implementation of Standards of Nursing Practice*. Washington, DC: Author, 1976.)

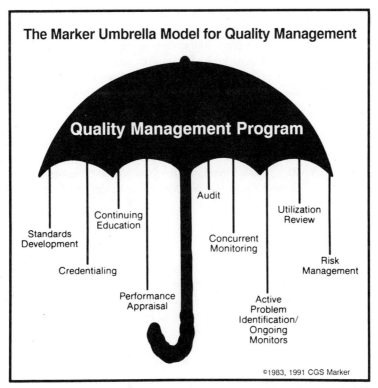

■ **Figure 13–5** Marker Umbrella Model. (From Marker, C. Journal of Nursing Quality Assurance, *1*(3): 52–63, 1987.)

3. Continuing education is vital to maintaining and updating knowledge and skills to support competent nursing practice, creating new competencies, and correcting deviations from noncompliance with existing standards. Methods to achieve this include providing for attendance at continuing education events for new or mandatory competencies and personal staff development. Tracking of learning events should be included.

4. Performance appraisal is essential to the managerial role and relates to quality assurance with respect to performance matched to standards. This is accomplished through use of an appraisal tool based on the employee's job description; performance standards that define specific expectations relative to a particular position; and monitoring, tracking, and documenting performance related to nursing care, which are then shared with the employee.

5. Audit procedures define a formal process of data collection from a representative sample of individuals or elements to determine compliance with specific care procedures and criteria for meeting standards. Audits should be carried out concurrently during the course of the work to examine structure, process, and outcome criteria rather than done retrospectively. Auditing procedures can include chart reviews, direct observations, and interviews with staff and employee clients.

6. Concurrent monitoring may be considered a minireview and usually occurs through a small nonrepresentative sample of observations. Its purpose is to spot-check a specific aspect of care at a designated point by a specific care-giver. Examples of concurrent monitoring activities include observation of physical assessment skills, occupational history taking, medication administration practices, research, and log recording practices.

7. Active problem identification/ongoing monitors involves reporting and documenting problems in order to identify approaches to improve performance. Report forms, where problems can be logged, and conferences, the results of which are recorded, are valuable data sources for problem identification and monitoring.

8. Utilization review involves monitoring and tracking resources for the health unit to determine adequacy and appropriate utilization. This can be done through reviewing budgeting records and workload logs.

9. Risk management involves activities designed to prevent loss such as through health hazard evaluations, safety inspections, and periodic health surveillance.

The ANA model defines a more traditional approach to quality assurance while the Marker Model focuses on integration of specific elements into the system and then monitoring compliance with the elements described.

Various tools for quality assurance are available and are often specific to meet the needs of the nursing specialty. Quality assurance tools in occupational health nursing are scarce. Examples include an instrument titled Standards, Interpretation, and Audit Criteria for Performance of Occupational Health Programs developed by the Department of Environmental Health, Kettering Laboratories, University of Cincinnati, Ohio (AAOHN, 1987); an Assessment Guide for Occupational Health Nursing Practice (Appendix 13–2) developed by Manchester and colleagues (1991), based on job descriptions and 1988 AAOHN practice standards, which uses structure and process and outcome criteria for evaluating occupational health programs and services; and a tool titled Quality Assurance in Occupational Health Nursing (Appendix 13–3) developed by Jarrett (1987) using the Marker Quality Assurance Umbrella Model.

In corporate settings with multiple nurses, a quality assurance program can be developed by this group and utilized in several different sites. However, establishing quality assurance programs is more difficult in occupational health nursing settings where nurses often work alone. One alternative is the development of a quality assurance review team by interested peers located within close proximity, or by occupational health nurses representing local AAOHN constituencies. Professional standards for practice from AAOHN can also be used and serve as the basis for specific criteria development.

Peer Review and Quality Circles

Peer review is a quality assurance technique and is also used as a method of employee evaluation. It is usually time consuming and costly; however, it generally provides an extensive and objective appraisal of the employee. The group or committee selected to perform the peer evaluation should be representative of and knowledgeable about the specialty, that is, occupational health nursing. In order to conduct the peer review, appraisal tools will need to be obtained and/or developed to measure the characteristics being evaluated (i.e., technical competence, organizational, leadership, and interpersonal relations skills) and a process must be established. The committee conducting the review must be oriented to the established process and procedure, which may include a review of the employee's self-evaluation, the manager's performance evaluation of the employee, a determination of the employee's contributions to occupational health nursing, a review of external letters critiquing the employee's work and any other supporting documentation (e.g., project reports, publications), and an interview with the employee. Once the review is completed, feedback is given to the employee to provide recognition for exceptional performance and information about areas for further growth and development.

Quality circles represent another approach to quality assurance wherein a small group of employees (5–10) meet generally on a weekly basis to solve problems related to the work (Marks, 1986). The group identifies common problems, and working on one problem at a time, concentrates on problem etiology and solutions. The solution is then presented to management for approval. If the proposal for change or correction is approved, the quality circle implements the action and evaluates the effectiveness.

Once quality assurance programs have been implemented it is important that all staff involved be given feedback about positive areas and areas needing change or correction (Brodbeck, 1992). Reports of favorable findings can serve to enhance and reinforce quality performance. For areas needing modification, strategies need to be determined, such as training, education, skill development and organization change.

It is important to recognize that quality assurance should be viewed as one mechanism for quality improvement. In many instances quality assurance is linked to risk management in an effort to identify causes of injury and help determine the best resolution to eliminate the problem. In addition, it should be emphasized that improvements in care and service must involve an interdisciplinary approach and commitment from all levels of the organization's structure. Quality health care services will be achieved as the result of positive interactions among professionals and departments working together to build a dynamic mechanism that continuously improves the processes and outcomes of service delivery (Dienemann, 1992).

■ QUALITY MANAGEMENT

Quality assurance programs should focus on quality work and preventive managing rather than satisfying accrediting bodies or as a method to detect employees who make errors. Quality assurance activities alone are considered by some as too restrictive and insufficient for contemporary health care and management needs, and need to be expanded to reflect improvement in client satisfaction based on quality service and management (Caper, 1988).

Total quality management was first developed in the United States and successfully integrated into the Japanese business structure through the work of Deming (Oberle, 1990). While the concept of quality management or continuous quality improvement is not foreign to the U.S. business industry, it is relatively new to the health care sector. The concept of quality management or improvement should be considered seriously as a method to enhance both management and productivity. Quality management incorporates and expands the traditional quality assurance functions while focusing efforts on continuous improvement with a more satisfying outcome. The idea is to do the right thing right the first time, on time, all the time, and to strive always for improvement and client/customer satisfaction (Deming, 1982; Hume, 1990; Masters & Schmele, 1991).

W. Edwards Deming, a leading expert in quality improvement, suggests that there must be a shift in management's thinking and managing which includes changing the philosophy of the organization to value quality; emphasizing empowering the worker to be more productive; and focusing on leadership and team building. Deming outlines a 14-point system encompassing these concepts (Table 13–14) (Walton, 1986).

■ TABLE 13–14   Deming's Guidepoints for Quality Improvement

1. Create constancy of purpose for improvement in product or service.
2. Adopt the new philosophy related to quality.
3. Cease dependence on inspections.
4. End the practice of awarding business on the price tag alone.
5. Improve constantly and forever the system of production and service.
6. Institute training and retraining on the job.
7. Adopt and institute leadership.
8. Drive out fear.
9. Break down barriers among staff and departments.
10. Eliminate slogans, exhortations, and targets for the workforce.
11. Eliminate quotas for the workforce (including numerical goals).
12. Remove barriers to pride in work performance.
13. Institute a program of education and self-improvement for everyone.
14. Implement the transformation through team effort.

Data from Deming, WE. Quality, productivity, and competitive position. Cambridge, MA: Massachusetts Institute of Technology, 1982.

It is important to note that quality management or improvement focuses on the system, not the employee. According to Deming, 15% of quality improvement focuses on people; the remaining 85% focuses on systems problems (Walton, 1986). Quality improvement can be considered preventive rather than reactive wherein the focus is to anticipate problems so they can be prevented and/or take corrective action to solve an identified problem in the system to prevent it from occurring again (Widtfeldt, 1992). The focus is on the process of doing the job right to ensure a quality outcome. Thus, time is spent on fixing the system versus fixing broken products. The notion of quality improvement that is prevention oriented shares the same philosophy as prevention versus cure in health care; that is, it is more cost-effective to prevent an illness than to treat the symptoms and illness.

Another important aspect of quality improvement is customer satisfaction (Casalov, 1991; Ervin, 1992; McLaughlin & Kaluzny, 1990). The occupational health nurse in the business setting is certainly familiar with total quality management with respect to goods and customer services, and this is or can be carried over into the occupational health unit. This means satisfaction by employees and other groups or departments who are served by the occupational health unit; satisfaction as demonstrated by staff morale; staff satisfaction with their own performance; and satisfaction from external groups (e.g., community). For example, Rogers et al. (1993) conducted a satisfaction survey of nearly 500 employees regarding the delivery and perceived quality of occupational health services in a pharmaceutical company. Results indicated high satisfaction with both services delivery indicators (e.g., waiting time) and quality indicators (e.g., provider interaction). One area noted for improvement was employees' inability to identify specific health care providers. This could potentially have an impact on continuity of care and thus reduce quality. Resolution of this problem was the institution and utilization of name tags.

Quality management shifts the focus from the individual to a team with a fundamental concept that if something goes wrong, it's usually not the people, it's the system at fault. It relies on input from employees as a source for change (Reilly, 1991). This management philosophy is basically consistent with that of McGregor's Theory Y and Herzberg's motivators.

Laza and Wheaton (1990) emphasize the importance of monitoring the system for improvement. This means that each work process is questioned and evaluated as to its usefulness, efficiency and effectiveness. For example, Widtfeldt (1992) describes one situation of a Fortune 500 company whose hypertension screening program had not been evaluated in several years, and also significant numbers of employees walked into the occupational health unit for blood pressure monitoring, thereby disrupting prearranged occupational health unit services. This was both a quality assurance and quality improvement issue. The problem was addressed through reviewing the current Joint National Committee on Detection, Evaluation, and Treatment of High Blood Pressure recommendations for screening high blood pressure and updating the occupational health service program standards and criteria for blood pressure monitoring (quality assurance). By doing this, high-risk individuals could more appropriately be identified and scheduled for blood pressure monitoring and disruption of prearranged occupational health service activities was reduced (quality improvement).

Before initiating a quality management program, it is important that the occupational health nurse assess the organization, including such elements as customer satisfaction planning, quality assurance, resource utilization, leadership, and teamwork. This is necessary to recognize strengths and weaknesses and to avoid potential pitfalls (Arikian, 1991; Thompson, 1988). Various tools such as flowcharts, Pareto charts, scatter diagrams, and cause and effect diagrams can be useful in analyzing work processes and problem areas (Hume, 1990).

Masters and Schmele (1991) point out that nurses often have more impact on the quality of care than any other member of the health care team, thus nursing is in a good position to implement quality management. Further, they describe advantages of quality management as

- increased quality
- increased productivity
- increased savings in time and money
- increased teamwork
- increased employee morale
- employee "ownership" of the organizational improvement process
- meeting of accreditation standards
- decreased rework
- decreased employee turnover
- decreased recruitment costs
- decreased costs

To implement quality management, top administration must commit to the philosophy of continuous improvement in all aspects of work. This will mean not only a change in thinking from the management perspective, but also from the staff. The solution to enhanced quality with cost savings should be embraced.

Occupational health nurses are often the decision makers with respect to occupational health indicators and unit functioning; thus their expertise is invaluable. More emphasis should be placed on incorporating a team philosophy that utilizes all skills with less focus on hierarchical occupational nursing decision making.

■ CHANGE

To be sure, the management of change is an integral component of the nurse manager's job. Change is a dynamic, inevitable phenomenon in life that provides a stimulus for growth. In health care, change provides an opportunity to improve the delivery and management of health care services. Although change is often initiated or allowed to occur in a random or haphazard fashion, it should be introduced in a planned, organized manner by one who is knowledgeable about change concepts, processes, and predicted outcomes.

Various theories seek to explain the concept of change (Olsen, 1978; Sullivan & Decker, 1988). For example, conflict theory of social change contends that the basis of most organizational change is due to some form of conflict experienced by individuals in the organization. Change is initiated to eliminate the conflict. Systems theory emphasizes that because of the interdependence and reciprocal relationship of one group or another, a change in one part of the system will result in a change in some other part of the system. Attitudinal change at the individual level is reported to be a function of the degree of internal conflict or disagreement between old and new information (Spradley, 1980). In addition, how one perceives a situation and her or his role in conformity to group pressure is a strong influencing factor.

In addition to the systems theory of change (interdependence of systems) previously described, the concepts of homeostasis and resistance are important to consider (Spradley, 1980). With respect to homeostasis, when change occurs, the system equilibrium is disturbed and stability is pursued, which follows after change has occurred. Resistance to change is common, and occurs frequently when change is introduced and should be anticipated. The occupational health nurse manager as a change agent should plan strategies to deal with expected changes.

Lippitt et al. (1958) point out that "as a change agent, the manager identifies the problem and helps others become problem aware; assesses the capacity and motivators of individuals for change; explores alternative change options with the individual or group; assesses resources needed; establishes and maintains a helping relationship; recognizes the phases of the change; and guides the process and techniques for the planned change" (p. 126). The classic process of change is well described by (Bennis et al., 1985) and involves three phases: unfreezing, moving, and refreezing. Unfreezing involves problem awareness or dissatisfaction with the status quo and recognition of the need for change. Moving involves working toward change through problem identification, exploring alternatives for problem resolution, developing a clear plan for change, and then implementing the plan. The nurse manager plays a critical role here and should be viewed as a facilitator and approachable expert who is available to help, not demand. The success of the change is positively related to the relationship the change agent has to the targeted individual or group (Kemp, 1986).

Assuming the change is accepted, refreezing is the integration of the change into one's life or performance and stabilization of the change, which probably will require reinforcement and/or practice. It's important to note that not all change will be accepted. If the change is rejected, the nurse manager or change agent must determine why this occurred and explore new alternatives and plans for accomplishing the task (Kemp, 1986). After the change has been introduced, the consequences should be evaluated both short-term and long-term to determine both the effects of the process and outcome.

Kurt Lewin's (1953) description of force-field analysis is a classic widely known approach to planned change. Lewin states that in any situation a dynamic equilibrium of simultaneously operating driving and restraining forces exists to maintain the status quo (Table 13–15). To create change, the status quo must be unfrozen, which requires either an increase in driving forces or decrease in restraining forces in the situation (Marriner-Tomey, 1991). Driving forces might

■ **TABLE 13–15** Forces of Change

Restraining forces Status quo	↓	↓	↓	↓	↓
Driving forces	↑	↑	↑	↑	↑

Concept from Lewin, K. Studies in group decisions. In Group dynamics. D. Cartwright & A. Zander, Eds. Evanston, IL: Row Peterson, 1953.

include pressure from or desire to please the manager, the desire to get ahead or for recognition, or a desire to improve working conditions. Restraining forces might include pressure to conform to group norms or lack of sufficient resources to accomplish unit goals and objectives. Haffer (1986) describes three change strategies:

1. The **empirical-rational strategy** is based on the assumption that people are rational and will adapt to a recommended change if it is justified and beneficial.
2. The **normative re-educative strategy** is based on the assumption that people will change their attitudes and behaviors if they share a part in problem identification and resolution, and planning for the desired change.
3. The **power-coercive strategy** is based on the assumption that those with less power will comply with directives for change from those who are more powerful.

Resistance to change is normal and comes primarily from those who oppose the change (Table 13–16). Change may represent a threat to the employee's

■ **TABLE 13–16** Factors Influencing Resistance to Change

Vested interests
Routines and habits
Risk of error
Fear of failure
Conflict with personal goals
Threats to employees'
    Role
    Economic/job security
    Self-esteem
    Social support
Excessive work pressure
Conflict with change agent
Institutional power structure
Clique forces of conformity

■ **TABLE 13–17** Strategies to Reduce Resistance to Change

Involve participants in the change process.
Start change process with those most receptive.
Gradually introduce changes.
Be sure information is clear.
Avoid attempts at coercion.
Employ consultant collaborator, if needed.
Identify resisters and try to understand reasons for resistance.
Involve the "resisters" with specific tasks to increase ownership.
Divide the "clique."
Provide avenue for compromises.
Provide rewards, incentives, and positive reinforcement for changes made.
Foster trusting relationship.

role, job security, or self-esteem, or the employee may simply have a low tolerance for change or the change may be misperceived as to its benefit or impact. Workers may perceive that the change implies (by management) inadequate work performance on their part. An experienced manager will recognize that individuals who complain the most about the change will actually prove to be less resistant than those who remain silent and refuse to discuss their objectives, or those who pretend acceptance but have no intention to modify their behavior (Gillies, 1989). Several strategies can be employed to reduce resistance to change (Table 13–17). Different strategies may be useful in different situations and multiple approaches may need to be deployed.

■ SUMMARY

The essence of management is to work with others to accomplish organizational goals. In order to achieve this, the manager must adapt and display management methods that help motivate and support the work performance.

While traditional management philosophy has assumed a more authoritarian management style, contemporary theory supports participative management with input from employees in the planning, doing, and evaluating of the work and work performance.

It seems appropriate that managerial functions and quality assurance activities be integrated within a total quality management philosophy with emphasis on continuous improvement. Within this framework, all workers share a common bond to not only assure but improve quality with a reduction in cost. Utilizing contemporary management approaches will also enhance worker self-esteem and ownership of the services and products produced.

References

American Association of Occupational Health Nurses. Occupational health nursing: The answer to health care cost containment. Atlanta: Author, 1989.

American Association of Occupational Health Nurses. Standards of occupational health nursing practice. Atlanta: Author, 1988.

American Association of Occupational Health Nurses. A comprehensive guide for establishing an occupational health nursing service. Atlanta: Author, 1987.

American Nurses Association. Standards of clinical nursing practice. Kansas City, MO: Author, 1991.

American Nurses Association. Suggested state legislation: Nursing practice act, nursing disciplinary diversion act, prescriptive authority act. Kansas City, MO: ANA, 1990.

Arikian, V. Total quality management. Journal of Nursing Administration, 21(6): 46–50, 1991.

Bennis, WG, Benne, KD, & Chinn, R. The planning of change. New York: Holt, Rinehart, & Winston, 1985.

Beyers, M. Getting on top of organizational change: The corporate nurse. Journal of Nursing Administration, 14(12): 32–37, 1984.

Bozman, A & Childres, F. The budgeting process. AAOHN Update Series, 4(8): 1–8, 1991.

Brodbeck, K. Professional practice actualized through an integrated shared governance and quality assurance model. Journal of Nursing Care Quality, 6(2): 20–31, 1992.

Caper, P. Defining quality in medical care. Health Affairs, 7: 50–61, 1988.

Casalov, R. Total quality management in health care. Hospital and Health Services Administration, 36(1): 134–146, 1991.

Decker, CM. Quality assurance: Accent on monitoring. Nursing Management, 16(11): 20–24, 1985.

Deming, WE. Quality, productivity and competitive position. Cambridge, MA: Massachusetts Institute of Technology, 1982.

Dienemann, J. Continuous quality improvement in nursing. Washington, DC: American Nurses Publishing, 1992.

Donabedian, A. Evaluating the quality of medical care. Milbank Memorial Fund Quarterly, 44(3): 166–206, 1966.

Douglas, L. The effective nurse. St. Louis: C.V. Mosby, 1988.

Drucker, P. The practice of management. New York: Harper & Row, 1982.

Dubnicki, C & Sloan, S. Excellence in nursing and management. Journal of Nursing Administration, 21(6): 40–45, 1991.

Ervin, D. Quality issues in group practice. MGM Journal, Jan/Feb: 25–31, 1992.

Finkler, S. Budgeting concepts for nurse managers. Philadelphia: W.B. Saunders Company, 1992.

Flarey, D. Redesigning management roles. Journal of Nursing Administration, 21(2): 40–45, 1991.

Gardner, D, Kelly, K, Johnson, M, McCloskey, J, & Maas, M. Nursing administration model for administrative practice. Journal of Nursing Administration, 21(3): 37–41, 1991.

Gillies, DA. Nursing management: A systems approach. Philadelphia: W.B. Saunders, 1989.

Goodstein, LD, Nolan, TM, & Pfeiffer, JW. Applied strategic planning. San Diego: Pfeiffer & Co, 1992.

Haffer, A. Facilitating change: Choosing the appropriate strategy. Journal of Nursing Administration, 16(4): 18–22, 1986.

Hein, E & Nicholson, MJ. Contemporary leadership behavior, 2nd ed. Boston: Little, Brown & Company, 1986.

Hersey, P & Blanchard, K. Management of organizational behavior, 6th ed. Englewood Cliffs, NJ: Prentice Hall, 1993.

Hume, SK. Total quality management. Health Progress, 71(8): 16–19, 1990.

Jarrett, M. Writing successful business proposals. AAOHN Update Series, 3(21): 1–8, 1989.

Jarrett, ME. A questionnaire to identify quality assurance activities in occupational health nursing. Chapel Hill: University of North Carolina, unpublished, 1987.

Jones, C. The money value of time. Harvard Business Review, July/Aug: 94–101, 1968.

Katz, RL. Skills of an effective manager. Harvard Business Review, Jan/Feb: 33–42, 1955.

Katz, D & Kahn, RL. The social psychology of organizations. New York: John Wiley, 1978.

Kemp, V. An overview of change and leadership. In Contemporary leadership behavior, 2nd ed. Hein, E & Nicholson, MJ, Eds. Boston: Little, Brown & Company, 1986.

Kerfoot, K. Thinking administratively: A must for the effective nurse manager. Nursing Economics, 6(3): 139–140, 1988.

Lang, NM. Issues in quality assurance in nursing: Issues in evaluation research. Kansas City, MO: ANA, 1976.

Laza, RW & Wheaton, PL. Recognizing the pitfalls of total quality management. Public Utilities Fortnightly, 125: 17–21, 1990.

Lewin, K. Studies in group decisons. In Group dynamics. D Cartwright & A Zander, Eds. Evanston, IL: Row Peterson, 1953.

Lieske, A. Standards, the basis of a quality assurance program. In C.G. Meisenheimer. Quality assurance: A complete guide to effective programs. Rockville, MD: Aspen, 1985.

Lippitt, R, Watson, J, & Westley B. Dynamics of planned change. New York: Harcourt, Brace, & Co, 1958.

Lorsch, J & Mathias, P. When professionals have to manage. Harvard Business Review, July/Aug: 78–83, 1987.

Mailbusch, R. Evaluation of quality assurance for nursing in hospitals. In Nursing quality assurance: A unit-based approach. P. Schroeder & R. Mailbusch, Eds. Rockville, MD: Aspen Publishers, pp. 3–18, 1984.

Manchester, J, Summers, V, Newell, J, Graughan, B, & Spitter, K. Development of an assessment guide for occupational health nurses. AAOHN Journal, 39(1): 7–12, 1991.

Marker, C. The Marker Umbrella model for quality assurance: Monitoring and evaluating professional practice. Journal of Nursing Quality Assurance, 1(3): 52–63, 1987.

Marks, M. The question of quality circles. Psychology Today, March: 36–42, 1986.

Marriner-Tomey, A. Guide to nursing management. St. Louis: C.V. Mosby, 1991.

Maslow, AH. Motivation and personality. New York: Harper & Row, 1954.

Masters, F & Schmele, J. Total quality management: An idea whose time has come. Journal of Nursing Quality Assurance, 5(4): 7–16, 1991.

Migliozzi, A. Quality assurance in occupational health nursing. Occupational Health Nursing, 33(2): 63–65, 1985.

Moss-Kanter, R. The new managerial work. Harvard Business Review, 67(6): 85–92, 1989.

McClure, M. Managing the professional nurse: Part I. Organizational theories. Journal of Nursing Administration, 14(2): 15–21, 1984.

McClure, M. Managing the professional nurse: Applying management theory to the challenges. Journal of Nursing Administration, 14(3): 11–17, 1984.

McLaughlin, CP & Kaluzny, AD. Total quality management in health: Making it work. Health Care Management Review, 15(3): 7–14, 1990.

Nightingale, F. Notes on nursing: What it is and what it is not. New York: Appleton, 1860.

Oberle, J. Quality gurus: The men and their message. Training, *Jan:* 47–52, 1990.

Olsen, ME. The process of social organization. New York: Holt, Rinehart & Winston, 1978.

Patz, J, Biordi, D & Holm, K. Middle nurse manager effectiveness. Journal of Nursing Administration, *21*(1): 15–24, 1991.

Poulin, M. The nurse executive role. Journal of Nursing Administration, *14*(2): 9–14, 1984.

Reilly, D. Can joy be found in the workplace? MGM Journal, *Jan/Feb:* 10–11, 1991.

Rogers, B, Winslow, B, & Higgins, S. Employee satisfaction and occupational health services. AAOHN Journal, *41:* 58–65, 1993.

Salmond, S. Supporting staff through decentralization. Nursing Economics, *3*: 295–300, 1985.

Simms, LM, Price, SA, & Pfoutz, SK. Nurse executives: Functions and priorities. Nursing Economics, *3*(4): 238–244, 1985.

Simyar, F & Lloyd-Jones, J. Strategic management in the health care sector. Englewood Cliffs, NJ: Prentice Hall, 1988.

Spradley, B. Managing change creatively. Journal of Nursing Administration, *11*(5): 32–37, 1980.

Sullivan, E & Decker, D. Effective management in nursing. New York: Addison-Wesley, 1988.

Tappen, R. Nursing leadership and management. Philadelphia: F.A. Davis, 1989.

Thompson, R. The six faces of quality. Healthcare Executive, *Mar/Apr:* 26–27, 1988.

Townsend, M. Creating a better work environment. Journal of Nursing Administration, *21*(1): 11–14, 1991.

Vestal, KW. Writing a business plan. Nursing Economics, *6*(3): 121–124, 1989.

Wallace, K & Ventura, M. Planning the interview for a clinical nurse researcher. Journal of Nursing Administration, *21*(12): 54–59, 1991.

Walton, M. The Deming management method. Putnam, NY: Dodd, Mead & Co., 1986.

Widtfeldt, A. Quality and quality improvement in occupational health nursing. AAOHN Update Series, *4*(3): 1–8, 1992.

Yukl, G. Leadership in organizations. Englewood Cliffs, NJ: Prentice-Hall, 1989.

Yura, H. Nursing leadership process. In Contemporary leadership behavior, 2nd ed. Hein, E & Nicholson, MJ, Eds. Boston: Little, Brown & Company. 1986.

13–1

Job Description for Department Head for Occupational Health Center

Example of Job Description for Department Head for Occupational Health Center

JOB DESCRIPTION
U 1300   5/92

Wellcome

INSTRUCTIONS ON HOW TO COMPLETE THIS FORM CAN BE FOUND IN THE SUPERVISORS MANUAL

Job Title	Unit	Dept.	Cost Center	
Health Center Department Head	OD	OH&S	5600	☐ RTP ☐ GVL ☐ Other

This job description supersedes all previous job descriptions for this position. Management retains the discretion to add to or change the duties at any time.	Compensation Dept. Use Only: Exempt ☐ Grade Code _____ Nonexempt ☐

JOB SUMMARY

Briefly state the main purpose of and basic responsibilities of the job.

> To plan, develop, and administer the policies and procedures of the RTP Health Centers and manage resources to meet Company needs. To provide health care to RTP and Field Staff employees that is directed toward the promotion, protection and restoration of worker health within the context of a safe and helpful work environment.

JOB DUTIES AND RESPONSIBILITIES

List in order of importance and/or frequency of occurrence each predominant and significant duty, task, or responsibility. Indicate if the job duty is essential (yes), which means that removing the function would fundamentally alter the job, or not essential (no). For each major job duty list the most important knowledge, skill, or ability (K, S, A) required to accomplish the duty.

JOB DUTIES	ESSENTIAL DUTIES (YES/NO)	REQUIRED K, S, A's
Assure completion and follow-up of pre-placement physical examinations complying with government regulations, environmental job demands and physical ability to perform work.	Yes	• Professional interdisciplinary knowledge base including the public health, occupational health, social and behavioral sciences, management and administration and nursing science. • Knowledge of EEO standards, handicap laws, ADA, and job demands • Decision making capabilities.
Manage the Company-sponsored periodic physical exams and medical surveillance programs. Promote employee health and life-style changes through individual counseling and referrals to Wellcome Health. Consult with Company physician to gain clarify regarding health related issues. Consult with Safety on environmental and safety concerns.	Yes	• Professional interdisciplinary knowledge base including the public health, occupational health, social and behavioral sciences, management and administration and nursing science. • Planning and organizing skills.
Verify eligibility of the employee within the sickness and accident/LTD plans. Monitor progress and coordinate community health services for rehabilitation purposes to assist the employee in return to work. Communicate appropriate information to immediate supervisor, Benefits, Human Resources, and Employee Relations.	Yes	• Professional interdisciplinary knowledge base including the public health, occupational health, social and behavioral sciences, management and administration and nursing science. • Working knowledge of job demands and ergonomics. • Working knowledge of B.W. Co. benefit plan. • Working knowledge of community health resources.

Courtesy of Burroughs-Wellcome

JOB DUTIES	ESSENTIAL DUTIES (YES/NO)	REQUIRED K, S, A's
Manage health services and reimbursement process for Field Staff.	Yes	• Professional interdisciplinary knowledge base including the public health, occupational health, social and behavioral sciences, management and administration and nursing science. • Working knowledge of B.W. Co. Flex Formula Insurance. • Working knowledge of accounting and budget.
Promote, supervise, and perform prompt and effective medical assistance to employees in acute and chronic situations.	Yes	• Professional interdisciplinary knowledge base including the public health, occupational health, social and behavioral sciences, management and administration and nursing science. • Working knowledge of job demands. • Skill in providing emergency care. • Working knowledge of B.W. Co. emergency response plan.
Supervise the development and maintenance of accurate up-to-date medical records and/or reports to track employee health/illness and provide the Company wit the needed data ensuring client confidentiality.	Yes	• Professional knowledge of medical terminology, attention to detail, skill in technical writing. • Confidentiality principles.
Manage Health Center operation and act as a resource and advisor to staff as health care services are rendered to the employee population. Evaluate performance, counsel, and coach as necessary.	Yes	• Professional interdisciplinary knowledge base including the public health, occupational health, social and behavioral sciences, management and administration and nursing science. • Leadership skills. • Oral and written communication skills. • Working knowledge of B.W. Co. policies and procedures.
Investigate illness and injury episodes and trends to determine health and safety needs of the employee population. Communicate this information to Safety and/or Wellcome Health Coordinator for program development.	Yes	• Professional interdisciplinary knowledge base including the public health, occupational health, social and behavioral sciences, management and administration and nursing science. • Working knowledge of B.W. Co. safety procedures. • Working knowledge of Wellcome Health program. • Communications skills
Represent the Health Center at B.W. Co. meetings and/or community affairs as requested.	Yes	• Leadership skills. • Oral communication skills. • Working knowledge of B.W. Co. policies and procedures.
Promote the Employee Assistance Program through individual and/or supervisor referrals.	Yes	• Professional knowledge of nursing process. • Working knowledge of B.W. Co. policies and procedures. • Counseling skills. • Oral communication skills.
Meets attendance requirements for the job. Other duties as assigned.	Yes	Ability to attend work regularly.

Courtesy of Burroughs-Wellcome

September 24, 1992

PROBLEM SOLVING AND DECISION MAKING

In the first column describe three or four of the <u>most important</u> problems that the job incumbent must solve or decisions that must be made to achieve the <u>primary objectives</u> of the job. For each problem, indicate in the second column the checks or controls that exist to help improve the quality or accuracy of the problem-solving/decision-making process. Then, in the third column, estimate the potential impact these problems/decisions can have on the department/unit <u>or</u> Company if handled <u>correctly</u> or <u>incorrectly</u>.

Problem/Decision	Checks/Controls	Potential Impact
Provide medical placement approval for existing or new employees in a job that matches their physical capabilities.	Medical opinions	Job turndowns, additional recruiting costs, lawsuits, increase WC cost and liability.
Approval of diagnosis for S&A benefit; judgment of potential long-term sequel on and need for LTD benefits.	Medical opinions	Improper use of benefit plan; increased liability to B.W. Co.
Ensure adequate job restrictions to protect B.W. Co. and facilitate employee rehabilitation.	Medical opinions	Increased WC cost and liability; illness/injury to other employees; increased lost work time, low productivity, lawsuits.
Interpret and comply with the medical requirements of regulations issued by ADA, OSHA, FDA and other government agencies.	Medical opinions Legal advise	Fines issued by government agencies for failure to comply or improper interpretation. Liability of employee lawsuits.

CONTACTS WITH OTHERS

List the most significant interactions that the job has within the Company (other than the immediate supervisor and the subordinates) and outside the Company. Under "Purpose of Contacts" indicate the reason why the contacts are made and why they are important to B.W. Co.

Title of Contact	Purpose of Contacts
Managers/Supervisors	To make recommendations to the manager on health related issues such as job restriction, job assignment, and/or job design.
Safety Department	To communicate potential health/safety hazards in the work place and ask for assistance in investigating.
Human Resources	To recommend the health ability or inability to perform a job as a pre-employment applicant or transfer through Operation Opportunity; to recommend job restrictions and/or job reassignment.
Employee Relations	To communicate the health status of employees when requested and advise Employee Relations of the need to drug test based on cause.
Employee Assistance Program	To refer and communicate the counseling needs of individual employees or groups of employees to the designated EAP counselor. Interact with counselor to resolve problems.
Physician's Contract	To ensure provisions of physician's contract are being carried out and monitor the medical services being rendered so that the highest standards of medical practice and services are being offered to B.W. Co. employees.

Courtesy of Burroughs-Wellcome

September 24, 1992

CREATIVE THOUGHT

What aspects of the position require the highest levels of creative thought (i.e., the conception and formulation of new ideas, techniques, procedures, programs, etc.)?

> Rendering decisions with regard to work area placement and restrictions based on the employee health status and capabilities.

WORKING CONDITIONS AND SPECIAL REQUIREMENTS

List any adverse working conditions, exposure to hazardous materials or conditions, travel requirements, requirements for working long hours, at night, weekends, rotating shifts, etc. **ALSO ATTACH A COMPLETED PHYSICAL AND ENVIRONMENTAL JOB DEMANDS FORM, U 294, IF A NORMAL SEDENTARY OFFICE ENVIRONMENT DOES NOT APPLY.**

X   none   see attached   list follows:
                     form U 294

JOB SPECIFICATIONS

Basic Background

Check the <u>minimum</u> education level and list the base level of experience required to successfully perform the job. Include the time length of experience required, if appropriate, as well as the nature of the experience required. If different combinations of education and/or experience could be considered equivalent, check and complete all that apply. Indicate they are alternatives by typing "OR" after each option.

> Education and Experience
>
> ☒   Four-year college curriculum with a major concentration in nursing.
>
>   PLUS: Be a Registered nurse in the State of North Carolina. Certification in audiometric and pulmonary function testing. Five year's experience in an Occupational Health nurse setting. Two year's supervisory experience.
>
> ☒   Other (special certification, licensure, etc., please specify) Certification as an Occupational Health Nurse.

Other Factors to be Considered in Selection Include:

List required KSAs not mentioned under Basic Background, Targeted Selection® Dimensions, and any <u>preferred</u> job related factors.

> • Professional image.
> • Experience in health/hygiene counseling; working with variety of patients in outpatient, adult health settings.
> • Skills: Oral and written communication, integrity, planning and organizing, problem analysis, decision making, leadership, team building.
> • Non-smoker.

APPROVALS & DATE	Signature	Date
Immediate Supervisor	_____	_____
Supervisor's Supervisor	_____	_____
Compensation	_____	_____
HR Manager	_____	_____

Courtesy of Burroughs-Wellcome

September 24, 1992

U 2196   5/92

REQUEST FOR JOB EVALUATION
(To be completed only when submitting the J.D. for Job Evaluation.
Submit to the Compensation Department RTP or Greenville when complete.)

☐ RTP
☐ GVL
☐ Other

Job Title: Health Center Department Head _____   Cost Center: 5600 _____

Initiating Supervisor: _____   Department: OH&S _____   Unit: OD _____

Supervisor's Supervisor: _____   Date of Request: _____

| Please complete checklist | An incomplete checklist will slow your request for job evaluation. |

1.   Please indicate the reason for job evaluation. (Check one)
  ☐ New Job
  ☐ Change in Existing Job Responsibility
  ☐ Other (Describe) _____

2.   ☐ This new job description (JD) makes obsolete the former JD with the
  title _____ in cost center _____
  -or-
  ☐ N/A.

3.   ☐ New JD attached.

4.   ☐ Physical and Environmental Job Demands form, U 294 attached.
  -or-
  ☐ N/A. Normal Sedentary office environment. No unusual physical and environmental demands involved.

5.   ☐ Organization chart attached.
  -or-
  ☐ Organization chart completed below.

```
                    +---------------------------------+
                    |   Immediate Supervisor's Title  |
                    |        Director of OH&S         |
                    |  _____  |
                    +---------------------------------+
                    +---------------------------------+
                    |        This Job's Title         |
                    |  Health Center Department Head  |
                    |  _____  |
                    +---------------------------------+
```

Title Occupational Health Nurses	Title Administrative Specialist	Title	Title	Title
Number of employees with this title 3	Number of employees with this title 2	Number of employees with this title	Number of employees with this title	Number of employees with this title

Total number of employees supervised (including employees who report in through the direct reports shown above).   5

―――――――――――――― FOR COMPENSATION DEPARTMENT USE ONLY ――――――――――――――

Job Code _____

Job Evaluation by/Date _____

Compensation Department Approval _____

☐ EXEMPT   ☐ NONEXEMPT

Current Grade

Revised Grade

GRADE

TOTAL POINTS

Courtesy of Burroughs-Wellcome

BW cc(lh)*/5

September 24, 1992

Assessment Guide for Occupational Health Nursing Practice

Date:

Evaluator:

Standard	Criteria	Level of Practice					Comments/ Recommendations
		All of the time	Most of the time	Some of the time	Not at all	N/A	
I. FUNCTION The OHN collaborates with management in developing objectives for the employee health service compatible with the company's corporate goals and objectives.	**STRUCTURE** 1. Functions: a. As manager for the health program and policymaker; b. under the supervision of a qualified occupational health nurse; c. as part of overall management in the development of policies for the health unit.						
	PROCESS 1. Develops philosophy and written goals and objectives for the occupational health program. 2. Conducts periodic reviews of Occupational Health Services to assure goals and objectives are being met. 3. Keeps informed of legal requirements of occupational health programs and assures compliance with same, i.e., medical surveillance, record keeping, etc. 4. Communicates findings to other members of management team and makes recommendations for programs and intervention strategies. 5. Conveys cost and benefits of occupational health programs in the workplace to management by: a. analysis of data; b. literature documentation.						
	OUTCOME 1. Occupational health programs are developed and implemented to: a. meet health needs of individual employees; b. assure optimal health and safety of all employees. 2. Occupational health programs are in compliance with federal and state laws. 3. The OHN is a member of the interdisciplinary team responsible for occupational health and safety.						

If not applicable N/A, please explain, i.e., This is not a responsibility of the OHN, this is responsibility of the supervisory nurse, corporate office, physicians, personnel, safety, etc.

Standard	Criteria	Level of Practice					Comments/ Recommendations
		All of the time	Most of the time	Some of the time	Not at all	N/A	
II. FUNCTION The OHN administers the employee health service	**STRUCTURE** 1. The health Service is managed by a qualified registered occupational health nurse. 2. The occupational health unit is of adequate size and quality and is suitably located to perform the nursing functions of the occupational health program. 3. The OHN is familiar with the products and processes of the company which affect health.						
	PROCESS 1. Develops and coordinates written policies and procedures with other members of the health team and management. 2. Determines the number and qualifications of nursing and paraprofessional staff that are required for a comprehensive on-site occupational health program. 3. Identifies and supervises the nursing care which can safely be performed by allied health workers. 4. Develops and monitors operating budget. 5. Collects data and prepares reports on the health status of the worker and the existing or potential health hazards in the work environment. 6. Provides management with data on trends in health-related statistics in order to inform them of the impact of occupational health program planning and implementation.						
	OUTCOME 1. The occupational health program is comprehensive and an integral part of the workplace. 2. The OHN is responsible for managing the occupational health department.						

If not applicable (N/A), please explain, i.e., This is not a responsibility of the OHN, this is responsibility of the supervisory nurse, corporate office, physicians, personnel, safety, etc.

Standard	Criteria	Level of Practice					Comments/
		All of the time	Most of the time	Some of the time	Not at all	N/A	Recommendations
III. FUNCTION The OHN defines nursing authority and responsibility based on standards of service and practice established by the nursing profession and collaborates with management in deter-mining the nurses' position in the organ-ization structure.	**STRUCTURE** 1. A written organizational chart is established for the health unit. 2. Written job descriptions are developed and available for all levels of nursing and allied staff. 3. Orientation programs and continuing educational plans are established for all nursing and allied personnel.						
	PROCESS 1. Functions with his/her level of preparation and experience in accordance with state and federal regulations for practice. 2. Attends educational and professional programs and meetings on a regular periodic basis in order to practice and promote state-of-the-art occupational health nursing.						
	OUTCOME 1. Evaluations to measure performance based on completion of activities defined in their job descriptions are conducted on an annual basis by the OHN manager.						

If not applicable N/A, please explain, i.e., This is not a responsibility of the OHN, this is responsibility of the supervisory nurse, corporate office, physicians, personnel, safety, etc.

Standard	Criteria	Level of Practice					Comments/ Recommendations
		All of the time	Most of the time	Some of the time	Not at all	N/A	
IV. FUNCTION The OHN administers nursing care and develops nursing care procedures and protocols with specific goals and interventions appropriate for employee's needs.	STRUCTURE 1. a. There is a written policy and procedure manual for nursing activities. b. A method exists for nursing care procedures and protocols to be communicated to appropriate personnel and health care providers. 2. Recordkeeping and reporting systems are in place which meet legal requirements, ensure continuity of care and confidentiality, and are coordinated with the company's systems. 3. Written, signed and dated medical directives or protocols are provided and updated at least annually.						

	PROCESS
	1. Identifies employee health needs and collaborates with health care providers, in establishing nursing care procedures and protocols.
	2. Actively participates in:
	  a. Preplacement assessments, periodic and special medical assessments; and
	  b. Determines health risk factors, employee and company needs in relation to job placement.
	3. Nursing care:
	  a. is individualized to meet the physical, emotional, social, and cultural needs of employees.
	  b. ensures optimal opportunities for employees with special needs.
	  c. is based on measures of prevention and health promotion.
	4. Demonstrates professional judgement and skill in patient assessment, nursing care, counseling, and evaluation techniques.
	5. Renders professional nursing care and follow-up of occupational and non-occupational illness and injuries within the scope of the company's Medical Directives and the Nurse Practice Act.						

	OUTCOME 1. Nursing care policies and procedures are recorded and available for review. 2. Nursing care policies and procedures are revised and periodically updated as goals are achieved or changed. 3. Accurate, complete and concise records of nursing activities are maintained. 4. Records are audited for appropriate treatment and/or referral.						

If not applicable N/A, please explain, i.e., This is not a responsibility of the OHN, this is responsibility of the supervisory nurse, corporate office, physicians, personnel, safety, etc.

Standard	Criteria	Level of Practice					Comments/ Recommendations
		All of the time	Most of the time	Some of the time	Not at all	N/A	
V. FUNCTION The OHN coordinates responsibilities in the health assessment program and promotes health maintenance and preventions of illness and injury.	**STRUCTURE** 1. The preventive approach to health care, which includes early detection, medical monitoring, health teaching and counseling with appropriate referral is a primary concern of the occupational health program. 2. Company sponsored health and wellness programs have been established by the OHN to assist employees in improving and maintaining their health. 3. A mechanism exists for the OHN to periodically reevaluate employee health and safety needs.						
	PROCESS 1. Plans, coordinates, implements, and evaluates on-site health education programs. 2. Intervenes appropriately on behalf of individuals and populations at risk of preventable, potential health problems. 3. Intervenes for an employee who evidences an acute illness, injury or temporary disabling condition. 4. Ensures that the employee is informed about his/her current health status. 5. Conducts or collaborates with other team members regular plant walk-throughs and health tours to assess potential or existing environmental, health and safety hazards. 6. Informs corporate personnel, when appropriate, about adaptations or interventions, of the work environment required to meet individual employee health needs. 7. Provides education, support and motivation in areas of health and safety.						
	OUTCOME 1. Health problems of employees are identified at an early stage. 2. Employees utilize information provided in making decisions and choice about promoting, maintaining, and restoring health, seeking and utilizing appropriate health care personnel and health care resources. 3. Employees demonstrate healthy lifestyle choices, knowledge of health care resources, and an understanding of the means of disease and accident prevention. 4. Employees, including handicapped, chronically and terminally ill, show evidence of participation in the workforce activities to the fullest extent possible in relation to each individual's health status.						

If not applicable N/A, please explain, i.e., This is not a responsibility of the OHN, this is responsibility of the supervisory nurse, corporate office, physicians, personnel, safety, etc.

Standard	Criteria	Level of Practice					Comments/
		All of the time	Most of the time	Some of the time	Not at all	N/A	Recommendations
VI. FUNCTION The OHN collaborates with other onsite members of the occupational health team to evaluate the work environment and utilizes outside resources when services are not available within company.	**STRUCTURE** 1. Functions as a member of the interdisciplinary health and safety team and as a resource person to other team members to establish parameters of service. 2. Coordinates the health care of the employees. 3. Is consulted, when appropriate, in selection of personal protection wear. 4. Coordinates and assists in development of safety education program, policies and procedures.						
	PROCESS 1. Utilizes States, Federal and private agencies and resources for assistance as needed. 2. Provides information to management to assist company in adhering to OSHA regulations, fire codes, SARA and Hazard Communication, recognizing safety as a priority.						
	OUTCOME 1. The OHN is part of a professional team, the goals of which are to provide a healthy and safe work environment for all employees. 2. The OHN defines his/her role and responsibility in contributing to the provision of a safe and health work environment.						

If not applicable N/A, please explain, i.e., This is not a responsibility of the OHN, this is responsibility of the supervisory nurse, corporate office, physicians, personnel, safety, etc.

Standard	Criteria	Level of Practice					Comments/
		All of the time	Most of the time	Some of the time	Not at all	N/A	Recommendations
VII. FUNCTION The OHN establishes and promotes working relationships with appropriate community agencies.	**STRUCTURE** 1. Acts as a member of management team and as a liaison to the community.						
	PROCESS 1. Establishes contact with agencies and services of the community that might be a reciprocal basis for a "good neighbor" policy (i.e., American Red Cross for Blood Drives, CPR, First Aid, Catastrophic Assistance etc.; American Cancer Society, Police with substance abuse assistance; Fire Department with Right to Know data, etc.) 2. Coordinates employee educational programs with appropriate community agencies.						
	OUTCOME 1. The OHN is an integral part of Management team by solidifying good public relations within the community. 2. Community health resources available for support are utilized in accomplishing health service goals and objectives.						

If not applicable (N/A), please explain, i.e., This is not a responsibility of the OHN, this is responsibility of the supervisory nurse, corporate office, physicians, personnel, safety, etc.

From Manchester et al. AAOHN Journal, *39*(1): 7–12, 1991.

13–3

Quality Assurance in Occupational Health Nursing

This questionnaire is divided into several small sections, each preceded by directions or comments to assist you in completing the questionnaire.

Standards of practice define and measure nursing accountability and the quality of patient care. The first series of questions addresses professional standards in the occupational health nursing unit where you are currently practicing.

1. Are there written standards of nursing practice for the occupational health nursing unit?
_____ Yes
_____ No

    2. If yes: What is the focus of the standards? (check those that apply)
    _____ Characteristics of the physical facilities
    _____ Type, quality, and quantity of equipment and supplies
    _____ Licensure, certification, and formal education
    _____ Staffing requirements
    _____ Continuing education
    _____ Policies and procedures
    _____ Job performance
    _____ Changes in health status of employees expected as a result of nursing care
    _____ Other, please specify: _____
    _____

Continuing education (CE) includes all professional developmental experiences occurring inside and outside the agency you are employed by. The following questions are concerned with the CE activities, with the exception of certification activities, associated with the occupational health nursing unit.

3. Do staff members have the opportunity to attend CE activities (either internal or external) directed at maintaining current competency in existing standards of nursing care?
_____ Yes
_____ No

    If yes: Please describe _____
    _____
    _____

4. Do staff members have the opportunity to attend CE activities that are directed at developing competencies when new standards are implemented?
_____ Yes
_____ No

    If yes: Please describe _____
    _____
    _____

5. Do staff members have the opportunity to attend CE activities that are directed toward correcting identified deficiencies in the knowledge or skills required in the particular practice setting?

_____ Yes

_____ No

        If yes: Please describe _____

        _____

        _____

Credentialing involves the validation of professional competency. The following questions are concerned with the subject of credentialing in the occupational health nursing unit you are currently practicing in.

6. Are annual licensure validations conducted and documented?

_____ Yes

_____ No

7. Is there periodic certification of staff members for competency in knowledge and skills identified in the unit standards of performance or job description?

_____ Yes

_____ No

        If yes, please identify the following that apply:

Certification	How often
_____ Pulmonary function testing	_____
_____ Hearing conservation	_____
_____ First aid	_____
_____ CPR	_____
_____ Other, please specify: _____	_____
_____	_____
_____	_____

8. Are there approval lists that identify those practitioners certified to practice in high-risk extended nursing roles such as suturing of wounds and prescribing of prescription medications?

_____ Yes

_____ No

_____ Not applicable

Performance appraisals can be utilized to provide staff members with feedback regarding their job performance and compliance to standards. Please answer the following questions dealing with the use of performance appraisals in your practice setting.

9. Is a job performance appraisal instrument used to evaluate your performance?

_____ Yes

_____ No

        10. Is the appraisal instrument based on the job description or performance standards for your position?

        _____ Yes

        _____ No

11. Is your job performance monitored and documented by your supervisor?

_____ Yes

_____ No

        12. If yes, please describe how performance is evaluated: _____

        _____

        _____

13. If yes: Does your supervisor discuss the results of these monitoring efforts with you on a periodic basis?

_____ Yes

_____ No

    If yes, how often? _____

14. If yes: Is information on your job performance obtained from these monitoring and review efforts utilized to identify problems and take corrective action?

_____ Yes

_____ No

I would like to gain knowledge of the use of audits in occupational health nursing programs. Please answer the following questions concerning the use of audits in your work setting for questions 15-20.

An audit is defined in the context of this questionnaire as a formal process of data collection from a representative sample.

15. Are audits of nursing practice conducted on site by internal or external reviewers?

_____ Yes (If yes, proceed to question # 16)

_____ No (If no, proceed to question # 21)

16. What is the position title of the person responsible for conducting the audits? _____

17. Is there a written schedule that specifies when audits are to be conducted?

_____ Yes

_____ No

    If yes, how often? _____

18. Please indicate how audits are utilized to obtain data. (place a check by those that apply).

_____ Chart reviews

_____ Direct observation of staff and clients

_____ Staff interviews

_____ Client interviews

_____ Other, please specify: _____

19. Please indicate the purposes for auditing in your unit (check those that apply).

_____ To review compliance to unit standards

_____ To determine how safe and effective a particular aspect of care is

_____ To determine the extent of a problem and which staff members, if any, are responsible

_____ To determine staff satisfaction

_____ To determine client satisfaction

_____ To evaluate staff documentation

_____ Other—please specify: _____

20. On the average, about how many audits are conducted each year? (please check one)

_____ 1-2

_____ 3-5

_____ 6-10

_____ 10-20

_____ more than 20

Risk management is concerned with the prevention of loss of human resources. The following questions have been included in order to obtain information on any risk management activities utilized in your occupational health nursing unit.

21. Does a preventive maintenance program exist in the unit to identify, take corrective action, and document safety hazards?

_____ Yes

_____ No

22. Are there standards, policies, and/or procedures that focus on infection control?

_____ Yes

_____ No

23. If yes: Is compliance to these standards reviewed on a periodic basis?

_____ Yes

_____ No

If yes, how often? _____

_____

Active problem identification refers to tools utilized by the manager as data sources for tracking events in the unit on a continuous basis. These tools serve a dual purpose in that they identify problems and monitor the results of actions taken to correct problems.

24. Please identify any of the tools listed below that are utilized for this purpose in your work setting. (check those that apply)

_____ Problem identification sheets—used by the staff to report complaints and perceived problems in a written manner.

_____ Problem log—a summarized list of problems identified in the unit, corrective actions (planned or implemented), and evaluations of short- and long-term results of the interventions.

_____ Shift report—provides a summation of the shifts' activities and communicates to the manager any problems or events that warrant immediate attention.

_____ Other—please specify: _____

_____

_____

_____ None utilized

The next two questions concern the quality assurance activities that review the utilization of resources in the occupational health nursing unit in which you are now practicing.

25. Are unit resources such as staffing, budget monies, equipment, facilities, and supplies monitored and evaluated to determine if they are adequate and are being used in an efficient manner?

_____ Yes

_____ No

26. If yes: What tools are used to monitor and evaluate resources? (please check those that apply)

_____ Unit log—used to record vital statistics on clients seen in the unit including any adverse events that occur.

_____ Unit record—used to record information on staff workload including volume indicators such as number of clients seen per day or number of procedures done per day.

_____ Budgetary record—used to track unit expenditures and compare the current budget status with predetermined budget goals.

_____ Other—please specify: _____

_____

_____

For the following question please check those responses that apply.

27. The results of quality assurance activities, if any, are communicated to whom?
_____ There are no quality assurance activities conducted
_____ Nurses working in the unit
_____ Corporate or supervisor nurse
_____ Medical director or corporate physician
_____ Personnel director/human resources manager
_____ Safety director
_____ General manager
_____ Other—please specify: _____

_____

When answering questions #28 and #29 please indicate the extent to which you agree or disagree by circling the appropriate response.

28. Quality assurance programs can assist in the maintenance or improvement of the quality of professional services by occupational health nurses.

| Strongly Agree | Agree | Uncertain | Disagree | Strongly Disagree |

29. A quality assurance program should be an integral part of all occupational health nursing units.

| Strongly Agree | Agree | Uncertain | Disagree | Strongly Disagree |

I would appreciate some information on the participants in this study and their practice settings. Please complete the following questions.

30. What is the total number of years you have practiced as a professional nurse? (check one)
_____ Less than 1 year
_____ 1-5 years
_____ 6-10 years
_____ 11-20 years
_____ More than 20 years

31. What is the total number of years you have practiced in an occupational health/employee health setting? (check one)
_____ Less than 1 year
_____ 1-5 years
_____ 6-10 years
_____ 11-20 years
_____ More than 20 years

32. Are you a Certified Occupational Health Nurse (COHN)?
_____ Yes
_____ No

33. What degrees/diplomas do you hold? (check those that apply)
_____ Associate Degree in nursing
_____ Hospital school of nursing Diploma Program
_____ Baccalaureate Degree in nursing

_____ Baccalaureate Degree other than nursing. Please specify:

_____

_____ Masters in nursing
_____ Masters in field other than nursing. Please specify:

_____

_____ Doctorate in nursing
_____ Doctorate in field other than nursing. Please specify:

_____

_____ Other, please specify: _____

_____

34. How many hours per week do you work on the average? (check one)
_____ 20 or fewer
_____ 21-39 hours
_____ 40 or more hours

35. Who is your immediate supervisor? (check one)
_____ Corporate or supervisor nurse
_____ Medical director or corporate physician
_____ Personnel director/human relations manager
_____ Safety director
_____ General manager
_____ Other—please specify: _____

36. Which of the following best describes your current position? (check one)
_____ Staff or general duty nurse
_____ Supervisor nurse or nurse manager
_____ Corporate nurse
_____ Nurse consultant
_____ Nurse educator
_____ Other—please describe: _____

37. How many registered nurses, including yourself, staff the occupational health nursing unit? (please check one)
_____ 1
_____ 2-4
_____ 5-10
_____ More than 10

38. If known, please identify your employer's Standard Industrial Classification: _____ If not known, please describe the major product or services of the agency: _____

39. Approximately how many people are employed at the facility? (please check one)
_____ Fewer than 250
_____ 250-499
_____ 500-999
_____ 1000-1999
_____ 2000-3999
_____ 4000 or more

Thank you for participating in this study.

From Jarrett, ME. A questionnaire to identify quality assurance activities in occupational health nursing. Chapel Hill: University of North Carolina, unpublished, 1987.

14

RESEARCH IN OCCUPATIONAL HEALTH NURSING

While the scope of occupational health nursing practice has expanded considerably in the last couple of decades, so too has there been increased emphasis on promoting and conducting occupational health nursing research and disseminating research findings. The conduct of research is necessary to support and expand the knowledge base that provides the foundation for practice. In an applied professional discipline such as occupational health nursing, research is needed to improve and foster the health and well-being of the worker and workforce, and improve working conditions to support this effort. Research and practice go hand in hand.

Nursing research is concerned with the systematic study and assessment of nursing problems or phenomena, finding ways to improve nursing practice and client care through creative studies, initiating and evaluating change, and taking action to make new knowledge useful in nursing. Treece and Treece (1982) have stated that in order to be answerable by research, questions must be conceived that will produce answers through some form of data collection from observation or explanation. In other words, a systematic, carefully designed approach must be used if true and meaningful answers are to be discovered. Research findings are intended to aid nurses to deliver quality health care services and help document the unique role that nursing has in the health care system (Polit & Hungler, 1991; Wilson, 1989).

This chapter has several purposes, including a discussion of the importance of occupational health nursing research and advances made in the field with a description of several examples. In addition, research preparation and training, the importance of research collaboration, and a brief discussion of the research process will be provided. It is important to emphasize that while this chapter presents an overview of the research process, it is only intended to provide the reader, who may have limited knowledge of and familiarity with the research process, with an appreciation for concepts and procedures involved in the conduct of research. Persons interested in becoming more involved in research are encouraged to acquire knowledge and skills to facilitate the experience.

■ RESEARCH PREPARATION

Research training and education is important in order to understand and utilize the research process, so that scientifically derived solutions to problems can be developed and implemented. Exposure to, appreciation for, and some application of nursing research occur at the undergraduate level, yet it is primarily at the graduate level that nurses become engaged in the knowledge and application of scientific processes and investigations. Many master's degree programs prepare nurses as beginning researchers; however, doctoral education is designed to prepare researchers who will:

- provide leadership for the integration of scientific knowledge with other sources of knowledge for the advancement of practice;
- conduct investigations to evaluate the contribution of nursing activities to the well-being of clients; and
- develop methods to monitor the quality of the practice of nursing in a clinical setting (ANA, 1981).

While many occupational health nurses may not have had formal academic preparation in nursing research, they are or have opportunities to be involved in research to varying degrees. Agnew and Travers (1990, p. 559) point out that "occupational health nurses have long been involved in research activities but have not always recognized them as such." The authors state that "it often is the nurse who identifies an outbreak of work-related illness, investigates the cause, and initiates the resolution." This underscores the need for being familiar with and understanding the research process and methods, and creating collaborative relationships with seasoned investigators who can provide primary investigative guidance and serve as mentors, when needed. Collaborative research has several advantages that include, but are not limited to, the following (Rogers, 1988):

- provides an opportunity to develop and expand clinical research skills in the work environment, including research mentorship;
- provides an opportunity for the clinician, researcher, and administrator to jointly discuss imperative questions or problems that need solutions;
- combines the expertise of the clinician and the researcher, thereby enhancing clinical integrity and scientific rigor to achieve a mutual benefit: quality, cost-effective health care;
- increases research skills through mutual learning and sharing; and
- provides for early dissemination of the research findings from both the research and clinical perspective, allowing for a recognition of a valuable partnership, which can lead to new nursing interventions.

Persons involved in research will find that collaborative efforts stimulate the mind, broaden the learning experience, and lay the foundation for future research opportunities.

■ ADVANCING OCCUPATIONAL HEALTH NURSING RESEARCH

A research-based practice is foundational to any professional discipline. Increasingly, research is being conducted by occupational health nurses to develop and expand knowledge in the field of occupational health nursing, and to test theories and ideas aimed at improving workers' and workplace health and safety.

A review of the literature in separate reports by Atkins and Magnuson (1990) and Rogers (1990) shows evidence of advances in occupational health nursing research. Atkinson and Magnuson report that for a five-year period from 1984 to 1989 more than 50% of research conducted by occupational health nurse investigators was concerned with health promotion and stress and coping topics related to worker health. Testing of theories and interventions to improve healthy lifestyles was apparent. Rogers reports that much of the occupational health nursing research in the early 1980s focused on programmatic activities, role delineation, and scope of practice, while more emphasis was placed on worker health promotion and protection research in the latter part of the decade.

The support for the conduct of nursing research is evidenced by congressional establishment of the National Center for Nursing Research in 1986, now (1993) the National Institute for Nursing Research, to help provide funding for research projects. In addition, funding support by other public, private, and professional groups has been established or enhanced. For example, the American Association of Occupational Health Nurses offers two research awards annually. Other examples of potential funding sources for occupational health nursing research are shown in Appendix 14–1.

Further evidence of support for occupational health nursing research has been the establishment of occupational health nursing research priorities by the AAOHN (Table 14–1). These priorities were identified through a sophisticated delphi-technique survey of a national random sample of occupational health nurses (Rogers, 1989). The priorities represent vital areas of importance to improve the health and safety of America's workforce and have been distributed to key agencies and groups (e.g., NIOSH, NINR, NIH) in order to focus attention on these areas for support in funding opportunities.

Many of the AAOHN research priorities for occupational health nursing are

■ **TABLE 14–1**   Research Priorities in Occupational Health Nursing

- Effectiveness of primary health care delivery at the worksite.
- Effectiveness of health promotion nursing intervention strategies.
- Methods for handling complex ethical issues related to occupational health (e.g. confidentiality of employee health records, truth telling.)
- Strategies that minimize work related health outcomes (e.g. back injuries).
- Health effects resulting from chemical exposures in the workplace.
- Occupational hazards of health care workers.
- Factors that influence worker rehabilitation and return to work.
- Mechanisms to assure quality and cost effectiveness of occupational health programs (e.g. effects of employee assistance programs or health surveillance programs on improving employee health).
- Effectiveness of occupational health nursing programs on employee productivity and morale.
- Factors that contribute to behavioral changes among health care workers for self-protection from occupational hazards (e.g. HIV/AIDS).
- Factors that contribute to sustained risk reduction behavior related to lifestyle choices (e.g. smoking, substance abuse, nutrition).
- Effectiveness of ergonomic strategies to reduce worker injury and illness.

From American Association of Occupational Health Nurses, February 1990.

being addressed. For example, in the area of health promotion, Christenson and Kiefhaber (1988) report an increase in health promotion activities offered by companies. Smoking control (35.6%), health risk assessment (29.5%), back care (28.6%), and stress management (26.6%) were cited as the types of activities/programs most frequently offered.

Taylor (1987) describes the successful implementation of a comprehensive health promotion program in a single-nurse unit aimed at reducing costs and absenteeism, and Conn and Barclay (1987) report on the value of creating health awareness in several lifestyle areas not only among employees but also at the organizational level. More research that documents the cost-effectiveness of these programs needs to be conducted to assist employers in making decisions about health interventions that will ultimately improve employee health.

Pilon and Renfroe (1990) provide evaluation data on significant reductions in cardiovascular risk factors in employees as a result of nursing interventions, including education classes and counseling. Also using education/counseling interventions directed at multilifestyle behaviors, Harrell et al. (1992) reported reductions in blood pressure among more than 500 textile workers. However, nonsignificant increases in cholesterol levels as well as variations in smoking behaviors were also found. The authors believed that a multibehavioral approach might be confusing and overwhelming and perhaps targeting a single behavior is most effective. This needs further study.

Within the scope of the AAOHN research priorities are several areas related to health protection that are being addressed by occupational health nursing researchers. Newlin (1984) implemented a stress reduction program for intensive care nurses after surveying the population for stress indicators. Pre- and post-test interviews and observations were completed. On completion of the program, subjects indicated reduction in feelings of stress and more ability to cope with stressful situations. Jung (1986) has reported an increase in somatic complaints such as headaches, gastrointestinal problems, fatigue, insomnia, nervousness, and decreases in work productivity in workers on rotating shifts. Jung recommends that occupational health nurses assess workplace shiftwork schedules to determine work patterns and shiftwork sequences in order to focus work assignments better, particularly for those at high risk (e.g., workers with diabetes, asthma, and other chronic diseases).

Rogers (1987) has done extensive work on the hazards to which nurses who handle antineoplastic agents are exposed. The results showed that nurses exposed to antineoplastic agents at work were significantly more likely to have urinary mutagenicity when compared to nonexposed nurses. This was also true in a comparison of on-duty vs. off-duty urine samples from exposed nurses. In addition, the author's investigation suggests that handling antineoplastic agents may be associated with potential health problems such as gastrointestinal symptoms, hair loss, and reproductive loss (Rogers & Emmett, 1987).

Garrett et al. (1992) examined risk factors related to back injuries among nursing personnel and found that more serious injuries were likely to occur on the nightshift. In addition, nurses who worked on long-term care units and nurses with excess weight were involved in more severe injuries, leading to increased absenteeism and disability.

Another study related to health care workers examined this groups' knowledge and acceptance of hepatitis B vaccination. In a survey of 480 health care workers in a large metropolitan hospital, McKenzie (1992) found that 45% of workers had not received the vaccine. Primary reasons given were fear of side effects (38%), feeling it was unnecessary (24%), and being unaware of vaccine availability (21%). Obvious implications are for improved education regarding vaccine protection, safety, and availability.

Studies related to cost-containment approaches, evaluation of primary care strategies, and ethics are less often reported. Rogers (1990) has investigated ethical problems facing occupational health nurses and has identified several recurring issues such as confidentiality of health information, exposure and right to know issues, and dealing with substance abuse. Conflicts often arise as to how such problems should be managed. Strategies for ethical effectiveness need to be developed.

With the continuing rise of health care costs and more emphasis placed on primary health care delivery at the worksite, strategies to evaluate the effectiveness and efficiency of primary care delivery at the worksite need to be evaluated. Occupational health nursing contributions in this research endeavor are imperative.

These are but a few examples of recent research conducted by occupational health nurse investigators. Knowledge development will help to identify strategies that will improve worker health and reduce hazard risk. In addition, designing studies to evaluate methods to reduce health care-related costs to the employer is vital.

■ FEASIBILITY OF CONDUCTING THE RESEARCH

The investigative process involves deliberate steps and activities within a carefully designed framework, or blueprint so to speak. Of clear importance in conducting research is whether the research can be done. Several factors should be considered for the successful completion of the project (Tornquist & Rogers, 1987).

- a research problem of some importance;
- research experience or collaboration with a seasoned researcher for consultation and/or co-investigation;
- a commitment from the researcher to complete the project, as it may take many months and sometimes years to finish;
- cooperation of organizational management, particularly if it requires employee time and company involvement;
- adequate time available to the researcher to conduct the study, which is particularly important if there are competing obligations such as job responsibility;
- accessibility and availability of research subjects;
- sufficient resources, including money, equipment, supplies, and additional personnel if needed, depending on the scope of the project;
- facilities, space, and equipment to conduct the research; and
- attention given to ethical considerations of the research, including issues related to risk/benefit, the potential for harm, informed consent, and maintenance of confidentiality.

Determining early on the feasibility of conducting the research will save time, money, and energy and help to avoid unnecessary frustration.

■ TERMINOLOGY

Scientific research has specific terminology with which the researcher must be familiar. Basic terms will briefly be discussed here.

Concepts are generally abstractions or ideas that are based on observations of certain behaviors or characteristics (e.g., stress, self-esteem, pain, health). When concepts are put into operation (operationally defined) or made amenable to measurement, they are usually referred to as variables.

A **variable** is something that varies such as weight, height, temperature, and attitude and takes on different values. For example, the variable gender has two values, male and female; whereas, age may have values from zero to more than 100. In the research context, if relationships between variables are presumed, variables are often labeled as dependent or independent. The dependent variable (DV), otherwise referred to as the outcome or *"presumed effect"* variable, is the variable under investigation; whereas, the independent variable (IV) is the *"presumed cause"* variable. For example, the researcher may investigate the extent to which lung cancer (DV) depends on smoking behavior (IV); the effects of teaching employees about diet and cholesterol (IV) on cholesterol reduction (DV); or the use of incentives (IV) to affect employee participation (DV) in health promotion programs; or the effect of peer influence (IV) on the use of protective equipment (DV). It is usually not too difficult to spot the difference between dependent and independent variables in a research study. The researcher needs to be cautioned, however, not to presume that the independent variable is, in fact, the cause of the dependent variable. There are many other factors that need to be taken into consideration before conclusions regarding cause and effect can be drawn, such as research design and sampling scheme, which will be discussed later. In addition, a variable can be purely descriptive, such as the attitudes about health.

An **operational definition** specifies what the researcher does to make the concept or variable measurable. For example, the variable weight will be operationally defined by measuring a subject's weight on scales, undressed after fasting for 10 to 12 hours. If anxiety related to overwork is being measured, then overwork needs to be defined, such as more than 60 hours per week, and anxiety measured, perhaps through use of a survey instrument, many of which are available. Defining variables operationally allows the researcher to collect data systematically and consistently from all subjects and to communicate exactly what the terms mean.

Other variables of note, termed *confounding* or *extraneous variables,* may have relevant effects on the dependent variable (other than the independent variable), and the research must take these into account in the design, analysis, and interpretation of the findings. For example, a researcher may be interested in studying whether women who work rotational shiftwork are at higher risk of having low-birth weight babies than are women who work regular daytime jobs. Although the key variables of interest are rotational shiftwork and low birth weight, the researcher may need to be concerned with the effects of other variables, such as age, diet, medications, and smoking. Because uncontrolled extraneous variables can lead to erroneous conclusions, the researcher will need to identify these extraneous variables and determine approaches within the design of the study to control for them. For example, control of the variable smoking can be accomplished through limiting participation of research subjects to nonsmokers; this eliminates or equalizes the effects of that variable.

Data are the pieces of information the investigator collects from the subjects, usually by means of *instruments* or *tools*. Instruments may include questionnaires; rating scales; paper and pencil tests; physiological and biological measurement devices such as thermometers, sphygmomanometers, or blood tests; and a variety of industrial hygiene sampling devices.

■ RESEARCH PROCESS

The major steps in the research process (Table 14–2) will be very briefly described. The description of the process will focus on quantitative rather than qualitative research, although the latter is a useful approach to in-depth descriptive or hypothesis-generating research.

1. Identifying and Limiting the Research Problem

Selecting the research problem can be the most challenging task of the research process, especially for the beginning investigator. The researcher may have some idea of what she or he is interested in studying, but may be unfamiliar with what is known about the subject, or concerned with whether the problem is in fact researchable. In addition, the researcher will want to study a problem that is of some significance, that is, that the research idea is important and will contribute to the knowledge base and practice in the discipline, in this case occupational health nursing.

Sources of Research Problems

When beginning to identify a research problem for study there are at least three sources from which ideas can be generated: work experience; trends and patterns in health, illness, injury, behavior, and so forth; and the literature.

Experience.   No matter what the work setting, there are always problems and one may wonder what could improve or alter the situation. For example, what makes some employees use protective equipment while others do not? Is a certain counseling approach more effective in helping employees lower cholesterol levels? Are nursing guidelines for practice effective in reducing costs? Whatever the problems, curiosity will help generate a research idea.

Trends and Patterns.   Practitioners can identify research problems from observations of individual cases that form a pattern of occurrence. For example,

---

■ TABLE 14–2   Steps in the Research Process

---

1. Identify problem
2. Conduct literature review
3. Identify theoretical/conceptual framework
4. Formulate hypothesis
5. Operationalize variables
6. Select research design
7. Ascertain and select sample
8. Conduct pilot study
9. Collect data
10. Analyze data
11. Interpret results
12. Disseminate information

---

when several workers from the same work area report to the occupational health unit with similar health complaints, or there is an increased incidence in spontaneous abortions over a period of time, a problem may be occurring that lends itself to investigation.

Literature. Ideas for researchable problems often come from published and unpublished reports. When reading the nursing, occupational health, or related literature fields, authors will often suggest problem areas for further research as an extension of their own work. Unpublished master's theses or doctoral dissertations also provide fruitful areas for research ideas. Furthermore, questions for study are often stimulated by contradictory results reported by different investigators about the same general area.

In addition, the AAOHN priorities in occupational health nursing previously discussed (Table 14–1) were identified in order to focus attention on critical areas needing research and support for funding (Rogers, 1989).

Problem Development

The development of a researchable problem requires creativity and thoughtfulness and the researcher may find herself or himself generating several ideas. Try not to be critical of the ideas; rather, write down the areas of interest and don't worry about the terms or structure used (e.g., job satisfaction among nurses, effective use of personal protective equipment, transmission of communicable diseases, and cost-effectiveness of prenatal care at the worksite).

Once a general topic of interest has been identified, the focus should be narrowed so a researchable problem or question can be developed. Discussing thoughts and ideas with fellow colleagues can help further define or clarify the question. A stem will need to be added to the topical statement, such as What types . . . ? What is the relationship between . . . ? or Why do . . . ? For example, one might ask, "What conditions promote the use of gloves when delivering employee health care?"

Brink and Wood (1988) describe three levels of research and respective types of questions, each based on the amount of knowledge and/or theory about the topic under study. Level I questions are developed when the topic has not been studied or there is limited information or knowledge gaps. Level I questions begin with the "what is/what are" stem; examples can be found in Table 14–3.

■ **TABLE 14–3**   Examples of Research Questions

Level I
- What is the prevalence of hypercholesterolemia in the worker population?
- What are the characteristics of employees who exercise regularly?

Level II
- Is there a relationship between eating worksite prepared foods and hypercholesterolemia in workers?
- What is the relationship between absenteeism and exercise?

Level III
- Why do employees resist or comply with using protective devices?
- Why is there an increase in violence in the workplace?

The researcher moves to Level II questions when information on the topic has already been described. Here the researcher focuses on relationships between at least two variables not previously examined together, such as pregnancy outcomes and extended work duty or shiftwork. At this level a good foundation for why two variables should be related is based on previous descriptive studies (Rogers, 1990, 1991). Level II questions may begin with the stem "what is the relationship" and are completed by relating two variables together (Table 14–3). At Level III, the question asks "why" there is a relationship between the variables, implying that one variable influences the other specifically. A cause and effect relationship is assumed and the researcher is able to manipulate the independent variables, such as an intervention (e.g., a learning experience) to predict an outcome. Examples are shown in Table 14–3.

The research problem normally identifies the key variables (independent and dependent), study subjects, and topic area. Although the problem is often stated as a question, it may be stated in a declarative form such as, The purpose of this research is to examine the relationship between pregnancy outcome and shift rotation.

2. The Literature Review

A literature review involves a comprehensive and systematic examination of available material in order to help find out more precisely what is known about the topic or investigative area. Depending on what the literature reveals, the level of inquiry of the question may change. For example, if the question asked "What are the characteristics of employees with back problems?" and several research and related articles dealing with that issue were discovered, moving to a second level of inquiry such as "What is the relationship between lifting techniques and back injuries?" would be in order. As the topic becomes clearer from the literature review, the question level will also become clearer.

There are several reasons to conduct a literature review. First, it is important to determine what is already known about the problem to avoid unnecessary duplication if the problem has had satisfactory research. Second, reviewing the literature helps to provide a context into which the problem fits; that is, it will help to establish links to existing research so there is a building of a body of knowledge. Third, the literature review helps to identify gaps in research, and will then enable the researcher to better define the problem. A study conducted in isolation cannot be clearly evaluated for significance and meaning, whereas a study that links up with previous research or theory provides a sense of context and history (Wilson, 1989). The more one's study is linked with other research, the more contribution it is likely to make.

Several sources and approaches can be used to conduct the literature review. The scope of the review should be comprehensive in breadth and depth and include the following:

Research Literature.   A review of relevant research literature from nursing and other related disciplines will provide a background for and document progress on a specific topic or problem.

Theoretical and Conceptual Literature.   This type of information will provide a theoretical or conceptual context for a research problem. This context or framework will help to extend the scope of one's knowledge.

Methodological Literature.   Articles concerning research similar to the topic area under investigation can be helpful when examining how a study was conducted, that is, what approaches were used, how variables were operationalized or measured, how samples were selected, and data analyzed. References dealing with statistical tests and instrumentation will also be useful.

Clinical Literature.   Nonresearch articles provide background information for the topic area; however, for a research study they are of limited value as they provide general information and often are subjective rather than objective in opinion. Nevertheless, they do help broaden the researcher's understanding of the problem.

Literature references are categorized as either primary or secondary sources. Primary sources are written by the investigator who conducted the study, while secondary sources provide summary descriptions, usually of several research studies, written by someone other than the original researcher. Secondary sources provide useful bibliographic information on primary sources; however, primary sources must be read by the researcher in order to obtain sufficient detail necessary about the problem. When the literature is reviewed, it is helpful to write critiques about each article and put them onto separate index cards. The researcher will then be able to systematically analyze the literature identifying not only the content but flaws, gaps, and methodological weaknesses. For example, if a study has a sample size of five volunteers and the author generalizes its findings to a workforce of a thousand, caution in interpretation should be exercised.

To begin the literature review use a computerized search (get help from the librarian, as there are many different types of searches and software available) and make notes on index cards as previously mentioned. It will be helpful to sort the cards into logical categories such as etiology of the problem, social and demographic characteristics, or attitudinal issues. This will help to organize thoughts conceptually.

3. Theoretical or Conceptual Context

Theory guides the researcher in understanding not only what happens related to certain phenomena (e.g., stress, pain, or anxiety) but why these phenomena occur. Theories help to link facts and concepts together and represent the scientist's best efforts to explain relationships between variables (e.g., anxiety and pain), predict what will happen (e.g., anxiety increases pain), and ultimately control or change the phenomena of concern (e.g., decrease pain through visualization or medication). The relationship between theory and research is reciprocal; theory guides and generates ideas for research and research from empirical data helps to validate or add to the theory.

Not all research conducted is done so within a theoretical context, as many nursing research studies are still at a descriptive point that may later serve as the basis for theory development. Although it is true that fitting a problem to a theory enhances its value, scientific meaning, and knowledge building, artificially cramming a problem into a theoretical framework serves no purpose; in other words, there is no point in fabricating a link if one does not exist (Polit & Hungler, 1991). Conceptual models are less well-developed attempts at organizing phenomena but for the beginning researcher provide an important step in beginning to establish factual links between variable relationships. An imaginative mind can create a conceptual model that later may be developed into a theory.

4. Formulating the Hypothesis

Once the problem has been identified, literature reviewed, variables conceptualized, and an appropriate theoretical or conceptual framework identified, the researcher will specify researchable questions to be answered or hypotheses to be tested. A research hypothesis is a tentative prediction or explanation of the relationship between two variables. A question often arises as to whether a hypothesis is always necessary or if a research question is sufficient. Descriptive research aimed primarily at describing phenomena generally proceed without hypotheses, and research questions are used to gather data and provide a beginning foundation for later research, which often is hypothesis generating. In these cases research questions will serve as the basis for inquiry.

Hypotheses, by setting direction and interconnecting and predicting relationships between two or more variables, help extend knowledge about the phenomena under investigation. Within the framework of previous research or theory, hypotheses usually flow from a researcher's observations or experiences. Hypotheses must be written clearly and specifically so that variables are identifiable and definable. Hypotheses may be simple or complex. A simple hypothesis predicts the relationship between one independent variable and one dependent variable, whereas a complex hypothesis predicts the relationship between two or more independent and two or more dependent variables. Examples of hypotheses are provided in Table 14–4.

The testing of hypotheses is the center of empirical research and must indicate an anticipated relationship between two or more variables. After hypotheses are developed, they are subjected to empirical testing through the collection, analysis, and interpretation of data. Not all investigations are designed to test hypotheses; rather, they may answer questions to provide a foundation for empirical hypothesis testing later.

■ **TABLE 14–4** Examples of Hypotheses

Hypothesis	Independent Variable	Dependent Variable	Simple or Complex
Women workers are more likely to frequent the occupational health unit than are male workers.	Gender (female versus male)	Occupational health unit visits	Simple
Nurses who randomly rotate shifts are more likely to have a higher number of sick days and decreased job satisfaction than nurses scheduled by block rotation.	Schedule method (random versus block secondary)	Absenteeism Job satisfaction	Complex
There is a relationship among worker age, sex, and work experience and knowledge about use of protective equipment.	Demographic characteristics (age, sex, experience)	Knowledge and use of protective devices	Complex
Younger workers are more likely to have on-the-job accidents than are older workers.	Age	Accidents	Simple

5. Operationalizing Variables

Once research questions or hypotheses have been stated, variables will need to be defined and measured in the research context, that is, operationally defined. Variables were previously discussed. The operational definition specifies a concrete definition of how a variable will be measured. For example, in a study involving an intervention aimed at blood pressure reduction, the variable blood pressure would be easy to define and measure. The operational definition might state that employee blood pressures of research subjects would be measured weekly at a specific location, with the employee at rest for five minutes, using a calibrated sphygmomanometer. It is important that the measurement of all variables be consistent for all study subjects.

Many variables measured in nursing research deal with attitudes and behaviors and psychological, social, or health quality concepts that may be less easily operationalized; however, many instruments exist that measure stress, coping, risk perception, social support, and so forth. The research will need to develop or choose an instrument that can validly measure the concepts under study. Issues related to reliability and validity of the instrument must be considered.

6. Selecting a Research Design

The research design is the blueprint or plan for conducting the research, the selection of which is guided by the purpose or research questions/hypotheses undertaken. There are many types of research designs; however, only commonly used designs will be briefly discussed, for purposes of example. Reference to a good research text will be helpful in determining which type of design is most appropriate to answer the research question(s).

Experimental Research

Experimental research is scientific investigation that is characterized by the properties of manipulation, randomization, and control. Manipulation occurs when the investigator does something (i.e., introduces the independent variable), often referred to as the treatment or intervention, to the experimental group(s). Randomization involves the random assignment of subjects to experimental or control groups. Randomization actually eliminates the systematic bias in the groups and equalizes attributes such as age, education, and marital status that may affect the dependent or outcome variable. The investigator will need to decide on a method to randomly assign subjects to groups; however, the most frequent approaches used are assignment by random number tables or computer-generated numbers.

Control involves carefully managing the experiment through manipulation, randomization, and use of at least one control or comparison group. For example, suppose 30 employees with high cholesterol are enrolled in a study to test the effectiveness of two types of nursing interventions in reducing blood cholesterol levels. One intervention involves individual counseling and the other utilizes individual counseling plus structured group teaching. The investigator will randomly assign (e.g., through use of a random table) 10 subjects to each intervention group and the third group (control group) will receive usual but no special treatment. The investigator will then compare all group outcomes, that is, cholesterol levels, to test the effectiveness of the interventions.

There are several types of experimental designs that can be used, such as pretest-posttest, posttest only, Soloman four-group, and factorial design; however, a discussion of these designs is beyond the scope of this text, and the reader should consult a research text for detailed discussion.

Quasi-experimental designs are similar to experimental research designs in that they involve manipulation of the independent variable but lack either randomization or a control group. These types of designs are obviously weaker but are useful if the researcher cannot randomly assign subjects to experimental or control groups, as happens when volunteer subjects are used. There are several types of quasi-experimental designs as well.

Nonexperimental Research

Much research that is conducted does not involve applying a treatment or intervention (i.e., manipulation of an independent variable) as previously described; the research may be purely descriptive in nature. Because the research is nonexperimental, cause and effect cannot be presumed. For example, descriptive research is designed to obtain information or facts about certain variables of interest. The purpose may be to describe the status or characteristics of the variables rather than the relationships between variables. It is important to conduct descriptive surveys when lack of knowledge about a variable or population precludes the use of a theoretical base for the study. Studies of a single variable or characteristic in one population do not mean it is the same in another population; therefore, further description of a variable in another population would be appropriate for study. In descriptive research there are no cause and effect relationships and no predictions can be made. For example, a survey of employees about their health beliefs, or a record review of the types and frequency of health visits to the occupational health unit are examples of descriptive research.

Another example of nonexperimental research is a correlational design where investigators suspect a relationship between variables based on previous research. The purpose of correlational research is to describe relationships among variables, rather than to test theory (although the findings may support existing research or theory). The investigator may be uncertain if one variable affects another or vice versa or whether there is any association at all. All variables are measured as they exist, and therefore the independent variable if known is not controlled. The study of the relationship between stress and premenstrual symptoms and disability, or examination of the relationship between length of employment or age and accidents would be examples of correlational research.

Other types of nonexperimental research include historical, methodological, or epidemiological research. Historical research involves examining and analyzing records or data concerning previous events through the use of historical evidence and is often undertaken to examine trends relating to past events that may relate to present behaviors or practices. For example, examining the historical roots of occupational health nursing related to the development and enhancement of independent functioning will help to further define and extend professional occupational health nursing roles and practice.

Methodological research is aimed at studying the development and validity of research approaches or tools used in research designs. It is concerned with internal aspects of research involved with obtaining, organizing, or analyzing data that impact on the validity of the research findings. For example, research dealing with the development of research instruments, validity and reliability testing of instruments, and studies related to increasing response rates of subjects, such as the timing of telephone calls when telephone interviews are used, are examples of methodological research.

Epidemiological research is population based and may use both experimental and nonexperimental types of research designs. However, the two most common types of research are nonexperimental in design and termed cohort and case-control studies. In cohort studies, sometimes referred to as prospective studies, subjects without disease or the health outcome of interest, are categorized with or without exposure, and followed forward in time for observation on the occurrence of the disease or problem. For example, in a classic cohort study, groups, with the characteristic under investigation such as workers exposed to a specific chemical (independent variable), are compared to unexposed workers and the incidence of disease or untoward health outcome (dependent variable) is statistically measured in both groups over time. Measurement may be through clinical examinations, self-reports of health effects, or standardized test measurements (Meininger, 1989).

Case-control studies, also referred to as retrospective studies, are conducted in the opposite direction. That is, subjects diagnosed with a disease or symptom (cases) are identified and compared with persons without the disease or symptom (controls), going back in time to determine if a certain exposure or risk occurred. The intent is to identify factors in the past that may account for or contribute to illness/symptom occurrence. For example, a certain type of cancer (dependent variable) which occurred in a worker population may be investigated by determining, through review of past exposure records, if a previous chemical exposure occurred (independent variable), and then comparing exposures with a similar worker population without cancer.

7. Sampling

When conducting research, in most cases data are not gathered from an entire population, rather from a sample or subset of the population. The target population is the total group of interest that meets defined criteria, to which the researcher would like to generalize her or his findings. The accessible population is the group from which the sample will actually be drawn. For example, a target population might be all employees who work for General Motors but the accessible population might be restricted to those in Michigan.

The process of sampling is intended to enable the researcher to make statements about the larger group based on a smaller group. The principle aim in sampling is to be concerned with how representative the sample is of the larger population. How does one go about doing this? Sampling plans are categorized into two major approaches: probability and nonprobability sampling. Probability sampling involves some form of random selection of subjects from the accessible population so that each subject has the same chance of being selected or included in the sample. Because this sampling procedure is a more rigorous approach, representatives of the population in samples is much more likely to occur, and generalizability of the findings is increased.

Nonprobability sampling involves selection of subjects (e.g., volunteers) in a nonrandom method, and thus there is no way to determine the probability or chance for each subject to be included in the selection. The results, therefore, are usually only representative of and generalized to the sample itself. However, many studies utilize nonprobability sampling. When using nonprobability sampling approaches, caution in interpreting the findings needs to be emphasized. The basic types of probability and nonprobability sampling follow.

Probability Sampling

Simple Random Sampling.   This type of sampling allows for each subject to have an equal chance of being selected into the sample. After the population has been defined, subjects or elements are consecutively numbered and, using, for example, a table of random numbers, randomly drawn from the population until the desired sample size is obtained.

Systematic Sampling.   Systematic sampling involves drawing subjects from a listing of names at a specified sampling interval, such as every 10th subject. Procedurally, the desired sample size *(n)* will need to be known in advance, as well as an estimate of the population size *(N)*. By dividing *N* by *n,* the sampling interval is established. For example, if you decided to interview 100 workers *(n)* from a population of 5,000 workers *(N)*, the sampling interval would be 50 (5,000/100); that is, every 50th employee from the list of 5,000 would be sampled for interviewing, resulting in 100 workers interviewed.

Stratified Random Sampling.   Stratified random sampling is similar to simple random sampling except that the population is first grouped together into strata such as age, gender, and occupation. Subjects are then selected randomly from each stratum either in equal numbers or proportionately depending on the size or number in each stratum. For example, using gender as the stratifying variable, if the worker population of 1,000 consisted of 70% women and 30% men, drawing a proportionate stratified sample of 100 employees would include 70 women and 30 men.

Cluster Sampling.   Because it is not always possible to obtain a list of all potential subjects or because the cost of doing so is prohibitive, especially in large-scale surveys, cluster or multistage sampling may be employed. Cluster sampling involves successive random sampling of units and elements. It requires that the population be divided into clusters or groups, and clusters are then randomly selected by either simple or stratified methods, after which subjects themselves are randomly selected from the clusters. For example, suppose a large corporation that employs 80,000 workers has 100 sites nationwide. A random sample of 20 sites might be drawn, which are then clustered into geographic regions. This is followed by random sampling the desired number of employees within each cluster group.

Nonprobability Sampling

Convenience or Accidental Sampling.   This type of sampling is used frequently by researchers and obtains subjects who are the most readily available. For example, asking for volunteers or distributing questionnaires to a classroom of students constitutes a sample of convenience. Because of the inherent bias associated with subjects obtained by this type of sampling scheme, convenience sampling has weaknesses; however, it is commonly used because of cost or population access issues.

Quota Sampling.   Quota sampling is not random but allows for some built-in representativeness in the sampling plan. The researcher first divides the population into groups or strata such as gender and selects the sample by convenience based on proportions of subjects in each stratum.

Purposive Sampling. Purposive sampling is accomplished by the researcher handpicking the subjects for the study based on certain criteria. Here the researcher uses her or his judgment to decide who is representative of the population. Although not usually recommended for obvious reasons of bias, this type of sampling approach is useful when the investigator may want to pretest an instrument with a handpicked sample of workers in order to refine the instrument for later use with the actual research subjects.

8. Pilot Study

In many cases it is advisable to conduct a pilot study in order to iron out any details or correct previously unforeseen problems with the project. The pilot study will help determine if any modifications need to be made in the design or data collection procedures. For example, the researcher may find out that individuals will not participate in the study because of the types of procedures employed to collect the data (e.g., subjects may be unwilling to have certain invasive tests performed or refuse to answer certain sensitive questions). In addition, the researcher will want to know if participants can understand the directions and questions on survey instruments, and if an interview is conducted, how much time is involved.

The pilot study should mimic as similarly as possible the actual study. Subjects selected for the pilot study should possess the same characteristics as subjects who will be selected for the actual study, and data collection procedures should be carried out in the same proposed manner. Once data are collected and examined, revisions or modifications should be incorporated in order to reduce or eliminate anticipated problems.

9. Data Collection

The actual data collection phase of the project will probably be the most time consuming, but also the most fun. This phase proceeds in an orderly, consistent, and systematic way to minimize confusion and bias, which could occur if data were collected haphazardly.

There must be a plan established to collect the data that will be dependent on the research questions or hypotheses and chosen design. The researcher will need to be concerned about several procedural aspects (depending on the type of design and variables to be measured), including determining measurement instruments (e.g., questionnaires, blood tests, weight scales, and reliability and validity testing), determining measurement approaches (e.g., mailed or telephone surveys, interviews, observations) and settings for data collection (e.g., home, clinic), training data collectors, establishing administrative and clerical procedures (e.g., coding questionnaires, scheduling appointments, mailing surveys, collecting specimens or responses, follow-up on nonrespondents), and implementing procedures for confidentiality and anonymity, as appropriate, including storing data securely. It is during this phase that the researcher begins to feel that the project is actually real.

■ 10. Data Preparation and Analysis

Preliminary steps to prepare the data for analysis are usually necessary. For example, if data are collected through use of open-ended questions, responses will need to be categorized and assigned a numerical form. For most types of quantitative data, computer analysis will be used. Coded data will need to be entered into the computer file with an individual record for each subject. Data will then need to be verified, which may entail rechecking the data entered in its entirety. Even after data verification, a few errors are likely to persist from input mistakes. Data cleaning, that is, checking for outliers, strange codes, and consistency checks, will be required to minimize any errors. Once the data have been cleaned, a duplicate file copy should be made and stored.

Data analysis techniques will be derived from the research question(s) (Rogers, 1991). The data analysis should be planned at the time the research questions, hypotheses, and design are formulated. Data are basically analyzed through descriptive and inferential statistics. Descriptive analysis summarizes the data through reporting the variable frequencies, measures of central tendency such as the mean, median, or mode, and examining relationships between variables.

Inferential analysis almost always involves using more sophisticated statistical measures to test for significance between variables or support or reject hypotheses. The statistical tests you choose will be dependent on the research questions and type of data you have collected. This should be planned "up front" when the study is designed, in consultation with a biostatistician.

11. Interpretation of Findings

The researcher will need to report the results of the statistical analyses with respect to the overall aims of the project, its theoretical underpinnings or conceptualization, specific questions being answered or hypotheses tested, existing body of research knowledge, and the limitations of the research methods used (Polit & Hungler, 1991).

It is always preferable to be cautious when reporting conclusions about research findings. The researcher must always remember that even when statistical significance is achieved it does not necessarily reflect a causal relationship, as when the research design is nonexperimental, or when tests of significance examined associations between variables rather than for causation. In addition, because statistical tests are based on probability, there is always a possibility that the results are due to chance. The researcher should always consider alternative explanations for the findings, particularly within the limits of the research design; if alternatives can be eliminated, the researcher may feel more confident about her or his interpretation of the findings. In addition, caution must be taken in generalizing the findings beyond the sample, particularly when nonprobability sampling has been used.

When the researcher is testing hypotheses, the hypotheses are either accepted or rejected rather than proved or disproved. Sometimes the results will be statistically nonsignificant; however, the researcher should not reword the hypotheses to obtain statistical inference. Rather, a consideration of alternative theories or explanations should be explored and considered for future research.

In addition, if a particular treatment or intervention was deemed successful, others may want to utilize it in other settings or with other populations. Therefore, the researcher will need to be careful about generalizing research findings within the context of the sampling scheme. The researcher also needs to report and interpret the findings within the context of what already is known. This will then impact on knowledge development and expansion, and identify areas for future research.

12. Dissemination of Research

When the researcher undertakes a research project, she or he should have a concomitant commitment to disseminating the results. There are a number of approaches that can be used to accomplish this task; however, the primary methods are through writing and speaking.

Written Presentation

Written reports of scientific work allow for information dissemination to a much broader audience and can be in the form of an article, abstract, technical report, thesis, dissertation, or book. Be aware that the written report is for someone else; therefore, material should be presented so that it is readable, understandable, and organized, emphasizes the important points, and is presented without using jargon or in a condescending fashion. Research papers are presented in a different format than clinical articles and generally include the major categories of introduction, background/literature review, theoretical/conceptual framework, methods, results, and discussion (Table 14–5).

If this is the first published paper, the researcher will want to refer to a writing reference, such as Strunk and White's (1979) *Elements of Style,* Tornquist's (1986) *From Proposal to Publication,* and the *Publication Manual of the American Psychological Association* (1987). In addition, other published works can be examined for style and format, and colleagues who have previously published might be asked if they would review and critique the manuscript.

■ **TABLE 14–5**   Typical Format for Research Article

1. Title page
   a. Title of study
   b. Authors' names
   c. Institutional affiliation
2. Abstract
   a. Summary of research purpose, methods, findings
3. Sections of the article
   a. Introduction
      (1) Statement and significance of the problem
      (2) Purpose of the study
   b. Background/Literature review
   c. Conceptual/Theoretical framework
   d. Methods
      (1) Design, variable definition, sampling, setting, instrumentation
      (2) Procedures for data collection
   e. Results
      (1) Descriptive, inferential
      (2) Tables, graphs
   f. Discussion
      (1) Interpretation of results and limitations, conclusions, implications for nursing and future research
4. References
5. Figures/Models (optional)
   a. Appropriate for further clarification of the study/findings

Oral Presentation

An oral presentation usually occurs at a professional society meeting. Although the research presentation usually follows a format similar to the research article, it will usually be presented more concisely and with more attention focused on the results. When presenting research it is important to be well organized. State the purpose and major objectives and only briefly mention the supporting literature, or provide this information in a handout. Provide sufficient detail about the study design, measurement instruments, and data collection procedures but do not dwell on this aspect of the talk.

Results of the study are the meat of the matter and the bulk of the time should be focused here. Explain the findings clearly and be sure to use visual aids especially when reporting numerical values and statistical tests. In presenting the findings it will be vitally important to discuss the implication of the findings with respect to practice.

The technical quality of visual aids is important as this will play a large role in conveying the message (Selby et al., 1989). The research presentation can be practiced before friendly colleagues in order to get constructive criticism and adjust the speech where necessary. In the actual presentation try to be calm, organized, field questions appropriately, and do not panic. The key point is to get the message across.

■ ETHICS IN RESEARCH

Protecting the rights of human subjects involved in the conduct of research is imperative. Human subject rights that must be protected include: the right to self-determination; the right to informed consent; the right to full disclosure; the right to privacy, confidentiality, and anonymity; and the right to protection from harm (American Nurses Association, 1985; Rogers, 1990). In self-determination, persons should have control over their own destiny and the freedom to voluntarily choose to participate in a research study without coercion or fear of recrimination. Research subjects should be given full disclosure of information, and deception by withholding of information is unwarranted. Informed consent, usually written, to participate in a study should be obtained when the research involves more than minimal risk (i.e., more than that encountered in everyday living).

Privacy is the right of a person to determine what information will be shared with or disclosed to others. An invasion of privacy occurs when private information, such as that collected through surveys or interviews, is collected under false pretenses. Confidentiality means that information divulged by a research subject will be guarded and not made public or shared with others. Breaches of confidentiality can be quite harmful emotionally and socially for the subject.

Anonymity occurs when the subjects' identities cannot be linked with their responses. Code numbers should be used on questionnaires rather than identifying information, and all data should be analyzed in the aggregate, with pseudonyms used to protect subjects. For example, names of hospitals or industries should not be used; rather, giving a geographic location such as an airline industry in the northeast would be more appropriate.

Research subjects should be protected from harm or discomfort whether it be physical, mental, or emotional. Any research that has the potential for inflicting permanent damage is highly questionable, regardless of the benefits.

In general, great care should be taken to ensure that research subjects' rights are fully protected. Ethics in research is a complex phenomenon when one is engaged in scientific inquiry for the betterment of society. However, the safeguards that exist to protect study subjects are designed to protect the researcher as well, and will enable the investigator to develop sensitivity to ethical considerations.

■ QUALITATIVE RESEARCH

Another approach to research is through the conduct of qualitative studies. Qualitative research has been described as holistic, that is, concerned with humans and their environment in all of their complexities, and based on the premise of describing the human experience (Polit & Hungler, 1991). It often involves the researcher trying to comprehend those experiences under study. The focus of investigations is process rather than structure oriented, and data analysis techniques are oriented toward description.

For example, if the research question is "How do workers feel about the consequence of a hazardous exposure and reproductive toxicity?", the investigator is trying to access personal feelings and experiences. Although these data could be obtained through a structured questionnaire, much would probably be lost in the translation. This type of research may be more suited for descriptions of relationships or hypothesis generation.

■ CONCLUSION

Occupational health nursing provides a rich field for the conduct of research focused on improvement of worker health through health promotion and protection strategies that need to be tested. In addition, use of theories and conceptual models in the development of occupational health nursing will need to be expanded to enhance the growing body of knowledge. Nurses need to be skilled in the conduct of research through education and the actual doing of the research. For those less skilled it is important to work with a mentor, doing collaborative research, in order to gain the experience needed to acquire and maintain scientific rigor. The AAOHN Research Priorities (Table 14–1) can provide ideas or topics for research; however, it is important to select a topic that is of interest (to you) as well as one that is significant to knowledge development. Additional ideas for research can be found in Chapter 17.

Finally, it is vital that research findings be disseminated, through publications and presentations, and to begin to determine and encourage the utilization of findings in practice as this reflects the ultimate success of research.

The process of doing research is one of rigor and requires thought and attention to concepts, design, and detail. The product, developing more effective approaches to manage employee health care, will clearly add to improving occupational health services and continue to expand our knowledge base.

REFERENCES

Agnew, J. & Travers P. Editorial: Occupational health nursing research. AAOHN Journal, 38(12): 509, 1990.

American Nurses Association. Guidelines for investigative functions of nurses. Kansas City, MO: 1981.

American Nurses Association. Human rights guidelines for nurses in clinical and other research. Kansas City, MO: Author, 1985.

American Psychological Association. Publication Manual. Washington, DC: Author, 1987.

Atkins, J & Magnuson, N. Occupational health nursing research. June 1984 to June 1989. AAOHN Journal, 38: 560–566, 1990.

Brink, B & Wood M. Basic steps in planning nursing research. Boston: Jones and Bartlett, 1988.

Christenson, GM & Kiefhober, A. National survey of worksite health promotion activities. AAOHN Journal, *36*(6): 262–265, 1988.

Conn, R & Barclay, L. Heath education in the workplace. AAOHN Journal, *35*(9): 407–412, 1987.

Garrett, B, Singiser, D, & Banks, S. Back injuries among nursing personnel: The relationship of personal characteristics, risk factors, and nursing practices. AAOHN Journal, *40*(11): 510–516, 1992.

Harrell, J, Cornetto, AD, & Stutts, W. Cardiovascular risk factors in textile workers: Prevalence and intervention. AAOHN Journal, *40*(12): 581–589, 1992.

Jung, F. Shiftwork: Its effect on health performance and well-being. AAOHN Journal, *34:* 160–164, 1986.

Meininger, J. In Brink, B, & Wood, M. Advanced design in nursing research. Newbury Park, CA: Sage Publications, 1989.

McKenzie, C. Hepatitis B vaccination: A survey of health care workers' knowledge and acceptance. AAOHN Journal, *40*(11): 517–520, 1992.

Newlin B. Stress reduction for the critical care nurse: A stress education program. Occupational Health Nursing, *32:* 315–319, 1984.

Pilon, BA & Renfroe, D. Evaluation of an employee health risk appraisal program. AAOHN Journal, *38*(5): 230–235, 1990.

Polit, D & Hungler, B. Nursing Research: Principles and Methods (4th ed.). Philadelphia: J.B. Lippincott, 1991.

Rogers, B. Ethics and research. AAOHN Journal, *38:* 581–585, 1990.

Rogers, B. The question and the answer: Part I: Levels of research questions. AAOHN Journal, *38:* 502–503, 1990.

Rogers, B. The question and the answer: Part II: Planning for data analysis. AAOHN Journal, *39:* 42–44, 1991.

Rogers, B. Research in occupational health nursing. Recent Advances in Nursing, *26:* 137–155, 1990.

Rogers, B. Establishing research priorities in occupational health nursing. AAOHN Journal, *37:* 493–500, 1989.

Rogers, B. Research and practice: Collaborating for improved nursing care. AAOHN Journal, *36*(10): 432, 1988.

Rogers, B & Emmett, E. Handling antineoplastic agents: Urine mutagenicity in nurses. IMAGE, *19:* 108–113, 1987.

Selby, M, Tornquist, E, & Finerty, E. How to present your research. Nursing Outlook, *37:* 236–238, 1989.

Strunk, W & White, EB. The elements of style (3rd ed.). New York: Macmillan, 1979.

Taylor, J. Health promotion in a single-nurse unit. AAOHN Journal, *34:* 518, 1987.

Tornquist, E. From Proposal to Publication. Menlo Park, CA: Addison-Wesley, 1986.

Tornquist, E & Rogers, B. Research proposals: The significance of the study. AAOHN Journal, *35:* 190, 1987.

Treece, L & Treece, J. Elements of research in nursing. St Louis: C.V. Mosby, 1982.

Wilson, H. Research in Nursing. (2nd ed.). Redwood City, CA: Addison-Wesley, 1989.

APPENDIX

14–1

Some Potential Funding Sources Relevant to Occupational Health and Occupational Health Nursing

Organization	Application Deadline*
Agency for Health Care Policy and Research Rockville, MD 301-443-3091	February 1, June 1, October 1; January 15, May 15, September 15 for small grants

*Subject to change

Organization	Application Deadline*
American Association of Occupational Health Nurses Atlanta, GA 1-800-241-8014	December 1
American Cancer Society New York, NY 404-320-3333	April 1, November 1
American Federation on Aging Research New York, NY 212-570-2090	January 15
American Foundation for AIDS Research Los Angeles, CA 213-857-5900	Two-step process: August and December
American Lung Association New York, NY 212-315-8700	November 1
American Nurses Foundation Washington, DC 202-789-1800	June 1
Association of Hospital Employee Health Professionals Sacramento, CA 916-443-2046	October 1 (every 2 years—even)
Diabetes Research and Education Foundation Bridgewater, NJ 908-658-9322	September 30
Ittleson Foundation New York, NY 212-838-5010	None
March of Dimes Foundation White Plains, NY 914-428-7100	Varies
Metropolitan Life Foundation New York, NY 212-578-7049	None
Ruth Mott Fund Flint, MI 313-232-3180	March, July, November
National Institute for Nursing Research Bethesda, MD 301-496-0526	February 1, June 1, October 1

Organization	Application Deadline*
National Institute for Occupational Safety and Health Atlanta, GA 404-262-6575	February 1, June 1, October 1
National Institutes of Health Bethesda, MD (Cancer; Eye; Heart, Lung, & Blood; Allergy/ Infectious Diseases; Arthritis/Musculo Skele- tal/Skin; Child Health; Diabetes/Digestive/ Kidney; Environmental Health; General Medical; Drug Abuse; Mental Health; Alco- hol; Neuro/Communicative Disorders; Nurs- ing) 301-496-7441—Inquire for contact for individ- ual Institute	February 1, June 1, October 1
National Library of Medicine Bethesda, MD 301-496-6131	February 1, June 1, October 1
National Science Foundation Washington, DC 202-375-7880	None
PPG Industries Foundation Pittsburgh, PA 412-434-2970	September
Prudential Foundation Newark, NJ 201-802-7354	None
Robert Wood Johnson Foundation Princeton, NJ 609-243-5957	None
Sigma Theta Tau International Indianapolis, IN 317-634-8171	March 1
Smokeless Tobacco Research Council New York, NY 212-697-3485	June, December

LEGAL RESPONSIBILITY IN OCCUPATIONAL HEALTH NURSING PRACTICE

During the last two decades, many changes have occurred in nursing that have resulted in an expanded definition of nursing. This expansion has led to more comprehensive and explicit standards of practice, increased the independent functioning of nurses in making nursing diagnoses and treatments, and broadened the legal scope of nursing practice. In addition, occupational health nurses have unique responsibilities related to legislative authority and regulations specific to worker health and safety. Thus, the occupational health nurse must be familiar with the Occupational Safety and Health Act (1970), recordkeeping requirements and record access, and various legislative mandates that govern occupational health and safety. This chapter will address the OSH Act (1970), major new legislative acts that have important implications for occupational health and nursing practice (i.e., Hazard Communication Standard, Bloodborne Pathogen Standard, Americans With Disabilities Act), Workers' Compensation Systems, and legal responsibilities within the practice framework. It is imperative that the occupational health nurse be knowledgeable about any changes, modifications, or addenda to any statute or regulation.

■ OCCUPATIONAL SAFETY AND HEALTH ACT

All workers are entitled to a safe and healthful work environment. In the last 20 years, several public laws have been enacted to promote and protect worker health and safety and major acts of legislation are summarized in Table 15–1. However, the most comprehensive federal legislation enacted is the Occupational Safety and Health Act of 1970 (Public Law 91-596, 91st Congress, S.2193, December 29, 1970, effective April 28, 1971). The purpose of the OSH Act is to "assure so far as possible every working man and woman in the Nation safe and healthful working conditions and to preserve our human resources." Comprehensive provisions to achieve this goal are embodied in the Act and presented in Appendix 15–1.

In general, coverage of the OSH Act, as provided through federal OSHA or an OSHA-approved state plan, extends to all employers and employees in the

■ **TABLE 15–1**   Major Federal Occupational and Environmental Health Legislation

Date	Legislation	Purpose
1936	Walsh-Healy Act	Authorized the federal government to establish occupational safety and health standards for businesses engaged in federal contracts.
1969	Federal Coal Mine and Safety Act DOL (Amendments, 1977)	Regulates mine health and safety through mandatory standards governing mine inspections, training, medical monitoring, and control of toxic exposures in the mines.
1970	Clean Air Act (amended) EPA	Regulates air quality through promulgation of standards to control emissions of hazardous air pollutants.
1970	Environmental Protection Agency	Develops regulations and standards pertinent to the protection of the environment.
1970	Consumer Product Safety Act CPSC	Requires consumer product manufacturers, distributors, and retailers to notify the Consumer Product Safety Commission if a product is unsafe or contains a defect that could create a substantial product hazard.
1970	Occupational Safety and Health Act DOL-OSHA	Requires employers to provide safe and healthful working conditions for all employees.
1972	Noise Control Act EPA	Regulates the identification and control of major noise sources.
1972	Clean Water Act EPA	Regulates pollutant discharge to surface water. Pollution sources are required to meet stringent waste treatment requirements through technology-based standards. Industries that discharge wastes to public treatment plants are required to install the best available treatment for toxic pollutant removal and may not discharge wastes that will interfere with or pass through public treatment works and cause them to violate their permits.
1972	Federal Insecticide Fungicide and Rodenticide Act EPA	Amended earlier legislation regulating the manufacture, distribution, and use of pesticides.
1973	Rehabilitation Act EEOC	Provides for civil rights of persons with respect to discrimination against any employee or candidate for employment on the grounds of physical or mental disability for any position for which the applicant is otherwise qualified.
1974	Safe Drinking Water Act EPA	Regulates water quality through setting of standards to control contaminants that may have an adverse impact on human health (both public drinking water and well water).
1976	Toxic Substances Control Act EPA	Regulates the production and use of potentially harmful chemicals using a premanufacturing notification (PMN) and standard-setting procedure. Requires EPA to establish an inventory of chemicals manufactured or processed in the U.S. (excluding those regulated by FIFRA, Food, Drug and Cosmetic Act, and the Atomic Energy Act) and to require chemical manufacturers, importers, or processors to perform health hazard testing.
1976	Resource Conservation and Recovery Act (RCRA) EPA	Regulates the storage, transport, and disposal of hazardous waste.

■ **TABLE 15–1** Major Federal Occupational and Environmental Health Legislation *Continued*

Date	Legislation	Purpose
1980	Comprehensive Environmental Response, Compensation, and Liability Act (CERCLA) or Superfund EPA	Remediates environmental releases from pre-RCRA hazardous waste disposal through clean-up procedures and enforcement.
1983	Hazard Communication Standard DOL-OSHA	Requires chemical manufacturers and importers to evaluate chemicals produced or imported with respect to health hazards and communicate information to employers, employees, and other appropriate parties. Employers must develop, implement and maintain a written hazard communication program including labeling, MSDS, training and record-keeping.
1986	Emergency Planning and Community Right to Know Act EPA	Establishes a program to deal with emergency situations involving hazardous substances at the local level. Requires facilities that store or use hazardous substances to notify local authorities and EPA's National Response Center of their existence.
1990	Americans with Disabilities Act EEOC	Mandates that employers may not discriminate against a qualified individual with a disability with regard to job application, hiring, termination, training, compensation/benefits, medical/job evaluations, advancements, or other conditions of work.
1991	Bloodborne Pathogens Standard DOL-OSHA	Requires employers to develop and implement procedures to prevent and control exposures to blood or other potentially infectious materials.

50 states, the District of Columbia, and all other territories under Federal Government jurisdiction. Those not covered under the OSH Act include self-employed persons; farms where only immediate members of family are employed; and working situations such as with the mining, nuclear, or civil aircraft industries, regulated by other federal agencies under other federal statutes. However, where a specific federal agency regulation does not cover a particular area, OSHA standards apply. In some instances, where the division of authority between OSHA and another agency has been unclear, OSHA has entered into agreements or memoranda of understanding to clarify the lines of jurisdiction.

Under the OSH Act, federal agency heads are required to comply with OSHA standards consistent with those issued for the private sector. In addition, they are required to record and analyze injury and illness data, provide personnel training to protect employees from on-the-job hazards, and to self-inspect the workplace at least annually (USDOL, 1991a). While OSHA has the authority to inspect federal workplaces under certain circumstances, it cannot level penalties against federal agencies for safety or health hazards (Blosser, 1992). OSHA requires that federal agencies investigate any accidents that result in a fatality or hospitalization of five or more employees.

OSHA provisions do not apply to state and local governments in their role as employers. The Act does provide that any state desiring to gain OSHA approval for its private sector occupational safety and health program must provide a program that covers its state and local government workers and that is at least as effective as its program for private employees. State plans may also cover only public sector employees (USDOL, 1991a).

States may seek authority to establish their own occupational safety and health programs by submitting a state plan to OSHA for approval. OSHA's approval will be contingent on the state's ability to demonstrate implementation of all program elements within three years, including program administration, standard setting, enforcement and appeals procedures, public employee protection, adequate funding for personnel to carry out the program, training and education programs, and reporting mechanisms (i.e., illness/injury data). Once a state plan is approved, OSHA funds up to 50% of the program's operating costs. State standards must be at least as effective as federal OSHA's program. When OSHA adopts a new standard, states with approved programs must also issue a corresponding rule (USDOL, 1991a).

To date, 25 state plans have been certified by OSHA (USDOL, 1991a): Alaska, Arizona, California, Connecticut, Hawaii, Indiana, Iowa, Kentucky, Maryland, Michigan, Minnesota, Nevada, New Mexico, New York, North Carolina, Oregon, Puerto Rico, South Carolina, Tennessee, Utah, Vermont, Virgin Islands, Virginia, Washington, and Wyoming. (Puerto Rico and the Virgin Islands fall within OSHA's definition of "states"; Connecticut and New York state plans cover public sector employees only.) States may withdraw from OSHA plan agreements or OSHA may withdraw approval of a state plan. To date, eight states have withdrawn from OSHA agreements, but OSHA has never withdrawn plan approval. However, in the wake of a catastrophic fire in which 25 workers were killed at a poultry processing plant in Hamlet, North Carolina, in 1991, OSHA threatened to withdraw its state approval. North Carolina OSHA developed a plan to correct its deficiencies, as identified by OSHA, increased its number of inspectors, and retained its authority to maintain the state plan.

There is some debate as to the effectiveness of state plans. Organized labor has contended that state program enforcement efforts are weak while state plan administrators believe their enforcement efforts surpass those of federal OSHA. For example, in fiscal 1989 state-plan agencies conducted 113,582 inspections and cited employers for 386,723 alleged violations compared with 54,557 OSHA inspections and 184,620 citations during the same period.

Within the context of the state programs, consultation may be provided to the employer, upon request, to help identify and correct hazards, provide technical assistance, education, and training. Consultation programs are kept separate from the enforcement program and information obtained from the consultative activities cannot be given to either state or federal OSHA enforcement personnel unless the employer fails to correct a dangerous deficiency or the employer wishes to request an exception from an OSHA general inspection for a period of one year (USDOL, 1991a).

Three separate bodies were established to administer the major requirements of the OSH Act, including the Occupational Safety and Health Administration (OSHA), the National Institute for Occupational Safety and Health (NIOSH), and the Occupational Safety and Health Review Commission (OSHRC). OSHA, administered by the Assistant Secretary for Labor, was created within the Department of Labor to carry out regulatory functions prescribed within the purposes of the OSH Act previously identified. NIOSH is an institute of the Centers for Disease Control and Prevention within the U.S. Department of Health and

Human Services and, as described later, is the leading federal occupational safety and health research agency.

The OSHRC is an independent, quasi-judicial review board, composed of three members or commissioners appointed by the President (with the advice and consent of the Senate) each for a six-year term. The Commission is separate from OSHA and hears challenges by employers about OSHA citations and proposed fines. If an employer decides to contest the citation, prescribed time period for abatement, or proposed penalty, a written Notice of Contest must be filed within 15 working days with the OSHA area director who then forwards the case to the OSHRC. The case is first assigned by the Commission to an administrative law judge who hears the case much like in a court of law, and upholds, modifies, or disallows the citation. This decision becomes final within 30 days, unless the commission deems it necessary to review the case report. Commission rulings may be appealed to a U.S. Court of Appeals (USDOL, 1991a).

At any stage of the hearing process, OSHA may withdraw the citation, the employer may withdraw its notice of contest, or a settlement agreement may be entered into by the two parties to resolve the dispute. More than 90% of all cases disposed of by OSHRC administrative law judges are terminated prior to case hearings by such actions (Blosser, 1992).

Standards

OSHA is the regulatory agency responsible for promulgating legally enforceable standards that employers must meet in order to be in compliance with the OSH Act. OSHA has issued hundreds of occupational health and safety standards covering a wide range of hazards, such as toxic chemicals, hazardous equipment, and working conditions. These standards require employers to use appropriate practices, means, methods, operations, or processes to protect employees from hazards on the job. For example, if an employee is working with a tool or machine that has the potential to harm or injure the worker, the employer must ensure that the equipment meets recognized safety design criteria, has proper guards and lockout features, is adequately maintained, and that the employee has received appropriate training to use the equipment. OSHA standards fall into four major categories: General Industry (29CFR-1910); Construction (29CFR-1926); Maritime (29CFR-1915); and Agriculture (29CFR-1928) (Table 15–2).

OSHA standards are developed and established through a public rule-making process. The OSHA rule-making process is laborious and cumbersome, often taking several years. However, it is deemed necessary to be designed this way so that all interested parties can be heard (McNeely, 1992). The conditions for OSHA's rule making are specified in statutory provisions and include a petition for rule making from individuals or groups, NIOSH, public officials, or within OSHA itself; advanced notice of proposed rule making; public comment period; notice of proposed rule making; public comment period; public hearing; posthearing comment period; and posting of the final rule (USDOL, 1991a). Some critics have stated that OSHA's standard setting agenda is too often set as a result of specific interest group pressures, and that the agency needs to examine its regulatory goals.

Once standards have gone through the rule-making process, final standards are published in the Federal Register as required by the OSH Act. While major standards may take two years or more to reach the final rule, under certain

■ **TABLE 15–2**   Industry Classifications for Standards

GENERAL INDUSTRY STANDARDS

The broadest category of OSHA regulations. Rules generally apply to all industries. Specific standards called vertical standards are applicable for certain industry segments (e.g., pulp, paper, and paperboard mills; textiles; telecommunications) and address unique conditions in these workplaces. Standards that cut across industry boundaries and apply to conditions in many different workplaces (e.g., toxic chemicals; hazardous materials; machine guarding; personal protective equipment) are called horizontal standards. Vertical standards take precedence over horizontal standards.

CONSTRUCTION STANDARDS

Govern safety and health conditions at building sites. Standards for ladders and scaffolding, excavations and trenches, explosives, and other conditions and equipment found in the building trade are included.

MARITIME STANDARDS

Standards that apply to workplaces involved in water-borne commerce conducted within the United States. Rules pertain to work at shipyards, operations at maritime terminals, longshoring activities, and gear certification.

AGRICULTURE STANDARDS

Govern safety and health rules for agricultural operations. Rules include standards for roll-over protective structures for tractors, field-sanitation rules for farm laborers, and guarding farm equipment.

The construction, maritime, and agricultural standards are considered vertical standards and take precedence over general industry rules that cover similar hazards.

conditions, OSHA has the authority to set emergency temporary standards that may be put into effect immediately until superseded by a permanent standard. The OSH Act authorizes emergency rulemaking if:

- employees are exposed to grave danger from exposure to substances or agents determined to be toxic or physically harmful or from new hazards; and
- that such emergency standard is necessary to protect employees from such danger.

The emergency temporary standard must be published in the Federal Register, where it also serves as a proposed permanent standard, subject to the usual standard adoption procedures. A final permanent standard must be issued no later than six months after publication of the emergency standard.

Employers may seek a temporary variance order from OSHA for a standard or regulation if the employer believes it cannot comply by the effective date. To qualify for such an order, the employer must show that she or he:

- is unable to comply by the effective date because necessary personnel, materials, or equipment are not available, or because needed workplace construction or renovation cannot be completed by then;
- is taking all available steps to protect employees from the hazard covered by the standard;
- has an effective program for coming into compliance as quickly as it can;

- has informed employees about the request for a temporary variance; and
- has posted a summary of the application (Blosser, 1992).

A temporary variance may be granted for the period needed to achieve compliance or for one year, whichever is shorter. It is renewable twice, each time for six months.

As OSHA standards are not all inclusive, OSHA may utilize the general duty clause of the OSH Act to address hazards not cited by a particular standard. The general duty clause imposes on employers the general obligation of furnishing workplaces that are "free from recognized hazards that are causing or are likely to cause death or serious physical harm." Sources of information on standards include the Federal Register, available in many public and university libraries and from the Superintendent of Documents, U.S. Government Printing Office, Washington, D.C.

OSHA Workplace Inspections

Under the OSH Act, OSHA is authorized to enter and inspect the workplace, without advance notice, in order to enforce its standards. Similarly, states with their own programs also conduct inspections. If an employer refuses to admit an OSHA compliance officer, a search warrant may be obtained with evidence for cause (Marshall v. Barlows, 1978).

The OSHA inspection process generally consists of three components: the opening conference, the inspection, and the closing conference (USDOL, 1991a). When a compliance official arrives at the worksite, official credentials from the U.S. Department of Labor should be presented to the employer. In the opening conference, the compliance officer explains the nature of the visit, why the establishment was selected for inspection, and the standards that apply. The employer or designated representative may accompany the compliance officer on the inspection, and an employee representative may also be given the opportunity to attend the opening conference and inspection.

The two primary components of the inspection are (1) a records check, in which records of illness, injury, medical surveillance, exposure documentation, and so forth are examined, and (2) a walkaround, in which work areas and conditions are examined and consultation with employees is conducted during the inspection. Employees may be asked about safety and health practices, and education and training opportunities and practices. Any unsafe or unhealthful conditions observed during the walkthrough will be pointed out to the employer. Depending on the nature of the visit, the occupational health nurse may or may not be involved. However, it is likely that any record reviews will involve the nurse and she or he should be prepared for this inspection and any questions the compliance officer may direct regarding the occupational health and safety program and related hazards.

After the inspection, a closing conference is held that is attended by the compliance officer, employer, and employee representative (optional), at which time any unsafe/unhealthful conditions observed, any apparent violations for which a citation may be issued, and methods to abate violations are discussed. In addition, employer and employee rights are discussed.

Priorities for inspections include imminent danger to employees, fatalities or catastrophies, employee complaints, programmed or planned inspections directed

■ **TABLE 15–3**   OSHA Inspection Priorities

1. IMMINENT DANGER

Any condition where there is reasonable certainty that a danger exists which can be expected to cause death or serious physical harm immediately, or before the danger can be eliminated through normal enforcement procedures.

Serious physical harm is any type of harm that could cause permanent or prolonged damage to the body or which, while not damaging the body on a prolonged basis, could cause such temporary disability as to require inpatient hospital treatment (e.g., simple fractures, concussions, burns, or wounds involving substantial loss of blood and requiring extensive suturing or other healing aids).

2. FATALITIES AND CATASTROPHIES

Employee deaths and catastrophies resulting in hospitalization of five or more employees. Such situations must be reported to OSHA by the employer within 48 hours. Investigations are made to determine if OSHA standards were violated and to avoid recurrence of similar incidents.

3. EMPLOYEE COMPLAINTS

Alleged violation of standards or of unsafe or unhealthful working conditions made by an employee.

The Act gives each employee the right to request an OSHA inspection when the employee feels he or she is in imminent danger from a hazard or when he or she feels that there is a violation of an OSHA standard that threatens physical harm.

4. PROGRAMMED HIGH-HAZARD INSPECTIONS

Planned inspections aimed at specific high-hazard industries, occupations, or health substances. Industries are selected for inspection on the basis of factors such as the death, injury and illness incidence rates, and employee exposure to toxic substances.

5. FOLLOW-UP INSPECTIONS

Conducted to determine whether previously cited violations have been corrected. Failure to abate alleged violations may result in additional proposed daily penalties while such failure or violation occurs.

From U.S. Department of Labor, Occupational Safety & Health Administration. All about OSHA. Washington, DC: OSHA Pub #2056, 1991.

toward high-hazard workplaces or occupations, and follow-up investigations (Table 15–3). A high-hazard industry is one whose injury rate is equal to or higher than the lowest average injury rate for industry as a whole, as determined by the Bureau of Labor Statistics; or one with a history of OSHA citations for serious health infractions (Blosser, 1992). Industries are selected for inspection on the basis of factors such as death, injury, or illness incidence rates, and employee exposure to toxic substances (USDOL, 1991a).

After the inspection and report are completed, OSHA may issue citations for violations discovered during the inspection process, and determine what penalties, if any, will be proposed. Citations must inform the employer and employees of the regulations and standards alleged to have been violated and the time-frame set for abatement. The citation must be posted at or near the location where the violation occurred for three days or until the violation is abated,

■ **TABLE 15–4** Types of Violations Cited by OSHA and Proposed Penalties

Violation	Proposed Penalty
OTHER THAN SERIOUS VIOLATION A violation that has a direct relationship to job safety and health, but probably would not cause death or serious physical harm.	Discretionary penalty of up to $7,000 for each violation as proposed
SERIOUS VIOLATION A violation where there is substantial probability that death or serious physical harm could result and that the employer knew, or should have known, of the hazard.	Mandatory penalty of up to $7,000 for each violation as proposed
WILLFUL VIOLATION A violation that the employer intentionally and knowingly commits. The employer either knows that what he or she is doing constitutes a violation, or is aware that a hazardous condition existed and made no reasonable effort to eliminate it.	Penalties of up to $70,000 may be proposed for each willful violation, with a minimum penalty of $5,000 for each violation
If an employer is convicted of a willful violation of a standard that has resulted in the death of an employee, the offense is punishable by a court-imposed fine or by imprisonment for up to six months, or both.	A fine of up to $250,000 for an individual, or $500,000 for a corporation, may be imposed for a criminal conviction.
REPEAT VIOLATION A violation of any standard, regulation, rule or order where, upon reinspection, a substantially similar violation is found.	A fine of up to $70,000 for each violation may be imposed
FAILURE TO CORRECT PRIOR VIOLATION A violation wherein a previous violation has not been abated.	A civil penalty of up to $7,000 for each day the violation continues beyond the prescribed abatement date
FALSIFYING RECORDS, REPORTS, OR APPLICATIONS	A fine of $10,000 or up to six months in jail, or both may be imposed
POSTING-REQUIREMENT VIOLATIONS	A civil penalty of up to $7,000 may be imposed
ASSAULTING A COMPLIANCE OFFICER OR OTHERWISE RESISTING, OPPOSING, INTIMIDATING, OR INTERFERING WITH A COMPLIANCE OFFICER IN THE PERFORMANCE OF HIS OR HER DUTIES	A fine of not more than $5,000 and imprisonment for not more than three years may be imposed

From U.S. Department of Labor Occupational Safety & Health Administration. All about OSHA. Washington, DC: OSHA Pub #2056, 1991.

whichever is longer. Categories of violations that may be cited and accompanying proposed penalties are shown in Table 15–4. An employer has 15 working days in which to contest a citation, which must be done in writing.

McNeely (1992) points out that OSHA's enforcement capabilities are limited in scope and force due to the insufficient number of personnel to conduct inspections and because the appeal process allows for citations to be overturned and penalties to be reduced. Only 2% of the nation's workplaces can be inspected in any given year by OSHA (Council on Occupational and Environmental Health, 1988), and it wasn't until 1990 that OSHA maximum penalties were increased. However, OSHA continues to adjust penalties on the basis of the company size, employer's good faith, and history of compliance (Blosser, 1992).

National Institute for Occupational Safety and Health

Included in the OSH Act is a provision that created the National Institute for Occupational Safety and Health (NIOSH). As previously stated, NIOSH is a unit within the Centers for Disease Control and Prevention in the Department of Health and Human Services and is authorized to:

- develop recommendations for OSHA standards;
- develop information on safe levels of exposure to toxic materials and harmful physical agents and substances;
- conduct research on new workplace safety and health problems;
- conduct on-site investigations to determine the toxicity of materials used in workplaces; and
- fund research/training by other agencies or private organizations through grants, contracts, and other arrangements.

NIOSH conducts research on various workplace safety and health problems, provides technical assistance to OSHA, and develops criteria documents for recommendations on standards for OSHA's adoption. While conducting its research, NIOSH may make workplace investigations, gather testimony from employers and employees, and require that employers measure and report employee exposure to potentially hazardous materials. NIOSH has the authority to enter a workplace to conduct an investigation based on probable cause for believing a problem exists. NIOSH does not have authority to issue citations and penalties. A health hazard evaluation may be requested by an employee or employee representative or as part of a planned research program (29USC 669 (a) (b)). NIOSH also may require employers to provide medical examinations and tests to determine the incidence of occupational illness among employees. However, when performed as part of a research program, the cost must be borne by NIOSH (USDOL, 1991a). NIOSH has identified 10 leading types of work-related illness and injuries on which their research focuses (CDC, 1983):

- Occupational lung disease
- Musculoskeletal diseases
- Occupational cancers
- Occupational cardiovascular disease
- Severe traumatic injuries
- Reproductive disorders
- Neurotoxic disorders
- Noise-induced hearing loss
- Dermatological conditions
- Psychological disorders

NIOSH also:

- develops other types of documents, such as Current Intelligence bulletins, to disseminate new information on workplace hazards; and

- maintains and annually revises the NIOSH Registry of Toxic Effects of Chemical Substances.

Under the OSH Act, NIOSH is authorized to conduct directly, or by grants/ contracts, education programs to provide an adequate supply of qualified occupational and safety personnel and to provide for consultation and the establishment and supervision of programs for the education and training of employers and employees related to occupational health and safety. NIOSH grants support academic programs through established Educational Resource Centers across the country. (See Appendix 2–1, Chapter 2.)

Recordkeeping and Access Requirements

The OSH Act of 1970 requires covered employers to prepare and maintain records of occupational illnesses and injuries. The Bureau of Labor Statistics (BLS) within the Department of Labor is responsible for administering the recordkeeping system established by the OSH Act (USDOL, BLS, 1986). The purposes of keeping records are to permit BLS survey material to be compiled, to help define high hazard industries, and to inform employees of the status of their employer's record.

The employers of 11 or more employees must maintain occupational injury/ illness records. Employers with 10 or fewer employees and several categories of employers, including religious, domestic household, and small employer establishments, are exempt from recordkeeping requirements unless they are selected by the BLS to participate in the annual survey of Occupational Injuries and Illnesses. Exempt categories of employers include those in retail trade, finance, insurance, real estate, and service industries—Standard Industrial Classification (SIC) 52-89 (except building materials and garden supplies, SIC 52; general merchandise and food stores, SIC 53 and 54; hotels and other lodging places, SIC 70; repair services, SIC 75 and 76; amusement and recreation services, SIC 79; and health services, SIC 80). Exempt employers must comply with OSHA standards, display the OSHA poster, and report to OSHA within 48 hours any accident that results in one or more fatalities or the hospitalization of five or more employees.

Where companies employ an occupational health nurse, OSHA recordkeeping responsibilities are usually managed by the nurse. Thus, the occupational health nurse must be thoroughly familiar with the regulatory requirements (29CFR 1904). Only two forms are used for OSHA recordkeeping. One form, the OSHA No. 200, serves two purposes: (1) as the Log of Occupational Injuries and Illnesses on which the occurrence, extent, and outcome of cases are recorded during the year and (2) as the Summary of Occupational Injuries and Illnesses, which is used to summarize the log at the end of the year to satisfy employer posting obligations. The other form, the Supplementary Record of Occupational Injuries and Illnesses, OSHA No. 101, provides additional information on each of the cases that have been recorded on the log.

The OSHA No. 200 log is used for recording and classifying recordable occupational injuries and illnesses, and for noting the extent and outcome of each case. For every injury or illness entered on the log, it is necessary to record additional information on the supplementary record, OSHA No. 101. The supplementary record describes how the injury or illness exposure occurred, lists the objects or substances involved, and indicates the nature of the injury or illness and the part(s) of the body affected. Substitute forms (for both the OSHA 200 and 101) are acceptable as long as required information can be detailed and is easily understood. Employers selected to participate in the BLS annual survey will receive from BLS form 200S, which must be completed and returned to BLS.

Many specific standards and regulations of the Occupational Safety and Health Administration (OSHA) have additional requirements for the maintenance and retention of records for medical surveillance, exposure monitoring, inspections, and other activities and incidents relevant to occupational safety and health. Reporting of certain information to employees and to OSHA is also specified. The occupational health nurse should also be familiar with these recordkeeping and reporting requirements within these specific standards.

In 1980 the Department of Labor issued a standard, Access to Exposure and Medical Records, which was revised in 1988. The purpose of this standard is to ensure employee, or a designated representative, access to employee exposure and medical records. Access must be provided within 15 working days of the request.

Employee exposure records include environmental monitoring or measurements of a toxic agent; biological monitoring results; material safety data sheets; and any other record that reveals the identity of a harmful or toxic substance (29CFR, Part 1910, 1988). If no exposure records exist, the employer must provide records of other employees with similar job duties.

Employee medical records are those concerning the health status of the employee and are maintained by health care personnel. These do not include physical specimens, health insurance claims maintained separately from the record, litigatory records, and separate voluntary employee assistance program records. Access to the medical records of another employee may be provided only with specific written consent of that employee.

The standard provides for special circumstances such as a terminal illness or psychiatric condition, under which the company physician may deny the employee direct access to record information. However, information must be given to the designated representative with written consent of the employee. This position is difficult to understand and smacks of paternalism.

The following requirements regarding retention of exposure and medical records are addressed in the standard:

- exposure records are to be retained for 30 years;
- medical records are to be retained for the duration of employment plus 30 years;
- background data for exposure records are to be retained for one year; and
- records of employees who have worked for less than one year and first-aid records of one-time treatment need not be retained.

The role of the occupational health nurse in recordkeeping requirements is both a legal and professional obligation. With respect to recordkeeping and disclosure practices, it is necessary to follow the law and document accordingly, and at the same time protect the employee's right to privacy (Mistretta, 1990; Simonowitz & Spencer, 1985). Legal requirements will dictate the release of occupational injury, illness, and exposure data to specific agencies or individuals. The nurse must have a full understanding of current statutory requirements for recordkeeping procedures and access, and should also have a policy in place for protection of employee health records and information disclosure. Only the occupational health nurse and physician should have access to the employee's personal health record and access by other individuals should not be released without the employee's written consent. In addition to the legal requirements, the occupational health nurse should utilize professional standards and ethical codes as guides to protect employee confidentiality and invasion of privacy. Understanding both the legal and ethical parameters of professional practice will help the nurse in the safe and effective recordkeeping practices. OSHA record-keeping requirements are currently under revision; thus a more detailed discussion is inappropriate at this time.

■ OSHA STANDARDS

While several standards have been promulgated by OSHA, it is beyond the scope of this chapter to discuss each one. Thus, two recent standards that have important implications for occupational health nursing practice will be described as examples. In addition, sample policy/procedure documents (Bloodborne Pathogens Compliance Program and Lockout/Tagout Procedure) are given in Appendixes 15–2 and 15–3.

Hazard Communication Standard

Hazard communication is designed to prevent work-related illness and injury through communicating information to workers about the hazards and the risks. The importance of designing and detailing a hazard communication program and involving health care professionals in the program planning, implementation, and evaluation cannot be underscored. McNeely (1990) states that:

> If the nurse, who sees the employee for health care and health education, is not collecting and disseminating the hazard information described in the Occupational Safety and Health Administration's Hazard Communication Rule, then employee health problems that arise from work exposures may go undetected at clinic visits. Furthermore, both the employee and the nurse may lack adequate understanding about the use of personal protective equipment or careful work practices to prevent work-related illness and injury.

According to OSHA, about 32 million workers are potentially exposed to one or more chemical hazards that may cause or contribute to many serious health effects, such as cardiovascular, hepato-renal, respiratory, reproductive and dermatological problems (USDOL, 1992a). Because of the seriousness of these health and safety problems, OSHA issued its Hazard Communication Standard (HCS) (29 CFR 1910, Subpart Z, Toxic and Hazardous Substances) on November 23, 1983, which initially applied to "affected employers and employees within the manufacturing sector." Since then, the HCS has been amended (1985; 1986) and was revised in August 1987 to state the purpose as:

> to ensure that the hazards of all chemicals produced or imported are evaluated, and that information concerning their hazards is transmitted to employers and employees. This transmittal of information is to be accomplished by means of comprehensive hazard communication programs, which are to include container labeling and other forms of warning, material safety data sheets, and employee training.

The HCS does not apply to hazardous waste (regulated by the Resource Conservation and Recovery Act and the Environmental Protection Agency); tobacco and wood products; consumer products packaged for consumer use (food, drugs, cosmetics, alcohol); any drug in solid, final form for direct administration to a patient (i.e., tablets, pills); or manufactured articles with a specific shape that does not release or result in a hazardous chemical exposure.

Meyer and Watson (1992) point out that the formal HCS has placed the emphasis on providing the worker with detailed information about each hazardous substance in the workplace. The authors state that this emphasis has fostered an environment where information is gathered on hazardous material more for the sake of HCS compliance rather than an integration of the information as a component of the total health and safety program. The occupational health and safety professional needs to consider all aspects of information collected and develop a hazardous communication and management program that will be purposeful as well as compliant.

Responsibilities of Manufacturers and Importers

The HCS requires chemical manufacturers and importers to evaluate chemicals they produce or import using available scientific evidence concerning such hazards, and to report such information to their employees and to employers who distribute or use their products. The determination of occupational health hazards is complicated by the fact that many of the effects or signs and symptoms occur commonly in nonoccupationally exposed populations, so that effects of exposure are difficult to separate from normally occurring illnesses. Occasionally, a substance causes an effect that is rarely seen in the population at large, such as angiosarcomas caused by vinyl chloride exposure, thus making it easier to ascertain that the occupational exposure was the primary causative factor. More often, however, the effects are common, such as lung cancer. Also, most chemicals have not been adequately tested to determine their health hazard potential, and data do not exist to substantiate these effects.

Regardless of the complexities involved in making a hazard determination, the chemical manufacturers, importers, and any employers who choose to evaluate hazards are responsible for the quality of the hazard evaluation undertaken. Each chemical must be evaluated for its potential to cause adverse health effects and physical hazards such as flammability. (The scope of health hazards covered and criteria related to completeness of the evaluation can be found in the appendix to the Hazard Communication Standard.) Chemicals that are listed in one of the following sources are to be considered hazardous in all cases:

- *29 CFR 1910, Subpart Z, Toxic and Hazardous Substances,* Occupational Safety and Health Administration (OSHA) and
- *Threshold Limit Values for Chemical Substances and Physical Agents in the Work Environment,* American Conference of Governmental Industrial Hygienists (ACGIH).

In addition, chemicals that have been evaluated and found to be a suspect or confirmed carcinogen in the following sources must be reported as such:

- National Toxicology Program (NTP), *Annual Report on Carcinogens* (see Chapter 6);
- International Agency for Research on Cancer (IARC), *Monographs;* and
- Regulated by OSHA as a carcinogen (USDOL, 1991b).

A written description stating the procedures used in the hazard determination must be made available to employees, their designated representatives, the Assistant Secretary of Labor for Occupational Safety and Health, and the Director of NIOSH.

Written Hazard Communication Program

Covered employers must develop, implement, and maintain at the workplace a written hazard communication program that contains provisions for:

- container labeling and other forms of warning;
- collection, availability, maintenance, and updating of Material Safety Data Sheets (MSDS);
- a list of hazardous chemicals in the work areas cross-referenced with the material safety data sheets;
- employee information and training;
- methods used to inform employees of the hazards of non-routine tasks (e.g., cleaning vessels) and hazards associated with chemicals in unlabeled pipes;
- methods to ensure that other employers with employees working on-site (e.g., construction employees working on-site) who may be exposed are provided with information regarding hazards, precautionary and protective measures for these employees, and the labeling system used in the workplace.

Labels

The chemical manufacturer, importer, or distributor must ensure that each container of hazardous chemicals leaving the workplace is labeled, tagged, or marked with the chemical identity, appropriate hazard warning, and name and address of the manufacturer, importer, or responsible party. In the workplace the employer must ensure that each container (i.e., bag, barrel, bottle, box, can, cylinder, drum, reactor vessel, storage tank) must be labeled, tagged, or marked with the identity of the hazard, by chemical or common name, including health and physical hazards. Hazard warnings may be in the form of words, pictures, or symbols that convey the hazard of the chemical(s) in the container. Labels and/or warnings must be legible, in English, and prominently displayed. Several exemptions for in-plant labeling requirements exist:

- pipes, piping systems, engines, fuel tanks and other vehicle operating systems do not require labeling;
- signs, placards, process sheets, batch tickets, operating procedures, or other written materials may be substituted for individual labels to stationary process containers (e.g., reactor vessel) if they contain the same information and are readily accessible to employees in the work area; and
- portable containers, into which hazardous chemicals are transferred from labeled containers and are intended only for the immediate use (within the workshift) of that employee who performs the transfer, do not require labeling.

Material Safety Data Sheets

Chemical manufacturers and importers must develop a material safety data sheet (MSDS) for each hazardous chemical they produce or import and must provide all MSDSs to distributors or employers with their initial shipment and after a MSDS is updated. Each MSDS must be in English and include the following information regarding the hazardous chemical(s):

- the specific identity and common name(s) (including designation as singular substance or mixture);
- physical and chemical characteristics (e.g., vapor pressure, flash point);
- physical hazards including the potential for fire, explosion, and reactivity;
- health hazards including signs and symptoms of exposure, acute and chronic health effects, and related health information;
- primary routes of entry;
- exposure limits (PELs; TLVs);
- whether the chemical is considered to be a carcinogen by NTP, IARC, or OSHA;
- precautionary measures for safe handling and use including hygiene practices and procedures for equipment maintenance, clean-up, and leaks;
- control measures, work practices, and use of personal protective equipment;
- emergency and first-aid procedures;
- date and preparation of the MSDS; and
- identification of the organization responsible for preparing the MSDS (name, address, telephone number).

Copies of required MSDSs for each hazardous chemical in the workplace must be maintained and made readily accessible during each workshift to all employees.

While the type of information to be provided was clearly established, the standard left a great deal of leeway regarding the format of MSDSs. In addition, in order to protect themselves from liability, chemical manufacturers have begun to use generic safety precautions within their MSDSs resulting in statements such as "use of respiratory protection required" for a wide range of materials regardless of whether the protection is warranted (Meyer & Watson, 1992). Chapter 6 appendix contains examples of MSDSs.

Employee Information and Training

One of the most important sections of the Hazard Communication Standard is the requirement that employers provide workers with training on hazardous chemicals in their work area. This training must be given before workers are assigned to do a job involving potential exposure to hazardous chemicals, and whenever a new hazard has been introduced. At a minimum, employees must be informed of the HCS and its requirements; operations in the work areas where hazardous chemicals are present; and the location and availability of the written hazard communication program, including the list of hazardous chemicals and MSDSs (USDOL, 1992a).

Under the HCS, employee training must include the following elements:

- the requirements of the Hazard Communication Standard;
- methods and observations workers can use to detect the presence or release of a hazardous chemical, such as air sampling, continuous monitoring devices, visual appearance, and the odor of hazardous chemicals;
- physical and health hazards of the chemicals in the work area;

- measures workers can take to protect themselves from exposures to hazardous chemicals, including proper work practices, ventilation controls, emergency procedures, and personal protective equipment; and
- details of the employer's hazard communication program, including an explanation of the labeling system and MSDSs and how workers can obtain and use hazard information (NCOSH, 1988).

The occupational health nurse can play a key role in this aspect of the risk communication program; however, in an interview study of 24 nurses employed by chemical industries, McNeely (1990) reported limited involvement of occupational health nurses in all aspects of the hazard communication program. Even though the sample size was small (n = 24), many of the nurses lacked knowledge about the hazardous substances at the worksites, health effects related to exposure, and control strategies. Only three nurses were involved in the formal training of employees. In addition, more than half the nurses believed that hazard communication was a safety rather than a health issue. Nurses who perceived hazard communication as part of their job were more knowledgeable about chemical exposures. Occupational health nurses need to be more involved in the hazard communication program, as they perhaps have the greatest opportunity to teach employees about the hazards both in group and individual encounters.

Trade Secrets

A provision is made in the HCS to protect "trade secrets." A trade secret is something that gives an employer an opportunity to obtain an advantage over competitors who do not know about the trade secret or who do not use it. For example, a trade secret may be a confidential device, pattern, information, or chemical make-up. Chemical industry trade secrets are generally formulas, process data, or a "specific chemical identity." The latter is the type of trade secret information referred to in the Hazard Communication Standard. The term includes the chemical name, the Chemical Abstracts Services (CAS) Registry Number, or any other specific information that reveals the precise designation. It does not include common names. Information regarding specific chemical identity may be withheld as a trade secret, provided that the MSDS contains information concerning the properties and effects of the hazardous chemical. However, when a treating physician or nurse determines that a medical emergency exists, the chemical manufacturer, importer, or employer must immediately disclose the specific chemical identity of the hazardous chemical. A written statement of need and confidentiality agreement may be required to be provided after abatement of the emergency.

In nonemergency situations, the specific chemical identity must be disclosed to health professionals (physicians, occupational health nurses, industrial hygienists, toxicologists, or epidemiologists) who provide medical or other occupational health services to exposed employees, and to employees or their own designated representatives providing the request is in writing. A reasonably detailed description of the need for the information that shall be used for one or more of the following purposes must be provided:

- to assess the hazards of the chemicals to which employees will be exposed;
- to conduct or assess sampling of the workplace atmosphere to determine employee exposure levels;

- to conduct pre-assignment or periodic medical surveillance of exposed employees;
- to provide medical treatment to exposed employees;
- to select or assess appropriate personal protective equipment for exposed employees;
- to design or assess engineering controls or other protective measures for exposed employees; and
- to conduct studies to determine the health effects of exposure.

In addition, the health professional, employee, or employee representative must explain why alternative information is insufficient, and detail procedures to be used to protect confidentiality of the information. A written confidentiality agreement not to use the information for any other purpose than the health need stated nor to release information under any circumstances, except to OSHA, must be given.

The occupational health nurse can play a major role in implementation and monitoring of the Hazard Communication Standard (Soloman, 1986). The occupational health nurse can coordinate activities with other team members to:

- assess hazardous workplace exposures;
- keep employees informed of the nature and effects of hazardous exposures;
- recognize signs and symptoms related to potential/actual exposures;
- develop strategies to contain exposures;
- communicate hazardous substance recognition and measures to control exposures to all workers;
- ensure emergency and disaster preparedness procedures are in place;
- make available appropriate and effective personal protective equipment, as necessary; and
- involve workers in the hazard communication program.

Observation of workers and collection and review of data, including MSDSs with respect to hazardous exposures, will aid in identifying, controlling, and eliminating hazardous substances.

Bloodborne Pathogens Standard

Exposure to bloodborne pathogens, such as the human immunodeficiency virus (HIV) and hepatitis B virus (HBV), has become a cause for serious concern among health care workers, who may be potentially exposed through contact with blood and other body fluids containing these pathogens. Even though the risk for occupational exposure is small, the potential for exposure remains due to the nature of the work. Two diseases are of primary concern. Acquired immunodeficiency syndrome (AIDS), caused by the HIV, was first recognized in the United States in 1981, and the incidence has since risen dramatically (CDC, 1991). Hepatitis B occurs in the United States at an estimated rate of 300,000 new cases annually. Of these, about 8,000 to 12,000 occur in health care workers, resulting in 200 to 300 deaths per year (USDOL, OSHA, 1991c). OSHA recognized the need for a regulation that prescribed safeguards to protect these workers against health hazards from exposure to blood and certain body fluids, including bloodborne pathogens. Thus, on December 6, 1991, the Occupational Safety and Health Administration (OSHA) published the final rule,

Occupational Exposure to Bloodborne Pathogens (29 CFR 1910–1030) with the aim to reduce the risk of occupational exposure to bloodborne diseases. The occupational health nurse needs to be fully familiar with this standard in order to better ensure employee health and safety and to assist management in compliance with the regulations (Goldstein & Johnson, 1991).

Scope of Application

OSHA's Bloodborne Pathogens Standard (BBPS) became effective March 6, 1992, and applies to all persons occupationally exposed to blood or other potentially infectious material (Table 15–5). These workers include, but are not limited to, physicians, dentists, dental employees, phlebotomists, nurses, morticians, paramedics, medical examiners, laboratory and blood bank technologists and technicians, housekeeping personnel, laundry workers, employees in long-term care facilities, and home care workers (USDOL, 1992b). Other workers who may be occupationally exposed to blood or other potentially infectious materials, depending on their work assignments, include research laboratory workers and public safety personnel (fire, police, rescue, correctional officers, etc.) (USDOL, 1992c).

As defined in the BBPS, an occupational exposure is a reasonably anticipated skin, eye, mucous membrane, or parenteral contact with blood or other potentially infectious materials that may result from the performance of an employee's duties. An exposure incident is a specific eye, mouth, other mucous membrane, non-intact skin, or parenteral contact with blood or other potentially infectious materials that results from the performance of an employee's duties. Under the BBPS, employers with occupationally exposed employees are required to develop a written exposure control plan (Table 15–6), which must be reviewed and updated annually and whenever new tasks or procedures affect occupational exposure. It is important to emphasize that an exposure determination must be

■ **TABLE 15–5**   Exposure Indicators: OSHA Bloodborne Pathogen Standard

---

Bloodborne pathogen (A pathogenic microorganism present in human blood that causes disease in humans)
Other potentially infectious material
1. Human body fluids
   Semen
   Vaginal secretions
   Cerebrospinal fluid
   Synovial fluid
   Saliva (dental procedures)
   Pleural fluid
   Pericardial fluid
   Peritoneal fluid
   Amniotic fluid
   Body fluids with visible blood
2. Any unfixed tissue or organ from a human (living or dead)
3. HIV-containing cell or tissue cultures, organ cultures, and HIV/HBV-containing culture medium or other solutions; blood, organs, or other tissues from experimental animals infected with HIV/HBV.

■ **TABLE 15–6**   Written Exposure Control Plan for Bloodborne Pathogens

Exposure determination
- List of job classifications with occupational exposure
- List of all tasks and procedures or groups of closely related tasks and procedures in which occupational exposure occurs and that are performed by employees in specified job classifications
- Exposure determined without regard to use of personal protective equipment

Schedule of procedure for implementing the standard covering:
- Methods of compliance
- HIV/HBV research laboratories and production facilities (as appropriate)
- Hepatitis B vaccination and post-exposure follow-up
- Communication of hazard to employees
- Recordkeeping

Procedure for evaluation of exposure incident:
- Documentation of the routes of exposure and how exposure occurred.
- Identification and documentation of the source individual, unless the employer can establish that identification is infeasible or prohibited by state or local law.
- Examination of the source individual's blood with consent as soon as possible to determine HIV and HBV infectivity and documentation of the source's blood test results. If the source individual is known to be infected with either HIV or HBV, testing need not be repeated to determine the known infectivity.
- Provision of the source individual's test results to the exposed employee, and information about applicable disclosure laws and regulations concerning the source identity and infectious status.
- Collection of exposed employee's blood, with consent, as soon as feasible after the exposure incident and testing the blood for HBV and HIV serological status. If the employee does not give consent for HIV serological testing during the collection of blood for baseline testing, preserve the baseline blood sample for at least 90 days.
- Provision of HIV and HBV serological testing, counseling, and safe and effective post-exposure prophylaxis following the current recommendations of the U.S. Public Health Service.
- Provision of information about the exposure incident to the evaluating health care provider as well as the regulation, exposed employee's duties, and medical records.
- Provision to the employee of a copy of the health care professional's written opinion.

based on an occupational exposure without regard to personal protective clothing and equipment.

Exposure Prevention and Minimization

To prevent and control exposure to blood or other potentially infectious materials, the BBPS identifies several precautions and control strategies that must be observed, the most important of which is utilizing universal precautions to prevent contact with blood or other potentially infectious materials. In addition:

- Engineering controls are designed to reduce employee exposure in the workplace by either removing or isolating the hazard or isolating the worker from exposure. Self-sheathing needles, puncture-resistant disposal containers for contaminated sharp instruments, resuscitation bags, and ventilation devices are examples of engineering controls. Engineering controls must be examined and maintained or replaced on a scheduled basis.
- Work practice controls are designed to alter the manner in which a task is performed and thereby minimize employee exposure. Examples of work practice controls include washing hands immediately after gloves are re-

moved and as soon as possible after skin contact with contaminant; restricting eating, drinking, smoking, applying cosmetics or lip balm, and handling contact lenses; prohibiting mouth pipetting; preventing the storage of food and/or drink in refrigerators or other locations where blood or other potentially infectious materials are kept; providing and requiring the use of handwashing facilities and/or equipment; and routinely checking equipment and decontaminating it prior to servicing and shipping.

Recapping and removing or bending needles is prohibited unless the employer can demonstrate that no alternative is feasible or that such action is required by a specific medical procedure. When recapping, bending, or removing contaminated needles is required by a medical procedure, this must be done by mechanical means, such as the use of forceps, or a one-handed technique. Shearing or breaking contaminated needles is also not permitted. Discarding contaminated sharps/needles into puncture-resistant containers is required as well as affixing appropriate biohazard labels to containers, specimens and so forth.

- Personal protective equipment is designed to help prevent occupational exposure to infectious materials. Protective equipment must not allow blood or other potentially infectious materials to pass through to workers' clothing, skin, or mucous membranes. Such equipment includes, but is not limited to, gloves, gowns, laboratory coats, face shields or masks, and eye protection.

The employer is responsible for providing, maintaining, laundering, disposing, replacing, and assuring the proper use of personal protective equipment, and for ensuring that workers have access to the protective equipment, at no cost, including proper sizes and types that take allergic conditions into consideration (USDOL, 1992c). Precautions for safe handling and using personal protective equipment, such as appropriate wearing and replacement of damaged or contaminated gloves, gowns, and other equipment, and removing and discarding of protective equipment before leaving the work area, is required.

- Housekeeping procedures are aimed at keeping the place of employment clean and sanitary and thus reducing the opportunity for exposure to potentially infectious materials. To do this, the employer must develop and implement a cleaning schedule that includes appropriate methods for cleaning and decontaminating all contaminated equipment, surfaces, and waste receptacles; handling and discarding broken glass, contaminated sharps, regulated waste; and handling and labeling contaminated laundry.

Labels

In order that workers recognize contaminated or potentially infectious material, strict labeling procedures are required. The standard requires that fluorescent orange or orange-red warning labels be attached to containers of regulated waste, to refrigerators and freezers containing blood and other potentially infectious materials, and to other containers used to store, transport, or ship blood or other potentially infectious materials. These labels are not required when 1) red bags or red containers are used, 2) containers of blood, blood components, or blood products are labeled as to their contents and have been released for transfusion or other clinical use, and 3) individual containers of

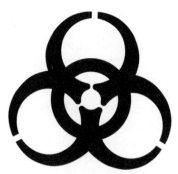

■ **Figure 15–1**   Biohazard Symbol

blood or other potentially infectious materials are placed in a labeled container during storage, transport, shipment, or disposal (USDOL, 1992c). The warning label must be fluorescent orange or orange-red, contain the biohazard symbol and the word BIOHAZARD (Fig. 15–1) in a contrasting color, and be attached to each object by string, wire, adhesive, or another method to prevent loss or unintentional removal of the label.

Preventive Measures and Post-Exposure Follow-up

HIV and HBV are spread through contact with blood and body fluids (see Table 15–5) and may be transmitted through sexual contact, needle sharing, contact with contaminated blood or blood products, and perinatally (USDOL, 1991c). Casual contact is not a mode of transmission. While there currently is no vaccine available to prevent HIV infection, HBV vaccine is available and effective in the protection of HBV infection.

According to the BBPS (USDOL, 1991c), the hepatitis B vaccination series must be made available within 10 working days of initial assignment to all employees with occupational exposure unless documentation is evident that the vaccination is not required or is contraindicated. An algorithm for hepatitis B vaccination requirements is shown in Figure 15–2 (Barlow & Handelman, 1993; USDOL, 1992d). In addition, a confidential, immediate postexposure evaluation and follow-up (Fig. 15–3) by a health care professional must be provided for all employees who have experienced an exposure incident. This health evaluation should include at a minimum documentation of the exposure route and circumstances; testing (with legal consent) and/or documentation of the source individual's blood as to HIV/HBV status and provision of test results to the exposed employee with information regarding maintenance of confidentiality and disclosure laws; baseline HIV/HBV serologic sampling from the employee with consent; counseling; and postexposure prophylaxis as currently recommended by the U.S. Public Health Service (Report of U.S. Preventive Services Task Force, 1989). If the employee elects to delay testing, the blood sample must be preserved for 90 days for future testing if desired.

The health care professional conducting the evaluation must be provided with a copy of the BBPS, a description of the employee's job duties and all information relevant to the exposure incident and source individual, if known, and employee's HBV vaccination status and medical history. Within 15 days after evaluation of

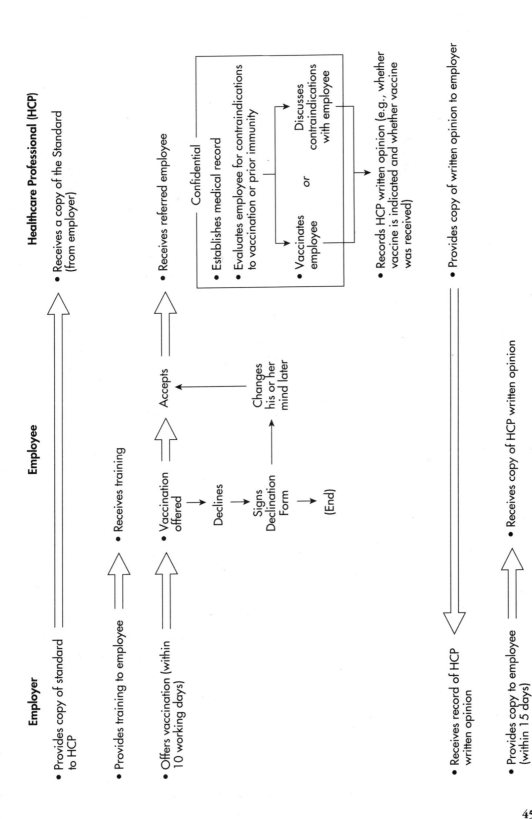

Figure 15-2 ■ Algorithm: Hepatitis B vaccination. (From U.S. Department of Labor, OSHA, 1991c.)

455

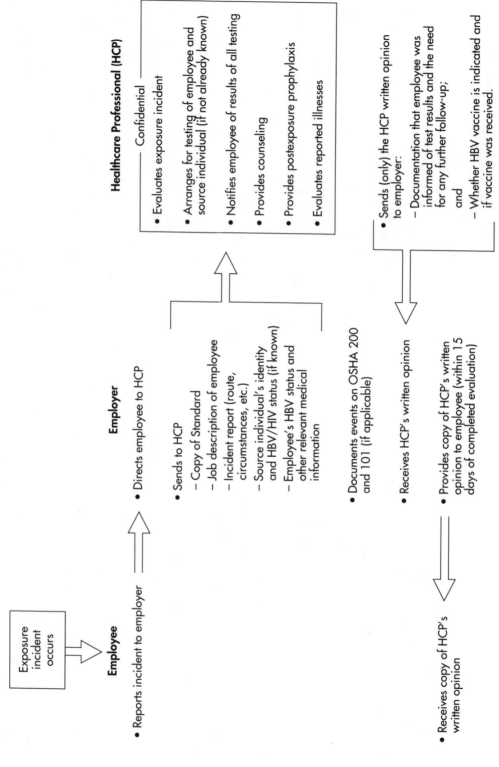

■ **Figure 15–3** Algorithm: Postexposure evaluation and follow-up. (From U.S. Department of Labor, OSHA, 1991c.)

Employee

- Reports incident to employer

Employer

- Directs employee to HCP

- Sends to HCP
  - Copy of Standard
  - Job description of employee
  - Incident report (route, circumstances, etc.)
  - Source individual's identity and HBV/HIV status (if known)
  - Employee's HBV status and other relevant medical information

- Documents events on OSHA 200 and 101 (if applicable)

- Receives HCP's written opinion

- Provides copy of HCP's written opinion to employee (within 15 days of completed evaluation)

Healthcare Professional (HCP)

Confidential

- Evaluates exposure incident

- Arranges for testing of employee and source individual (if not already known)

- Notifies employee of results of all testing

- Provides counseling

- Provides postexposure prophylaxis

- Evaluates reported illnesses

- Sends (only) the HCP written opinion to employer:
  - Documentation that employee was informed of test results and the need for any further follow-up; and
  - Whether HBV vaccine is indicated and if vaccine was received.

Exposure incident occurs

- Receives copy of HCP's written opinion

the exposed employee, the employer must provide the employee with a copy of the health care professional's written opinion. The written opinion is limited to whether the vaccine is indicated and if it has been received. The written opinion for postexposure evaluation must document that the employee has been informed of the results of the medical evaluation and of any medical conditions resulting from the exposure incident that may require further evaluation or treatment. All other diagnoses must remain confidential and not be included in the written report.

Vaccines, vaccinations, and follow-up evaluations must be provided at no cost to the employee, provided at a reasonable time and place, and performed by or under the supervision of a licensed physician or another licensed health care professional whose scope of practice allows her or him to independently perform activities (see BBPS). Vaccinations also must be administered according to current recommendations of the U.S. Public Health Service (Report of the U.S. Preventive Services Task Force, 1989). Employees who decline the vaccination must sign a declination form. The employee may request and obtain the vaccination at a later date and at no cost, if she or he continues to be exposed. All information regarding the exposure incident, evaluation and follow-up must be documented in accordance with the regulations, kept confidential, and maintained for the duration of employment plus 30 years.

Communicating Hazards to Employees

It is the responsibility of the employer to provide information and training as described in the standard to each occupationally exposed employee, at the time of initial assignment, when new tasks involve occupational exposures and annually thereafter (taking into consideration vocabulary, educational level, and literacy of the employee). Training records must be maintained for a minimum of three years.

In addition to the required technical information provided with respect to the bloodborne pathogens, that is, exposure and transmission, work practice controls, labeling, personal protective equipment, preventive measures, emergency and reporting procedures and postexposure follow-up, the employer must explain the BBPS and the exposure control plan, make copies of each available to the employee, and provide an opportunity for an interactive question and answer session.

The occupational health nurse can assist management in complying with the standard (Goldstein & Johnson, 1991) through:

- developing an effective plan to protect employees from potential exposures to bloodborne pathogens;
- establishing effective control strategies and compliance measures to reduce exposures;
- developing and implementing a vaccination and postexposure follow-up program;
- communicating, through employee training and education programs, information about the nature of the problem and exposure, prevention, and control measures;
- recording information, maintaining and storing records as required, and maintaining confidentiality; and
- evaluating and monitoring program performance.

In order to do this, the occupational health nurse will need to be thoroughly knowledgeable about OSHA regulations and other relevant state laws, and collaborate with other departments and disciplines to develop, implement, and evaluate the program. The occupational health nurse, working with other health care professionals, can help to identify and implement appropriate control strategies, as well as monitor compliance with strategies recommended or required.

The occupational health nurse should be involved in counseling exposed employees about the risk of infection, the need for screening, and methods to prevent transmission of viruses. As the employee's anxiety level may be heightened, the nurse needs to be astute to the needs of the worker and provide anticipatory guidance. In addition, the nurse can coordinate the education and training program and help develop methods and materials appropriate to the needs and educational levels of the workers.

Maintenance of confidentiality of employee health information is of paramount importance as employees may fear the loss of employment or alienation from coworkers if information is misreported or divulged. The occupational health nurse will need to devise a policy and procedure for handling health and medical information and records.

Program evaluation should be conducted annually to determine if changes in policies, work practices, education and training, and monitoring procedures are in order. The occupational health nurse will need to work closely with workers, management, and other health care professionals to create an effective and efficient program.

■ AMERICANS WITH DISABILITIES ACT

In 1990, Congress passed the Americans With Disabilities Act (ADA), which is designed to protect an estimated 43 million disabled individuals from discrimination. The ADA addresses requirements to end discrimination against persons with disabilities under five separate titles (Table 15–7).

Emphasis will focus on Title I of the ADA, Employment, which has the most

---

■ **TABLE 15–7**   Americans with Disabilities Act

Title I: Employment
Prohibits entities from discriminating against a qualified individual with a disability in all aspects of employment.

Title II: State and Local Government Services
Prohibits discrimination against individuals with disabilities in providing government services including public transportation.

Title III: Public Accommodations
Requires access to private businesses by individuals with disabilities, thus requiring, where needed, degrees of alteration, modification, and new construction.

Title IV: Telecommunications
Requires that telecommunications services in varying forms be made available, to the extent possible, to the hearing impaired.

Title V: Miscellaneous Provisions
Requires varying provisions for accessibility to recreational and other public areas.

---

impact for occupational health nursing practice. It is important for the occupational health nurse to understand the provisions of the ADA in order to determine how to best assist management in implementing these provisions. For example, the occupational health nurse can help review job descriptions for any physical requirements of a function identified as essential (Kaldor, 1992). In addition, the nurse will want to be actively involved in identifying reasonable accommodations for disabilities, protecting the confidentiality of the employee's health record, identifying and coordinating outside resources for internal implementation of the ADA, and educating employees and management regarding the health and medical implications of the Act (Feutz-Harter, 1992). The occupational health nurse must seize the opportunity to participate with management as a member of the business team in defining effective approaches to disability management in the workplace.

Coverage

Title I of the ADA states that a "covered entity," which includes private employers, state and local governments, employment agencies, labor unions, and joint labor-management committees (hereinafter referred to as employer) cannot discriminate against qualified applicants and employees on the basis of disability. The ADA's requirement applies to all employers with 15 or more employees. Coverage began July 26, 1992, for employers with 25 or more employees and begins July 26, 1994, for employers with 15 or more employees.

Nondiscrimination

Under the ADA, no employer may discriminate against a qualified individual with a disability with regard to job application and testing procedures, hiring assignments and termination, training, compensation, fringe benefits, medical and job evaluations, advancement, or any other term or condition of work (EEOC, 1991, 1992). The ADA specifies types of actions that may constitute discrimination:

1. Limiting, segregating, or classifying a job applicant or employee in a way that adversely affects employment opportunities for the applicant or employee because of his or her disability.
2. Participating in a contractual or other arrangement or relationship that subjects an employer's qualified applicant or employee with a disability to discrimination.
3. Denying employment opportunities to a qualified individual because she or he has a relationship or association with a person with a disability.
4. Refusing to make reasonable accommodation to the known physical or mental limitations of a qualified applicant or employee with a disability, unless the accommodation would pose an undue hardship on the business.
5. Using qualification standards, employment tests, or other selection criteria that screen out or tend to screen out an individual with a disability unless they are job-related and necessary for the business.
6. Failing to use employment tests in the most effective manner to measure actual abilities. Tests must accurately reflect the skills, aptitude, or other factors being measured, and not the impaired sensory, manual, or speaking skills of an employee or applicant with a disability (unless those are the skills the test is designed to measure).

7. Discriminating against an individual because she or he has opposed an employment practice of the employer or filed a complaint, testified, assisted, or participated in an investigation, proceeding, or hearing to enforce provisions of the Act.

Disabled Individual

A qualified individual with a disability is defined within the ADA as an individual with a disability who meets the skill, experience, education, and other job-related requirements of a position held or desired, and who, with or without reasonable accommodation, can perform the essential functions of a job. The ADA definition of an individual with a disability is very specific. A person with a disability is an individual who:

- has a physical or mental impairment that substantially limits one or more of his or her major life activities;
- has a record of such an impairment; or
- is regarded as having such an impairment.

A physical impairment is defined by the ADA as:

a(ny) physiological disorder, or condition, cosmetic disfigurement, or anatomical loss affecting one or more of the following body systems: neurological, musculoskeletal, special sense organs, respiratory (including speech organs), cardiovascular, reproductive, digestive, genitourinary, hemic and lymphatic, skin, and endocrine.

A mental impairment is defined by the ADA as:

a(ny) mental or psychological disorder, such as mental retardation, organic brain syndrome, emotional or mental illness, and specific learning disabilities.

A person's impairment is determined without regard to any medication or assistive device that she or he may use. Such conditions that would be considered a physical or mental impairment would include orthopedic, visual, speech, or hearing impairments, cerebral palsy, epilepsy, muscular dystrophy, multiple sclerosis, HIV infection, cancer, heart disease, diabetes, drug addiction, and alcoholism (Feutz-Harter, 1992). A physical condition that is not the result of a physiological disorder, such as pregnancy, or a predisposition to a certain disease would not be an impairment. Similarly, personality traits such as poor judgment, quick temper, or irresponsible behavior are not themselves impairments.

An impairment is only a disability under the ADA if it substantially limits one or more major life activities; that is, the individual must be unable or significantly limited in performing an activity compared to an average person in the population. Factors to consider in making this determination include the nature and severity of the impairment, duration or expected duration, and its permanent or long-term impact (EEOC, 1992). Major life activities include such activities as caring for oneself, walking, breathing, performing manual tasks, seeing, hearing, learning, speaking, and working.

An employer may require that an individual not pose a "direct threat" to the health or safety of herself, himself, or others. A health or safety risk can only be considered if it is "a significant risk of substantial harm." Employers cannot deny an employment opportunity merely because of a slightly increased risk. An assessment of "direct threat" must be strictly based on valid medical analyses and/or other objective evidence, and not on speculation. This requirement must apply to all applicants and employees, not just to people with disabilities. If an individual appears to pose a direct threat because of a disability, the employer must first try to eliminate or reduce the risk to an acceptable level with reasonable accommodation. If an effective accommodation cannot be found, the employer may refuse to hire an applicant or discharge an employee who poses a direct threat (EEOC, 1992).

Essential Job Functions

Essential job functions are those fundamental rather than marginal to the job duties. The ADA Title I regulations provide guidance on identifying the essential functions of the job. The first consideration is whether employees in the position actually are required to perform the function. For example, a job announcement or job description for a secretary or receptionist may state that typing is a function of the job. If, in fact, the employer has never or seldom required an employee in that position to type, this could not be considered an essential function (EEOC, 1992).

The next consideration is whether removing that function would fundamentally change the job. According to the regulations, examples of reasons why job functions could be considered essential include:

1. the position exists to perform the function;
2. there are a limited number of other employees available to perform the function, or among whom the function can be distributed; and
3. a function is highly specialized, and the person in the position is hired for special expertise or ability to perform the function.

Whether a particular function is essential is a factual determination that must be made on a case-by-case basis. In making this determination various types of evidence will be considered, such as:

- the employer's judgment;
- written job descriptions prepared before advertising or interviewing applicants for the job;
- the amount of time spent performing the function;
- the consequences of not performing the function;
- the terms of a collective bargaining agreement; and
- the work experience of those who previously held the job and of those who currently perform similar jobs.

Nothing in the ADA prohibits employers from defining physical and other job criteria and tests for a job as long as the criteria and tests are job-related and equally applied (Cross, 1992).

The occupational health nurse can perform a valuable service in reviewing and collaborating on the identification of requirements of a function stipulated as essential. Kaldor (1992) points out that recognizing that the job description provides the foundation for any subsequent discussions and decisions around reasonable accommodations, the occupational health nurse should select a tool or process which facilitates a systematic approach to the job analysis. Data collected in that analysis should include: task and process list; "essential functions" identified; description of how the job is done currently; physical, emotional, intellectual requirements of the "essential functions"; and comments on what influence the tools, work postures, work environment have on the incumbent employee. Once documented, the analysis provides proof of an employer's determination of essential functions for a given position, without regard to a specific applicant. Figure 15–4 is an example of a job description questionnaire with specific reference to essential and marginal functions.

Reasonable Accommodation

Reasonable accommodation is a key nondiscrimination requirement of the ADA. While many individuals with disabilities can perform jobs without any need for accommodation, many others are excluded from jobs that they are qualified to perform because of unnecessary barriers in the workplace and work environment, such as physical barriers, communication problems, rigid work schedules, and unfounded fears and stereotypes. Under the ADA, when an individual with a disability is qualified to perform the essential functions of a job, except for functions that cannot be performed because of related limitations and existing job barriers, an employer must try to find a reasonable accommodation that would enable this person to perform these functions. The reasonable accommodation should reduce or eliminate unnecessary barriers between the individual's abilities and the requirements for performing the essential job functions. Reasonable accommodation is any modification or adjustment to a job, an employment practice, or the work environment that makes it possible for an individual with a disability to enjoy an equal employment opportunity. Legal obligations include:

- An employer must provide a reasonable accommodation to the known physical or mental limitations of a qualified applicant or employee with a disability unless she or he can show that the accommodation would impose an undue hardship on the business.
- The obligation to provide a reasonable accommodation applies to all aspects of employment. This duty is ongoing and may arise any time that a person's disability or job changes.
- An employer does not have to make an accommodation for an individual who is not otherwise qualified for a position.
- Generally, it is the obligation of an individual with a disability to request a reasonable accommodation.
- A qualified individual with a disability has the right to refuse an accommodation. However, if the individual cannot perform the essential functions of the job without the accommodation, she or he may not be qualified for the job.
- If the cost of an accommodation would impose an undue hardship on the employer, the individual with a disability should be given the option of providing the accommodation or paying that portion of the cost which would constitute an undue hardship.

A reasonable accommodation applies only to accommodations that reduce barriers to employment related to a person's disability, and need not be the best accommodation available, as long as it is effective for the purpose. It is not required primarily for personal use (EEOC, 1992). Some examples of reasonable accommodation include:

Job Description Questionnaire

Job Title:

Department:

Supervisor:

1) What Essential Functions do you perform?

Essential Function	% of time E	Constant E	Frequent E	Occasional E	Is This Function Essential?	Would the Job Change if not done?

2) What Marginal Functions do you perform?

Marginal Function	% of time M	Constant M	Frequent M	Occasional M	Is This Function Marginal?	Would the Job Change if not done?

3) What education, training, experience, licenses are required for satisfactory performance?

4) What machines or equipment are you responsible for operating?

5) List working conditions such as heat, cold, dust, etc.

6) Do you supervise other employees? If YES, give job titles and description of jobs.

7) If you were unable to perform your function, what effect would it have on management?

8) Do you have authority in training others? If YES, describe.

■ **Figure 15–4** Example of job description questionnaire. (From Goldenthal, N. Understanding the Americans with Disabilities Act. Beverly, MA: OEM Press, 1993.)

- making facilities readily accessible to and usable by an individual with a disability;
- restructuring a job by reallocating or redistributing marginal job functions;
- altering when or how an essential job function is performed;
- providing for part-time or modified work schedules;
- obtaining or modifying equipment or devices;
- modifying examinations, training materials, or policies;
- providing qualified readers and interpreters;
- allowing for reassignment to a vacant position;
- permitting use of accrued paid leave or unpaid leave for necessary treatment;
- providing reserved parking for a person with a mobility impairment; and
- allowing an employee to provide equipment or devices that an employer is not required to provide.

The role of the occupational health nurse can be vital in this process. It is important to critically analyze the job involved and collaborate with the individual involved to determine what types of accommodations will help the employee perform the job. The occupational health nurse can then help assist in selecting the accommodation that is most appropriate.

As stipulated, an employer is not required to make a reasonable accommodation if it would impose an undue hardship on the operation of the business; that is, an action requiring "significant difficulty or expense" in relation to the size of the company, resources available, and nature of the operation. This will be decided on a case-by-case basis. When determining undue hardship the following factors are considered in the regulations:

1. the nature and cost of the accommodation;
2. the overall financial resources of the specific facility where the accommodation is considered and the effect of the accommodation on the expenses and resources of the company facility;
3. the overall financial resources of the company, including the total size of the parent company, the number of employees, and type of company; and
4. the type of operations of the business, including the business's structure, administrative organization, geographic separateness, and fiscal relationship of the facility to the entire company.

It has been suggested that proving undue hardship will be a difficult defense by the employer (Frierson, 1992).

Medical Examinations

Another provision of the ADA is with respect to medical examinations and inquiries. Certain restrictions are placed on the employer regarding preemployment examinations and inquiries. An employer may not require a job applicant to take a preemployment medical examination and may not ask the applicant about the existence, nature, or severity of a disability. For example, an employer may not ask about the applicant's workers' compensation history or about any conditions that might prevent the applicant from doing the job. Applicants may be asked to describe how or demonstrate their ability to perform specific job functions.

An employer may condition a job offer on the satisfactory result of a postoffer medical examination or inquiry if this is required of all entering employees in the same job category. After making a conditional job offer, before a person starts work, an employer may make unrestricted medical inquiries but may not refuse to hire an individual with a disability based on results of such inquiries unless the reason for rejection is job related and justified by business necessity (EEOC, 1992). After employment, any medical examination or inquiry required of an employee must be job-related and justified by business necessity. Exceptions are voluntary examinations conducted as part of employee health programs and examinations required by other federal laws. Information about the medical condition or history of the applicant/employee must be collected and maintained on separate forms and in separate medical files and be treated as a confidential medical record, except that:

- supervisors and managers may be informed regarding necessary restrictions and necessary accommodations;
- first aid and safety personnel may be informed, when appropriate, if the disability might require emergency treatment;
- government officials investigating compliance with the ADA must be provided relevant information on request; and
- the result of such physical examination is not used to identify a disability, which is then the basis of withdrawing the offer of employment.

An employer may conduct voluntary medical examinations and inquiries as part of an employee health program (such as medical screening for high blood pressure, weight control, and cancer detection), providing that:

- participation in the program is voluntary;
- information obtained is maintained according to the confidentiality requirements of the ADA; and
- this information is not used to discriminate against an employee.

Kaldor (1992) describes the role of the occupational health nurse in this phase of the ADA process to:

1. review existing preplacement examination requirements for compliance;
2. work with appropriate resources to construct preplacement examinations that accurately test for the essential function-related physical requirements;
3. coach the consulting physician regarding the ADA prohibition against predictions about future incapacities of an applicant; and
4. protect the confidentiality of these testing results.

Testing for illegal drugs is not considered a medical examination; therefore, employers may continue to conduct drug screening in order to maintain a drug-free workplace (Cross, 1992).

Equal Employment Opportunity Commission

The Equal Employment Opportunity Commission (EEOC) is the federal agency responsible for enforcing the employment requirements of the ADA. Thus, an individual must file a complaint of an alleged violation with the EEOC within 180 days of the alleged discrimination act. If employment discrimination is found, various remedies are available. Several resources that provide assistance in implementing the ADA are listed in the Resource Directory section of the

EEOC Technical Assistance Manual. However, several examples of federal agency resources are found in Appendix 15–2. National nongovernmental technical assistance resources (nearly 75) and regional and state locations of federal programs are also listed in the *Technical Assistance Manual.*

■ WORKERS' COMPENSATION

With the advent of the Industrial Revolution, the number and severity of workplace injuries increased, bringing about the need for changes in providing financial and medical support for employees with work-related injuries. Workers' compensation is a system by which individuals who sustain physical or mental injuries due to their jobs are compensated for their disabilities, medical costs, some rehabilitation costs, and by which the survivors of workers who are killed receive compensation for lost financial support (Nackley, 1987). Excepting federal civilian employees, who are covered by federal laws, primarily the Federal Compensation Act, workers are covered under the various state laws.

While the first state workers' compensation law was passed in New York in 1910, it was later determined to be unconstitutional; Wisconsin's 1911 law was the first viable law passed (Howard & Davies, 1985). Currently, each of the 50 states and the District of Columbia have a workers' compensation law, and while the law is specific to each jurisdiction, commonalities exist across statutes. In general, workers' compensation laws provide that in exchange for paying workers' compensation for damages, the employer receives immunity from lawsuits. However, under certain circumstances, this immunity may not apply, such as:

- injuries not covered by workers' compensation;
- injuries sustained by an employee of a noncomplying employer;
- injuries caused by the employer's intentional act;
- injuries sustained while the employer and employee entered into a separate relationship or "dual capacity" independent of their master/servant relationship; and
- discharge, demotion, or other punitive action by an employer taken in retaliation for employees' filing workers' compensation claims or otherwise pursuing workers' compensation rights (Nackley, 1987).

Work-related Injuries and Diseases

In order to be compensable, occupational injuries and diseases must be work-related. The most common type of workers' compensation claim is the injury that is an unexpected event in the sense that it is unintended (Nackley, 1987). The traditional terms "in the course of" and "arising out of employment" may be used to determine if an injury is work-related and thus compensable. However, it is important to remember that because workers' compensation systems are state administered, determinations of similar situations or cases may vary from state to state. Thus, regardless of the terms or language, the determining factor as to whether an injury is compensable should be whether the injury is work related.

With respect to workers' compensation, the definition of occupational disease varies from state to state. However, the obvious application of the definition is one where the illnesses are associated with particular industrial occupations or processes. Virtually any disease that is caused by an industrial trade or process can be recognized as an occupational disease. In those jurisdictions in which occupational diseases are distinguished from injuries, coverage is provided by statutes that generally recognize occupational diseases or by statutes that list certain "scheduled" ailments as recognized occupational diseases associated with certain trades or industrial processes, or by both.

The statutory provisions for coverage of occupational diseases also vary from state to state. Some provide schedules of such diseases, others do not. States that have schedules may also include a catch-all provision. The "schedules" of some states may contain only one disease, listed separately from the general accident or injury provision, while New York's schedule lists 29 diseases, and Ohio's and North Carolina's, 27 each. The diseases most often occurring on such schedules include the various pneumoconioses, which are associated with exposure to dusts (including coal dust), silicosis from exposure to silica, asbestosis, and radiation illness (Nackley, 1987).

Compensation and Benefits

Awards made to injured workers in workers' compensation systems vary from state to state and are usually designed to compensate the disabled worker or dependent survivor, in the case of the death of an employee, for economic or wage loss, or for lost earning capacity. In addition, medical care costs and related expenses, funeral and burial costs, and in most cases, some form of rehabilitation costs are included. Most workers' compensation systems make some effort to compensate injured workers for permanent medical impairment. These awards are usually paid irrespective of any actual or prospective loss of wages and are divided into so-called scheduled awards, usually for loss of limb, eyesight, hearing, or for other defined categories of impairments, disability, or impairment awards.

One reason for establishing these awards was to give injured workers some incentive to return to work; another reason was simply to give the worker some quasi-damage award for the physical impairment endured. The basis of the award is related to the extent of the disability, or impairment. Extent of disability is concerned with duration and degree. Duration of disability is concerned with permanent or temporary disability, while degree is concerned with total or partial disability (Table 15–8). As determined by individual state worker's compensation systems, compensation is usually paid weekly and is calculated as a fraction of the workers' weekly wage at the time of injury or death (e.g., two thirds, three fourths), usually with an upper and lower limit. Compensation payments usually start on the date of the injury and continue until the employee returns to work, or as permitted within the workers' compensation system's defined schedule.

In most U.S. jurisdictions, workers' compensation systems are administered by specific agencies usually referred to as industrial commissions or boards, workers' compensation bureaus, or industrial accident boards. The state agency is almost always given general power over the workers' compensation system. This power includes the authority to investigate claims, to collect and disburse funds, to employ sufficient staff to perform its statutory duties, and to compel employers and insurance carriers to comply with the workers' compensation act.

The National Commission on State Workers' Compensation Laws identified seven primary obligations of workers' compensation systems:

■ **TABLE 15–8**   Workers' Compensation Disability Awards

Duration of Disability	Degree of Disability	
	Total	**Partial**
Permanent	1. Disability caused by work-related injury or occupational disease that completely removes claimant from substantially re-munerative employment (in some juris-dictions) 2. Loss or loss of use of designated part or parts of the body (e.g., loss of both legs, loss of vision of both eyes).	Disability caused by work-related injury or occupational disease that does not remove claimant from substantially remunerative employment but that has left the claimant with residual medical impairment expected to be of indefinite duration. For example, loss of limb, hearing, or other de-fined categories of impairment.
Temporary	1. Disability caused by work-related injury or occupational disease that does not appear to be of indefinite duration but keeps the claimant from gainful em-ployment; 2. Disability caused by work-related injury or occupational disease that keeps claimant from returning to regular em-ployment. This is the most commonly awarded disability compensation under workers' compensation. It is payable during the acute post-injury phase of disability, while the claimant is in the hospital or recuperating from an injury, and so long as the injury keeps the claimant who has an expectation of re-turning to the job or to the job market from work. It is intended to compensate a worker for loss of wages during re-covery.	Disability caused by work-related injury or occupational disease that does not appear to be of indefinite duration and that is not keeping the claimant from gainful employment (e.g., frac-ture).

From Nackley, JV. Workers' compensation. Washington, DC: Bureau of National Affairs, 1987.

- taking the initiative in administering the law;
- continually reviewing the performance of the program with a willingness to change its procedures and to request the state legislature to make needed amendments;
- advising workers of their rights and obligations and assuring that they receive the benefits to which they are entitled;
- apprising employers and carriers of their rights and obligations;
- informing other parties in the delivery system such as health care providers of their obligations and privileges;
- assisting in voluntary and informal resolution of disputes that are consistent with law and prohibiting inappropriate agreements; and
- adjudicating claims that cannot be resolved voluntarily (Larson, 1983).

Increasingly, occupational health nurses are becoming more involved in the management and administration of workplace safety programs, whether it be counseling the injured worker about injury management and worker rights, or administration of worker injury claims. The occupational health nurse should be thoroughly familiar with the workers' compensation laws and system, as these will vary from state to state. It is important that records be kept accurately and that injuries be reported and documented promptly so that claims and defenses can be handled effectively.

■ LEGAL PRACTICE OF NURSING

In the United States, each state has a licensure law, generally called the Nurse Practice Act, which defines and regulates the practice of nursing. In most states, the law is implemented, interpreted, and enforced by an administrative agency, usually termed the Board of Nursing. While nursing licensure laws may differ slightly from state to state, each Nurse Practice Act contains a legal definition of nursing practice that determines the legal scope of nursing practice and provides the legal authority to perform those functions, which are generally defined as "nursing" (Keener, 1985).

La Bar (1984) states that the definition of nursing practice should be broad to allow for flexibility and utilization of appropriate skills of the professional nurse. In addition, a broader rather than narrower definition can then be interpreted to reflect the expansion of nursing practice as the scope of practice evolves. La Bar collected, reviewed, and analyzed the statutory definitions of nursing practice with respect to certain ANA principles and suggested the following definition of professional nursing practice:

The practice of nursing means the performance for compensation of professional services requiring substantial specialized knowledge of the biological, physical, behavioral, psychological, and sociological sciences and of nursing theory as the basis for assessment, diagnosis, planning, intervention, and evaluation in the promotion and maintenance of health; the casefinding and management of illness, injury, or infirmity; the restoration of optimum function; or the achievement of a dignified death. Nursing practice includes but is not limited to administration, teaching, counseling, supervision, delegation, and evaluation of practice and execution of the medical regimen, including the administration of medications and treatments prescribed by any person authorized by state law to prescribe. Each registered nurse is directly accountable and responsible to the consumer for the quality of nursing care rendered.

Unfortunately, legal boundaries defining the scope of nursing practice are neither clearly delineated between the practice of nursing and the practice of other health professions, nor do they comprehensively differentiate the "expanded" role of the nurse from nursing practice in general. However, nursing professional groups and state legislatures seem to be moving toward legal definitions of nursing that adequately reflect specialization and advanced practice (Yorker, 1989). La Bar (1984) states that it is the function of the professional association to upgrade practice, to certify individuals in special areas, and to establish the scope and qualifications of each practice area.

Each nurse has the responsibility to obtain and be familiar with the nurse practice act that governs nursing practice within the state where she or he practices. In addition, she or he must know the rules and regulations that further specify nursing functions as set forth by the respective state board of nursing. Keener (1985) lists several points the nurse should consider when making a determination regarding the legal authority (i.e., nurse practice act) to perform specific nursing functions:

- How does the state nurse practice act define professional nursing? Is it a broad, open-ended statutory definition that authorizes all nursing functions and contains language such as "including but not limited to?" Does it specifically provide for nursing diagnosis and assessment? Does the act contain specific authorization for the expanded scope of nursing practice? Is such practice limited only to certain types of practitioners or specialists with particular credentials?
- Do the Board of Nursing rules and regulations specifically define or limit the scope of nursing practice? Is there a "laundry list" of functions that nurses are legally permitted to perform? Do the rules and regulations recognize practitioners or specialists? Are there specific credentials or certifications required?
- Is there a limitation regarding practicing within the guidelines of medical standing orders and protocols?

If there are questions or if clarification is needed regarding the statute and/or regulations, the nurse may contact the state nursing board and/or state nurses' association to determine what common practices are accepted regarding the use of such protocols and standing orders in her or his state and whether there have been any statutory, regulatory, or judicial opinions issued recently concerning the nurse's legal authority to perform such functions. The nurse should also check other practice acts, such as medicine and pharmacy, where overlapping functions may exist by interpretation, to determine if any statutory prohibitions exist.

Nurses have a duty of care that requires the nurse to conform to a standard of care for protection of the patient or client against unreasonable risk of injury (Creighton, 1988). As a professional, the nurse is required to possess and exercise the knowledge and skill as a member of the profession in good standing in the same or similar communities, that is, the nurse's conduct will be measured against that of the "reasonably prudent nurse" in a similar situation (Locklear-Haynes, 1989, 1990). Thus, the care the occupational health nurse renders to an employee will not be measured against that of a physician. When the nurse's actions or conduct do not meet the required standard, the legal duty of care may be breached, which may be grounds for a case of negligence or malpractice (Kramer, 1986; Keener, 1985).

While very few malpractice suits have been filed against occupational health nurses, the following case is of interest. When a nurse cleaned and bandaged a puncture wound sustained by an employee after a piece of metal pierced the employee's forehead, the court said the nurse would be expected to also probe the wound. In this particular case, it was company policy that employees could only see a physician if the occupational health nurse made a referral.

The nurse continued to treat the reddened area over the next 10 months until it became swollen. By the time the nurse referred the employee to a physician, a basal-cell carcinoma had developed. The nurse and the employer were held liable for his damages. The court reasoned that a prudent occupational health nurse would have explored the wound for potential metal slivers, knowing that failure to heal is a warning sign of cancer, and further, the nurse should have referred the employee to a physician much earlier (Cooper v. National Motor Bearing Co., 288 P.2d 581 [Cal. 1955]) (Yorker, 1989; Wolff, 1984).

Recent case law regarding advanced nursing practice has focused on the practice of two nurses who provided services in a women's health clinic in Missouri. The suit was filed by physicians on the medical licensing board who claimed that the nurses were practicing medicine. As a part of their practice, "the nurses performed a variety of diagnostic and treatment functions, including breast and pelvic examinations, pregnancy testing, Pap smears, gonorrhea cultures, and blood serology; the administration of all kinds of contraceptive methods, including intrauterine devices and oral contraceptives; and the counseling and education of patients." All these functions were performed according to signed physician protocols.

While lower courts found the nurses guilty of engaging in the practice of medicine, the Supreme Court of Missouri unanimously reversed the decision, stating that nurses who could demonstrate appropriate specialized skill, education, and judgment were practicing within the Nurse Practice Act as set forth in the state's statutory definition of nursing. Yorker (1989) emphasizes several important points with respect to this decision. First, the court placed considerable emphasis on the nurses' graduate education. Second, the court was impressed by the overwhelming response of professional groups and private citizens in support of the nurses' expanded role. Third, the court recognized the prevailing trend of independence in nursing practice, even to the point of conceding that the functions of diagnosis and prescription no longer fall within the exclusive territory of the medical doctor.

Rowe (1989) describes an opinion issued by the Attorney General of Georgia, which stated that no statutory authority existed for public health nurses to prescribe medications such as birth control pills (for public health clients) by reference to a protocol; therefore, the activity was considered unlawful even though it had been performed by public health nurses by protocol since 1973. The Attorney General interpreted Georgia's Nurse Practice Act to authorize (by physicians) only the administration of medications.

Because many medical and nursing functions overlap, nurses need clear statutory authority regarding the use of protocols and the functions that may be delegated by protocols in order to prevent nurses from being confronted with charges such as practicing medicine without a license (Rowe, 1989). Occupational health nurses working under protocols should be aware of the permissible scope of nursing practice in their state and determine that the functions delegated to them by protocol fall within that permissible scope. All protocols with delegatory functions should be dated and signed by a physician with defined tasks clearly authorized. The educational preparation a nurse must have to perform tasks should be identified (Northrop, 1988; Wold, 1990). The company policy should distinctly authorize nurses to practice by protocol.

With duties such as recording laboratory results, history taking, physical assessments, screening examinations, and health counseling, the occupational health nurse must comply with the accepted standard of care generally expected of any nurse when performing such procedures. It is particularly important to keep accurate records and to report all observations regarding the client's physical and mental condition, as well as all information given to him or her (Kramer, 1986). However, additional types of recording such as the keeping of OSHA logs are specific to occupational health nursing duties and must conform to the accepted practice therein.

Sometimes the occupational health nurse may be faced with a dilemma when an ethical decision conflicts with a legal requirement. This may be the case with confidentiality of health information versus disclosure of information when others may be at risk (Yorker, 1988; Rogers, 1988). However, the nurse can utilize ethical codes, frameworks, and standards for practice that will help to guide decisions for safe and effective occupational health nursing practice (AAOHN, 1987, 1992).

Nurse Practice Acts were developed because state governments are concerned with protecting their citizens from unsafe nursing practice. These laws govern all nursing practice within each state, and violation of these laws is a crime. For example, if dispensing medications at the worksite is outside the scope of nursing practice, performance of this function by the occupational health nurse would be in violation of the law. There is little potential for criminal violation in the practice of nursing if one is adequately trained and educated, and then conducts oneself in a reasonable manner (Kramer, 1986).

■ CONCLUSION

In summary, the occupational health nurse is responsible to be knowledgeable about federal, state, and local statutes and regulations affecting the occupational health and safety of workers and to implement appropriate practice strategies to comply with these mandates. The nurse must be thoroughly familiar with the state nurse practice act where she or he practices, recognizing the legal parameters for professional nursing practice. As the scope of occupational health nursing evolves and expands, the nurse will assume greater responsibility in the overall management and delivery of occupational health services. Accountability for legal and professional nursing practice is of paramount importance in ensuring safe and effective health care for all workers.

References

American Association of Occupational Health Nurses. Role of government, business, and professional societies. In Proceedings of the Occupational Safety & Health Summit. Des Plaines, IL: American Society of Safety Engineers, p. 175, 1992.

American Association of Occupational Health Nurses. A comprehensive guide for establishing an occupational health service. Atlanta: Author, 1987.

Americans With Disabilities Act. P.L. 101–356, 42USC 12101–12213, 1990.

Barlow, R & Handelman E. OSHA's final bloodborne pathogens standard: Part II. AAOHN Journal, 41(1): 8–15, 1993.

Blosser, F. Occupational safety and health. Washington, DC: Bureau of National Affairs, 1992.

Centers for Disease Control. The HIV/AIDS Epidemic: The first 10 years. MMWR, 40(22): 357–363, 1991.

Centers for Disease Control. Prevention of leading work-related diseases and injuries. MMWR, 1983.

Council on Occupational & Environmental Health. National Association for Public Health Policy: Organizational safety and health legislative agenda, 1989. Journal of Public Health Policy, Winter: 544–555, 1988.

Creighton, H. Laws every nurse should know. Philadelphia: W.B. Saunders, 1988.

Cross, LJ. Americans With Disabilities Act: Meeting the requirements. AAOHN Journal, 40(6): 284–286, 1992.

Equal Employment Opportunity Commission. Rule for Individuals with Disabilities, 29 CFR, part 1630. Washington, DC: Author, 1991.

Equal Employment Opportunity Commission. A technical assistance manual on the employment provisions (Title I) of the Americans

With Disabilities Act. EEOC-M-1A. Washington, DC: Author, 1992.

Feutz-Harter, S. The Americans With Disabilities Act: How it impacts on occupational health nursing. AAOHN Update Series, 5(1): 1–8, 1992.

Frierson, J. Employer's guide to the Americans With Disabilities Act. Washington, DC: Bureau of National Affairs, 1992.

Goldstein, L & Johnson, S. OSHA Bloodborne pathogens standard: Implications for the occupational health nurse. AAOHN Journal, 39(4): 182–188, 1991.

Howard, PH & Davies, W. Workers' compensation: An overview. AAOHN Update Series, 2(3): 1–8, 1985.

Kaldor, CS. The Americans With Disabilities Act: An invitation for occupational health nurse intervention. AAOHN Update Series, 5(2): 1–8, 1992.

Keener, ML. Legal boundaries of nursing practice. AAOHN Update Series, 1(24): 1–8, 1985.

Kramer, LC. Professional responsibility: The legal and ethical issues. AAOHN Update Series, 2(1): 1–8, 1986.

La Bar, C. Statutory definitions of nursing practice and their conformity to certain ANA principles. Kansas City: ANA, 1984.

Larson, A. The law of workmens' compensation. New York: Matthew Bender & Company, 1983.

Locklear-Haynes, T. Public health in the workplace. AAOHN Journal, 38(2): 78–79, 1990.

Locklear-Haynes, T. Public health in the workplace. AAOHN Journal, 38: 475–477, 1989.

Marshall v. Barlows, Inc. 436 U.S. 307(1978) 54, 55, 114.

McNeely, E. Tracking the future of OSHA: Regulatory policies into the 90s. AAOHN Journal, 40(1): 17–23, 1992.

McNeely, E. An organizational study of hazard communication: The health provider perspective. AAOHN Journal, 38(4): 165–173, 1990.

Meyer, AF & Watson, DL. Hazard communications: A process beyond mere compliance. In Proceeding of the Occupational Safety & Health Summit. Des Plaines, IL: American Society of Safety Engineers, pp. 49–58, 1992.

Mistretta, E. Health care records and the law. AAOHN Journal, 38(11): 545–547, 1990.

Nackley, JV. Workers' compensation. Washington, DC: Bureau of National Affairs, 1987.

North Carolina Occupational Safety & Health Project. Right to know handbook. Durham, NC, 1988.

Northrop, C & Kelley, M. Legal issues in nursing. St. Louis: C.V. Mosby, 1988.

Occupational Safety and Health Act. P.L. 91-596, 64USC 1590-1620, 1970.

Report of the U.S. Preventive Services Task Force: Guide to clinical preventive services. Baltimore: Williams & Wilkins, pp. 369–374, 1989.

Rogers, B. Ethical dilemmas in occupational health nursing. AAOHN Journal, 36(3): 100–105, 1988.

Rowe, BB. Expanding the nurse's role to diagnosis and treatment: Understanding the legal significance. AAOHN Journal, 37(5): 198–199, 1989.

Simonowitz, J & Spencer, JA. The role of the occupational health nurse in OSHA compliance. AAOHN Update Series, 2(5): 1–8, 1985.

Soloman, C. Hazard communication and right-to-know. AAOHN Journal, 34(6): 264–268, 1986.

U.S. Department of Labor, Bureau of Labor Statistics, Washington, DC: O.M.B. #1220-0029, 1986.

U.S. Department of Labor, Occupational Safety & Health Administration. Occupational safety and health standards Subpart Z—Toxic and hazardous substances hazard communication standard. 29CFR part 1910.1200. Federal Register, 52: 31877–31892, 1987.

U.S. Department of Labor, Occupational Safety & Health Administration. Access to employee exposure and medical records. 29CFR Part 1910-20. Federal Register, 53: 38162–68, 1988.

U.S. Department of Labor, Occupational Safety & Health Administration. All about OSHA. Washington, DC: OSHA Pub. #2056, 1991a.

U.S. Department of Labor, Occupational Safety & Health Administration. Hazard communication guidelines for compliance. Washington, DC: OSHA Pub #3111, 1991b.

U.S. Department of Labor, Occupational Safety & Health Administration. Final rule. Occupational exposure to bloodborne pathogens. 29CFR Part 1910.1030. Federal Register 56(235): 64004–64182, 1991c.

U.S. Department of Labor, Occupational Safety & Health Administration. Chemical hazard communication. Washington, DC: OSHA Pub. #3084, 1992a.

U.S. Department of Labor, Occupational Safety & Health Administration. Occupational exposure to bloodborne pathogens. Washington, DC: OSHA, Pub #3127, 1992b.

U.S. Department of Labor, Occupational Safety & Health Administration. Bloodborne pathogens and acute care facilities. Washington, DC: OSHA Pub. #3128, 1992c.

U.S. Department of Labor, Occupational Safety & Health Administration. Enforcement procedures for the occupational exposure to bloodborne pathogens standard, 29CFR 1910.1030. OSHA Instruction CPL 2-2.44C: 1-71. Washington, DC: Office of Health Compliance Assistance, 1992d.

Wold, JL. Workers' compensation law and the

occupational health nurse. AAOHN Journal, 38(8): 385–387, 1990.

Wolff, M. Court upholds expanded practice for nurses. Law, Medicine & Health Care, 12: 26–29, 1984.

Yorker, BA. Scope of practice: Case law. AAOHN Journal, 37(2): 80–81, 1989.

Yorker, BA. Confidentiality—an ethical dilemma. AAOHN Journal, 36(8): 346–347, 1988.

APPENDIX

15–1

Occupational Safety and Health Act of 1970

To assure so far as possible every working man and woman in the Nation safe and healthful working conditions and to preserve our human resources.

1) by encouraging employers and employees in their efforts to reduce the number of occupational safety and health hazards at their places of employment, and to stimulate employers and employees to institute new and to perfect existing programs for providing safe and healthful working conditions;

2) by providing that employers and employees have separate but dependent responsibilities and rights with respect to achieving safe and healthful working conditions;

3) by authorizing the Secretary of Labor to set mandatory occupational safety and health standards applicable to businesses affecting interstate commerce, and by creating an Occupational Safety and Health Review Commission for carrying out adjudicatory functions under the Act;

4) by building upon advances already made through employer and employee initiative for providing safe and healthful working conditions;

5) by providing for research in the field of occupational safety and health, including the psychological factors involved, and by developing innovative methods, techniques, and approaches for dealing with occupational safety and health problems;

6) by exploring ways to discover latent diseases, establishing causal connections between diseases and work in environmental conditions, and conducting other research relating to health problems, in recognition of the fact that occupational health standards present problems often different from those involved in occupational safety;

7) by providing medical criteria which will assure insofar as practicable that no employee will suffer diminished health, functional capacity, or life expectancy as a result of his work experience;

8) by providing for training programs to increase the number and competence of personnel engaged in the field of occupational safety and health;

9) by providing for the development and promulgation of occupational safety and health standards;

10) by providing an effective enforcement program which shall include a prohibition against giving advance notice of any inspection and sanctions for any individual violating this prohibition;

11) by encouraging the States to assume the fullest responsibility for the administration and enforcement of their occupational safety and health laws by providing grants to the States to assist in identifying their needs and responsibilities in the area of occupational safety and health, to develop plans in accordance with the provisions of this Act, to improve the administration and enforcement of State occupational safety and health laws, and to conduct experimental and demonstration projects in connection therewith;

12) by providing for appropriate reporting procedures with respect to occupational safety and health which procedures will help achieve the objectives of this Act and accurately describe the nature of the occupational safety and health problem;

13) by encouraging joint labor-management efforts to reduce injuries and disease arising out of employment.

─────────── APPENDIX ───────────

15–2

Bloodborne Pathogens Compliance Program

PURPOSE
To eliminate or minimize exposure to bloodborne pathogens or other potentially infectious materials.

POLICY
GoodMark Foods, Inc., Garner Operation, establishes, maintains and enforces work practices and standard operating procedures to eliminate or minimize contact with blood or other potentially infectious materials.

DEFINITIONS
Bloodborne pathogens: Pathogenic microorganisms that are present in human blood and can cause disease in humans. These pathogens include, but are not limited to hepatitis B virus (HBV) and human immunodeficiency virus (HIV).

Other potentially infectious materials: Includes the following human body fluids: semen, vaginal secretions, cerebrospinal fluid, synovial fluid, pleural fluid, pericardial fluid, peritoneal fluid, amniotic fluid, saliva in dental procedures, and any body fluid that is visibly contaminated with blood.

Occupational exposure: Actual or potential parenteral, skin, eye or mucous membrane contact with blood or other potentially infectious materials that may result from the performance of an employee's duties.

Universal blood and body fluid precautions: An approach to infection control. According to the concept of universal precautions, all human blood; body components including serum; other body fluids containing visible blood; semen; vaginal secretions; tissues; and cerebrospinal, synovial, pleural, peritoneal, pericardial, and amniotic fluids are treated as if they are infectious for HIV, HBV, and other bloodborne pathogens.

North Carolina regulated medical waste: Blood and body fluids in individual containers in volumes greater than 20 ml.; microbiological waste, such as laboratory cultures and stocks; and pathological waste such as human tissue, organs, or body parts.

Sharps which are considered regulated medical waste: Contaminated needles, scalpels, plastic slides and cover slips, broken glass and capillary tubes, ends of dental wires, and other contaminated objects that can penetrate the skin.

EXPOSURE DETERMINATION
GoodMark Foods, Inc., Garner Operation, has developed written exposure determinations and maintains a list of all job classifications in which employees have occupational exposure to bloodborne pathogens. All job tasks are classified into one of three categories to facilitate exposure determination:

Category I: Tasks that involve potential for mucous membrane or skin contact with blood, body fluids, or tissues, or potential for spills or splashes of them.
  • Occupational Health Nurse

Courtesy GoodMark Foods, Inc., Garner Operation, Garner, North Carolina.

Category II: Tasks that involve no exposure to blood, body fluids, or tissues, but employment may require performing unplanned Category I tasks.
- None at this time

Category III: Tasks that involve no exposure to blood, body fluids, or tissues, and Category I tasks are not a condition of employment.
- All other employees

PROCEDURE
Preventive measures

1. *Hepatitis B vaccinations:* Employees who have occupational exposure to bloodborne pathogens are required to have hepatitis B vaccine. The vaccination series is provided to employees at no charge.
   a. The first dose of vaccine is to be made available to employees within 10 working days of initial assignment. Subsequent doses are to be administered according to current Centers for Disease Control and Prevention recommendations.
   b. Employees who decline hepatitis B vaccine are required to sign a Hepatitis B Vaccine Declination Form (See BPCP Attachment I), and have the option of taking the vaccine at a later date if occupational exposure continues.
2. *Universal blood and body fluid precautions:* Universal Precautions must be observed. This method of infection control requires the employer and employee to assume that all human blood and specified human body fluids are infectious for HIV, HBV, and other bloodborne pathogens. Where differentiation of types of body fluids is difficult or impossible, all body fluids are to be considered as potentially infectious.

METHODS OF CONTROL
Engineering and work practice controls

1. Engineering and work practice controls are used as the primary method to eliminate or minimize employee exposure. Where occupational exposure remains after institution of these controls, personal protective equipment will also be used.
2. Handwashing facilities are readily accessible to employees. Additionally, appropriate antiseptic towelettes are provided in each department's first aid kit.
3. There is no potential for contaminated needles at this site because no needles are used.
4. Contaminated instruments are decontaminated with wipes and placed in a puncture-resistant container that is leakproof on the sides and bottom and labeled. This container does not require employees to reach by hand into the container where the sharps have been placed.
5. All procedures involving blood or other potentially infectious materials will be performed in such a manner as to minimize splashing, spraying, spattering, and generation of droplets of these substances.

Personal protective equipment

1. When there is occupational exposure, appropriate personal protective equipment such as, but not limited to, gloves, gowns, aprons, masks, and eye protection will be provided at no cost to the employee.
2. Appropriate personal protective equipment in appropriate sizes will be available to employees.
3. Use of personal protective equipment by the employees will be monitored and enforced.
4. Hypoallergenic gloves, glove liners, powderless gloves, or other similar alternatives will be readily accessible to those employees who are allergic to the gloves normally provided.
5. Personal protective equipment will be cleaned, laundered, and disposed of at no cost to the employee.
6. Personal protective equipment will be replaced as needed to maintain its effectiveness at no cost to the employee.
7. If a garment(s) is penetrated by blood or other potentially infectious materials, the garment(s) will be removed immediately or as soon as feasible.
8. All personal protective equipment will be removed before the employee leaves the work area. When personal protective equipment is removed, it will be placed in an appropriately designated area or container for disposal.
9. Gloves will be worn when it can be reasonably anticipated that the employee may have had contact with blood, other potentially infectious materials, mucous membranes, or nonintact skin; when touching contaminated items or surfaces.
10. Disposable (single use) gloves will be replaced as soon as practical when contaminated or as soon as feasible if they are torn or punctured. They will not be washed or decontaminated for reuse.

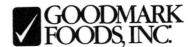

4851 JONES SAUSAGE ROAD
GARNER, NORTH CAROLINA 27529
(919) 772-1511

HEPATITIS B VACCINE DECLINATION FORM

I understand that due to my occupational exposure to blood or other potentially infectious materials that I may be at risk of acquiring hepatitis B virus (HBV) infection. I have been given the opportunity to be vaccinated with hepatitis B vaccine at no charge to myself. However, I decline hepatitis B vaccination at this time. I understand that by declining this vaccine, I continue to be at risk of acquiring hepatitis B, a serious disease. If in the future I continue to have occupational exposure to blood or other potentially infectious materials and I want to be vaccinated with hepatitis B vaccine, I can receive the vaccination series at no charge to me.

Name: _____

Signature: _____ Date: _____

Witness: _____ Date: _____

10/4/92

11. Masks in combination with eye protection devices, such as goggles or glasses with solid side shields, or chin-length face shields will be worn whenever splashes, spray, spatter, or droplets of blood or other potentially infectious materials may be generated and eye, nose, or mouth contamination can be reasonably anticipated.
12. Appropriate protective clothing such as, but not limited to, gowns, aprons, lab coats, clinic jackets, or similar outer garments will be worn in occupational exposure situations.

Housekeeping
1. Any contaminated equipment or work surfaces will be decontaminated immediately after contact with blood or other body fluids with an EPA-approved disinfectant such as 1:10 dilution of bleach or Isolyser.

2. Contaminated disposable items, such as dressings or drapes, that would release blood or body fluids in a liquid or semiliquid state if compressed or items that are caked with dried blood are regulated waste as defined by OSHA. Regulated waste does not require treatment and may be disposed of as general solid waste. However, while onsite, blood-soaked or caked items must be discarded, stored, and transported in closable, leakproof, biohazard-labeled containers.

POSTEXPOSURE PROCEDURE
Following a report of an exposure incident:
1. An Incident Report, "Employee Exposure to Bloodborne Pathogens," will be obtained from the Occupational Health Nurse and completed and returned to the supervisor or Occupational Health Nurse before the end of the shift.
2. A confidential medical evaluation and follow-up will be made immediately available to the employee.
3. The Occupational Health Nurse will assess the employee's exposure, his/her hepatitis B vaccination and vaccine response status, whether the source of the blood is available, and the source's HIV and HBsAG status. This is done by interviewing the employee; reviewing the completed Incident Report Form, the employee's confidential medical record, and the source's record; contacting the source's physician, and talking with other employees as indicated.
4. Individualize postexposure management and treatment of exposed employee(s) on a case by case basis, following current communicable disease rules.
5. Make arrangements for HIV and HBsAG testing and counseling of source person, if known, according to the communicable disease rules [15A NCAC .0202 (4)(a)(i) and .0203(b)(3)(A)], unless already known to be infected.
6. Conduct HIV and HBV pretest counseling before obtaining laboratory tests from the exposed employee. Obtain consent for confidential HIV testing from the employee.
    a. If the employee consents to a baseline blood specimen collection but does not give consent at that time for HIV serologic testing, the serum sample must be preserved for at least 90 days. If within 90 days of the exposure incident the employee elects to have the baseline sample tested, such testing will be done as soon as feasible.
7. Consult with Garner Family Physician if hepatitis B immune globulin or hepatitis B vaccine is indicated, and if any other evaluation or treatment is required. To ensure that the physician is adequately informed, a copy of the OSHA Bloodborne Pathogens Standard, applicable communicable disease rules, GoodMark Foods, Inc., Garner Operation, exposure plan, a description of the specific exposure incident, route of exposure, related job duties, the infection status of the source, the vaccination and immunity status of the exposed employee.
8. Conduct postexposure counseling on return of laboratory results. All employees will receive their laboratory results.
9. Provide prophylactic treatment or immunizations as ordered by the physician and as required by the communicable disease rule [15A NCAC .0203(b)(3)(B) and (C)] and provide the employee with a copy of the health care professional's written evaluation.
10. If the source person is HIV-positive or is unknown, conduct follow-up HIV testing and counseling for the exposed employee at 3 and 6 months.
11. Completed Incident Report Form should be filed in individual's medical file and in personnel.
12. Record the route(s) of exposure, circumstances of exposure, and postexposure management on the employee's confidential medical record.
13. If medical treatment is administered to the exposed employee (e.g., HBIG or a booster hepatitis B immunization is given), record the exposure incident as an injury on the OSHA 200 Log.

TRAINING/HAZARD COMMUNICATION
GoodMark Foods, Inc., Garner Operation, will ensure that all employees with occupational exposure participate in a training program which must be provided at no cost to the employee and during working hours.

Because the Occupational Health Nurse is currently the only employee whose job tasks fit into Categories I and II, the annual educational contact hours she receives will include annual training regarding the Bloodborne Pathogen Standard. Documentation of training will be maintained.

RECORDS

All health information collected regarding the exposure, recommended treatment and follow-up, and information provided to the employee will be documented and kept confidential and stored securely for the duration of employment plus 30 years.

Original Date: _____

Annual Review Date: _____   Signature: _____

Annual Review Date: _____   Signature: _____

Annual Review Date: _____   Signature: _____

APPENDIX
15–3

GoodMark Foods Lockout/Tagout Procedure

PURPOSE

To establish the minimum requirements for the lockout and tagout of hazardous energy isolating devices to prevent the unexpected energization or startup of equipment or release of stored energy. Lockout/Tagout is an effort to protect the employee from injury when he or she is performing maintenance on equipment. Lockout/Tagout is an OSHA-mandated safety requirement for all manufacturing environments.

SCOPE AND APPLICATION

These requirements apply to the maintenance and operation of equipment where the unexpected energization, startup, or release of stored energy could result in injury to an employee. Generally applies anytime an employee is required to put any portion of his or her body in an area of the machine or equipment where moving parts or energy such as electricity and steam can cause injury. Also applies to tools being used by an employee working on the equipment such as scrapers, shovels, or pitch forks. These requirements DO NOT apply to the following:

1. Normal production operations where the employee IS NOT required to place any portion of his or her body in the danger area of moving parts or where the employee bypasses safety guards and devices.
2. Work on cord or plug connected devices for which exposure to hazards can be effectively controlled by unplugging or disconnecting the device from its sole power source and keeping the plug under the EXCLUSIVE control of the person performing the maintenance.

EMPLOYEE CLASSIFICATIONS

1. *All employees:* Every employee at the manufacturing site, regardless of his or her work assignment or position, shall be instructed about the procedures and requirements of the lockout/tagout program.
2. *Affected employees:* Every employee whose work assignments require that he or she operate equipment or work in an area where lockout/tagout devices are used. Affected employees are not charged to apply lockout/tagout devices but are charged with thoroughly understanding the procedures in order to effectively monitor the process and take corrective actions when they are violated.
3. *Authorized employees:* Every employee who has been given the authority, responsibility, and training to implement the lockout/tagout procedure on specified pieces of equipment. Authorized employees are required to thoroughly understand the lockout/tagout procedures and be certified on each piece of equip-

ment by his or her supervisor or manager. Every authorized employee will be issued a lock and tag specifically identified to be used for lockout/tagout.

GENERAL REQUIREMENTS

1. Lockout and tagout: Every energy-isolating device capable of being locked out must have both a lock and tag applied according to the procedures.
2. Energy-isolating devices NOT capable of being locked out must be tagged out according to the procedures. Every precaution should be taken for tagging out a piece of equipment in order to reduce the chance of inadvertent re-energization of the equipment. The tag must be applied in such a manner that it will withstand any environmental conditions for whatever period of time necessary and retain the required information. Additional precautions such as pulling fuses, locking a breaker box or door to a panel room, or applying additional tags around the work site should be taken.
3. Whenever equipment is installed, relocated, or undergoes major modification or repair, energy-isolating devices capable of being locked out must be installed.
4. Locks and tags used for lockout/tagout must be singularly identified and issued to authorized employees. They shall not be used for any other purpose and must be standardized in color, shape, and size. Locks and tags must be capable of withstanding the environment to which they will be exposed for the maximum time that they are to be applied. Application of a lock or tag or both must be substantial enough to prevent their removal without the use of excessive force or unusual techniques.
5. A lockout/tagout device shall be applied only by the authorized employee to whom it was issued. Locks and tags CANNOT be loaned to another authorized employee. Each authorized employee performing maintenance on a piece of equipment must apply his or her own lock and tag prior to placing his or her body in a danger area. Affected employees (those who ordinarily work on the equipment) MUST NOT perform or help perform any maintenance on equipment even if it has been locked out by an authorized employee.
6. Outside personnel or contractors are required to follow GoodMark Foods lockout/tagout procedures even though their lockout and tagout devices may be different in size, shape, and color from GoodMark's. It is the departmental or area managers' responsibility to ensure that the outside personnel or contractor understands and adheres to GoodMark Foods procedures.

PROCEDURE FOR APPLYING LOCKOUT/TAGOUT

Only an authorized employee certified to lockout and tagout a specific piece of equipment shall be allowed to perform the lockout/tagout procedure.

1. Notification of employees: The authorized employee must notify all affected employees in the area that a lockout/tagout of a piece of equipment is going to take place.
2. Preparation for shutdown: The authorized employee shall locate and identify all energy sources for that piece of equipment and the means to release any stored energy.
3. Equipment shutdown: If the piece of equipment is being operated, it should be shut down according to normal stopping procedures.
4. Equipment isolation: Energy-isolating devices for that piece of equipment shall be switched to the OFF position to isolate it from ALL sources of energy.
5. Lockout/Tagout application: The specified lock shall be applied to the energy-isolating device in such a manner as to safely hold the device in the OFF position. The specified tag shall be clearly filled out with the authorized employees' name, the date, the equipment name or number or both, and a brief description of the maintenance being performed. The tag or tags must be affixed in such a manner that they are readily visible at the isolation device and will withstand the environmental conditions for the necessary length of time. Additional tags may also be placed at the work site or any other area deemed necessary.
6. Release stored energy (try): All potentially hazardous stored energy must be released by pushing the normal start buttons to verify the isolation of energy. Opening of valves might also be necessary with pneumatic, hydraulic, vacuum, or pressurized water systems to release stored energy. When the isolation is verified and the stored energy is released, the normal STOP buttons should be activated.
7. Verification of isolation: Before starting maintenance on the equipment, the authorized employee must take a moment to verify that the equipment has been properly isolated—locked and tagged out—and that all affected employees are clear of the danger area.

RELEASE FROM LOCKOUT/TAGOUT

1. Inspection of area: The work area must be inspected by the authorized employee to ensure that all tools and nonessential items are put away. All guards and equipment components must be operationally intact on the equipment.
2. Notification of employees: The authorized employee must notify the affected employees in the area where the equipment is about to be reenergized. He or she must make a visual check of the area to ensure noone is in the danger area.
3. Removal of lockout/tagout devices: The authorized employee must remove his or her lock and tag. The energy-isolating device should then be switched back to the ON or energized position.

LOCKOUT/TAGOUT REMOVAL BY SOMEONE OTHER THAN THE AUTHORIZED EMPLOYEE

If for some reason the authorized employee who applied the lockout/tagout device is not available to remove it, the device can only be removed according to the following procedure:

1. Verify that the authorized employee who applied the lock is not on site and cannot be reached. Every effort must be made to contact the employee to have him or her return to remove the lockout/tagout device.
2. Contact the manager of the affected area and inform him or her of the situation. The manager will verify that the employee cannot be contacted and will fill out the required form: Lockout Removal Notice. The manager will verify that it is safe to have the lockout/tagout device removed. The manager can then remove the lockout/tagout device.
3. The manager must ensure that the authorized employee is notified about the lockout/tagout device removal before he or she begins work the following day.

SHIFT OR PERSONNEL CHANGES

While maintenance work is in progress and shift or personnel changes occur, the continuity of lockout/tagout protection must be maintained. The incoming employee must notify the working employee of his or her intention to assume the maintenance on that piece of equipment. The working employee must give the incoming employee a complete update of the status of that piece of equipment. The incoming employee must apply his or her lockout/tagout devices according to the procedure. When he or she has completed that function, the working employee can remove his or her lock and tag according to the procedure.

TROUBLESHOOTING

Certain conditions require that maintenance be performed while the equipment is in an energized state. Troubleshooting equipment in an energized state is very hazardous and must be performed only by an Authorized Troubleshooter. A list of authorized troubleshooters will be posted in each area. The equipment and area must be adequately secured during troubleshooting in such a fashion so as to maintain operations and still protect the troubleshooter while he or she is working. The authorized troubleshooter must lockout and tagout equipment to perform functions that do not require that the piece of equipment be in an energized state for repair.

──────────── APPENDIX ────────────

15–4

Examples of Federal Agency Resources for Assistance with the ADA

American Foundation for the Blind (AFB) and Gallaudet University–National Center for Law and the Deaf (NCLD)
1615 M St., N.W., Suite 250, Washington, D.C. 20036
(202) 651-5343 (NCLD) or (202) 223-0101 (AFB)

American Speech-Language-Hearing Association
10801 Rockville Pike, Rockville, MD 20852
Consumer Help (301) 897-5700 or (800) 638-8255 (Voice)
Consumer Help (301) 897-0157 (TDD)

The Association on Handicapped Student Service Programs in Postsecondary Education (AHSSPPE)
P.O. Box 21192, Columbus, OH 43221-0192
(614) 488-4972
ADA Hotline (800) 247-7752 (Voice/TDD)

The Association for Retarded Citizens of the United States (ARC)
500 East Border, S-300, Arlington, TX 76010
(817) 261-6003

Centers for Independent Living Program
Rehabilitation Services Administration
U.S. Department of Education
Mary E. Switzer Building, 330 C St., S.W., Washington, DC 20202

Clearinghouse on Disability Information
Office of Special Education and Rehabilitation Services
U.S. Department of Education
Switzer Bldg., Rm. 3132, Washington, DC 20202-2524
(202) 732-1241 or (202) 732-1723 (Voice/TDD)

Developmental Disability Councils
Administration on Developmental Disabilities
U.S. Department of Health and Human Services
200 Independence Ave., S.W., Rm. 349-F, Washington, DC 20201
(202) 245-2890 (Voice/TDD)

Education and Assistance Program for Farmers with Disabilities
USDA Extension Service
U.S. Department of Agriculture
Washington, DC 20250-0900
(202) 720-3377

Federal Communications Commission
1919 M St., N.W., Washington, DC 20554
(202) 632-7260 (Voice) or (202) 632-6999 (TDD)

Foundation on Employment and Disability
3820 Del Amo Blvd., #201, Torrance, CA 90503
(213) 214-3430

Information Access Project
National Federation of the Blind
1800 Johnson St., Baltimore, MD 21230
(301) 659-9314

Job Accommodation Network
P.O. Box 6123, 809 Allen Hall, Morgantown, WV 26506-6123
(800) 526-7234 (Accommodation Information) (Out of State Only/Voice/TDD)
(800) 526-4698 (Accommodation Information) (In State Only/Voice/TDD)

Job Training Partnership Act (JTPA) Programs
Office of Job Training Programs
Employment and Training Administration
U.S. Department of Labor
200 Constitution Ave., N.W., Rm. N-4709, Washington, DC 20210
(202) 535-0580

National Council on Disability
800 Independence Ave., S.W., Suite 814, Washington, DC 20591
(202) 267-3846 (Voice) or (202) 267-3232 (TDD)

National Institute on Disability and Rehabilitation Research
400 Maryland Ave., S.W., Washington, DC 20202-2572
(202) 732-5801 (Voice) or (202) 732-5316 (TDD)

National Rehabilitation Hospital
102 Irving St., N.W., Washington, DC 20010
(202) 877-1000 (Voice) or (202) 877-1450 (TDD)

The President's Committee on Employment of People with Disabilities
1331 F St., N.W., Washington, DC 20004
(202) 376-6200 (Voice) or (202) 376-6205 (TDD)

State Vocational Rehabilitation Services Program
Rehabilitation Services Administration
Office of Special Education and Rehabilitative Services
U.S. Department of Education
Switzer Building, 330 C St., S.W., Rm. 3127, Washington, DC 20202-2531
(202) 732-1282 (Voice/TDD)

U.S. Department of Justice
Civil Rights Division
Office on the Americans with Disabilities Act
P.O. Box 66118, Washington, DC 20035-6118
(202) 514-0301 (Voice) or (202) 514-0381 (TDD)
(202) 514-6193 (Electronic Bulletin Board)

U.S. Equal Employment Opportunity Commission
1801 L St., N.W., Washington, DC 20507
ADA Helpline (800) 669-EEOC (Voice) or (800) 800-3302 (TDD)

16

ETHICAL PERSPECTIVES IN OCCUPATIONAL HEALTH NURSING PRACTICE

In recent years the practice of occupational health nursing has expanded dramatically, bringing with it complex ethical issues that health care providers must face. These issues impact the health and welfare of the worker, workplace, society, workers' and health care providers' rights, and the economic position and, in some cases, survivability of the company.

This chapter will provide a discussion of ethical theories and principles and related ethical dilemmas in occupational health nursing practice. In addition, a model for ethical decision making will be presented with application to a case example.

▪ ETHICAL ISSUES AND PRACTICE

Much attention has been paid to societal ethical issues such as right to life or right to die, organ transplantation, and the use of scarce health care resource dollars for expensive technological advances; however, ethical issues in occupational health settings have received far less attention in part because they are somewhat different in nature, and are often subtle and insidious rather than overt (Rogers, 1988). Based on recent research, issues related to the balancing of costs and benefits, confidentiality of employee health records, truth telling, worker notification and right to know, exposure considerations, screening of employees, mandatory AIDS testing for health care workers, substance abuse by both employees and health care providers, workplace discrimination, worker and employer compliance with health protection and surveillance, professional competence and unethical/illegal acts (e.g., fraudulent credentials), and whistle-blowing are challenges occupational health professionals and managers face in an effort to protect and improve worker health (Rogers, 1991, 1992). In addition, language understanding in the face of illiteracy and cultural differences (Aroskar, 1989) present ethical complexities related to effective transmission of information necessary to protect workers from hazardous substance exposures.

In corporate environments where the primary mission is to produce a successful product while ensuring corporate survival and profitability, conflicts may be created if health and safety issues compromise that goal (Walsh, 1987). Issues related to the employee's right to know about exposure to hazardous substances may result in company liability, economic loss, and survival jeopardy. In addition, long-term consequences for the worker, family, and community resulting from potentially hazardous workplace exposures have yet to be fully explored.

Davis and Aroskar (1983) state that the nurse as a moral agent is concerned with values, choices, priorities, and duties for the "good" of the individual, the profession, and society. In the face of these concerns, what is needed is a more systematic way of approaching ethical issues confronting nursing at all levels, from the clinical provider/client encounter to the level of policy making for the delivery of health and nursing care.

In most occupational health settings the occupational health nurse bears the primary responsibility for management of the occupational health unit and provision of direct health services. Thus, the occupational health nurse acts as an agent of the company but also acts as an advocate for the worker with responsibility to uphold professional standards and codes. Characteristics of a professional are shown in Table 16–1.

Professions develop codes of ethics that indicate collective philosophies about what constitutes professional practice. Ethical principles that help health care professionals to deal effectively with ethical dilemmas are embodied in established professional codes of ethics. These codes provide for an expression of values and beliefs reflected in a framework to guide professional practice and ethical obligations and for professional responsibility and accountability to the health care consumer and society. Rather than to define rules and regulations for conduct, codes are generally intended to create an awareness of ethical considerations and to provide a framework for ethical decision making by the health care professional. The codes of ethics from the American Association of Occupational Health Nurses and the American Nurses Association are displayed in Tables 16–2 and 16–3 respectively.

■ ETHICAL THEORIES AND PRINCIPLES

The word ethics, derived from the Greek *ethos,* originally meant customs, habitual usages, and conduct of character. The word morals, derived from the Latin *moralis,* means customs or habits. These terms are often used interchangeably to describe acts related to conduct, character, and motives that are described as good, desirable, or right or, conversely, as bad, undesirable, or wrong (Davis & Aroskar, 1983). Socrates, in the Crito dialogue, argued that we must let reason determine our ethical decisions rather than emotion (Jameton, 1984). In order

■ **TABLE 16–1** Characteristics of a Professional

- Possesses expertise, formal education, or special technical competence
- Has a unique degree of autonomy that entitles her or him to exercise judgment
- Consciously conforms to a code or standard
- Feels a sense of service to humanity
- Acknowledges a higher responsibility for more than making a living
- Instills public trust

■ **TABLE 16–2** Code of Ethics: American Association of Occupational Health Nursing

- The occupational health nurse provides health care in the work environment with regard for human dignity and client rights, unrestricted by considerations of social or economic status, national origin, race, religion, age, sex, or the nature of the health status.
- The occupational health nurse promotes collaboration with other health professionals and community health agencies in order to meet the health needs of the workforce.
- The occupational health nurse strives to safeguard the employee's right to privacy by protecting confidential information and releasing information only upon written consent of the employee or as required or permitted by law.
- The occupational health nurse strives to provide quality care and to safeguard clients from unethical and illegal actions.
- The occupational health nurse, licensed to provide health care services, accepts obligations to society as a professional and responsible member of the community.
- The occupational health nurse maintains individual competence in occupational health nursing practice, recognizing and accepting responsibility for individual judgments and actions, while complying with appropriate laws and regulations (local, state, and federal) that impact the delivery of occupational health services.
- The occupational health nurse participates, as appropriate, in activities such as research that contribute to the ongoing development of the profession's body of knowledge while protecting the rights of subjects.

From American Association of Occupational Health Nurses, 1991.

■ **TABLE 16–3** American Nurses Association Code for Nurses

1. The nurse provides services with respect for human dignity and the uniqueness of the client, unrestricted by considerations of social or economic status, personal attributes, or the nature of health problems.
2. The nurse safeguards the client's right to privacy by judiciously protecting information of a confidential nature.
3. The nurse acts to safeguard the client and the public when health care and safety are affected by the incompetent, unethical, or illegal practice of any person.
4. The nurse assumes responsibility and accountability for individual nursing judgments and actions.
5. The nurse maintains competence in nursing.
6. The nurse exercises informed judgment and uses individual competence and qualifications as criteria in seeking consultation, accepting responsibilities, and delegating nursing activities to others.
7. The nurse participates in activities that contribute to the ongoing development of the profession's body of knowledge.
8. The nurse participates in the profession's efforts to implement and improve standards of nursing.
9. The nurse participates in the profession's efforts to establish and maintain conditions of employment conducive to high quality nursing care.
10. The nurse participates in the profession's effort to protect the public from misinformation and misrepresentation and to maintain the integrity of nursing.
11. The nurse collaborates with members of the health professions and other citizens in promoting community and national efforts to meet the health needs of the public.

Reprinted with permission from *Code for Nurses with Interpretive Statements,* © 1985, American Nurses Association, Washington, D.C.

to accomplish this we must have factual information regarding the situation and keep our minds clear as we deliberate the issue. It is not enough to appeal to what people generally think, since they may be wrong. We must find an answer by informed reasoning that we regard as correct and not by what will happen to us as a consequence, or what others will think of us, or how we feel about the situation. Each society and professional group has its principles or standards of conduct, and as persons concerned with being reasonable in our conduct, we rely on these standards for guidance.

Even though standards or ethical codes and principles provide us with guidance regarding acts of care, we still face tough ethical dilemmas and choices. A dilemma involves a choice between equally unsatisfactory alternatives; sometimes one might think it is a choice of selecting the worst of two evils. For example, in a situation where the ethical code guides us to maintain confidentiality, one may decide to break confidentiality in order to protect the health of others. This example shows that in honoring one ethical principle (i.e., beneficence) we can violate another (i.e., autonomy). Hence, although ethical principles can guide decision making, they can never be complete enough to anticipate all possible situations involving moral decisions. Nevertheless, we may be faced with conflicting principles and will need to determine which choice brings the most benefit and least risk. Furthermore, one needs to understand that answers to ethical dilemmas will not be arrived at easily or quickly (Omery, 1989).

The study of ethics falls within the broader domain of philosophy and is defined as a value, a standard adhered to by an individual, group, or organization in an attempt to define principles to decide which actions are desirable or undesirable (Beauchamp & Childress, 1988; Fry, 1986). Ethical theories and principles guide ethical decision making; thus, it is important to be familiar with these tenets. Teleological and deontological theories (Table 16–4), are the most widely discussed ethical theories and provide the foundation for application of principles (Beauchamp & Childress, 1988). Decisions about ethical dilemmas in occupational health nursing can be formulated within these theories and principles.

■ **TABLE 16–4**   Major Ethical Theories

Teleological (consequentialist) theory

The rightness or wrongness of an action is determined by the results of that action . . . by its consequences. One ought to do that which is conducive to one's goals. The end justifies the means.

Utilitarianism is the most common teleological theory. It is often thought of as the greatest happiness principle, or the greatest good for the greatest number.

John Stuart Mill, philosopher

Deontological (formalist) theory

The rightness or wrongness of an action is based on the nature of the action, or the motives behind the action, but not on the results or consequences of the action. One can determine the rightness of an action based upon principles.

Every individual is worthy of respect and must be honored and revered. It means doing your duty. One deserves respect for one's action only if that action was done for the sake of doing the moral thing i.e. from a respect for one's moral duty.

Immanuel Kant, philosopher

Utilitarianism (teleological) focuses on the consequences of an action and gauges the worth of the action by the end or results rather than the means to achieve the end. It focuses on providing the greatest good or least harm for the greatest number. Policy formulation based on cost-benefit analysis, wherein the greatest benefit is achieved by the most for the lowest cost, and the provision of health services to those who will benefit the most from the services are examples of utility (Fry, 1986; Rest & Patterson, 1986).

Deontological theory focuses primarily on the action itself and asserts that rightness and wrongness are inherent in the act independent of the consequences of the act. For example, deontologists assert that truth telling is always essential and should never be violated for any reason. Utilitarians on the other hand may argue that when truth telling does more harm than good (e.g., telling a psychiatric patient information that may severely jeopardize her or his mental health), the obligation to tell the truth may not need to be honored.

Ethical principles extend from deontological theory and the most widely observed principles as shown in Table 16–5 are autonomy, nonmaleficence, beneficence, and justice. Autonomy is a form of personal liberty where the individual deliberates about and chooses a plan that determines her or his own course of action. Inherent in this principle is the right to self-determination. Adherence to this principle requires that the individual's values and goals be considered in major decisions that affect her or his welfare (Childress, 1990; Evans, 1989). This rules out paternalism (when one claims to know what is best for another) in decision making and thereby precludes health professionals or others' making decisions for employees without their input and consent.

Autonomy as characterized by self-determination relates to issues such as

■ **TABLE 16–5**   Examples of Ethical Issues Facing Occupational Health Nurses

---

Autonomy: the right to self-determination; a form of personal liberty
Confidentiality
Right to know
Paternalism
Informed consent

Nonmaleficence: the duty to do no harm
High-risk jobs
Second party–induced hazard
Incompetent, unethical, illegal practices

Beneficence: actions that contribute to the welfare of others
Screening for potential health hazards
Health promotion activities
Breach of confidentiality (to protect others)
Walk-throughs
Research

Justice: fairness or giving persons what is due them
Discrimination
Distribution of benefits and burdens
Cost containment vs. quality

---

informed consent, confidentiality and right to privacy, right to refuse treatment, right to know about potential workplace health hazards, and worker inclusion in decision making. Potential dilemmas include the use of hazard pay for dangerous jobs; access/denial of exposure information by employees, which may reinforce knowledge gaps about toxic exposures and their long-term consequences; access to medical records by management personnel, which may result in denial of promotion or loss of job or other forms of punitive or coercive behavior; and the maintenance of confidentiality of a substance-abusing employee who handles heavy equipment that can harm other workers.

The second principle, nonmaleficence, is often referred to as the "no harm" principle. Foundational to most professional ethical codes, this precept encompasses the concepts of both harm and risk of harm avoidance. For example, an employee with a known hearing loss should not be placed in a job situation that will further compromise hearing, and a pregnant employee should not be exposed to potential or known teratogens that may jeopardize her health and endanger the offspring. The performance of preplacement, periodic, and mandatory examinations aids in identifying work-related hazards and helps occupational health professionals in their decision making to protect the health of the employee.

Occupational health nurses are widely recognized as employee advocates as evidenced by their contributions to employee health and welfare. Beneficence, the third ethical principle, requires that health care professionals act in the best interest of the worker. Interventions aimed at health promotion and health protection, such as wellness, screening, and health surveillance programs that benefit the employee through primary and secondary prevention efforts, exemplify this principle. The identification of potential health hazards or employees at increased risk of illness and injury and recommendations for risk reduction represent positive health interventions aimed at worker protection. Examples include the installation of engineering control devices such as needle/sharps container boxes in patient rooms or clinic areas or the development of a back injury prevention program for workers with back problems or previous injury. Walk-throughs by the occupational health nurse to identify health and safety hazards and recommend risk reduction programs are also included under the rubric of this principle.

Although screening and health surveillance programs benefit the employee through early detection of potentially serious occupational and nonoccupational disease, care should be taken to observe ethical principles related to screening and to select an appropriate screening test, secure reliable testing procedures and laboratories, and protect individuals' rights (Table 16–6). Mandatory screening programs and the access and availability of test results demand cautious evaluation

■ **TABLE 16–6** Prerequisites for Ethical Screening Programs

1. The purpose of the screening must be acceptable ethically.
2. The means used to obtain information must be appropriate to its intended use.
3. High-quality laboratory services must be used.
4. Notification of screening must be given.
5. Individuals screened have a right to be informed of results.
6. Appropriate counseling programs to interpret results and referral options for treatment must be available before and after screening.
7. Confidentiality must be protected.

to ensure worker autonomy and to protect confidentiality and right to privacy. For instance, some serious concerns center on whether urine drug screening should be required, how data should be obtained and stored, and the repercussions based on results of unreliable testing procedures.

Increasingly, biomedical tests such as urine drug screening are being used in ways that reveal social and personal information. Although the tests seem simple, there may be problems of test sensitivity and specificity as a result of operator errors and scientific inaccuracy. This type of screening may place the employee in the position of proving innocence, may result in erroneous job loss, has the potential for discriminatory usage, and can be viewed as a method of social control that might offend societal expectations of privacy (Engleking, 1986; Hofner, 1988; Panner, 1986).

The fourth principle, justice, is directed toward treating employees fairly, equally, and without discrimination. This includes providing equal opportunity for disabled persons regarding job availability and promotion, and assuring that individuals will not be discriminated against because of a health condition, such as acquired immunodeficiency syndrome or other chronic disease, when they are able to perform the job. This concept is embodied in the Americans With Disabilities Act (1990). Sexual or alcohol history as well as the general health status of employees may be considered risk information with respect to the potential for discrimination. Singling out individuals or work groups to perform unpleasant or hazardous jobs would also violate this principle.

In many instances, ethical principles provide us with a guide to weigh the risks and benefits with respect to individual health and welfare and the development of policies and procedures to safeguard individuals' rights and protect their health (Aroskar, 1987). It is incumbent upon the occupational health nurse to examine the situation with respect to the guiding principles and assure that the benefits of the action clearly outweigh the risks.

As health care practitioners or providers we are placed in positions that require moral considerations, that is, questioning what ought to be done in a health situation from an ethical standpoint. Dilemmas are difficult problems that have no easy solutions; however, understanding and utilizing ethical theories and principles will help in the decision-making process to arrive at a resolution. Based on original research funded by NIOSH, recurring ethical problems in occupational health nursing were identified by a national random sample of approximately 200 certified occupational health nurses (Table 16–7). These dilemmas were then analyzed, and alternative recommendations for resolution, as determined by practicing occupational health nurse experts in the field, were delineated at a national invitational workshop (Rogers, 1991). The dilemmas and alternative responses were then formatted into survey instruments, which were pilot tested and then mailed to more than 300 practicing occupational health nurses to obtain their reactions/responses to these dilemmas. Examples are shown in Table 16–8.

▪ ETHICAL DECISION MAKING

To resolve ethical problems it is important that the occupational health nurse recognize and understand both personal and corporate values, and know that these values may often compete. Nielsen (1989) points out that the consequences of addressing organizational ethics issues can be unpleasant . . . one can be punished or fined; one's career can suffer; or one can be ostracized. Within the context of the corporate environment two approaches to addressing ethical prob-

■ **TABLE 16–7** Recurring Ethical Issues Relevant to Occupational Health
Nursing Practice

- Incompetent/illegal nursing practice
- Substance abuse (drugs/alcohol) by health care providers
- Nonlicensed personnel practicing professional nursing
- Withholding information/truth about hazardous substance exposure
- Screening for illness (e.g., HIV) and/or drugs without informed consent
- Confidentiality of health records/Invasion of privacy
- Substance abuse by workers potentiating personal/coworker harm on the job
- Employees placed in unsafe jobs by management
- Worker exposures to hazardous substances resulting in fetal harm/reproductive toxicity
- Incompetent medical practice
- Employee health condition or dangerous behavior at work posing safety threat to other workers
- Whistleblowing related to deceptive practice by health care professional
- Health risk to selected groups of workers (e.g., older employees, pregnant employees) without adequate risk assessment
- Breaching confidentiality related to communicable disease exposure
- Inappropriate decisions by management regarding employee health status

lems in the workplace may be considered: (1) intervening as an individual to work against others and organizations who perform unethical acts and (2) leading an ethical organizational change by working with others and the organization to promote integrity. Acting individually will probably require some form of whistleblowing and can entail significant risk, particularly if the company culture demands conformity; however, if the individual knows how to lead, the corporate management is reasonable, the degree of risk and severity of risk is understood, and changes can be made within a reasonable timeframe, trying to lead an organizational change may be a more effective and safer approach.

When one encounters a dilemma, the answer is not clear cut, and often one principle conflicts with another. For example, how long should a substance abuse problem be dealt with if others are at potential risk of harm? Should the burden of a potential toxic exposure, no matter how small, be shared by all or only a few? Should all health care workers be informed of the HIV status of a patient or an employee? Should mandatory testing for HIV be required for all health care workers? Ethical problems raise awareness and questions as to how problems can be resolved, what criteria should be used in decision making, and what ethical principles influence the decision to resolve (Fowler, 1989; Rogers, 1989).

Notifying workers about exposures to toxic substances is clearly embodied in the 1970 Occupational Safety and Health Act, the 1976 Toxic Substances Control Act, more recently in the 1983 Hazard Communication Standard, and now extended to the public by Community Right to Know provisions of Superfund Amendment Reauthorization Act (SARA). Underlying the legal requirements of these acts is the ethical imperative of autonomy, wherein workers have the right to participate in decisions to minimize risk and limit exposure through workplace controls. For example, issues related to "right to know" include short-term and latent effects on personal health, reproductive toxicity, concern about the physical and mental integrity of future offspring, appropriate and scientifically and technically sound test measurements, who should be notified and what constitutes the content, and the appropriateness of notification without causing unnecessary fears and anxiety.

■ **TABLE 16–8**   Description of Responses to Ethical Dilemma

Ethical Dilemma	Nursing Action	Likely Response Yes	No	SA	A	U	D	SD

Percentage of Nurses Indicating the Likely and Ideal Response to the Dilemma — Likely Response / Ideal Response

HAZARDOUS SUBSTANCE EXPOSURE DURING PREGNANCY

A pregnant employee is concerned about exposure to hazardous substances in her work and reports this to the OHN. The nurse plans an investigation to assess risk. The supervisor becomes aware of the proposed investigation and reports this as unnecessary to the nurse manager, who agrees. The supervisor says "he knows best" and this type of investigation will unduly alarm all employees.

1. Educate supervisor/management regarding the Hazard Communication Standard (OSHA).
2. Proceed overtly with the investigation and document the findings.
3. Proceed covertly with the investigation and document the findings.
4. Notify OSHA.
5. Tell the employee management's decision so she can make informed choice.
6. Ask other health personnel (i.e., safety officer, industrial hygienist, employee's obstetrician) to support your position.
7. Do nothing.

SCREENING FOR HIV WITHOUT INFORMED CONSENT

All job applicants are being screened for HIV without their knowledge or informed consent. The OHN discusses with management the need to inform employees; however, management does not agree and instructs the OHN to continue the screening.

1. Develop policy regarding HIV testing (with nursing input) and live with the policy.
2. Obtain external legal counsel and give information to management.
3. Refuse to screen workers under these circumstances.
4. Do HIV screening with informed consent but without management knowledge and give results to applicant without management knowledge.
5. Continue to screen employees without informed consent.
6. Resign your position.
7. Educate management regarding legal implications of testing without consent and fair employment practices.

		Percentage of Nurses Indicating the Likely and Ideal Response to the Dilemma						
		Likely Response		**Ideal Response**				
Ethical Dilemma	**Nursing Action**	**Yes**	**No**	**SA**	**A**	**U**	**D**	**SD**

CONFIDENTIALITY OF HEALTH RECORDS/INVASION OF PRIVACY

Management requests information on personal illness health conditions of employees. When the OHN refuses, management breaks into the record file and removes health records. The OHN is threatened with job loss if record access is refused again. In addition, safety personnel (and other health colleagues) walk into OH unit ad lib and review health records for what they say are "employee health and safety reasons" to determine causes for absenteeism. OHN objects but is not supported by management.

1. Follow company policy/procedure on confidentiality access to records regardless of what it is.
2. Educate management/safety/personnel about access to records and under what circumstances information can be released; do not release information without employee consent.
3. Contact company legal department for advice and proceed according to counsel.
4. Refuse access to records and resign if necessary.
5. Go public with information.
6. Do nothing and allow record access.

RISK OF EXPOSURE TO HIV/CONFIDENTIALITY

Employee is positive for HIV and tells the OHN he has exposed two coworkers and his spouse, but he refuses to tell them and instructs the OHN not to reveal the information.

1. Verify HIV test and assess the exposure and high-risk behavior.
2. Establish policy to handle HIV/AIDS.
3. Educate and counsel employee of risks to self, others, and so forth without breaching confidentiality.
4. Counsel employee to notify those who are exposed within a timeframe and advise that if he does not you will do so.
5. Develop and implement AIDS education program but say nothing to those exposed.
6. Provide support and counseling to all parties involved, breaching confidentiality.
7. Do nothing, maintain confidentiality.

Key: SA = strongly agree; A = agree; U = uncertain; D = disagree; SD = strongly disagree.

constitutes the content, and the appropriateness of notification without causing unnecessary fears and anxiety.

To arrive at a rational, deliberate resolution to an ethical problem, within the parameters of leading an ethical organizational change, a model for ethical decision making is presented (Fig. 16–1) (Rogers, 1991). This framework includes the following steps: (1) problem statement, (2) value awareness, (3) data gathering, (4) clarification of the ethical problem, (5) identification of involved parties, (6) determination of alternative courses of action, (7) application of ethical principles, (8) reaching resolution, (9) resolution implementation, and (10) feedback or outcome evaluation. An actual case example is used to illustrate the model from conceptual and applied points of view (Rogers, 1990).

■ ■ ■ **CASE EXAMPLE:**   A pregnant employee is concerned about exposure to chemical hazardous substances in her work and reports this to the staff occupational health nurse. The nurse plans an investigation to assess the risk. The worker's supervisor becomes aware of the proposed investigation and reports this activity as unnecessary to the nurse manager, who agrees. The supervisor says "he knows best" and this type of investigation will unduly alarm all employees.

Problem Statement.   The problem identified should be clearly stated and validated. In this case example the problem as identified by the employee is a complaint of hazardous exposure. Validation of the problem can be done initially through employee interviews, walk-through observations, and sampling.

Value Awareness.   Values clarification enhances understanding and analysis of one's personal belief system and how one ideally should act toward others as compared to real actions. In the workplace setting, value awareness should also include recognition of the corporate value system. In this case example, the

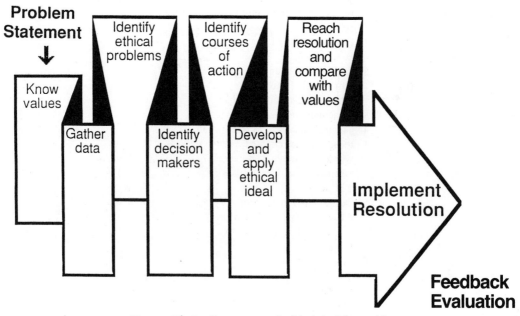

■ **Figure 16–1**   Components of ethical decision-making.

following types of questions should be considered: What constitutes risk and how is it perceived by different parties? Is there an acceptable risk level? Who should have access to information and what should be disclosed? Is there a difference in opinion about the risk among health care professionals, employees, management, peers, and so forth? Who, if anyone, will be harmed from the exposure?

Data Gathering.   To develop an informed decision, as much information as possible should be collected about the problem and any contributory factors. In this case example, data regarding the type, concentration, and duration of exposure will be helpful. Recent literature as well as Material Safety Data Sheets should be reviewed along with pertinent information obtained from observations and environmental monitoring. Determination of who are the high-risk groups, identification and validation of potential and actual adverse health effects, and knowledge of control measures and compliance with recommended safety standards should be evaluated.

Clarification of the Ethical Problem.   An ethical problem is complex, and the solution will have far-reaching effects on many areas of human concern. It is important to assess which ethical principles (autonomy, nonmaleficence, beneficence, and justice) are being compromised or violated in order to determine the associated benefits and risks. In this case example all principles are involved. For example, problems related to this hazardous exposure include: What are the exposure limits and who should receive exposure notification (autonomy)? What level of risk will be allowed and tolerated (nonmaleficence)? Is there a causal relationship between exposure and disease or outcome (nonmaleficence)? Are protective controls and monitoring systems in place and if not, why not (beneficence)? What are the implications of crude or unreliable monitoring measurements (nonmaleficence, beneficence)? Are there select groups at risk of exposure (justice)?

Once these issues are delineated, other types of ethical concerns can also be determined. For example, is it a case of withholding the truth about a hazardous substance, or an issue of uninformed voluntary consent? What type of harm will be imposed (i.e., physical or psychological) and who will be affected (i.e., employee, unborn child)? The more clearly one can identify the ethical problem, the more precise can be the analysis.

Identification of Involved Parties.   All persons involved in the decision making along with how they are involved should be known, such as the worker or workers, managers, health care professionals, labor union officials, and family members, if appropriate (Hardwig, 1990; Rogers, 1991). In this case example, the employee, occupational health care professionals, and private physician/ obstetrician should be involved in discussion of the problem. Management should be involved with respect to notification of the exposure, its impact and work-related recommendations. Other involved parties may include family members, coworkers, or other employee supports, as determined by the employee.

Information about worker-manager relationships and control mechanisms and about factors affecting the individual's ability or freedom to make a decision should be obtained. Failure to deal with this component of ethical analysis could lead to the wrong persons' making the wrong decisions for the wrong reasons. Paternalism in decision making may interfere with the reasoning process and should be avoided.

Determination of Alternative Strategies.   In any given situation there are usually several courses of action available. The employee and health care professionals, with consultation from the private physician, should discuss the situation and recommendations should be communicated to management. The purpose of the proposed actions and related potential or probable consequences of these actions should be explored fully. Sometimes none of the solutions seem desirable, and one may need to choose the option that will produce the most good (or least harm). In addition, the issue of feasibility needs to be considered; that is, can a strategy be implemented and what is the cost? For example, alternative strategies determined in this case example might include the following:

- control of hazardous exposures through engineering redesign of the work station, which will have cost implications;
- use of appropriate protective devices to minimize exposure and the institution of a monitoring and surveillance program that may be less costly; and
- institution of administrative controls through job rotation or temporary reassignment.

Research regarding the effectiveness of exposure minimization will be important data to consider in the development of alternative courses of action.

The issue of exposure and protection of the unborn fetus, and resultant corporate liability from possible harm is of concern. How this is handled, if the worker believes she should be allowed to continue working in the environment because the financial rewards are greater, will be an important consideration. If temporary reassignment is recommended and instituted, stable pay should be maintained.

Application of Ethical Principles for Resolution.   Herein, the ethical principles (autonomy, nonmaleficence, beneficence, justice) should be reexamined: Are the worker's right-to-know and right to make an informed decision compromised (autonomy)? Is the employee at risk of a potential or known toxic exposure without appropriate disclosure or from withholding of information (nonmaleficence and autonomy)? Are the company and health care professional assuming a position of "knowing what is best" for the worker (autonomy/paternalism)? All ethical principles should be weighed in terms of benefits and risks. Principles should be addressed within the framework of benefit maximization and risk minimization. Once the principles and any violations are addressed, resolutions to deal with the problem can be identified.

Reaching Resolution.   In deciding the course of action to take, carefully think through the problem, weigh the ethical principles in the balance and recommend a resolution that is rational, feasible, and defensible. In all decision making, we have limited capabilities and must select the most beneficial option. One can, of course, be wrong in the choice; however, it is imperative to act with integrity according to the knowledge possessed in keeping with one's obligations and values in search of a satisfactory outcome.

Resolution Implementation.   Once the appropriate resolution is determined, details of the action should be stated, that is, what is to be done, by whom, and under what conditions, and implemented. In this case example costly engineering controls may not be needed if administrative transfer is an effective resolution.

Feedback/Outcome Evaluation.   Once a resolution is recommended and implemented, obtain feedback as to the outcome of the decision: Who benefitted? What were the costs? Was the resolution acceptable or should another course of action be tried? There may be no real solution to the problem, but a resolution that reduces harm and affords some measure of autonomy and beneficence and that is just may be acceptable.

Although not common in the occupational health setting, ethics committee, which are used frequently in hospital environments, are helpful in dealing with ethical issues (Blake, 1992). These committees are usually multidisciplinary in composition and thereby bring a variety of expertises for problem delineation and problem solving. Establishment of these types of bodies can help in the overall problem solving and evaluation.

■ CONCLUSION

Ethical problems related to occupational health are becoming more numerous and increasingly complex. Occupational health nurses, other health care professionals, and corporate managers must be knowledgeable about the issues, differentiate ethical imperatives, develop approaches to handle these problems, and evaluate the impact of decisions made. The nurse as a moral agent is concerned with values, choices, and duties related to the "good" of individuals and larger societies, and with upholding and advancing the standards of the profession. In this role, the occupational health nurse not only brings a special expertise to occupational health dilemmas but also needs to be able to structure the issues so that sound and deliberate decisions are made using a reasoned approach. Knowledge of ethical theories and principles and understanding their application to occupational health problems is essential to the decision-making process. The nurse must acquire, enhance, and utilize these skills to provide effective leadership and guidance in the ethics of health care.

References

American Association of Occupational Health Nurses. Code of ethics. Atlanta, 1991.

American Nurses Association. Code for nurses. Kansas City, MO, 1976.

Americans With Disabilities Act, 1990.

Aroskar, M. The interface of ethics and politics in nursing. Nursing Outlook, *35:* 268–272, 1987.

Aroskar, M. Community health nurses: Their most significant ethical decision-making problems. Nursing Clinics of North America, *24:* 967–975, 1989.

Beauchamp, TC & Childress, JE. Principles of biomedical ethics. New York: Oxford University Press, 1988.

Blake, D. The hospital ethics committee. The Hastings Center Report, *22*(1): 6–12, 1992.

Childress, J. The place of autonomy in bioethics. The Hastings Center Report, *20*(1): 12–16, 1990.

Davis, A & Aroskar, M. Ethical dilemmas and nursing practice. Norwalk, CN: Appleton-Century-Crofts, 1983.

Engleking, PR. Employee drug screening. AAOHN Journal, *34:* 416–419, 1986.

Evans, D. Private lives of employees: How much should employers know? Occupational Health & Safety, *57:* 36–41, 1989.

Fowler, M. Ethical decision-making in clinical practice. Nursing Clinics of North America, *24:* 955–965, 1989.

Fry, S. Moral values and ethical decisions in a constrained economic environment. Nursing Economics, *4:* 160–164, 1986.

Hardwig, J. What about the family? The Hastings Center Report, *20*(2): 5–10, 1990.

Hofner, K. Testing for drug use: Handle with care. Business Week, *65:* 28, 1988.

Jameton, A. Nursing practice—the ethical issues. Englewood Cliffs, NJ: Prentice-Hall, 1984.

Nielsen, R. Changing unethical organizational behavior. The Academy of Management, *3:* 123–130, 1989.

Omery, A. Values, moral reasoning, and ethics.

Nursing Clinics of North America, *24:* 499–508, 1989.

Panner, M & Christabis, N. The limits of science in on-the-job drug screening. The Hastings Center Report, *16:* 7–12, 1986.

Rest, K & Patterson, W. Ethics and moral reasoning in occupational health. Seminars in Occupational Medicine, *1:* 49–57, 1986.

Rogers, B. Ethical dilemmas in occupational health nursing. AAOHN Journal, *36:* 100–105, 1988.

Rogers, B. Ethical decision-making. Continuing Professional Education, *3*(20): 1–7, 1989.

Rogers, B. Making the case for ethics in occupational health. Dangerous Properties of Hazardous Materials, *10:* 2–8, 1990.

Rogers, B. Ethical decision-making in occupational settings. NIOSH Grant-K 010H0072, 1991.

Rogers, B. Ethics and cost containment. Continuing Professional Education, *4*(26): 1–8, 1992.

Walsh, D. Corporate physicians. New Haven, CT: Yale University Press, 1987.

17

FUTURE PERSPECTIVES IN OCCUPATIONAL HEALTH NURSING

In recent years, occupational health nurses have expanded their scope of practice to include more emphasis on health promotion activities, worker surveillance and counseling activities, management of occupational health services and program planning, standard setting, and research. Occupational health nursing has evolved significantly and dramatically into a highly specialized practice. However, as we celebrate our accomplishments of the past, we face a future that will bring a mixture of familiar and new challenges, problems, and opportunities. According to the Bureau of Health Professions, nearly 22,000 nurses provide health care to workers (USDHHS, 1990a). The goal is to prevent work-related illness, injury, and disability, and to help workers maintain and improve their overall health status.

As we move into the 21st century, increased emphasis will be placed on health promotion and primary health care at the worksite, with intervention strategies directed at enhancing healthy lifestyle changes and reducing risk. The vision for the future is characterized by enhanced quality of life, reduction in preventable death and disability, and health care cost containment. Occupational health nurses will play a major role in this vision through delivery of cost-effective, quality-driven programs at the worksite.

The nature and scope of practice of occupational health nursing has been discussed in Chapter 3 and emphasized throughout the text. This chapter will focus on trends affecting the work and health of society, strategies for health enhancement at the worksite, and nursing's role as cost-effective health care providers. The collection, analysis, and interpretation of data are vital in preparing for the future in occupational health and safety.

■ **TRENDS AND CHALLENGES**

What kinds of information do we need in order to make some rational projections about current and future services that will most benefit the American workforce and public? What are the trends that affect the future of health and work in the United States? How will the concept of an improved healthy workforce be realized? In order to answer these questions, available data need to be examined to try to plan for the future.

Information has been provided from several sources, which describe demographic and workplace trends, health status of the population, workplace hazards, and health care delivery systems (ANA, 1991; APHA, 1992; Bezold et al., 1986; NLN, 1992; USDHHS, 1990b). These factors suggest an increasingly important role for nurses who can provide innovative health promotion and health care services at the workplace.

Demographic and Workplace Trends

The elderly population, particularly women, continues to grow (age 65 or older), and it is predicted that by the year 2010 older adults will comprise 14% of the population. Chronic diseases will be more prevalent in the population as a whole and this will be reflected in the workforce as well. This will require new and expanded occupational health and safety programs targeted toward chronic disease monitoring and disability management.

Family structures will continue to change with more single parent households and more women in the workforce. In 1950, approximately 34% of women were in the workforce compared to nearly 50% in the workforce in 1985. In contrast, men comprised 87% of the workforce in 1950 compared to approximately 60% in 1985. Divorce rates are steadying at approximately 50% but out-of-wedlock pregnancies are increasing. While many women are taking professional positions, their earning power continues to be approximately two thirds that of their male counterparts. Therefore, their health needs and those of their families from an economic standpoint may be strained.

U.S. immigration trends will increase and within the next 20 years ethnic youths will provide the largest pool of workers. The poverty level for individuals and families, which now exceeds 20%, will increase to 25% by 1995 without a change in the economy (Bezold 1986).

The labor force will increase from approximately 110 million in 1988 to nearly 150 million by the year 2010 with most new jobs occurring in the service sector, such as banking, insurance, health, education, and social services. Manufacturing sector jobs will need major economic and technologic revitalization in order to remain competitive. Computers will become more commonplace in the workplace and human qualities may become devalued. Technological advances will increase our information-sharing capabilities but will bring the risk of invasion of privacy.

Worker personal values will become more important with increasing emphasis on creativity, autonomy, equality of life, concern for community and environment, social justice, international health, and greater participation in decision making. However, with more corporate emphasis on technology, management and labor values may conflict and tension will proliferate, resulting in greater physical and mental health problems.

Health Trends and Work-Related Health Care Delivery

A major issue of concern today in the corporate environment is the control of health care costs primarily through health insurance coverage. As discussed in Chapter 1, although heart disease and stroke are declining, they remain leading causes of death. Cancer rates continue to rise, and smoking rates, which have decreased for the nation as a whole, continue to rise for young women. Lung cancer now exceeds breast cancer as the leading cause of death in women.

Because of the demographic shift in the workforce, illnesses such as hypertension, cancer, cirrhosis of the liver, diabetes, homicide, and accidents will be more prevalent. AIDS will also impact the workplace not only in terms of the impact of the illness on quality of life but also issues regarding invasion of privacy, maintenance of confidentiality, potential exposure of the health care worker to HIV, and health care costs.

Benefits such as hospice care and living wills may become part of the health package and the occupational health nurse will need to become familiar with these options in order to offer appropriate counseling. New strategies will need to be developed to address disparities in health status, decrease morbidity and premature mortality rates, and increase positive self-health practices. In addition, family health services at the worksite will become more prevalent to help reduce health care costs. Increased gaps will be seen in the types of health services offered to workers in small businesses compared to large companies. Efforts will need to be aimed at closing the gap through alternative health programs or a change in the health care structure as proposed under Health Care Reform.

Although the number of work-related fatalities has been falling steadily during the last decade, it remains consistently elevated. The risk of injury for younger workers is five times greater than for older workers and this will increase with more younger workers in the workforce. Worldwide, some 50 million accidents occur every year (an average of 160,000/day) in industry alone. Each year industrial accidents and illnesses disable millions of workers for the rest of their lives. Farm-related accidents continue to lead the nation's injuries and little has been done to provide safety and health programs for farmers. Strategies will need to be developed to address health needs of the agricultural community. In addition, injuries and illnesses are caused by thousands of toxic chemicals, particularly new chemicals whose effects are not immediately obvious. A 1980 survey by the California Department of Industrial Relations found that the semiconductor industry had a worker illness rate three times that for the general manufacturing industry, possibly related to arsenic, a prime component of super chips (Bezold et al., 1986). Electronic and other high-tech manufacturing operations involve a host of potentially toxic substances, the interactions of which are yet to be known.

Forty-five percent of workers are employed in offices and this proportion will significantly increase. Musculoskeletal problems related to poorly designed work stations and stress related to human devaluation and increased productivity pressures will increase.

In recent years, the delivery of health care has shifted from hospitals to clinics, homes, and the workplace and this trend is expected to continue. It is evident that alternative health care and preventive programs such as aging programs, corporate health programs, prenatal, family, child and infant care programs at the workplace, and home visiting will become increasingly prevalent. As increased emphasis is placed on the delivery of these preventive and health promotion programs, health monitoring and surveillance will become more important and physicians and other health care providers will want to be seen as health care managers in direct competition with the occupational health nurse.

Self-care or self-help, which often involves participation in health promotion programs, is the preferred choice of health intervention for many, and this particular approach to health care at the worksite is increasing. Some corporations view health promotion programs, such as smoking cessation and improved nutrition programs, as a method to improve their cost savings and increase worker productivity during the initiation and building of corporate wellness efforts. Many, however, still do not see the connection between health and productivity and, as a result, health promotion programs may be fragmented, disjointed, or nonexistent. Increased efforts must be aimed at focusing management and worker thinking to develop and participate in health promotion programs. Integration of health into all aspects of work life that meet worker individual needs based on their health profile will increase the overall quality of life.

There will be an increased need for occupational health nurses to work in hospital employee health centers in order to focus more services on hospital workers, an underserved population at significant risk of various occupational health hazards. Health care workers are particularly threatened by musculo-skeletal injuries, stress, chemical toxins, and infectious diseases related to contact with blood or body fluids. In addition, few comprehensive health promotion programs are offered in hospital-based settings (Rogers & Haynes, 1991).

In future years, then, data indicate:

- an aging of the workforce with concomitant health problems that accompany this population;
- an increase of women in the workforce with concerns regarding prenatal, infant, and parenting programs, and increased flexibility in work schedules to accommodate child care needs;
- an increase in the number of immigrant workers in the labor market along with issues related to cultural diversity and communication;
- a displacement of human power by technological power;
- an increase in occupational health problems brought on by work-related exposures from advances in technology;
- an increase in mental or emotional problems, or addictive behaviors influenced by personal and work-related stress;
- the potential for invasion of privacy and restriction of rights related to infectious diseases and occupational illness;
- an increase in employer health care costs related to high cost health conditions for small numbers of individuals; and
- a need to increase alternative occupational health programs and professionals in nontraditional occupational health work settings such as hospitals and farm communities.

If there is some idea of what is coming, occupational health professionals can capitalize and expand on past successes to plan relevant programs for the future; the task is not only to succinctly plan and organize programs to address the health needs of the workforce but to imagine and create.

■ STRATEGIES FOR HEALTH ENHANCEMENT

In order for American industry and the occupational health nurse to effectively and efficiently meet the challenges in the work environment, strategies will center primarily on:

- developing new health benefit options for employees and alternative health services and programs;

- increasing programs that enhance the mental and physical well-being of the worker;
- increasing primary care and health promotion efforts at the worksite, including an option for family involvement;
- expanding occupational health nursing roles, including case management, and enhancing multidisciplinary collaboration;
- focusing a cost-effectiveness atmosphere at the worksite;
- improving quality management and assurance mechanisms;
- fostering environmental health;
- encouraging the generation of new knowledge through research and education; and
- developing and operationalizing a concept of health at the worksite.

New Health Benefit Options

The development of new health benefit options will be based on the availability of selection options for the employee. For example, older workers may choose packages that include increased health program offerings, or home care services. The occupational health nurse may then be more involved with community agencies, nurses, physicians, and other health care professionals with respect to referrals, planning care at home, and return-to-work programs. Working mothers may want to choose day care services at the worksite or programs aimed at child development and parent bonding. For workers who speak another language as their primary language, bilingual health and safety programs will need to be developed. Within the spectrum of new health benefits the occupational health nurse will and must play an integral role. This may require additional continuing education in unfamiliar areas, such as infant care programs, literacy counseling, and expanding and increasing managerial skills to better develop cost-effective and measurable program outcomes. Lifelong learning will be a necessity.

New programs will need to be developed to maximize worker health and keep the employee at work. For example, one sixth of all workers are women in childbearing years. The establishment of prenatal programs can be viewed as cost saving as well as health promotive and the occupational health nurse will serve as the catalyst to accomplish this goal. Data related to illness and pregnancy, neonatal illness, absenteeism, risk factors, and educational needs of mothers/fathers will need to be collected and analyzed by the occupational health nurse to determine the need for such programs as nutrition, stress, labor/delivery, and lifestyle risk factors. Programs can be offered on site, or referrals will need to be made. The nurse will either need to retool to provide prenatal care/education or develop a listing of community resources necessary to meet the needs and the challenges.

Mastroianni (1992) describes the importance of child care arrangements in reducing stress, anxiety, and potential illness in working mothers. The occupational health nurse will be instrumental in developing postnatal services for mothers who return to work and who may need to find day care accommodations, resolve conflicts about separation, breastfeeding, and so forth, and arrange for infant health care, which necessitates off-work time. If on-site day care is not feasible, establishment of a resource book for area day care facilities would be extremely helpful. Other helpful areas include establishing parental support groups, parenting programs, options for maintaining breastfeeding needs, and providing childhood immunizations.

As the population ages, more elder care will become a necessity. Approximately 75% of those over 65 live independently with a spouse or alone in their homes; 80% of those over 85 do not have a spouse, and 75% of those over 65 have at least two chronic diseases (USDHHS, 1990b). The increasing number of older adults has had an impact on employees of all ages in terms of caregiving, which can range from minimal to episodic care, personal care, or to total elder care management. The emotional impact of caregiving has been a problem identified by the caregiver, citing physical strain and family disruption as causing more burden than financial strain (Hart, 1992).

The occupational health nurse will be a valuable resource in helping employees maintain emotional, social, and personal functioning for the older family member, and also in providing a degree of comfort to the employee. The occupational health nurse's role will increase as counselor and teacher in helping employees conduct assessments and providing interventions needed to help the elderly maintain activities of daily living. From the organizational perspective, employees have reported cutting back on hours, altering work schedules and taking time off work without pay to meet caregiver obligations. The occupational health nurse will need to become increasingly familiar with community resources to help employees obtain necessary and new services for their older family members. Companies may want to consider flexible scheduling, job sharing, caregiver leaves, respite care, and adult day care as part of employee benefits.

Mental and Physical Well-Being

With the advancement of technology, computers will have an even more profound impact on people's lives especially at the workplace; employee livelihood may be threatened. This in turn may create enormous stress for the affected workforce, not only because of displacement but because of human devaluing. Displacement programs that include counseling and support groups will need to be designed for employees, managers, and families. Employee assistance programs should be expanded to employee and family assistance programs. Job retraining and placement will become critical elements to reckon with and the occupational health nurse will be a key figure in the development of these programs, which will serve to reassess and replace workers within the company environment.

Musculoskeletal injuries comprise the largest percentage of work-related injuries in the American workforce. Back injuries alone account for at least 25% of the compensable injuries (Chenoweth, 1988). When returning an injured worker back to the job, the health care provider should know the physical job demands the worker is expected to perform. The occupational health nurse will design prevention programs to decrease musculoskeletal injuries, including ergonomic training programs for body mechanics and back injury prevention programs. This will require job task analyses and recommendations for hazard control. The longer an employee is off the job, the less likely she or he is to return to work. For example, only 50% of employees return to work after six months off duty, 25% after one year, and almost none after work absence for two years (Bigos et al., 1986).

In disability management the employer must be prepared to allocate resources and support. Occupational health professionals must have access to physical therapy and rehabilitation programs to enable workers to return to productive and satisfying employment. People restricted by an injury for a prolonged period undergo role changes that are not well understood. Rehabilitation programs should be designed to help impaired employees retain a sense of self-worth.

Primary Care and Health Promotion

Primary care delivery will be increased at the worksite not only for workers but for their families. Many health care services provided by nurses and nurse practitioners, such as monitoring chronic conditions and worker health assessments, have been demonstrated to be effective, efficient, and of good quality (Jacox, 1987; McCloskey et al., 1987). In addition, extended services to family members, particularly in health promotion and prevention, will be part of a health concept.

Incorporating components of *Nursing's Agenda for Health Care Reform* (ANA, 1991), the American Association of Occupational Health Nurses and the American Nurses Association collaboratively developed five models for primary health care delivery at the worksite (Table 17-1). These models emphasize expanding the traditional focus of occupational health services and incorporating strategies to deal with current problems. Each model incorporates five criteria essential to providing quality care in a cost-conscious environment: (1) availability of qualified providers, (2) consumer involvement, (3) use of practice guidelines, (4) accountability for quality care and costs, and (5) case management (Burgel, 1993). The development of nurse-managed occupational health and primary health care centers at the worksite is an important strategy for health care cost containment and health care reform.

Expanded Occupational Health Nurse Roles and Collaboration

The role of the occupational health nurse will continue to expand. In collaboration with other professionals, the occupational health nurse will assume increased responsibility for case management to help determine safe and effective levels of worker physical and mental capacity necessary to perform the job. For example, as case manager, the nurse will help coordinate extended health care services to employees with complex illnesses or injuries, and work with community agencies to find the most appropriate and cost-effective services. The occupational health nurse will play a more prominent role in education and training not only for the worker but for management. This will entail developing both general and specific programs to increase awareness, knowledge, and understanding of risk factors and interactive effects associated with health, illness, and injury. Coupled with this, the nurse will be responsible for data analysis regarding the incidence/prevalence of injury and illness, epidemiological trends and patterns, and work practices related to the injury/illness events.

The nurse's management role must be enhanced as more occupational health nurses are engaged by businesses to operationally and programmatically manage occupational health services. The occupational health nurse will need to have a greater depth of understanding of managerial concepts and principles, financial management including cost-effective and cost-benefit analyses, and enhanced negotiation skills. In addition, more companies are pursuing contractual arrangements for occupational health nursing services. If this trend continues, these

■ **TABLE 17–1** Models for Primary Health Care Delivery at the Worksite

MODEL 1: ONE-NURSE UNIT, ON SITE

This model may be best suited for worksites with a small workforce, few workplace hazards, or those with limited resources. The occupational health nurse in this setting acts as the in-house expert on health-related issues. This includes assistance with policy development—for example, establishing a nonsmoking workplace—and providing consultation on health benefit design, thus ensuring an emphasis on wellness, preventive services, and managed care approaches. The on-site nurse has the opportunity to develop influential relationships with people—the employee, supervisors, the CEO, employees' families, and referral sources in the community. Using these relationships as vehicles, the nurse can underscore the importance of health and safety, emphasizing primary prevention for the reduction of both work-related and non-work-related illnesses and injuries. It is not feasible in this setting to offer all essential services on site. However, based on the demographics and the health needs of the employees, their dependents, and available community resources, the occupational health nurse can develop a network of quality community-based referrals—including HMOs and preferred provider contracts—with such groups as nurse midwifery services, nurse practitioners, psychiatric clinical-nurse specialists, community nursing centers, and physical and occupational therapists.

Service Components include:
- Direct-care services
- Compliance with regulations
- Case management
- Health surveillance
- Worksite analysis
- Preplacement evaluations
- Employee assistance programs
- Health promotion and disease prevention

MODEL 2: MULTIPLE NURSE UNIT, ON SITE

The goal of this model is to offer the majority of essential services on site, thus requiring additional health-care provider expertise. This would involve a nurse managed care center, focusing on primary care as well as work-related illnesses and injuries. Such an arrangement is ideal for medium to large employers.

This unit is staffed by registered nurses with specialty preparation—which specialties depend on the demographics of the workforce and the nature and extent of workplace hazards. Families could access this center for expanded case management services, EAP educational offerings, and wellness programs. Model 2 provides for a broader scope and depth of service components delivered on site. The strength of this model is the accessibility of health care at the worksite, its expanded case management approach, and its more comprehensive health promotion program. The challenge will be to expand personal health services with continued emphasis on occupational health and safety.

MODEL 3: CONSORTIUM MODEL: COMPANY COALITIONS

This model is designed for groups of small employers, enabling them to gain access to the service components in a centralized location (e.g., an industrial park). The strength of this model is its establishment of a nurse-managed, free-standing clinic that targets small employers, who traditionally have been underserved in occupational health and safety services and in personal health services as well. Family care also is more feasible in Model 3.

Unique to this model are the expanded operational hours, providing 12 or more hours of service daily, and a preferred provider agreement, with a local hospital providing services during off hours. Families have easier and more confidential access to this off-site, but convenient, location. Older employees can receive care here, too, once they have retired.

MODEL 4: LARGE EMPLOYERS WITH OUTREACH TO SMALL EMPLOYERS

This model's goal is to provide the strength of on-site delivery of essential services to those small employers who may not have sufficient employee/dependent numbers and/or resources to provide an efficient and high-quality health service. This model expands the service components adding a component of

■ **TABLE 17–1**   Models for Primary Health Care Delivery at the Worksite *Continued*

outreach to neighboring small employers. Not only does this model service small employers near the larger employer with convenient and accessible health care for employees and their family members, it also provides an incoming revenue stream to help support the larger employer's on-site health services.

MODEL 5: OCCUPATIONAL HEALTH NURSING CONSULTANT

Because a centralized clinic may not be feasible in rural communities and sparsely populated areas, this model utilizes outreach by an occupational health nursing consultant. The occupational health nurse contracts with the local hospital and small employers, in turn, contract with the hospital for the core of essential service components. The occupational health nurse visits each employer at least once every two weeks.

---

models should be managed and financed by nurses (Miller, 1989). As health care managers, nurses must expand their expertise and function in policy-making roles in all aspects of occupational health and safety ranging from the development of programs to resource acquisition and deployment.

Cost Effectiveness and Quality Enhancement

As discussed in Chapter 1, health care costs continue to rise. The occupational health nurse as the health care manager will be in a position to provide for quality cost-effective care through overseeing high-cost cases, and getting ill or injured employees who have been hospitalized back home and to work in safe jobs. Within the realm of cost savings, the occupational health nurse manager will need to target workers who are vulnerable to specific risks and recommend specific actions to reduce risks, including job reassignment and new or redesigned tools and work stations. Collaborative efforts will be required to achieve this purpose. The nurse will need to be able to communicate effectively and know what types of resources are readily available to provide for multidisciplinary collaboration.

The occupational health nurse will need to demonstrate both efficient and effective employee health services through measuring outcomes of nursing interventions. Quality improvement and assurance mechanisms such as satisfaction surveys, audit tools, and peer reviews will need to be implemented as a measure of accountability for cost-effective services. This may need to be company-specific, depending on the makeup of the workforce and concomitant health needs.

Environmental Health

Occupational health nurses will become more involved in environmental health as environmental agents, alone or in conjunction with lifestyle and genetic factors, increasingly cause adverse effects resulting in disease, dysfunction, disability, and death. Issues that need to be addressed include impaired reproductive and developmental health, such as occurs with lead exposure; air pollution and respiratory health; worker exposure to agricultural chemicals; the effects of chemical runoff into soil and drinking water; skin and other cancers associated with sun exposure; and waste management.

The National Institute of Environmental Health Sciences (1992) reports that a growing number of studies show that minorities and the poor suffer more than their share from pollutants. By living in residences near industrial worksites or hazardous waste dumps, in smog-filled inner cities, or simply in older houses containing lead paint, some face a higher risk just by staying home. In addition, minorities show greater incidences of specific diseases such as asthma, and are more likely to experience higher chemical and ergonomic exposures because of their high representations in certain occupations such as meatpacking and farm work.

Research and Education

The development of new knowledge or validation of old knowledge in occupational health nursing is a relatively new area for most nurses, yet one that will focus and develop the profession. The professional discipline, nursing, and the specialty, occupational health nursing, is very young in research; however, the creation of new knowledge is the cornerstone of a viable discipline. The rewards of conducting research are far reaching and long lasting. As a professional discipline, it is necessary to generate and disseminate knowledge and be responsive to rigorous scientific and professional accountability. Research brings the discipline to the forefront of a new era and helps to build and expand a body of knowledge. Several areas are ripe for investigation. In addition to AAOHN research priorities (Chapter 14), examples include:

- designing effective health promotion strategies to reduce morbidity and premature mortality in at-risk populations of workers; for example, measuring the effectiveness of self-esteem building on reducing stress;
- determining patterns of behavior that hinder or promote health such as factors that influence the use of personal protective equipment;
- designing and testing cost-effective interventions to reduce workplace injuries;
- developing and testing strategies to improve health literacy;
- examining organizational influences that create and reduce workplace stress; and
- determining factors that will enhance the image of the occupational health nurse.

In order to be well prepared for the future, occupational health nurses will need to expand their knowledge base through academic and continuing education. Knowledge, skills, and competencies need to be acquired for providing advanced clinical care, managing health care programs, and conducting research in the discipline. As we move in this direction, we must consider alternative options for educational experiences, for example, more independent and self-directed learning experiences such as computer-assisted instruction and teleconferencing; more flexibility in program scheduling to meet the needs of part-time students; and enhanced progression programs for individuals with diploma/associate degrees who desire to obtain graduate degrees.

Occupational health nursing content within nursing school curricula must be upgraded. Only minimal content in occupational health nursing concepts, practice, and related fields of knowledge is included in undergraduate programs with limited practicum experiences for students (Olson & Kochevar, 1989; Rogers, 1991). Well-prepared field preceptors are critically needed to work independently with undergraduate students to provide quality learning experiences based on achievement of objectives. At the graduate level more emphasis needs to be placed on development of curricular content consistent with workplace trends and with emphasis on cost containment and effectiveness of health programs. Occupational health nursing faculty with knowledge and expertise in the field of occupational health and safety, and who can engage in collaborative research to answer questions, evaluate interventions, and build knowledge are urgently needed.

Nursing curricula need to be reformed to include more socially relevant concepts that are reflective of a diverse and changing society. The "art of thinking" to recognize and solve problems, rather than learning through pedagogic lecturism, as well as multidisciplinary approaches for providing a broad and integrated knowledge base, need to be enhanced. Educational content must include critical thinking, skills in collaboration, shared decision making, social epidemiological viewpoints, and analyses and interventions at the systems and aggregate levels (NLN, 1992). Analysis of ethical issues should have a prominent role in the curriculum.

■ DEVELOPING AND OPERATIONALIZING A CONCEPT OF HEALTH

Developing and operationalizing a concept of health at the worksite will create a challenge for the occupational health nurse. This should be seized as an opportunity not only to influence the management of health, but to shape the health of the work environment with expansion beyond the corporate walls (Rogers, 1990). Workplace safety and health issues in the broad sense, that is, the inclusion of equitable health services for the employee, family, and community is the concept of health for which to strive. The occupational health nurse is in a unique position to guide and direct this effort. This concept, depicted in Figure 17–1, encompasses:

- self-help and the encouragement of individual responsibility for health behavior;
- integration of positive health behaviors such as nutrition and exercise into work life;

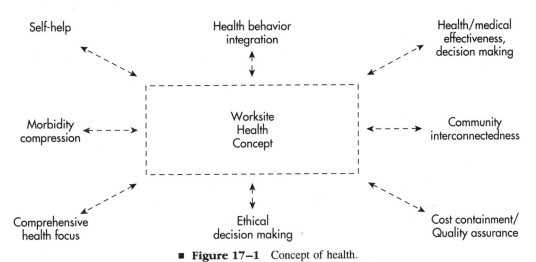

■ **Figure 17–1** Concept of health.

- decisions based on health and medical care effectiveness rather than medical technological imperatives;
- community involvement through collaborative provision and utilization of resources, and an organized effort to improve the health of the community and environment through research and education;
- corporate and employee activism aimed at reducing health care costs and improving quality;
- ethical decision making to guard worker rights;
- comprehensive health care services for all employees including targeted programs such as stress management and self-esteem building, with effectiveness measurement; and
- increased research efforts directed toward the compression of morbidity, that is, compressing or delaying chronic illness to the end of the life span through health-promoting behavior and disease prevention.

Within this concept, policy and planning decisions leading to nursing actions must be made by nurses, although often they are made by nonnurses. This means influencing policy decisions at federal, state, and local levels and in the corporate environment.

■ HEALTH CARE REFORM

We are on the threshold of new policy directives with health care reform as proposed by the administration in the American Health Security Act. It is anticipated that nurses will have an even larger role in the delivery of health care services, particularly primary health care services (USA Today, 1993). This is consistent with what occupational health nurses already do. We must seize the opportunity to continue to advance health care for American people.

■ SUMMARY

The future is filled with challenges for the profession and the individual occupational health nurse. There is much to do and it can be done with pride and enthusiasm, recognizing there will be struggles. The process of growth and change is inherent to a viable profession, and we can look for opportunities to be challenged rather than wait for them to happen.

References

American Nurses Association. Nursing's agenda for health care reform. Washington, DC: Author, 1991.

American Public Health Association. A national health program for all of us. Washington, DC: Author, 1992.

Bezold, C, Carlson, R, & Peck, J. The future of work and health. Dover, MA: Auburn Publishing, 1986.

Bigos, S, Spengler, DM, Martin, NA et al. Back injuries in industry: A retrospective study. Spine *11:* 246–251, 1986.

Burgel, B. Innovations at the worksite: Delivery of nurse-managed primary health care services. Washington, DC: American Nurses Publishing, 1993.

Chenoweth, DH. Health care cost management: Strategies for employers. Indianapolis, IN: Benchmark Press, 1988.

Hart, BG & Moore, PV. Aging work force: The challenge for the occupational health nurse. AAOHN Journal, *40*(1): 36–40, 1992.

Jacox, A. The OTA report: A policy analysis. Nursing Outlook, *35:* 262–267, 1987.

Mastroianni, K. Child day care arrangements and employee health. AAOHN Journal, *40*(2): 78–83, 1992.

McCloskey, J, Gardner, D, & Johnson, M. Costing out nursing services. Nursing Economics, *5:* 245–253, 1987.

Miller, MA. Social, economic and political forces affecting the future of occupational health nursing. AAOHN Journal, *37:* 361–366, 1989.

National Institute of Environmental Health Sciences. Health through environmental research. Research Triangle Park, NC: Author, Pub. #992, 1992.

National League for Nursing. An agenda for nursing education reform: In support of nursing's agenda for health care reform. New York: Author, 1992.

Olson, D & Kochevar, L. Occupational health and safety content in baccalaureate nursing programs. AAOHN Journal, *37:* 33–38, 1989.

Rogers, B. Occupational health nursing education: Curricular content in baccalaureate programs. AAOHN Journal, *39*(3): 101–108, 1991.

Rogers, B & Haynes, C. A study of hospital

employee health programs. AAOHN Journal, *39*(4): 157–166, 1991.

Rogers, B. Occupational health nursing practice, education and research: Challenges for the future. AAOHN Journal, *38:* 536–543, 1990.

U.S. Department of Health and Human Services, Health Resources and Services Administration, Bureau of Health Professions, Division of Nursing. The registered nurse population, 1988. Rockville, MD: Author, p. 52, 1990a.

U.S. Department of Health & Human Services. Healthy people 2000: National Health Promotion & Disease Prevention Objectives (DHHS Pub No 91-50212, 94–110). Washington, DC: U.S. Government Printing Office, 1991.

U.S.A. Today. Expanded nurses' role probable with new plan. pp. 1A, 8A, Sept 24, 1993.

INDEX

Note: Page numbers in *italics* refer to illustrations; page numbers followed by t refer to tables.

A

Abrasions, clinical nursing guidelines for, 263
Access to Exposure and Medical Records, of Department of Labor, 444
Accident(s). See also *Safety, workplace.*
　classification of, 124, 125t
　investigation of, 134
　rate of, 7
　trends in, 501
Accidental sampling, 424
Accountability, definition of, 365
Acetone, biological monitoring for, 237t
Achievement culture, 178t
Acquired immunodeficiency syndrome (AIDS). See also *Bloodborne Pathogens Standard (1991).*
　counseling on, 257
　virus causing. See *Human immunodeficiency virus (HIV).*
Administration, 44. See also *Management.*
Administrator role, 53–55
Adult learning, 311–314, 312t
African-Americans, in workforce, 2
Age, chemical toxicity and, 116
　in descriptive epidemiology, 74
Agent(s), chemical, 71, 76t. See also *Chemical(s).*
　in epidemiology, 67, 68, 70t, 71, 76t
　physical, 71
　psychosocial, 71
　transmission of, 68, 71
Agent factors, in epidemiology, 67, 68, 70t, 71, 76t
Aging, national resources on, 345
Agricola, Georgius, 18, 66
Agriculture standards, 438t
Air, sampling of, 101
Alcohol, deaths from, *5*
　per capita consumption of, 4
Alcoholism, economic impact of, 281t
Algorithm, 254, *256*
Aluminum, organ effects of, 106t
American Association of Industrial Nurses, 25–27
American Association of Occupational Health Nurses, 27
　code of ethics of, 486t

American Association of Occupational Health Nurses *(Continued)*
　practice standards of, 378, 379t
American Board for Certification of Industrial Nurses, 2
American College of Occupational and Environmental Medicine, 10
American Nurses Association, 24
　Code for Nurses of, 486t
　practice standards of, 378, 379t
American Public Health Association, 25
Americans With Disabilities Act (1990), 22, 435t, 458–466, 458t, 490
　coverage under, 459
　disabled individual under, 460–461
　enforcement of, 465–466
　essential job functions under, 461–462, *463*
　federal agency resources for, 481–483
　medical examinations under, 464–465
　nondiscrimination under, 459–460
　reasonable accommodation under, 462, 464
　undue hardship under, 464
4-Aminobiphenyl benzidine, as carcinogen, 76t
p-Aminophenol, biological monitoring for, 238t
Ammonia, health surveillance procedures for, 230t
Anaphylactic shock, clinical nursing guidelines for, 264
Anesthetic agents, reproductive toxicity of, 118t
Anilene, reproductive toxicity of, 118t
Aniline, biological monitoring for, 238t
　health surveillance procedures for, 230t
Anonymity, in research, 428
Anthropometry, 141
Antineoplastic agents, reproductive toxicity of, 118t
　urinary mutagenicity and, *114*, 413
Arsenic, as carcinogen, 76t
　biological monitoring for, 237t
　organ effects of, 106t
　reproductive toxicity of, 118t
　toxicity of, 106t, 112t, 118t
Arthritis, prevalence of, 5, *6*
Asbestos, 71
　as carcinogen, 76t
Asphyxiants, toxicity of, 114
Asthma, toluene and, 123

ISBN 0-7216-7588-3

90038

9 780721 675886